Beyond These Walls

Readings in Health Communication

Linda C. Lederman
Arizona State University

Foreword by
Gary L. Kreps

George Mason University

New York Oxford
OXFORD UNIVERSITY PRESS
2008

Oxford University Press, Inc., publishes works that further Oxford University's objective of excellence in research, scholarship, and education.

Oxford New York
Auckland Cape Town Dar es Salaam Hong Kong Karachi
Kuala Lumpur Madrid Melbourne Mexico City Nairobi
New Delhi Shanghai Taipei Toronto

With offices in
Argentina Austria Brazil Chile Czech Republic France Greece
Guatemala Hungary Italy Japan Poland Portugal Singapore
South Korea Switzerland Thailand Turkey Ukraine Vietnam

Published by Oxford University Press, Inc.
198 Madison Avenue, New York, New York 10016
http://www.oup.com

ISBN 978-0-19-533250-6

Printing number: 9 8 7 6 5 4 3 2 1

Printed in the United States of America on acid-free paper

Contents

Part II: PATIENT-PROVIDER COMMUNICATION

Part III: THE CHANGING ROLE OF PATIENTS IN HEALTH CARE

Part IV: HEALTH COMMUNICATION IN ORGANIZATIONS, GROUPS, AND TEAMS

Part V: BEYOND HEALTH-CARE PROVIDERS: SOCIAL SUPPORT

Part VI: HEALTH PROMOTION

FOREWORD
By Gary L. Kreps

I am very pleased with *Beyond These Walls* as a most provocative collection of relevant readings about health communication inquiry and application. The book provides a broad and encompassing view of health communication that illustrates the many relevant social settings and participants in health care and health promotion. This anthology demonstrates that health care and health promotion are primary survival activities that occur at home, at work, at school, and in recreational and social settings, and not just in doctors' offices, medical clinics, and hospitals. *Beyond These Walls* guides its readers through the complex multi-level, multi-media communication influences on health that occur within individuals (such as influences on health beliefs, values, and attitudes), within dyads (including promoting relational support and cooperation), in groups (such as families, health-care teams, support groups, ethics committees), organizations (clinics, hospitals, managed care systems), and within larger social systems (such as communities, cities, and countries). Readers will be empowered to serve simultaneously as informed health-care providers and consumers, using communication to help accomplish their many health goals.

Beyond These Walls helps us to recognize that we are all health consumers, even those of us who serve as health-care providers. We must actively resist the natural entropy caused by disease, injury, and aging that threatens well-being. Communication is a primary tool we can use to help overcome the myriad and insidious threats to our health and the health of our loved ones. Effective health communication is both a self-preservation tool and an advocacy tool that can be used to promote informed health decision-making, elicit required cooperation in the delivery of care, influence the adoption (and cessation) of relevant health behaviors, and facilitate needed social support.

Beyond These Walls also helps us realize the complexity of achieving important health goals. Health communication efforts must be strategic, sensitive, timely, informative, dramatic, and persuasive to be effective. Relevant information and support must be provided to individuals when they most need it, through channels they can effectively access, and in ways they can understand and incorporate into their lives. Effective health communication should be reinforced over time through coordinated communication channels, credible information sources, and complementary message strategies. Good health communication does not just happen; it must be carefully nurtured, supported, and planned.

Readers of this book will learn that rigorous communication inquiry can help explicate the complexities of effective health communication. Research can guide development of training programs to help consumers and providers establish needed health communication competencies for optimal care and health promotion. It can help us understand the demands of coordinating health preserving efforts within complex and often overly bureaucratic health-care systems, guide the development of influential health communication interventions, and direct the implementation of sensitive health-care policies and practices. It can also help us adapt information technologies to preserve, analyze, and disseminate relevant health information for guiding health promotion.

There are many thorny challenges in modern health care that must be addressed. These challenges include tremendous disparities in health outcomes between both well-resourced and vulnerable populations, problems with access to high-quality health-care services, inadequate cooperation and coordination between key participants within the health-care system, a plethora of serious errors and mistakes that regularly occur within health-care delivery systems, unmet emotional and psychosocial support for many individuals facing significant health challenges, ethical challenges to effective health-care decision-making and resource allocation, and the dire need to promote disease prevention, risk avoidance, and early detection of health problems. *Beyond These Walls* helps us recognize the potential contributions of health communication research and intervention in overcoming these serious challenges to health care and health promotion. It is my hope that this book will inspire readers to use communication strategically as a tool for promoting health and well-being, as well as to help overcome the major challenges to modern health care and health promotion.

***Gary L. Kreps**, Ph.D.*
Eileen and Steve Mandell Professor of Health Communication
Professor and Chair, Department of Communication, George Mason University

PREFACE
To the Instructor

Beyond These Walls: Readings in Health Communication was written to demonstrate that health communication is a complex and multi-faceted endeavor that incorporates a wide variety of theories, methods, sites, and concepts. The volume begins with an overview chapter, "Outside the Boundaries That Divide," and concludes with "A Final Word: Framing the Future of Health Communication." I wrote the last chapter in conjunction with a doctoral candidate and two doctoral students who are all health communication researchers. Thus, the volume ends by looking at the contents of the reader and current studies in health communication through the eyes of those who are in the process of becoming the next generation of health communication scholars. We wrote the chapter as a platform on which to predict the near future and what it is likely to hold for those of us interested in the role of communication in health issues.

Between these two chapters, readers will find a collection of exemplary research articles and essays that are designed to accompany and supplement leading overview textbooks in health communication. Health communication is one of the most rapidly growing areas of study in the discipline of communication. As an area of scholarly inquiry and applied research, health communication has historically had two major aspects: (1) interpersonal approaches to health communication (e.g., doctor-patient communication, self-disclosure of health-related information, social support and wellness) and (2) mediated approaches (e.g., promoting public health and wellness through persuasive campaigns and examining the Internet as a source of health-related information).

Within each of these areas there are books that focus on highly specific topics. For example, books on health-care provision tend to take a particular disease or health issue and focus on the role of communication in the care and treatment of individuals with that disease (e.g., Johnson, 1997). Books on public health campaigns often address the efficacy of using mediated messages to prevent the spread of HIV/AIDS, reduce cigarette smoking, prevent drug abuse among the general population (e.g., Rice & Atkin, 2001) or focus on more specific populations such as college students and the reduction of alcohol use (e.g., Lederman & Stewart, 2005). Researchers continue to examine the effectiveness of various health communication campaigns and suggest particular methodologies for evaluating them (e.g., Salmon & Murray-Johnson, 2001; Snyder, 2001). Thus, the examination of the effectiveness of health messages is also a vital part of the literature on health communication.

However, recent years have seen a burgeoning of new areas of study and newer ways of studying the role of communication in health. This volume is written to accompany a text in either an advanced undergraduate or graduate course in health communication. For undergraduate study, the health communication literature tends to consist of two types of books. The first type includes books on a specific health issue (e.g., HIV/AIDS, cancer, college drinking, breast cancer, or heart disease) and the role of communication in addressing that issue. These books address a variety of ways in which interpersonal and mediated communication can affect the information available to individuals about an issue of concern. Most often, these books are written as textbooks on the specific health issue or illness. For example, Greene, Derlega, Yep, and Petronio (2003) focus on privacy and disclosure of HIV in interpersonal relationships. Other books in this category are collections of essays. These cover either a variety of subjects that are subtopics of the area or a set of case studies in a variety of areas (e.g., Ray, 2005).

The second major category of health communication books read by college students is health communication textbooks that provide an overview of the area of health communication rather than focusing on one illness or area. These books have a number of topics in common with one another, much like most textbooks in public speaking have a specific set of topics that are covered (e.g., speech, speaker, audience, occasion). In health communication, these topics are generally health communication theories and perspectives, doctor-patient interaction, gender, culture, organizational contexts, mediated health communication messages, and public health campaigns. Some of these books (e.g., Thompson, Dorsey, Miller, & Parrott, 2003) are advanced texts that encompass theoretical and conceptual issues relevant to graduate students and more senior researchers, while others (e.g., du Pré, 2000; Kreps and Thornton, 1992) are texts designed for lower-level college students as introductions to the area of study. Other books in this category are directed toward health-care professionals (or potential professionals) and focus on skill development (e.g., Northouse & Northouse, 1998; van Servellen, 1997; Witte, Meyer, & Martell, 2001).

While overview textbooks are excellent resources for teaching a wide variety of topics in health communication, there are currently few books that are compilations of general articles that can be used in conjunction with these texts. *The Handbook of Health Communication* (Thompson, Dorsey, Miller, & Parrott, 2003) in many ways may be the only book before *Beyond These Walls* that bridges both of these areas. Thus, there is a need for a book of readings that can be used specifically with the leading textbooks in health communication. This reader is designed to meet this need. *Beyond These Walls* was compiled for advanced undergraduate students, at a plausible length to be read within one semester.

Beyond These Walls is organized into seven different parts. These parts and their contents are described in the overview chapter of the reader. Each chapter begins with a brief introduction to give you and your students a sense of the chapter in the context of health communication in general as well as the section of the book in particular. At the end of each chapter there is a series of discussion questions. The thrust of the questions is to prompt thoughtful discussions about the importance of the issues raised in the chapter itself.

I particularly want to call to your attention the Health Communication Grid, which you will find towards the end of the overview. I have included this grid to illustrate that many of the chapters can be read for a variety of topics. For example, while Chapter 19 is in Part VI of the book because it deals with health promotion, you will see on the grid that it also addresses several other health communication topics including ethical issues, health-care behaviors, and media. The grid is organized alphabetically for greater ease in finding topics across the reader.

Teaching health communication is a vibrant experience. Students bring to the course their own real world experiences with health issues in their lives, as well as in their family and friendship circles. Their experiences provide those of us teaching the course with a supply of relevant issues with which to help them make connections between the readings, the course theories, and individual practices. The readings in *Beyond These Walls* have been selected to add to your students' interests in a wide variety of topics. They are original research; therefore, these readings present the students with challenges that you can help them address as they learn about the ways that scholars in our discipline address health issues in our culture. I have done some cutting of the original versions of the chapters to make them more accessible to students without detracting from the work presented by the authors.

Beyond These Walls is a reader that I put together because it helps me to teach the course in health communication, either at the undergraduate or graduate level, in a better way. I have tried to include in it only those readings that enhance what you can find in the current textbooks. It is written to provide you with materials to help make the course you offer your students as dynamic and challenging as the area of health communication is itself today.

It is my hope that *Beyond These Walls* contributes to the rich learning experience you provide in your classroom as you and I work with our students to educate them about the role of communication in health issues.

References

du Pré, A. (2000). *Communicating about health: Current issues and perspectives.* Mountain View, CA: Mayfield Publishing.

Greene, K., Derlega, V. J., Yep, G. A., & Petronio, S. (2003). *Privacy and disclosure of HIV in interpersonal relationships: A sourcebook for researchers and practitioners.* Mahwah, NJ: Lawrence Erlbaum Associates, Inc.

Johnson, J. D. (1997). *Cancer-related information seeking.* Cresskill, NJ: Hampton Press.

Kreps, G. L., & Thornton, B. C. (1992). *Health communication: Theory and practice*(2nd ed.). Prospect Heights, IL: Waveland Press.

Lederman, L. C., & Stewart, L. P. (2005). *Changing the culture of college drinking: A socially situated health communication campaign.* Cresskill, NJ: Hampton Press.

Northouse, P. G., & Northouse, L. L. (1998). *Health communication: Strategies for health professionals* (3rd ed.). Stanford, CT: Appleton & Lange.

Ray, E. B. (Ed.). (2005). *Health communication in practice: A case study approach.* Hillsdale, NJ: Lawrence Erlbaum.

Rice, R. E., & Atkin, C. K. (2001). *Public communication campaigns* (3rd ed.). Thousand Oaks, CA: Sage.

Salmon, C. T., & Murray-Johnson, L. (2001). Communication campaign effectiveness. In R. E. Rice & C. K. Atkin (Eds.), *Public communication campaigns* (3rd ed., pp. 168–180). Thousand Oaks, CA: Sage.

Snyder, L. B. (2001). How effective are mediated health campaigns? In R. E. Rice & C. K. Atkin (Eds.), *Public communication campaigns* (3rd ed., pp. 180–190). Thousand Oaks, CA: Sage.

Thompson, T. L., Dorsey, A. M., Miller, K. I., & Parrott, R. (Eds.). (2003). *Handbook of health communication.* Mahwah, NJ: Lawrence Erlbaum.

van Servellen, G. (1997). *Communication skills for the health care professional: Concepts and techniques.* Gaithersburg, MD: Aspen.

Witte, K., Meyer, G., & Martell, D. (2001). Effective health risk messages: A step-by-step guide. Thousand Oaks, CA: Sage. ✦

Acknowledgments

As with any book that one writes or edits, there are so many people who have made the project possible. I want to thank each one of the people whose help has been essential to me as I have worked to put together *Beyond These Walls* as a contribution to the health communication literature. First, and of course most important, I thank those health communication scholars whose work I have included in this volume. It is their research and the ways in which they have shared it with the rest of us that advance this area of study. I hope that each will be pleased to find his or her work included in this collection. While I have done some minor cutting of some of the material to make it accessible to undergraduate students, I have tried to respect each piece in its entirety and to be true to its purpose and thrust.

When I began the project, I worked with my colleague and friend, Lea Stewart, at Rutgers University. Words are inadequate to express how fortunate I am to have had all the years of working collaboratively with Lea. She is a colleague and friend par excellence. My move to Arizona State University has only strengthened my appreciation of Lea, and I want to acknowledge her importance to me in this work as in all the work we have done and will do collaboratively.

While I was at Rutgers University, I also worked with many dedicated and excellent students. I thank all of the students who studied in various health courses with me for strengthening my own interest in, and commitment to, health communication. In particular I want to thank Cynthia (Cia) Bates and Jen Greenberg, my graduate assistants who helped me get this project started. Working with them in the Center for Communication and Health Issues Office was an important part of my Rutgers experience over the last few years. Cia in particular worked closely with me to get this collection started, and I thank her.

At Arizona State University I have had the pleasure of working on the book with three graduate students, Marianne LeGreco, Tara Schuwerk, and Emily Cripe. I thank each of them for their individual contributions and for creating the final chapter of the collection with me.

Marianne LeGreco and Tara Schuwerk have also served as editorial assistants on the final version of the entire manuscript. Because of the time demands on me as the Director of the Institute of Social Science Research at Arizona State, I would not have been able to complete this project in a timely fashion if Marianne and Tara had not assisted in this project along with the other many research projects on which they have been invaluable. I thank them for their dedication and all of their hard work.

Claude Teweles was the person who conceptualized this reader and brought the idea to me, and I can truly say that without him this reader would not be possible. He has also done a fine job of selecting reviewers to help with its development. I have never worked on a project that had as many reviewers. They represent diverse areas of interest, methodological preferences, and perspectives. I am most appreciative of what they brought to my attention. I thank him and Christine S. Davis, University of North Carolina at Charlotte; Darlene K. Drummond, University of Miami; Elissa Foster, San Jose State University; Heather L. Gallardo, University of North Carolina at Charlotte; Kathryn Greene, Rutgers University; Martha Haun, University of Houston; Karyn Ogata Jones, Clemson University; Kelly McNeilis, Southwest Missouri State University; Jennifer Peterson, University of Wisconsin; Esther Rumsey, Sal Ross State University; David Sachsman, University of Tennessee, Chattanooga; Meg Sargent,

Southern Connecticut State University; Pam Secklin, St. Cloud State University; Karin-Leigh Spicer, Wright State University; Teresa L. Thompson, University of Dayton; Pamela Whitten, Michigan State University. *Beyond These Walls* is a far better collection because of the reviewers' comments and suggestions. And of course, Renee Ergazos, our off-site editor, was invaluable in bringing her careful eye to the editing of the final manuscript.

I am most appreciative of Bud Goodall, director of the Hugh Downs School of Human Communication and of my colleagues at ASU working in the health area, in particular, Kory Floyd. I also want to thank Alan Artibise, Dean of Social Sciences and Executive Director of the Institute for Social Science Research, for his unswerving support at the Institute, including time to complete *Beyond These Walls*. And I thank all of the managers at the Institute, Steven Sepnieski, Jana Hutchins, Pam Hunter, Phil Puleo, and Katrina Walls, on whom I rely.

There are always those special people in our lives who contribute to everything we do, even when it is not a direct contribution. I thank Mel Fishman for his profound understanding of communication and health issues. And most especially, I thank Robert D. Kully and Josh Lederman on whom I count and appreciate beyond these words. ✦

Linda C. Lederman
Arizona State University

About the Editor

Linda Costigan Lederman is the director of the Institute for Social Science Research at Arizona State University and professor of communication in the Hugh Downs School of Human Communication. Her research focuses on the relationship among the domains of human interaction, experiential learning, and various health issues, including alcohol and other drugs, tobacco, and domestic violence. Her recent research has been funded by grants from the U.S. Department of Education, National Institute on Drug Abuse (NIDA), the U.S. Department of Justice, and the New Jersey Consortium, totaling more than $7.5 million. She is the author of 12 books and 65 journal articles, including the entry on *Alcohol Abuse and College Students* in the *Encyclopedia of Communication and Information* (2001). She is the creator of dozens of simulation games, including *Imagine That* and *RU SURE*, simulations of college students' alcohol-related decision-making, both of which are used at more than 360 institutions of higher education nationally. Her most recent books are *Changing the Culture of College Drinking* (2005 with Lea Stewart) and *Voices of Recovery* (with Lisa Laitman and Irene Silos), a collection of stories by people who began their recovery from alcoholism while undergraduates at Rutgers. ✦

About the Contributors*

Julie Abramson (Ph.D., Bryn Mawr College) is a professor emeritus and management consultant.

Paul Arnston (Ph.D., University of Wisconsin) is a professor of communication studies at Northwestern University and fellow at the Center for Medicine and Communication at Northwestern University Medical School.

Jacqueline Barnett (Ph.D.) was a member of the Department of Communication Studies and Theatre Arts at Bloomsburg University, Pennsylvania, at the time of the original publication.

Ellen W. Bonaguro (Ph.D., Ohio University) is the director of academic advising and retention at Western Kentucky University in Bowling Green, Kentucky.

Mollyann Brodie (Ph.D., Harvard) is the vice-president and director of public opinion and media research for the Kaiser Family Foundation.

Alex Broom (Ph.D., La Trobe University) is a postdoctoral fellow for the School of Social Sciences at the University of Queensland, Australia.

Patrice Buzzanell (Ph.D., Purdue University) is a professor in the Department of Communication, Purdue University, IN.

Donald J. Cegala (Ph.D., Florida State University) is a professor in the School of Communication at The Ohio State University.

Russell C. Coile, Jr. (MBA in Health Services, George Washington University) was a health-care management consultant. He was also a past president of the Society for Healthcare Strategy and Market Development of the American Hospital Association.

Emily T. Cripe (B.A., Purdue University) is a doctoral student and graduate teaching associate for the Hugh Downs School of Human Communication at Arizona State University.

Christine S. Davis (Ph.D., University of South Florida) is an assistant professor in the Department of Communication Studies at the University of North Carolina at Charlotte.

Laura Ellingson (Ph.D., University of South Florida) is an assistant professor of communication at Santa Clara University, California.

Vicki S. Freimuth (Ph.D., Florida State University) is a professor in the Department of Speech Communication and Grady College of Journalism and Mass Communication at the University of Georgia.

Fern Walter Goodhart holds a Master's of Science in Public Health and is a Certified Health Education Specialist. She is the director of health education at Rutgers University.

Nurit Guttman (Ph.D., Rutgers University) is a professor in the Department of Communication at Tel-Aviv University, Israel.

Stephen Haas (Ph.D., The Ohio State University) is an associate professor and graduate director in the Department of Communication at the University of Cincinnati, Ohio.

Michael Hardey is a reader in sociology at Hull/York Medical School.

Annette Harres (Ph.D., Monash University) is an assistant lecturer in the Department of European Languages and Studies at The University of Western Australia.

Kristen Harrison (Ph.D., University of Wisconsin-Madison) is an associate professor of communication at the University of Illinois—Urbana Champaign.

Krista Hirschmann (Ph.D., University of South Florida) is a medical educator with the Department of Medicine at Lehigh Val-

*The information listed for each author was the most recent available at the time of the publication of this volume.

ley Hospital and Health Network in Allentown, Pennsylvania.

Tina Hoff is the vice-president and director of Entertainment Media Partnerships for the Kaiser Family Foundation.

Jong Geun Kang (Ph.D., University of Massachusetts at Amherst) is a professor of communication at Illinois State University in Normal, Illinois.

Nina Kjellson is a partner at InterWest Partners, a diversified venture capital fund based in Menlo Park, California.

Gary L. Kreps (Ph.D., University of Southern California) is a professor and chair of the Department of Communication at George Mason University (GMU) in Fairfax, Virginia, where he holds the Eileen and Steve Mandell Endowed Chair in Health Communication.

Robert D. Kully (Ph.D., University of Illinois) is a professor emeritus at California State University, Los Angeles and the executive director of the California State University Emeritus and Retired Faculty Association.

Lisa Laitman (M.S.Ed., C.A.D.C.) is the Director of Alcohol and Other Drug Assistance Program for Students (ADAPS) at Rutgers University.

Joshua Lederman (MFA, Boston University) is a special instructor of writing in the Department of English at Emmanuel College in Boston.

Marianne LeGreco (M.A., Arizona State University) is a doctoral candidate and research associate in the Hugh Downs School of Human Communication at Arizona State University. She is also a faculty associate with the College of Nursing and Health Innovation at Arizona State University.

Kelly S. McNeilis (Ph.D., The Ohio State University) is an associate professor and assistant department head of the Department of Communication at Missouri State University.

Katherine Miller (Ph.D., University of Southern California) is a professor of communication at Texas A&M University in College Station, Texas.

Michelle Miller-Day (Ph.D., Arizona State University) is an associate professor in the Department of Communication Arts and Sciences and a faculty affiliate with the Center of Human Development and Family Research at the Pennsylvania State University.

Merle Mishel (Ph.D., RN, FAAN) is the Kenan Professor of Nursing at the University of North Carolina at Chapel Hill.

Terry Mizrahi (Ph.D., University of Virginia) is a professor and director of the Education Center for Community Organization in the School of Social Work at Hunter College, New York.

Molly Parker-Tapias (Ph.D., University of California, Berkeley) is a consultant for Bain and Company, Inc.

Michael Pfau (Ph.D., University of Arizona) is a professor of communication at the University of Oklahoma.

Jim L. Query, Jr. (Ph.D., Ohio University) is an associate professor of communication at the University of Houston in Houston, Texas.

Scott C. Ratzan (M.D., M.P.A.) is an associate clinical professor of the Department of Public Health and Family Medicine at Tufts University, Massachusetts.

Rajiv N. Rimal (Ph.D., Stanford University) is an assistant professor of the Bloomberg School of Public Health at Johns Hopkins University, Maryland.

Daniel J. Ryan (Ph.D., Texas A & M University) is a litigation consultant for Trial Analysts, Incorporated.

Kathleen A. Salkin (B.A., St. Andrews College and B.S., Gardner-Webb University) is an HRIS Specialist at Hanesbrands, Inc. in Winston-Salem, North Carolina.

Tara J. Schuwerk (M.A., University of Central Florida) is a doctoral student and graduate research associate for the Hugh Downs School of Human Communication at Arizona State University.

Barbara Sharf (Ph.D., University of Minnesota) is a professor in the Department of Communication at Texas A&M University.

Deborah Socha McGee (Ph.D., The Ohio State University) is a visiting associate professor and director of the Speaking Lab in the Department of Communication at the College of Charleston, South Carolina.

Lea P. Stewart (Ph.D., Purdue University) is a professor of communication at Rutgers University.

Rebecca W. Tardy (Ph.D, Ohio University) was a member of the Department of Communication at the University of Louisville, Kentucky at the time of original publication.

Steve Van Bockern (Ph.D., The University of South Dakota) is a professor of education at Augustana College and the Director of the Augustana Center for Reclaiming Youth.

Marsha Vanderford (Ph.D., University of Minnesota) is the associate director for communication at the Centers for Disease Control and Prevention.

Eben Weitzman (Ph.D., Columbia University) is an associate professor in the graduate program in dispute resolution and an adjunct instructor in the Master of Science in Public Affairs program at the University of Massachusetts, Boston.

Patricia Flynn Weitzman Ph.D., is an assistant professor of psychology in the Department of Psychiatry at Harvard Medical School.

Kim Witte (Ph.D., University of California) is a Professor of Communication at Michigan State University. ✦

OVERVIEW
Outside the Boundaries That Divide

I was diagnosed with sciatic nerve damage in my right leg some time ago and have been undergoing physical therapy and pain treatment. About a month ago, I noticed a different pain in the same leg and notified my doctor. He said it was related to the sciatic issue. My pain doctor told me not to worry. So I didn't.

Then about three weeks ago, I was playing golf when shortness of breath and disorientation overcame me. I went to the ER, and the doctor there initially diagnosed a heart attack. They put me on blood thinner and ran an angiogram. The results showed my heart was in good shape. The heart doctor told me not to worry. So I didn't.

But the pain in the right calf got worse and the calf got swollen. In a routine follow-up exam to my ER visit, the doctor who had never met me said that I probably had a blood clot and to go to the ER. He said I needed to start worrying.

Back at the ER, they discovered that I had not only one blood clot, but three that extended the length of my entire right leg. They examined my organs for cancer (one cause of blood clots) and mistakenly discovered that each of my lungs had a blood clot of impressive profile—my right lung is 50% blood clot. But they did not suspect clots in the lung because at the time I was not displaying symptoms (remember the shortness of breath and disorientation?). So by mistake they learned I had a pulmonary embolism and quickly started monitoring me more carefully.

So what happened? The pain doctor was looking for the cause of my pain in terms of his training; he thought it was due to the back problem. Likewise, the heart doctor determined my symptoms were due to a heart attack and when no heart problems were found, well, all was fine. Even the ER people who saw the blood clots in the leg did not suspect the lungs were at risk until they ran a CT scan for what they thought might be the cause of the leg blood clot.

When relating this event to my family physician, he said, "None of us know everything. We see through the eyes of our specialization. Sailors go to the sea, and farmers go to the field."

When I received an email from a friend with the above story, I realized more than ever the role of communication in health issues. My friend's email revealed how vitally important it is for effective communication to move beyond the boundaries that divide specialties in medicine, doctors from one another, doctors from patients, patients from friends, and families from researchers and practitioners. I also knew that I had to begin this chapter by sharing this story and arguing that the best hope for our individual and collective health is for those of us who are studying health communication to do our best to break through those boundaries. We have ample opportunities to do so.

Beyond These Walls explores communication beyond the divisions between traditional health-care research and delivery. Health communication is one of the most rapidly growing areas of study in the discipline of communication. As an area of scholarly inquiry and applied research, health communication emerged in the 1980s from two very different areas of communication study. The first area was interpersonal approaches to health communication, exemplified primarily in the analysis of communication between doctors and patients. The second was mediated approaches to communication, which were the foundations of promoting public health that grew out of theories of mass media campaigns and strategies. From its inception, health communication has been concerned with providing sophisticated understandings of the complex processes and practices that construct major health issues and the role of human communication in the design and delivery of various health-care practices. It is no surprise that in the last 20 years the topics studied in health communication and the approaches to those topics have gone far beyond the initial areas that bounded health communication from other areas of study, even in communication. A recent analysis by Thompson (2006) of articles published in *Health Communication* from 1989 to 2003, in fact, reported that 20.7% of the pieces have focused on patient-physician interaction, 13.4% on health campaigns, 11.8% on risk, 8.4% on aging, 7% on language (focusing on language that creates or does not create shared meaning), and 5.9% on media issues. Thompson went on to report that other topics that have been covered in more recent years include social support, inter- or multicultural concerns, technology, families, health information, and end-of-life concerns (p. 118).

Beginnings of Health Communication and Beyond

The title of the book, *Beyond These Walls,* was chosen to reflect how the growth of interest in issues in everyday life that involve health has provided the impetus for communication scholars to move beyond the original boundaries of health communication, and even beyond academia to expand what in the early days of the area of study was far more contained. As Thompson (2006) noted in reflecting on the first 75 issues of *Health Communication,* the broadening of focus in health communication work is perhaps the most notable trend in the area of study (p.118). Interpersonal scholars once concerned themselves primarily with how doctors conveyed to patients the health information to get them to comply with the doctors' prescriptions for restoring them to health. In recent years, health communication research has burst out of that tightly defined focus to include studies of the role of health care in the family, friends, and social networks as well as the whole range of health-care providers in which the doctor is included: nurses, social workers, health aides, insurance companies, hospital administrators, and case managers. For example, given the impact of insurance companies in determining what procedures are covered for patients by their plans, and the limits placed on doctors in terms of the services that they can provide for a patient who is covered, it is easy to see why it has become important to study the complex context in which the doctor/patient interaction takes place to understand its meaning.

Researchers studying health campaigns have also moved outside of traditional health promotion campaigns to include other mediated forms, including Internet sources of public information. In fact, the Internet's influence in health communication is dramatic. The Internet allows patients to seek out and find health information and to talk in chat rooms with others facing, or who have faced, the same health issues. This infusion of information through the Internet illustrates the ways in which the use of websites, chat rooms, email, blogs, and wikis (websites that allow visitors to contribute and edit content, creating a collaboratively authored site) break through once clear definitions of what constitutes "interpersonal" or "mass" communication. In a variety of ways, the boundaries that have until now divided interpersonal from mediated communication are being dismantled.

The Impact of the Internet on Health Communication

While the Internet has changed the ways in which doctors and patients themselves communicate, including email exchange as a source of doctor/patient communication, so too has the role of the patient itself seen rapid changes in current times. In many ways, I see this shift in the role of the patient-provider relationship as being akin to the change in paradigms in communication theory in which the prevailing notions of communication as linear, sender-centered, and sender-powered have been replaced by more interactive notions of communication in which the meaning and power in interactions are constitutive transactions (Lederman, 1996).

In the patient-provider relationship, the

role of doctor as an expert has been replaced by the doctor as a partner in health solutions. Viewed this way, the medical professional (doctor or other provider) has the expert medical knowledge and the patient has the expert knowledge of self and an empowered voice to express that knowledge in order to work collaboratively with the health-care provider. Communication between provider and patient is constitutive. The provider is responsible for the most current knowledge and best-practices experience. The patient's responsibility is to be versed well enough in his or her own health and health issues to be able to ask the right questions, provide the best self-based information, and listen carefully enough to decide on the value of the advice he or she is being given.

Utilizing the above view, medicine is no longer limited to the art of getting the patient to take medications. It is the art of communicative competence in which both the medical professional and the person seeking medical treatment are *partners* in effectively working collaboratively with one another. In a sense, it is a different dance. The old designated roles of leader and follower are replaced by dance partners each of whose performance enhances the other's. More practitioners are adopting a role in which they see their practice as a patient-centered practice.

Not all doctors are prepared to share responsibility with patients, nor are all patients looking for relationships with doctors that are collaborative. For some, there is comfort in doctor as expert. But for many doctors today, as well as patients, partnering on health issues is complex. And this discussion of the changing roles in doctor/patient communication would be incomplete if the health insurance companies and their demands were not a kind of invisible partner in the dance. Joel Cohen, who has been a doctor for 25 years, told me in an interview recently, "Insurance forms refer to me as the 'provider,' robbing me of my identity as a doctor, and the patient as the 'insured life.' How dehumanizing is that to all of us?"

In this new enactment of the role relationship, both partners must be comfortable with the shift in power and the concomitant shift in responsibility. The health-care provider must be a better listener and interviewer than ever before, assessing the patient's ability to provide honest and adequate information about his or her own health. The patient is more responsible than ever before for providing health-related information and must, therefore, be skilled in appropriate levels of self-disclosure. And both are affected by third parties like the medical context in which the interaction occurs (hospital, HMO, private practice, ER).

A vibrant example of this change is the story that introduced this chapter. You can be sure that the man who had the experience related there will enter each new medical interaction far more aware of his need to provide any doctor who sees him with whatever medical information he has about himself. Another example is a woman I interviewed with a history of alcoholism who had been in recovery for many years. When she moved to a new town, she had to find a dentist, an internist, and a surgeon to address her various health needs. One of her criteria for the selection of her new doctors was the providers' attitude toward the discussion of pain relief medications with her.

More patients are entering the interaction with their health-care providers armed with questions for which they need answers. Often, those questions are more informed and educated because patients have multiple sources of and access to information other than the doctor. But this is not always true, and doctors, at times, are faced with patients who have heard or read of medications that they want prescribed for them that are not what the doctors would recommend. While fewer boundaries separate those with medical knowledge from the rest of the population, doctors' education and training still give them a level of expertise that patients must rely on.

Additionally, patients also have their own self-information. This is particularly true of people suffering from chronic illness who may have a long history of medical interventions. Sometimes, it has been found that patients really want information that will help their understanding of their disease or illness, or regarding its treatment (Nelson,

2000). But other times what patients want from their doctors is reassurance and emotional support. Nelson called these "relational needs." In her work she found that health-care providers themselves often differed in terms of their method of dealing with patients. Some of them were more likely to provide patients with information; others tried to address their relational needs. The most satisfying interactions, she found, were when there was a match between the patient's need for information or relationship needs and the doctor's provision of that information or relational support.

Another example is the exceedingly slender woman I know who sees a health-care provider who knows nothing of her history with bulimia. More than ever, person-specific variables, such as education, intellect, emotional wellness, analytic ability, listening skills, and rhetorical sensitivity shape the interaction. Nowhere is this more true than with people suffering from chronic illness. Many of these patients have a long history of medical interventions and consequently a different experience in their relationships with their doctors. These patients often have not only a great deal of information about themselves but also about treatments and the effectiveness of those treatments for them. In fact, you could create a grid to exemplify what this means for communication between doctors and patients today.

As illustrated in the figure, satisfaction is the match between what the doctor or other health-care provider gives the patient and the patient's needs. When they match, there is satisfaction. Dissatisfaction occurs when there is a disparity between what the medical person provides and what the patient needs. Nelson (2000) was able to use a similar display of her data regarding patients suffering from diabetes.

Doctor Provides \ ***Patient Needs***	Information	Relational Comfort
Information	Satisfaction	
Relational Comfort		Satisfaction

As mentioned previously, these person-specific variables increasingly shape the interaction. This is true not only in the need for information versus relationship discussed above but also in terms of a range of other characteristics associated with doctors and patients. In public health, many scholars study the impact, for example, of health literacy, or the ways in which patient's level of education and the readability of medical instructions are harmonious, or not. For those with college educations, it may be hard to imagine what it is like for someone who cannot read to follow the instructions written on medications. Even for those of us who are educated, this is sometimes not easy. Leading health communication scholars, like Gary Kreps (2006), increasingly refer to patients as *consumers*. There is frequent discussion of the challenges of the transformation of health-delivery systems and the information technologies that make them possible. These discussions often address the need to sort out the rhetoric of access for all populations, and more communication scholars are bringing to light the reality of the communicative differences between those needing medical information and those providing it.

The topic of consumerism grows out of a reexamination of the communicative role relationship between doctors and patients. Thinking of patients as consumers is a way of emphasizing the power the patient has in amassing health information. Talking of health-care recipients as consumers suggests that individuals have the capacity to make a difference through their ability to make choices in the selection of the ways in which they engage in their own healthy well-being.

Added to the provider-patient relationship itself, health communication today is influenced by the impact of social support, both in terms of family and friends and mediated support through Internet-based support groups. This statement includes Floyd's work (2006) on human affection exchange and neuron-endocrine stress recovery, which examines the role of affection in wellness. As health communication and public health scholars have come closer together in terms of perspectives and the type of work conducted, there is more focus on health outside of the medical context and outside of planned intervention. Sometimes this focus is in talk about health in everyday life (Cline, 2003). Other instances are the ways in which patients involve their social networks in their health issues. Most of us spend much more time discussing health issues in everyday talk than we do in medical interactions or experiencing deliberate health intervention efforts (Cline, 2003), which is just one more way that the boundaries between health care and everyday life are disappearing.

Patients today often enter into their medical visits having talked first with others who have dealt with the same health issue. Beyond family and friends, these others may be Internet-based contacts at websites designed to pool and share information on a health issue. In addition, more patients are bringing relatives or other companions to serve as their advocates in the health interaction. Health communication researchers have begun to examine the impact of these circles of influence on what the patient brings to the interaction as well as the provider's response to it. One of the first dissertations written on this topic was an examination of online chat rooms and patterns of participation on a computer-mediated cancer site (Rumsey, 2001). Responsive health care has begun to take into account competent communication among all involved: the provider, client, family, community, and nation. This marks the ways in which health communication has gone beyond the traditional boundaries of doctor-patient communication.

Health and Wellness Are Socially and Culturally Constructed Issues

Even beyond the interaction level of patient-provider communication is the role of society in the construction of images of health and wellness. Included in these images are definitions of the rights and responsibilities of individuals, groups, and communities in dealing with the whole range of issues surrounding illness and disease. Chapter Four is included in the volume especially to draw attention to the notions of reality construction and what counts as "real" in health communication.

In the early days of the study of health communication, the literature tended to focus on the biomedical approaches that are prevalent within the mainstream culture of the United States. But as constructivist approaches suggest, these boundaries have shifted. Research on HIV/AIDS, for example, moves beyond the biomedical model (understanding the nature of the disease and how it is transmitted) to include study of the social stigma attached to it and the impact of stigmatization of advancing treatment for the disease as well as recognition of protective factors to prevent it or its spread. Drug abuse is another example of the complex sets of conflicting social values that surround how a health issue is handled in a society. Addicts are understood in the health community to be sick people with a disease; a disease that can be treated, that can be put into remission but cannot be cured. But drug use and abuse is also the focus of the nation's "war on drugs," in which drug users (addicts) and their affliction (addiction) are the targets of social disapproval. It is only as nicotine has become recognized as a heavily addictive drug that tobacco companies have been held accountable to smokers who die of lung cancer. But because nicotine is not socially constructed as a "drug" any more than caffeine, another socially acceptable addictive substance, there are no laws against buying cigarettes (for adults) or coffee (for anyone). While there are those who would argue that powerful economic forces drive what becomes legal and what does not, addictiveness in and of itself does not drive the decision to allow something to be legally acceptable. The social construction of addictions is what distinguishes between legal and illegal engagement in these behaviors.

Finally, as managed care and the role of health organizations are taken into account in health communication, the picture grows in terms of the complexity of health care and the vital role that communication plays throughout the doctor/patient relationship.

Health Campaigns and Beyond

In addition to doctor/patient communication, health communication has concerned itself with another major tributary: health campaigns and health promotion. An examination of the journals *Health Communication* and the *Journal of Health Communication* shows that much of the field of health communication has always had an impact on health campaigns and health promotion. The driving force behind health campaigns and health promotion tends to be problem solving: addressing a particular health issue in order to prevent its occurrence. Lapinski and Witte (1998) divide the theories underlying these campaigns into macro-level theories of change and micro-level theories of change. The macro-level theories include the health belief model, theory of reasoned action, social cognitive theory, stages of change model, fear appeals (risk communication), elaboration likelihood model, and inoculation theory. The micro-level approaches include social marketing, diffusion of innovation theory, and community empowerment. While these are a wide array, what is most critical is that all are concerned with how and why campaigns are effective or ineffective in influencing health attitudes and behaviors.

There is also considerable evidence that there has been an increasing trend in health campaigns and promotion toward theory testing. While there is less evidence of new theory development, there are campaigns that help in the development of communication theory. Lederman and Stewart (2005), in their work on college drinking, have advanced a conceptual framework, socially situated experiential learning that provides a conceptual basis and grounded theory approach to the ways in which learning takes place around a health issue with implications for many issues beyond college drinking.

There is other work that takes a critical and cultural approach to creating health campaigns. Examples include plain language websites for parents of deaf children, studies that look at pro-eating disorder websites, interactive safer-sex websites, drug resistance strategies, recall of anti-drug public service announcements, media literacy and smoking in adolescents, SARS (Severe Acute Respiratory Syndrome) in the media, telemedicine, and wording in health Internet sites (Thompson, 2006). Much of the research in health communication that is theory driven rests on grounded theory. Those theories that are used in health communication are theories that explain communicative phenomena, not just health communication behavior.

Outside the Boundaries

Research in health communication began with the coming together of two different streams: the study of the ways in which doctors tried to compel their patients to comply with "doctor's orders" and campaigns designed to influence public health issues. Each of these areas of studying and evaluating the role of communication in health reflected the scientific approach of the health sciences. While these ways of studying health issues and the role of communication in them continue, health communication researchers have begun to increasingly use other methods, primarily qualitative, in their approach. Some of these began with case studies. Others began with the study of critical incidents. More recently, researchers have used rhetorical, interpretive and ethnographic, critical, and participatory methods or perspectives.

I see these methodologies continuing to expand in their impact in health communication, and this is further discussed in the conclusion of this book. Expanding methodologies will allow for researchers to access the lived experiences of practitioners and patients in a wide variety of contexts, continuing to move health communication beyond doctors' offices and into the everyday realms where health practices are shaped. Perhaps no more striking an example of this exists than in the work being done in addiction medicine and presented at the conferences of the American Society of Addiction Medicine (ASAM) (Sucher, 2006).

Medical researchers and physicians work together with treatment specialists steeped in the practices of Alcoholics Anonymous to arrive at blended ways of addressing alcoholism. Communication researchers are just beginning to add their perspectives and training to the mix.

These changes in the study of health communication and the areas that have grown over the last 20 years are reflected in how *Beyond These Walls* was compiled and organized.

Organization of *Beyond These Walls*

Beyond These Walls: Readings in Health Communication provides a collection of research articles and essays written by leading scholars that address specific instances of research, theory, and practice. The text represents a variety of methodological approaches (e.g., surveys, interviews, narratives) and was designed specifically to accompany and supplement leading overview textbooks in health communication. All of the chapters are original research that has been published previously in leading journals and books in health communication. Each addresses a topic that falls within the rubric of one of the designated foci of the reader. Chapters have been selected for this anthology because they provide specific application of research and theory that is part of the broader topic. *Beyond These Walls* integrates relevant articles on the current challenges and opportunities presented by health communication information communicated via the Internet into each of the parts of the book. While at first the volume was going to have a separate parts on the Internet, so many areas of health communication are increasingly affected by the Internet that it seemed important to integrate its influence into each of the sections of the reader.

Beyond These Walls begins with the most current version of the classic chapter by Kreps, Query, and Bonaguro, which paints the picture of where the field of health communication began and how it has grown over the years. *Beyond These Walls* concludes with *A Final Word: Framing the Future of Health Communication* by the editor, LeGreco, Schuwerk, and Cripe, who are respectively a doctoral candidate and two doctoral students in human communication and health. Together we conjecture about the likely trends that will continue or emerge in the next decade. The majority of chapters in between these two are devoted to expanding the vision of the field by going beyond the original divides that demarked "health communication" and examining important new aspects of health communication that already have emerged in the past few years or earlier.

In addition, *Beyond These Walls* goes outside the academy, including pieces from health experts concerned with communication who write about it in collaboration with health-care professionals. To include all these, the reader is divided into seven related but different parts, each of which provides readings on the area that are exemplars of health communication studies.

These seven parts are (1) Health Communication: History and Contemporary Challenges; (2) Patient-Provider Communication; (3) The Changing Role of Patients in Health Care; (4) Health Communication in Organizations, Groups, and Teams; (5) Beyond Health-Care Providers: Social Support; (6) Health Promotion; and (7) Media Literacy and Health Issues. Each chapter is framed by an introduction that contextualizes the piece and its role in health communication and in the reader. After each chapter there is a list of discussion questions that focus on major themes in the chapter.

The areas of study within health communication continue to expand beyond what one volume could contain. To address this issue, I have created a topic grid, which is included on the following page, that shows many chapters address multiple topics. See the section that follows.

Health Communication Grid

In the grid, I have listed on the top row each of the chapters. In the most left-hand column, I have listed all of the topics covered in various ways in the reader. If you look at the *X* that appears in the various boxes in the grid, you will see which of the chapters deals with which of those topics. The grid has been created so that if there is a

Topics	Chapters												
	1	2	3	4	5	6	7	8	9	10	11	12	13
Aging			X						X				
Alcohol Prevention													
Body Image													
Cancer								X		X			
Chronic Care													
College Drinking													
Culture				X	X	X			X	X	X		
Disability													
Drug use													
e-Health	X		X					X				X	
Ethical Issues		X									X		
Family Communication													
Groups	X					X				X	X		
Health Campaigns	X										X		
Health-Care Behaviors	X	X	X	X						X	X	X	X
History	X			X									
HIV/AIDS													
Internet	X		X					X				X	
Managed Care		X	X										
Media	X		X				X	X	X	X	X	X	X
Organizations	X	X	X			X							
Patient-Centered Communication	X			X					X	X	X	X	
Patient-Provider Communication	X	X	X		X	X	X	X	X	X	X		X
Patients' Perspectives	X	X		X			X			X	X	X	
Qualitative Methods					X	X	X	X		X		X	
Quantitative Methods							X						
Role of Patient	X	X	X	X			X	X	X	X	X	X	X
Social Support				X				X		X	X		X

Topics	Chapters												
	14	15	16	17	18	19	20	21	22	23	24	25	26
Aging													
Alcohol Prevention							X					X	
Body Image				X							X		
Cancer	X												
Chronic Care					X								
College Drinking							X					X	
Culture		X	X	X	X		X	X	X	X	X	X	X
Disability				X									
Drug use									X				X
e-Health													X
Ethical Issues						X	X			X	X		
Family Communication				X	X								
Groups	X	X	X	X			X			X			
Health Campaigns						X	X	X	X	X			X
Health-Care Behaviors	X		X	X		X	X	X	X	X			X
History													
HIV/AIDS					X								X
Internet													X
Managed Care		X											
Media	X					X	X	X		X	X	X	X
Organizations	X	X	X							X			
Patient-Centered Communication			X										
Patient-Provider Communication	X												
Patients' Perspectives			X	X	X								X
Qualitative Methods	X	X	X	X	X		X		X				
Quantitative Methods		X						X			X		
Role of Patient													
Social Support			X	X	X								

particular topic of interest to you, you can scan this grid to see which chapters deal with that topic.

Conclusion

Much has changed since health communication began in the early 1980s as more and more communication researchers have taken their areas of communication training and methodological expertise and focused on health issues. The blurring of lines between academic and medical research and everyday considerations of health, disease, and wellness have contributed to these changes. The changes of the last 20 years have been reflective of both societal influences and changing notions of the ways in which communication works and its role in health issues. This reader provides you with a selection of important research pieces that will enhance your understanding of how far the study of health communication has come beyond the original boundaries that demarked it.

References

Cline, R. J. (2003). Everyday interpersonal communication and health. In T. L. Thompson, A. M. Dorsey, K. I. Miller, & R. Parrott (Eds.), *Handbook of health communication* (pp. 285–313). Mahwah, NJ: Lawrence Erlbaum Associates, Inc.

Floyd, K. (2006). Human affection exchange: XII. Affectionate communication is associated with diurnal variation in salivary free cortisol. *Western Journal of Communication, 70,* 47–63.

Kreps, G. (2006). *Information based healthcare practice as transformational tools: Separating rhetoric from reality.* Presentation at the national symposium, Transforming American Healthcare Over the Next Decade: Pathways to Change, Phoenix, AZ.

Kreps, G. L., Query Jr., J. L., & Bonaguro, E. W. (in press). The interdisciplinary study of health communication and its relationship to communication science. In A. Schorr (Ed.), *Gesundheits-Kommunikation (Health Communication).* Göttingen, Germany: Hogrefe-Huber Publishers.

Lapinski, M. K., & Witte, K. (1998). Health communication campaigns. In L. D. Jackson & B. K. Duffy (Eds.), *Health communication research* (pp. 139–161). Westport, CT: Greenwood.

Lederman, L. C., & Stewart, L. P. (2005). *Changing the culture of college drinking: A socially situated prevention campaign.* Cresskill, NJ: Hampton Press.

Lederman, L. C. (1996). Internal muzak: An exploration of intrapersonal communication. *Information and Behavior, 5,* 197–214.

Lupton, D. (1994). Toward the development of critical health communication praxis. *Health Communication, 6*(1), 55–67.

Nelson, M. (2000). *The diagnostic moment and the development of patterns of communication: Retrospective accounts of interactions between persons with chronic illness and their healthcare providers.* Unpublished doctoral dissertation, Rutgers University, New Brunswick, NJ.

Rumsey, E. (2001). *Making sense of health and illness online: A study of patterns of participation and use on one computer-mediated cancer support site.* Unpublished doctoral dissertation, Rutgers University, New Brunswick, NJ.

Sucher, M. (2006). *Current issues in addiction medicine.* Presentation at the national meeting of the American Society of Addictive Medicine, San Diego, CA.

Sharf, B. F., & Street, R. L. (1997). The patient as a central construct in health communication research [Special issue]. *Health Communication, 9*(1).

Thompson, T. L. (2006). Seventy-five (count 'em—75!) issues of Health Communication: An analysis of emerging themes. *Health Communication, 20*(2), 117–122. ✦

Part I

HEALTH COMMUNICATION: HISTORY AND CONTEMPORARY CHALLENGES

Chapter 1 The Interdisciplinary Study of Health Communication and Its Relationship to Communication Science

Gary L. Kreps, Jim L. Query, Jr., and Ellen W. Bonaguro

This chapter was chosen to begin this volume because it was one of the earliest articles to describe health communication as a field of study. Moreover, this chapter illustrates how health topics fit into the communication discipline, as well as which traditions informed the development of health communication as an area of inquiry. The authors demonstrate that, from the beginning, the area of health communication went outside the walls of academia to study the ways in which communication theories and practices could contribute to areas of everyday life. Health communication scholars frequently draw from interpersonal, group, and organizational communication theory as well as research in public health, medical sociology, healthcare economics, and epidemiology. This chapter focuses on the interdisciplinary features that underlie most health communication scholarship. The history of health communication is discussed to demonstrate the contexts, processes, and outcomes associated with health, health-care delivery, and health promotion.

Related Topics: e-health, groups, health campaigns, health-care behaviors, history, Internet, media, organizations, patient-centered communication, patient-provider communication, patients' perspectives, role of the patient

Health communication inquiry (research, education, and outreach) has developed over the last thirty years as a vibrant and important interdisciplinary area of study concerned with the powerful roles performed by human and mediated communication in health care delivery and health promotion (Kreps, Bonaguro, & Query, 1998). Health communication is an exciting applied behavioral science area of inquiry that examines the ways communication influences health, health care delivery, and health promotion. Research concerning health communication is often problem-based, focusing on identifying, examining, and solving health care and health promotion problems (Kreps, 2001). Health communication scholars typically examine the pragmatic influences of human and mediated communication on health care and public health, often using the data they gather to enhance the delivery of health care and direct health promotion efforts.

Health communication is a sub-field within the broader academic discipline of communication sciences. Communication science itself is a broad discipline, represented by a wide-range of interest groups and divisions within professional communication associations, such as the International Communication Association (ICA) and the National Communication Association (NCA). The breadth of the communication discipline is also reflected in the different academic programs that house the communication sciences, with school and department titles such as Communication Studies, Mass Communication, Media Studies, Journalism, Speech Communication, and Information Studies.

The study of health communication is interdisciplinary and combines and applies important theories, concepts, and methods from diverse areas of communication science (such as the study of language and behavior, interpersonal communication, group/organizational communication, persuasion, media studies, intercultural communication, and new communication technologies), as well as from the diverse academic fields of public health, health education, health psychology, medical sociology, medical anthropology, health economics, epidemiology, and medical informatics. Health communication also draws liberally from the literature and theories of the health professional fields, including medicine, nursing, social work, and clinical psychology. In this chapter we examine the interdisciplinary development of the study of health communication, identify key health communication topics and issues, and outline the future development of this important area of inquiry.

The Multi-Level, Multi-Channel, Multi-Site Nature of Health Communication

Health communication is an extremely broad research area, examining many different levels and channels of communication in a wide range of social contexts. The primary levels for health communication analysis include intrapersonal, interpersonal, group, organizational, and societal communication (Kreps, 1988; 2001). Intrapersonal health communication inquiry examines the internal mental and psychological processes that influence health care, such as the health beliefs, attitudes, and values that predispose health care behaviors and decisions. Interpersonal health communication inquiry examines the relational influences on health outcomes, focusing on the provider/consumer relationship, dyadic provision of health education and therapeutic interaction, and the exchange of relevant information in health care interviews. Group health communication inquiry examines the role communication performs in the interdependent coordination of members of collectives, such as health care teams, support groups, ethics committees, and families, as these group members share relevant health information for making important health care decisions. Organizational health communication inquiry examines the use of communication to coordinate interdependent groups, mobilize different specialists, and share relevant health information within complex health care delivery systems to enable effective multidisciplinary provision of health care and prevention of relevant health risks. Societal health communication examines the generation, dissemination, and utilization of relevant health information communicated via diverse media to a broad range professional and lay audiences to promote health education, health promotion, and enlightened health care practice.

Health communication inquiry involves examination of a broad range of communication channels. Face-to-face communication between providers and consumers, members of health care teams, and support group members are the focus of many health communication studies. A broad range of personal (telephone, mail, fax, e-mail) and mass (radio, television, film, billboards) communication media are also the focus of health communication inquiry. Increasingly, the use of new communication technologies are also examined as important health communication media for disseminating health information and connecting interdependent members of the health care system.

The settings for health communication inquiry are also quite diverse. They include all the many different settings where health information is generated and exchanged, such as homes, offices, schools, clinics, and hospitals. Health communication research has examined such diverse issues as the role of interpersonal communication in developing cooperative health care provider/consumer relationships, the role of comforting communication in providing social support to those who are troubled, the effects of various media and presentation strategies on the dissemination of health information to those who need such information, the use of communication to coordinate the activities of interdependent health care provides, the presentation of risk information to increase public recognition of health risks, the development of persuasive communication campaigns to help those who are at-risk avoid health threats, and the use of communication for administering complex health care delivery systems.

Information and Health Communication

Health information performs a central role in health communication inquiry (Kreps, 2001, 1988). Within the health communication field, communication is conceptualized as the central social process for generating, gathering, and sharing relevant health information in the provision of health care delivery and the promotion of public health. Health information is essential in health care and health promotion because it provides both direction and rationale for guiding strategic health behaviors, treatments, and decisions (Kreps, 1988).

Health information is the knowledge gleaned from patient interviews and laboratory tests that is used to diagnose health problems. It is the precedents developed from clinical research and practice used to determine the best available treatment strategies for a specific health threat. Health information is the data gathered in checkups used to assess the efficacy of health care treatments. It is the input needed to evaluate bioethical issues and weigh consequences in making complex health care decisions. Health information is the recognition of warning signs needed to detect imminent health risks and direct health behaviors designed to avoid these risks. Health care providers and consumers use their abilities to communicate to generate, access, and exchange relevant health information for making important treatment decisions, for adjusting to changing health conditions, and for coordinating health-preserving activities. The process of communication also enables health promotion specialists to develop persuasive messages for dissemination over salient channels to provide target audiences with relevant health information that influence health knowledge, attitudes, and behaviors. While communication is certainly a powerful process in health care, the dynamics of communication in health contexts are also very complex, the communication channels used are numerous, and the influences of communication on health outcomes are powerful. Health communication inquiry has developed to demystify the complexity of the multifaceted roles performed by communication in health care and health promotion. Such inquiry is conducted to increase knowledge about the influences of communication on health outcomes and direct the knowledge gained toward helping participants in the modern health care system use communication strategically to accomplish their health goals.

Communication in Health Care Delivery and Health Promotion

Health communication inquiry focuses both on health care delivery and the promotion of public health. These areas of health communication inquiry are distinct in many ways, yet are also increasingly interrelated within the modern health care system. Health communication research that focuses on health care examines the ways communication is used by health care consumers and providers in seeking and delivering health care services. Health communication research and applications on health care delivery is often concerned with the organization and coordination of health care services, the development of effective consumer/provider communication relationships, the process of health care decision-making, and the communication of social support. Traditionally, health communication research from the health care delivery perspective has adopted a human communication (interpersonal, group, organizational) focus.

Health communication research and applications that have focused on health promotion typically examine the persuasive uses of messages and media to promote public health, the diffusion of health innovations, the dissemination of health information, and the development and evaluation of communication campaigns. Traditionally, most health communication research from the health promotion approach has adopted a mediated communication (mass communication, campaign delivery, and new media) focus.

There are many points of overlap between the health care delivery and health promotion focuses on health communication. For example, modern health care delivery systems are increasingly adopting mediated channels for delivering health care, such as the use of telemedicine technologies as tools for diagnosing and treating patients. Health care delivery settings often serve as primary sites for health promotion efforts, with health care providers counseling their clients about prevention and screening opportunities, providing health education, and delivering health promotion messages in person, on-line, or with relevant publications. Indeed, health promotion efforts are increasingly utilizing human communication channels in health campaigns for disseminating health information, such as the use of support groups, personal appeals, family involvement programs, neighborhood, workplace, and government interventions. It is clear that health care delivery and health promotion are closely related activities, with health care providers devoting increasing energy towards health education, and health promotion efforts that are increasingly being coordinated with the many related activities and programs of the health care delivery system (Kreps, 1996a; 1990; Kreps, Bonaguro, & Query, 1998).

Development of the Health Communication: Social Scientific Influences

There were many starting points in the development of the field of health communication. One influential starting point was rooted in the communication discipline's adoption of theories and methods from other social sciences, such as psychology and sociology, which were actively studying the health care system (Kreps, Bonaguro, & Query, 1998). Scholars in these social science fields were beginning themselves to examine communication variables in health care (Bandura, 1969; Feldman, 1966; Kosa, Antonovsky, & Zola, 1969; McGuire, 1969; 1984; Tichenor, Donohue, & Olien, 1970; Zola, 1966), which encouraged communication scholars to follow suit.

The field of psychology generated a large body of literature that was very influential in the development of health communication inquiry. The humanistic psychology movement of the 1950s and 1960s, for example, pioneered by scholars such as Carl Rogers (1951, 1957, 1961, 1962, 1967), Jurgen Ruesch (1957, 1959, 1961, 1963), and Gregory Bateson (Ruesch & Bateson, 1951), stressed the importance of therapeutic communication in promoting psychological health and was most influential in the development of the health care delivery perspective to health communication inquiry. This exciting body of psychological literature captured the imagination of many communication scholars. In fact, the *Journal of Communication* devoted an entire issue in 1963 to the topic of "Communication and Mental Health."

The powerful book, *The Pragmatics of Human Communication* by Watzlawick, Beavin, and Jackson, published in 1967, builds upon the literature of humanistic psychology, indelibly tying together humanistic psychology and human communication. This book was very influential in the development of the fields of interpersonal communication and health communication. Written from an interactional family therapy perspective, the book examined the ways communication defines and influences interpersonal relations, clearly illustrating how the quality of relational communication can lead to therapeutic or pathological outcomes. This book, along with other humanistic psychology literature, provided a very influential springboard to the development of current interests in the field of health communication in provider/consumer relations, therapeutic communication, and the provision of social support.

The psychological literature about persuasion and social influence (Bandura, 1969; 1971; Festinger, 1957; Fishbein & Ajzen, 1975; Hovland, Janis, & Kelley, 1953; Katz & Lazarsfield, 1955; Rokeach, 1973) also provided a broad theoretic foundation for the field of health communication, influencing the development of the health promotion approach to health communication inquiry. The persuasion literature, in combination with the complementary sociologically-based diffusion of innovations literature (Rogers & Shoemaker, 1971; Rogers, 1973), social scientific theories about mass media influence (McCombs & Shaw, 1972–1973; Tichenor, Donohue, & Olien, 1970; Klapper, 1960; Wade & Shramm, 1969) and emerging literature about social marketing (Kotler, 1972; Kotler & Zaltman, 1971) encouraged communication scholars to study the role of communication in health promotion and develop persuasive communication campaigns to promote public health. A notable example of an early health communication campaign based upon a combination of social scientific theories is the Stanford Heart Disease Prevention Program. This landmark study illustrated the role of communication in health promotion with a longitudinal field experimental evaluation of a multi-city health promotion intervention program. This study, initiated in the early 1970's as a collaboration between cardiologist, Jack Farquhar, and communication scholar, Nathan Maccoby, clearly demonstrated the powerful influences of communication campaigns on public health promotion.

The medical sociology literature (Freeman, 1963; Jaco, 1972; Mechanic, 1968) was also influential in the development of the field of health communication. Medical sociologists have long been interested in the doctor-patient relationship and the social structure of health care delivery systems. Zola (1966) for example, in a now famous study, examined the ways that culture influences patients' presentations of health problems to health care providers, illustrating the need for practitioners to understand the backgrounds and orientations of their client and develop situationally specific strategies for communicating with individual patients. Kleinman's (1980) moving book, *Patients and Healers in the Context of Culture*, further reinforced this lesson about cultural influences on doctor-patient interactions and has encouraged current work on culture and health communication (see for example, Kreps & Kunimoto, 1994).

There were also important literature from the field of medicine that increased interest is health communication. Korsch and Negrete's (1972) influential article "Doctor-Patient Communication," published in the prestigious international journal, *Scientific American*, made communication in health care delivery an important academic and public issue that communication scholars raced to address. Several important books about doctor-patient communication, such as Bird's (1955) *Talking With Patients*, Blum's (1972) *Reading Between the Lines: Doctor-Patient Communication*, Bowers' (1960) *Interpersonal Relations in the Hospital*, Browne and Freeling's (1967) *The Doctor-Patient Relationship*, Ley and Spelman's (1967) *Communicating With Patients*, Starr's (1982) *The Social Transformation of American Medicine*, Verwoerdt's (1966) *Communication With the Fatally Ill*, and Vorhaus's (1957) *The Changing Doctor-Patient Relationship*, also set the stage for development of the field of health communication.

Institutionalization of the Field of Health Communication

A field of study is largely defined by the body of literature it generates, and the field of health communication has a rich and varied literature. The first books concerning health communication written by communication scholars began appearing in the 1980'[s] with Kreps and Thornton's (1984) introductory survey text written for an interdisciplinary audience of health care providers and consumers, *Health Communication: Theory and Practice*. Sharf's (1984) succinct text for medical students and practicing physicians, *The Physician's Guide to Better Communication*, and Northouse and Northouse's (1985) survey text geared towards nursing students and other health care professionals, *Health Communication: A Handbook for Professionals*. These first three texts were followed by a rapid succession of important health communication books, edited volumes, and a burgeoning literature of journal articles (too numerous to list here), solidifying and enriching the field of health communication.

As literature concerning the role of communication in health care and health promotion began to increase, there was a growing need for academic legitimization for communication scholars studying the role of communication in health. In response to this growing need, communication scholars interested in health care and health promotion banded together in 1972 to form the Therapeutic Communication interest group of the International Communication Association (ICA). The formation of this professional group is one of the most influential moments in the genesis of the modern field of health communication because it provided an academic home for an eclectic group of scholars, communicated to the rest of the communication discipline that health was a legitimate topic for communication research, and encouraged scholars in the discipline to consider health-related applications of their work.

The annual ICA conventions were very important sites for an emerging group of health communication scholars to meet, present their research, and generate new ideas and new directions for this new field of study. At the 1975 ICA convention, held at the LaSalle Hotel in Chicago, another important milestone in the development of this field of study transpired. The members of the Therapeutic Communication Division voted at this conference to change the name of the group to the broader title of "Health Communication," recognizing the many ways that communication influences health and health care. This was an important change because the new name represented a much larger group of communication scholars than the title therapeutic communication did. The therapeutic communication title was most attractive to interpersonally-oriented communication scholars, while the name health communication appealed broadly to scholars interested in persuasion, mass communication, communication campaigns, and the organization of health care services, as well as those interested in interpersonal communication.

The ICA Health Communication Division not only provided academic legitimization for a growing body of college faculty and graduate students, but the conference programs encouraged other communication scholars to conduct health communication research and submit it for presentation at ICA conferences. The ICA Health Communication Division began publishing the ICA Newsletter in 1973, communicating relevant information about health communication research, education, and outreach opportunities to a growing body of scholars. In 1977 the ICA began publishing the influential *Communication Yearbook* annual series, which included very important chapters about the emerging field of health communication.

In the first four volumes of the *Communication Yearbook* annual series each of the divisional interest groups (including the Health Communication Division) was allotted dedicated sections of the book to present research overviews and exemplar studies. In each of the first four volumes, Health Communication Division officers wrote important definitional overview chapters about the nature, purposes, and scope of health communication inquiry (see Cassata, 1978; 1980; Costello, 1977; Costello & Pettegrew, 1979). These overview chapters along with the accompanying research reports provided an excellent showcase for the developing field of health communication. Later issues of *Communication Yearbook* moved to a revised format of showcasing major review chapters along with accompanying responses from accomplished scholars representing the different ICA Divisions. The major review chapters concerning health communication were instrumental in defining this field of inquiry and the chapter responses helped to frame the major issues in the field for a large audience of scholars (see Kreps, 1987; Reardon, 1987; Pettegrew, 1987, for an example of a series of important health communication chapters in *Communication Yearbook* 11).

In 1985 the number of communication scholars interested in the field of health communication had grown enough that a groundswell of interested scholars formed the Commission for Health Communication within the Speech Communication Association (SCA, now renamed as the National Communication Association, NCA), the largest of the communication discipline's professional societies. Many of the members of the ICA Health Communication Division also became members of the NCA Commission on Health Communication and a large body of communication scholars who had limited exposure to health communication because they did not participate in the ICA, now learned more about this field of inquiry, in an uncommon example of cooperation between ICA and NCA, the two groups decided to share the publication of the *Health Communication Newsletter*, now renamed as *Health Communication Issues*. Within a few years the Commission for Health Communication had grown so rapidly that it surpassed the size of the ICA Health Communication Division and qualified to become the NCA Health Communication Division. Since 1992 the ICA and the NCA Health Communication Divisions have joined forces to present annual outstanding health communication dissertation and thesis awards to both the graduate student candidate and to the student's graduate advisor, rewarding and encouraging outstanding health communication scholarship.

Health Communication Conferences and Mini-Conferences

The health communication conference programs at ICA and NCA became increasingly popular within the field, and in the mid-eighties several health communication mini-conferences were founded to meet the burgeoning scholarly interest in this area. One of the first of these conferences was the "Medical Communication Conference" held at James Madison University in Virginia and hosted by Anne Gabbard-Alley. This mini-conference was quickly followed by a "Summer Conference on Health Communication" held at Northwestern University in July of 1985, hosted by Paul Arntson and Barbara Sharf. This very successful conference, which included a proceedings volume of contributed conference papers, began a popular trend of small research conferences focusing on health communication inquiry.

The Northwestern conference was followed by the first of several very effective annual "Communicating With Patients" conferences sponsored by the Communication Department of the University of South Florida and hosted by David Smith, Loyd Pettegrew, and others. Two important international conferences were organized in 1986, the "Oxford University/ICA Conference on Health Education in Primary Care," held at Oxford University (UK) and hosted by David Pendleton and Paul Arntson, as well as the "International Conference on Doctor-Patient Communication," held at the University of Western Ontario (Canada) and hosted by Moira Stewart. Since then there have been several additional international health communication conferences, which has expanded international interest in health communication inquiry.

In 1989 a series of "ICA Mid-Year Conferences on Health Communication" held at Monterey, California, and hosted by Marlene Friederichs-Fitzwater was started. Under the leadership of Jim Applegate, Eileen Berlin Ray, and Lew Donohew, the University of Kentucky began a series of successful health communication conferences held in Lexington, Kentucky. In 1994 a "Conference on Health Communication, Skills, Issues, and Insights" was held at the State University of New York at New Paltz and NCA held a Summer Conference on Health Communication in Washington, D.C., Emerson College, under the direction of Scott Ratzan, also has initiated a series of conferences on health communication. These health communication mini-conferences spurred the growth of health communication inquiry both by serving as channels for disseminating health communication research information to a very large and often diverse audience of scholars and also by providing health communication scholars with attractive outlets for presenting their work.

Dedicated Health Communication Journals

In 1989 a momentous occasion occurred in the life of the field of health communication. The first refereed scientific quarterly journal, *Health Communication*, dedicated exclusively to health communication inquiry, was introduced by its Founding Editor, Teresa Thompson. The publication of this journal marked the coming of age of this young field of study and encouraged scholars from around the globe to take this field of study seriously.

The first issue of *Health Communication* showcased five important invited essays by noted health communication experts evaluating the current status of the field of health communication and recommending directions for future development of the field. The lead article, by Barbara Korsch (1989), reviewed current knowledge about doctor-patient communication and identified fruitful directions for future inquiry. The next article, by Gary Kreps, describes the theory-building, theory-testing, discipline building, and pragmatic health care delivery system benefits of rigorous and relevant health communication inquiry. The third article, by David Smith, examines the ways health communication research has debunked the traditional medical model of doctor control and patient compliance, and advocates a sophisticated view of communication in future communication inquiry. The next invited essay, by Paul Arntson, argues for a focus on developing citizens' health competencies in future health communication research, empowering citizens to make active and enlightened health care decisions. The final invited essay in this inaugural issue of *Health Communication*, written by Jon Nussbaum, provides a charge to scholars to conduct important, sophisticated, and influential health communication research. This first issue of *Health Communication* marked an important point in the academic maturation of the field of health communication inquiry, and over the years the journal has provided the field with a respected outlet for health communication research.

In 1996 a second dedicated refereed quarterly health communication journal, the *Journal of Health Communication*, was introduced, under the Founding Editorship of Scott Ratzan. This journal differs from the established journal, *Health Communication*, by taking a more international orientation and health care practice perspective to health communication. While the important journal, *Health Communication*, is a rigorous research journal, the new journal, the *Journal of Health Communication*, is more of a research and practice journal. The two journals complement each other and provide important scholarly outlets for health communication scholarship, indicative of the growth and maturation of this field of study.

Curricular Growth in Health Communication

Along with the growth of health communication literature and professional organizations came the introduction of both undergraduate and graduate health communication courses. Some of the earliest health communication courses were housed in Departments of Speech Communication at large research universities such as the University of Minnesota (taught by Don Cassata), Pennsylvania State University (taught by Gerald M. Phillips), and the University of Southern California (taught by Gary Kreps). Several medical schools also began offering health communication courses focusing on interviewing skills for physicians at the University of Illinois (taught by Barbara Sharf), Southern Illinois University (taught by Susan Ackerman-Ross), University of North Carolina (taught by Don Cassata), and the University of Calgary (taught by Suzanne Kurtz). These courses were precursors to the development of many more undergraduate and graduate health communication courses in colleges both nationally and internationally.

Several undergraduate and graduate health communication majors are now offered at colleges (such as the University of Maryland, Emerson College, the University of Toledo, Bowling Green State University, the University of South Florida, the University of Florida, Northwestern University, Indiana University-Purdue University at Indianapolis, Rutgers University, Ohio University, the University of Georgia, Michigan State University, Stanford University, the University of Pennsylvania, and the University of Oklahoma). The Emerson College health communication graduate program is unique. It is a collaboration between Emerson's communication program and Tufts University's School of Medicine, enrolls students from both Emerson and Tufts, and offers courses taught by faculty from both institutions. This level of innovative interdisciplinary (and for that matter, interprofessional and inter-institutional) collaboration is unique and offers the students in this program an opportunity for a health communication education that emphasizes the intricacies of both the communication process and the health care delivery system.

Future Directions in Health Communication Inquiry

Health communication inquiry has come a long way and is moving in a very positive direction. Current research on health communication clearly illustrates the powerful influences of communication on health (see for example Kreps & O'Hair, 1995). Health communication inquiry has become increasingly sophisticated and directed towards addressing significant social issues. With the growing sophistication of health communication has come increasing interdisciplinary and institutional credibility for health communication scholars.

Health communication scholars are more likely now than in any time in the past to attract federal research funding. Federal agencies in the USA, such as the Centers for Disease Control (CDC), the National Cancer Institute (NCI), and the National Institute for Drug Abuse (NIDA) have become increasingly involved with sponsoring and conducting health communication research. For example, the NCI, the largest institute of the National Institutes of Health (NIH), recently identified cancer communications as one its scientific priorities for cancer research and outreach (1999). The NCI has designed and has begun implementing a comprehensive research and outreach strategy for introducing powerful new communication initiatives that promise to expand health communication knowledge and influence public health policies and practices. Responsibility for developing many of these new research and outreach initiatives rests with the new Health Communication and Informatics Research Branch (HCIRB), a part of NCI's Behavioral Research Program within the Division of Cancer Control and Populations Sciences that is dedicated to research about the influences of communication and informatics (computer-mediated communications) in cancer prevention and control. The introduction of the HCIRB coincides with and complements the NCI's identification of cancer communications as an area of extraordinary opportunity and institutional investment.

The CDC has also established an Office of Communications with a Division of Health Communication dedicated toward emphasizing the development of rigorous message-based communication interventions across the CDC's many important health risk prevention initiatives. Similarly, the US Agency for Health Care Research and Quality (AHRQ) has increasingly emphasized the importance of health communication research and interventions in their many publications, conferences, and outreach programs.

Communication scholars are receiving increasingly more respect from more established social sciences, with health communication scholars invited to participate in interdisciplinary research teams and edit interdisciplinary social scientific journals, such as the *American Behavioral Scientist*. See, for example, the November, 1994 issue of the *American Behavioral Scientist* edited by Scott Ratzan that is devoted to "Health Communication: Challenges for the 21st Century" and the July/August 1991 issue devoted to "Communicating to Promote Health," co-edited by Gary Kreps and Charles Atkin. Similarly, Kreps edited a special issue of the *Journal of Health Psychology* (Volume 1(3), 1996) devoted to "Messages and Meanings: Health Communication and Health Psychology" that showcased state-of-the-art health communication research by respected communication scholars. Kreps is currently editing another special issue of the *Journal of Health Psychology* on "E-Health: Computer-Mediated Health Communication," scheduled for publication in 2003. This level of interdisciplinary respect and credibility marks the growing maturation of the field of health communication.

There is a growing emphasis on public advocacy, consumerism, and empowerment in health communication research that will help revolutionize the modern health care system by equalizing power between providers and consumers and relieving a great deal of strain on the modern health care system by encouraging disease prevention, self-care, and making consumers equal partners in the health care enterprise (see Arntson, 1989; Kreps, 1993; 1996a; 1996b). We believe that communication research will increasingly be used to identify the information needs of consumers and suggest strategies for encouraging consumers to take control of their health and health care. Ideally, health communication research should help identify appropriate sources of relevant health information that are available to consumers, gather data from consumers about the kinds of challenges and constraints they face within the modern health care system, as well as develop and field test educational and media programs for enhancing consumers' medical literacy. Such research will help consumers negotiate their ways through health care bureaucracies and develop communication skills for interacting effectively with health care providers.

Current and future health communication research will increasingly focus on the effective dissemination of relevant health information to promote public health. Modern health promotion efforts will recognize the multidimensional nature of health communication, identify communication strategies that incorporate multiple levels and channels of human communication, and implement a wide range of different prevention messages and campaign strategies targeted at relevant and specific (well-segmented) audiences (Maibach, Kreps, & Bonaguro, 1993). Modern campaigns will become increasingly dependent upon integrating interpersonal, group, organizational, and mediated communication to effectively disseminate relevant health information to specific at-risk populations.

Health communication inquiry is becoming increasingly concerned with the role of culture on health and health care. We believe that communication scholars will work to end the prejudicial treatment of marginalized cultural groups within the modern health care system, such as prejudicial treatment of people with AIDS, the poor, minorities, women, and the elderly (Kreps, 1996a). Future research will examine the health communication needs of marginalized cultural groups and identify strategies for enhancing health communication with members of these groups.

We believe the field of health communication is moving toward a sophisticated multidimensional agenda for applied health communication research that will examine the role of communication in health care at multiple communication levels, in multiple communication contexts, evaluate the use of multiple communication channels, and assess the influences of communication on multiple health outcomes. We are hopeful that future health communication inquiry and education will provide relevant information about the development of cooperative relationships between interdependent participants in the modern health care system, encourage the use of sensitive and appropriate interpersonal communication in health care, empower consumers to take charge of their own health care, enhance the dissemination of relevant health information and the use of strategic communication campaigns to promote public health, facilitate the development of pluralistic ideologies for effective multicultural relations in health care, and suggest adaptive strategies for using health communication to accomplish desired health outcomes.

References

Arntson, P. (1989). Improving citizen's health competencies. *Health Communication*, 1(1), 29–34.

Bandura, A. (1971). *Social learning theory*. Morristown, NJ: General Learning Press.

Bandura, A. (1969). *Principles of behavior modification*. New York: Holt, Rinehart, & Winston.

Bandura, A., & Walters, R.H. (1963). *Social learning and personality development*. New York: Holt, Rinehart, & Winston.

Bird, B. (1955). *Talking with patients*. Philadelphia: J.B. Lippincott.

Blum, L.H. (1972) *Reading between the lines: Doctor-patient communication*. New York: International Universities Press.

Bowers, W.F. (1960). *Interpersonal relations*

in the hospital. Springfield, IL: Charles C. Thomas.

Browne, K., & Freeling, P. (1967). *The doctor-patient relationship*. Edinburgh: E & S Livingstone.

Cassata, D. (1980). Health communication theory and research: A definitional overview. In D. Nimmo (Ed.), *Communication Yearbook* 4, 583–589. New Brunswick, NJ: Transaction Press.

Cassata, D. (1978). Health communication theory and research: Overview of the communication specialist interface. In B. Ruben (Ed.), *Communication Yearbook* 2, 495–504. New Brunswick, NJ: Transaction Press.

Costello, D. (1977). Health communication theory and research: An overview. In B. Ruben (Ed.), *Communication Yearbook* 1, 555–567. New Brunswick, NJ: Transaction Press.

Costello, D., & Pettegrew, L. (1979). Health communication theory and research: An overview of health organizations. In D. Nimmo (Ed.), *Communication Yearbook* 3, 607–623. New Brunswick, NJ: Transaction Press.

Feldman, J. (1966). *The dissemination of health information*. Chicago: Aldine.

Festinger, L. (1964). *Conflict, decision, and dissonance*. Stanford, CA: Stanford University Press.

Festinger, L. (1957). *A theory of cognitive dissonance*. Evanston, IL: Row Peterson.

Fishbein, M., & Ajzen, I. (1975). *Belief, attitude, intention, and behavior: An introduction to theory and research*. Reading, MA: Addison-Wesley.

Freeman, H.E. (1963). *Handbook of medical sociology*. Englewood Cliffs, NJ: Prentice Hall.

Hovland, C, Janis, I., & Kelley, H. (1953). *Communication and persuasion*. New Haven, CT: Yale University Press.

Jaco, E.G. (1972). *Patients, physicians, and illness: A sourcebook in behavioral science and health*, 2nd. ed. New York: Free Press.

Janis, I., & Feshback, S. (1953). Effects of fear-arousing communications. *Journal of Abnormal and Social Psychology*, 48, 78–92.

Katz, E., & Lazarsfeld, P. (1955). *Personal influence*. New York: The Free Press.

Klapper, J. (1960). *The effects of mass communication*. New York: The Free Press.

Kleinman, A. (1980). *Patients and healers in the context of culture*. Berkeley: University of California Press.

Kosa, J., Antonovsky, A., & Zola, I.K. (1969). *Poverty and health: A sociological analysis*. Cambridge: Harvard University Press.

Korsch, B.M. (1989). Current issues in communication research. *Health Communication*, 1(1), 5–9.

Korsch, B.M., & Negrete, V. (1972). Doctor-patient communication. *Scientific American*, 227, 66–74.

Kotler, P. (1972). A generic concept of marketing. *Journal of Marketing*, 36, 46–54.

Kotler, P., & Zaltman, G. (1971). *Social marketing: An approach to planned social change. Journal of Marketing*, 35, 3–12.

Kreps, G.L. (2001). The evolution and advancement of health communication inquiry. In W.B. Gudykunst, Ed., *Communication Yearbook* 24 (pp. 232–254). Newbury Park, CA: Sage.

Kreps, G.L. (1996a). Communicating to promote justice in the modern health care system. *Journal of Health Communication*, 1(1), 99–109.

Kreps, G.L. (1996b). Promoting a consumer orientation to health care and health promotion. *Journal of Health Psychology*, 1(1), 41–48.

Kreps, G.L. (1993). Refusing to be a victim: Rhetorical strategies for confronting cancer. In B.C. Thornton & G.L. Kreps (Eds.), *Perspectives on health communication* (pp. 42–47). Prospect Heights, IL: Waveland Press.

Kreps, G.L. (1990). Communication and health education. In E.B. Ray & L. Donohew (Eds.), *Communication and health: Systems and applications*, 187–203. Hillsdale, NJ: Lawrence Erlbaum.

Kreps, G.L. (1989). Setting the agenda for health communication research and development: Scholarship that can make a difference. *Health Communication*, 1(1), 11–15.

Kreps, G. L. (1988). Relational communication in health care. *Southern Speech Communication Journal, 53*, 344–359.

Kreps, G. L. (1987). The pervasive role of information in health care: Implications for health communication policy. In J. Anderson (Ed.), *Communication Yearbook 11*, (pp. 238–276). Newbury Park, CA: Sage.

Kreps, G.L., Bonaguro, E.W., & Query, J.L. (1998). The history and development of the field of health communication. In L.D. Jackson & B.K. Duffy (Eds.). *Health communication research: A guide to developments and direction* (pp. 1–15). Westport, CT: Greenwood Press.

Kreps, G.L., & Kunimoto, E. N. (1994). *Effective communication in multicultural health care settings*. Thousand Oaks, CA: Sage.

Kreps, G.L., & O'Hair, H.D. (1995). *Communication and health outcomes*. Cresskill, NJ: Hampton Press.

Ley, P., & Spelman, M.S. (1967). *Communicating with patients*. London: Staples Press.

Maibach, E.W., Kreps, G.L., & Bonaguro, E.W. (1993). Developing strategic communication campaigns for HIV/AIDS prevention. In S. Ratzan (Ed.), *AIDS: Effective health communication for the 90's*. Washington, D.C.: Taylor and Francis.

McCombs, M., & Shaw, D. (1972–1973). The agenda-setting function of mass media. *Public Opinion Quarterly*, 36, 176–187.

McGuire, W.J. (1984). Public communication as a strategy for inducing health promoting behavioral change. *Preventive Medicine*, 13, 299–319.

McGuire, W.J. (1969). Attitude and attitude change. In G. Lindzey & E. Aronson (Eds.), *Handbook of social psychology* (2nd. ed., pp. 136–314). Reading, MA: Addison-Wesley.

Mechanic, D. (1968). *Medical sociology: A selective view.* New York: The Free Press.

Mendelsohn, H. (1973). Some reasons why information campaigns can succeed. *Public Opinion Quarterly*, 37, 50–61.

National Cancer Institute. (1999). *The nation's investment in cancer research: A budget proposal for fiscal year 2001*. Washington, DC: NCI.

Nussbaum, J.F. (1989). Directions for research within health communication. *Health Communication*, 1(1), 35–40.

Pettegrew, L.S. (1987). Theoretical plurality in health communication. In J. Anderson (Ed.), *Communication Yearbook* 11, (298–308). Newbury Park, CA, Sage.

Reardon, K.K. (1987). The role of persuasion in health promotion and disease prevention Review and commentary. In J. Anderson (Ed.), *Communication Yearbook* 11, (276–297). Newbury Park, CA, Sage.

Rogers, E.F., & Shoemaker, F.F. (1971). *Communication of innovations: A cross-cultural approach.* New York: Free Press.

Rogers, E.M. (1973). *Communication strategies for family planning*. New York: Free Press.

Rokeach, M. (1973). *The nature of human values*. New York: The Free Press.

Ruesch, J., & Bateson, G. (1951). *Communication: The social matrix of psychiatry.* New York: Norton.

Smith, D.H. (1989). Studying health communication: An agenda for the future. *Health Communication*, 1(1), 17–27.

Starr, P. (1982). *The social transformation of American medicine*. New York: Basic Books.

Tichenor, P.J., Donohue, G.A., & Olien, G.N. (1970). Mass media flow and differential growth in knowledge. *Public Opinion Quarterly*, 34(2), 158–170.

Verwoerdt, A. (1966). *Communication with the fatally ill*. Springfield, IL: Charles C. Thomas.

Vorhaus, M.G. (1957). *The changing doctor-patient relationship*. New York: Horizon Press.

Wade, S., & Schramm, W. (1969). The mass media as sources of public affairs, science, and health knowledge. *The Public Opinion Quarterly,* 33, 197–209.

Zola, I.K. (1966). Culture and symptoms: An analysis of patients presenting complaints. *American Sociological Review*, 3, 615–630.

Discussion Questions

1. How does an interdisciplinary approach enrich the study of health communication? What are the specific contributions of fields like psychology and social influence, and how have these fields aided the development of health communication scholarship?
2. What topics are important for health communication scholars to consider? Why do we need an entire sub-field of health communication to study these topics? Would there be an advantage if fields like epidemiology and health-care economics were to subsume the study of communication and health?
3. What institutions and organizations are involved in the study of health communication? What conclusions can we draw from the authors' description of key moments in health communication? ✦

Chapter 2 Communication in the Age of Managed Care

Introduction to the Special Issue

Katherine Miller and Daniel J. Ryan

In Chapter 2, Katherine Miller and Daniel J. Ryan shine a light on managed care and its impact on the whole realm of health care and health. The purpose of including the chapter in Part I is to remind us that we cannot talk about communication in the context of health without recognizing the increasing role of managed care. In a sense, managed care organizations represent new walls that potentially shape and thus divide health-care providers from the patients seeking their care. Managed care institutions, like HMOs, have significantly changed the ways in which Americans offer, receive, and discuss health-related issues. In this chapter, Miller and Ryan illustrate the ever-changing intersections between communication and managed care. Both organizations and human relationships are implicated in these changes; therefore, health communication scholars and practitioners must attend to the interpersonal, group, organizational, legislative, and mass-mediated elements of managed care.

Related Topics: ethical issues, health-care behaviors, managed care, organizations, patient-provider communication, patients' perspectives, role of the patient

---

From "Communication in the Age of Managed Care: Introduction to the Special Issue," Katherine Miller and Daniel J. Ryan, 2001, *Journal of Applied Communication Research*, Vol. 29:2, pp. 91–96.

Two decades ago, one would be hard-pressed to find a single scholarly article on managed care, let alone a special issue of a journal devoted to the topic. Hacker and Marmor (1999) claim that the term "managed care" was still being introduced and explained to the public in the *New York Times* as recently as 1989. Managed care, though, has quickly become the predominant method of providing health care in the United States. In 1996, managed care organizations had enrolled between 80 and 90% of individuals who had health insurance (Brider, 1996). This is remarkable considering that fee-for-service health care was clearly the system most people were familiar with in the 1970s and the start of the 1980s. Traditional fee-for-service, where a patient acts as a bill-payer and is reimbursed through an indemnity insurance plan, is no longer the dominant method of payment—indeed, fee-for-service now accounts for just 2% of private health plans (Hacker & Marmor, 1999). Thus, in just 20 years, the way Americans offer, receive, and discuss medical treatment has radically changed. Managed care, along with its many acronyms (the two most widely used are probably HMOs—health maintenance organizations—and PPOs—preferred provider organizations), has found its way into the lexicon of everyday life.

While the roots of managed care can be traced back to just after World War II, this delivery and payment system did not gain in popularity until the mid-1980s when health care costs skyrocketed and companies searched for ways to reduce costs (Lammers & Geist, 1997). The soaring costs were a result of a variety of factors, including the increasing life expectancy of Americans and increasing technological sophistication of medicine. And, when government health care programs like Medicare and Medicaid offered no real incentive to providers for keeping costs down, it is little surprise that health care costs spiraled out of control. As a result, employers supplying health insurance for their employees were struggling to keep up. A survey of 300 companies in New England between 1983 and 1985 found that health plan costs had risen an average 20 percent annually (Karpoff, 1986). Reducing benefits would only serve to hurt employee health care and morale, so many companies faced a choice: either continually increase deductibles of employees or implement managed care plans. Most organizations chose the latter.

Managed care plans have been in existence since the passing of the 1973 Health Maintenance Organization Act that began the proliferation of prepaid health care plans (Wilkerson, Devers, & Given, 1997). As a result of ever-increasing health costs and the factors outlined above, managed care quickly became a part of the vernacular of health care. One method of cost control was the elimination of fee-for-service indemnity insurance as a basis of health care reimbursement. To supporters of managed care, such a change effectively eliminated the system of giving doctors and hospitals blank checks with which to serve their patients. Managed care imposed managerial authority onto a system that was out of control (at least in the eyes of those paying the bills). This authority would do two things: it would first restrain costs but it would also "rationalize an allegedly archaic structure of medical finance and delivery" (Hacker & Marmor, 1999). To opponents of managed care, these plans were seen as an attempt by those who pay the medical bills to limit care to only those who absolutely need the care (Cohn, 1989).

The actual structures and processes of managed care are seen by proponents as mechanisms that will bring doctors and hospitals back in touch with realistic expectations for medical treatment. In doing so, the hope has been that costs will be controlled and also that access to care will increase and the quality of that care will improve. The use of utilization review, critical pathways, and gatekeeping, along with other processes, has enabled managed care systems to be somewhat successful in their goals. Utilization review, involves the precertification of medical procedures to ensure that the procedure is warranted, critical pathways are the day-by-day plans specifying the least costly procedures for a patient's recovery, and gatekeeping is where the physician controls all referrals within the system in order to keep costs down and limit needless referrals. Other structures and processes have been instituted as well, including the increased use of nurse practitioners and physician assistants, and the institution of "provider profiling" to track treatment choices and expenses. Opponents of managed care, however, argue that the goal of cost reduction is honored far more than the goals of quality and access. As a result, these structures and processes have the potential to decrease the level of care received by patients in today's health care system.

Influence of Communication in Managed Care

Institutions and human relationships are both changing as a result of the influx of managed care in our health care system, and communication is playing an ever-increasing role in these developments. These changes can be seen on a number of levels including interpersonal, group, organizational, legislative, and mass media. At the interpersonal level, managed care is changing one of the most fundamental relationships of health care, that between the provider and the patient. Often, the provider-patient relationship involves disclosing the most intimate details of one's life. This relationship may be less personal as medical personnel hurry from patient to patient as they contend with a burgeoning caseload (though a recent study—see Mechanic, McAlpine, & Rosenthal, 2001—concludes that managed health care has not been associated with a reduction in the length of office visits). Continuity of care may also be compromised if individuals must find a new physician when employers change health plans. Further, managed care introduces the possibility that confidentiality could be breached, as sensitive information is shared among a variety of health care workers (Allen, 1998).

In addition to a shift in the provider-patient relationship, managed care is also necessitating an interdisciplinary team approach to health care. Researchers have suggested that effective interdisciplinary health care teams are needed to meet the challenges of rapidly changing economic and competitive forces facing health care organizations (Hansen & Hayes, 1998; LaVallee & McLaughlin, 1994; Whorley, 1996). The study of health care teams is not new; research in this area has existed for over 50 years (e.g. Wilson, 1954). Managed care, however, has increased the use of health care teams and communication is critical in the success of these teams. Health care teams have evolved from being a set of "silos" with little overlap to a more integrative approach that emphasizes the collaborative nature of care (Abramson & Mizrahi, 1996; Fagin, 1992). Communication is key as health care professionals negotiate what it means to be involved on different teams, how to work with persons from different areas of health care and how all of this flux influences their professional identity.

At the organizational level, managed care has shaped both the tasks people play inside the organization as well as the messages companies are sending to their employees. The role of physicians and nurses now includes both providing treatment as well as attending to the forms and other administrative duties associated with managed care (e.g., Harrison, 1999; Miller, Joseph, & Apker, 2000). The increased documentation and coding procedures of treatment is necessary for reimbursement but may also take time away from seeing patients. Changes can be seen beyond the confines of health care organizations as well. A variety of industries are now increasingly concerned with reducing health care costs through the promotion of wellness programs, on-site fitness opportunities, and organizational assistance programs.

The legislative arena, where the real impetus for managed care began with the passing of the 1973 Health Maintenance Organization Act, has had considerable influence on managed care. Most states have introduced legislation that regulate health plans as well as attempt to protect the rights of people enrolled in the plans. Protections for emergency room patients, creation of panels for those denied care, and removing extreme financial incentives for physicians have all been methods legislatures have used to mold health care. The debate over the right to sue HMOs has been hotly contested, and this dialogue will undoubtedly modify the state of managed care in this country.

Finally, as modifications are continually being made to the system, managed care remains highly visible in the mass media. Almost daily newspaper articles can be found regarding the latest changes in health care policy or about lawsuits filed by disgruntled consumers. News magazine shows like *Dateline* and *60 Minutes* have aired stories regarding the subject of managed care and political advertising is rife with references to health care reform. Indeed, the 1993 health care reform debate was marked by the well-known "Harry and Louise" commercials, in which a couple discussed health care reform with the tag line "there must be a better way." Even in entertainment venues, managed care references abound. Theater audiences are reputed to have stood up and cheered when Helen Hunt's character in *As Good as it Gets* spoke in a derogatory way about HMOs.

With all of these notions in mind about the intersection between communication and managed care, a two day conference in early May 2000 was held on the campus of Texas A&M University. The title of the conference was "Communication in the Age of Managed Care" and the conference focused on the multitude of ways in which communication impacts this health care process. The conference brought together scholars, practitioners, and policy-makers to engage in discussion and debate on various aspects of communication, from patient provider interaction to organizational communication to public health and policy. The format included a mixture of workshops, roundtable discussions, and paper presentations given by persons from all over the country and abroad.

Highlighting the conference were three distinguished speakers: Ron Pollack, the Executive Director of Families USA—a national organization for health care consumers, and Jim Rohack, the president of the Texas Medical Association, gave the two plenary speeches. Theodore Marmor provided the keynote address. Pollack is a frequent guest on national television and radio programs and spoke on empowering consumers and physicians in a managed care environment. Rohack, who is also a senior staff cardiologist at Scott and White Clinic, presented "Competency, Communication and Cash" which focused on some of the economic realities of a managed care system. Finally, Dr. Theodore Marmor, Professor of Public Policy and Management at the Yale School of Management and director of the Robert Wood Johnson Foundation post-doctoral program in health policy gave the keynote address. Marmor's riveting talk tackled the current language being used in health care and its effect on how we view managed care.

The other highlight of the conference was the presentation of scholarly papers and participation in panel discussions by a range of researchers in the fields of communication, public health, medicine, journalism, and others. These papers ran the gamut of issues discussed above, including considerations of confidentiality in patient care, stress and burnout in managed care professionals, coverage of managed care in the media, communication within interdisciplinary health care teams, the influence of managed care in the treatment of specific patient populations, and the role of the community in managed care systems. Because of our excitement with the discussions at this conference, a call for papers was distributed to conference participants and the wider academic communities in communication and health, soliciting papers for this special issue of *Journal of Applied Communication Research.* The special issue you see before you, then, is the outcome of this conference and wider call.

The submissions to the special issue were evaluated by an editorial board that was both efficient and insightful. Our thanks go out to those reviewers: Chuck Atkin of Michigan State University, Ellen Bonaguro of Ithaca College, Eric Eisenberg of University of South Florida, Debra Ford of Creighton University, Patricia Geist of San Diego State University, Kathryn Greene of Rutgers University, Ruth Guzley of California State University at Chico, Linda Larkey of University of Arizona, Roxanne Parrott of Pennsylvania State University, Jim Query of Loyola University, Eileen Berlin Ray of Cleveland State University, Kevin Real of Texas A&M University, Rajiv Rimal of the University of Texas, Barbara Sharf of Texas A&M University, Sandi Smith of Michigan State University, Rick Street of Texas A&M University, Teresa Thompson of the University of Dayton, and Pam Whitten of Michigan State University.

The five articles that are included in this special issue represent the breadth of interest that can be stimulated when considering the intersection of managed health care and communication. Indeed, the articles represent a wide range of substantive issues, levels of analysis, and methodological choices and serve to stimulate our thinking about managed care in a number of areas. The first article, *The Politics of Breathing: Asthmatic Medicaid Patients under Managed Care* by S. Renee Gillespie takes a critical look at the discourse of asthmatic patients and their caregivers who rely on Medicaid. Her reading shows these patients actively struggling in the midst of a disciplinary logic created by the rules and regulations of managed care and by norms for self-care. The second article, *Role Development in the Managed Care Era: A Case of Hospital-Based Nursing* by Julie Apker moves our attention to the care provider working within a managed care environment. In a qualitative analysis of interviews and observation of a hospital nursing unit, Apker confronts the challenges that nurses face in trying to "make sense" of a role that faces many changes in a managed care environment. With the third article in this special issue, *Tensions in Community Health Improvement Initiatives: Communication and Collaboration in a Managed Care Environment* by Caryn E. Medved and colleagues, we confront the fact that managed care relationships and organizations are embedded within larger communities and that those communities are often active stakeholders in systems of health care provision. Medved, et al., examine Comprehensive Community Health Models in three counties, and reveal five tensions that characterized collaboration within these initiatives. The final two articles continue this "macro" view of managed care by pointing our attention to debates over managed care policy, both in legislative bodies and in public discourse. In *Confronting Free Market Romanticism: Health Care Reform in the Least Likely Place,* Charles Conrad and Brad Millay examine the 1997 debate in the Texas Legislature regarding Senate Bill 386, or the Texas "HMO Patient's Bill of Rights." Their examination of narratives of "good and evil," "hero[e]s and vill[ai]ns," and symbolic purification illustrate the rhetorical creation of health care reform, even in the "least likely" of places. Finally, in *Managing Health Care in Oregon: The Search for a Civic Bioethics,* Sharon L. Bracci reminds us of the role of the public in health care debate, and of the complexity of the bioethical issues that confront us in these debates. Her analysis of Oregon's attempt to engage in public deliberation regarding access to health care and allocation of scarce resources provides an important analysis of the difficult processes involved in fashioning a policy of "collective compassion."

References

Abramson, J. S., & Mizrahi, T. (1996). When social workers and physicians collaborate: Positive and negative interdisciplinary experiences. *Social Work,* 41, 270–281.

Allen, K. (1998). Maintaining patient confidentiality in today's health care environment. *Imprint,* 45, 37–39.

Brider, P. (1996). Huge job loss projections shock health professionals. *American Journal of Nursing,* 96, 61–64.

Cohn, V. (1989, November 21). Someone besides you and the doctor may be deciding how you get treated; welcome to "managed care." *The Washington Post,* pp. Z12.

Fagin, C. M. (1992). Collaboration between nurses and physicians: No longer a choice. *Academic Medicine,* 67, 295–303.

Hacker, J. S., & Marmor, T. R. (1999). How not to think about "managed care," *University of Michigan Journal of Law Reform,* 32.

Hansen, M. C, & Hayes, P. A. (1998). Integrating students into interdisciplinary teams: Extending the caring circle. *Seminars for Nurse Managers,* 6, 4, 214–218.

Harrison, J. K. (1999). Influence of managed care on professional nursing practice. *Image: Journal of Nursing Scholarship,* 31, 161–166.

Karpoff, S. (1986, January 5). Second opinions on benefit plans. *The Record,* pp. B01.

Lammers, J., & Geist, P. (1997). The transformation of caring in the light and shadow of "managed care." *Health Communication,* 9, 45–60.

LaVallee, R., & McLaughlin, G P. (1994). Teams at the core. In G P. McLaughlin & A. D. Kaluzny, (Eds.). *Continuous quality improvement in health care.* Gaithersburg, MD: Aspen.

Mechanic, D., McAlpine, D. D., & Rosenthal, M. (2001). Are patients' office visits with physicians getting shorter? *New England Journal of Medicine,* 344.

Miller, K., Joseph, L., & Apker, J. (2000). Strategic ambiguity in the role development process. *Journal of Applied Communication Research,* 28, 193–214.

Whorley, L. W. (1996). Evaluating health care team performance: Assessment of joint problem-solving action. *The Health Care Supervisor,* 14, 4, 71–76.

Wilkerson, J., Devers, K., & Given, R. (1997). *Competitive managed care: The emerging health care system.*

Wilson, R. N. (1954). Teamwork in the operating room. *Human Organization,* 12, 9–14.

Discussion Questions

1. How does managed care operate? Why would health communication scholars be interested in studying managed care?

2. Miller and Ryan highlight five areas in which communication and managed care intersect: interpersonal, group, and organizational communication, legislation, and mass media. Which of these five areas is most important to understand in order to improve individual health?

3. Are there better alternatives to managed care? If so, what are the communication opportunities and problems that these alternatives must consider? If not, how might communication improve the operation of managed care organizations? ✦

Chapter 3
E-Health

Reinventing Healthcare in the Information Age

Russell C. Coile, Jr.

Chapter 3 addresses yet another contemporary force impacting health communication dramatically: the Internet. Perhaps no other single factor accounts for more boundary-breaking ways in which health information and communication flow in the twenty-first century. The Internet is becoming the newest industry in health care. This chapter outlines nine strategies for health-care providers doing business on the Internet. There is great potential and opportunity for health-related businesses to become involved in e-health and the information age.

Related Topics: aging, e-health, health-care behaviors, Internet, managed care, media, organizations, patient-provider communication, role of the patient

The Internet is the next frontier for healthcare. Some consumers turn to local hospitals or health plans for health information, but many employ the web to search on a global basis for the latest medical research and evaluated treatment data. Healthcare consumers are flooding into cyberspace, and an Internet-based industry of health information providers is springing up to serve them. Last year more than 18 million Americans went online seeking health information and advice, according to Cyber Dialogue, a New York-based Internet market research organization (Santiago 1998). As Internet traffic continues to soar, even that 1998 estimate may be low. A January, 1999 poll by the Pew Research Center for People and the Press found that 74 million adults had logged onto the Internet, and 40 million of them had used it at least once for health reasons (Weber 1999).

Rapidly rising web traffic on health sites is only the beginning. A recent study by Northwestern University and KPMG in Chicago affirms that baby boomers are the quintessential generation to demand what they want, fueled by medical information that is available on the Internet (Howgill 1998). Healthcare providers with well-developed web sites, such as Houston's M. D. Anderson and the Cleveland Clinic, will reinforce their brand identity and gain customer loyalty by providing easy Internet access to detailed health information. Many hospitals and health systems are just beginning to focus resources on web-enabled e-commerce (i.e., electronic commerce) and business applications, such as marketing, physician directories, and employee recruitment, according to national data from the Health Information Management Systems Society.

Nine Strategies for Healthcare Providers and Businesses Doing Business on the Web

Although pharmaceuticals and over-the-counter remedies are widely splashed across the web, many healthcare providers, health insurers, and managed care plans have yet to climb on the Internet bandwagon. Market observer Robert Schaich recently commented that the use of the Internet to support true electronic commerce is accelerating in most industries while the health industry and managed care seem to be stuck in first gear (Schaich 1999).

Healthcare is a knowledge-based business, but knowledge has not been a part of the business model (Reuthe and Allee 1999). Knowledge is not perceived as a part of the value proposition of healthcare. That limited mindset is now being turned on its

From "E-Health: Reinventing Healthcare in the Information Age," Russell C. Coile, Jr. Used with permission from *Journal of Healthcare Management,* Vol. 45:3, pp. 206–210. (Chicago: Health Administration Press, 2000).

head. There are dozens of potential applications and e-commerce opportunities for web-enabled business in the health field, which range from information display and advertising to online commercial transactions and payments.

1. Advertising

Internet advertising may be the most cost-effective method for reaching healthcare consumers. Pharmaceutical companies that spend 50 percent of their marketing budgets on direct-to-consumer advertising are expected to invest heavily in the web. The web can connect healthcare consumers and providers at a mouse click, thus expanding healthcare to be a truly global enterprise. Michael Spector, MD, of the University Hospital in Cleveland, Ohio, reports: "When you talk to a patient about something major [health problem], they may remember 10 percent. The Internet allows them to ask questions again and get information that was once hard to get without access to a medical library" (Santiago 1998).

2. Choosing Providers

Many consumers do not have a regular source of health information or medical care until they get sick. Hospitals and health plans are employing the Internet to match patients with providers. A growing number of HMOs and health plans offer physician directories, which can be searched by zip code as well as clinical specialty. Most web-browsing healthcare consumers will ultimately choose a local provider, but some patients will use the Internet to find world-class medical organizations with top physicians and research projects. The Internet allows nationally recognized hospitals to advertise both nationally and internationally.

Health plans and hospitals have been the first to offer provider directories, but other healthcare services are catching up. Consumers seeking information on long-term care providers can now turn to Senior Place.com, a Portland-based firm. We are "building electronic bridges between acute care and long-term care," believes Jeff Pentacost, M.D., founder of SeniorPlace (Brock 1998). Offerings from SeniorPlace will include a patient referral network, listings of providers, and service profiles, with links to web sites of long-term care providers.

3. Customer Information and Referral

Internet-based "help desks" assist consumers with navigating the health system, finding a physician, and checking their health plan's benefits. United Healthcare offers Optum Health Forum, a sophisticated web site where United enrollees can search for information, ask about benefits, or check their doctors status as a participating provider. Other large health insurers are investing heavily in providing consumer information and referral through the web. Intelli Health, one of the most popular consumer web sites for health information, is a joint venture of Aetna with Johns Hopkins, which provides much of the site's medical content.

4. Online Shopping

The web is the biggest shopping mall on the planet. During the holiday season in December, 1998, online shoppers spent $3.5 billion over the Internet. Forrester Research predicts total online market sales may reach $200 billion a year by 2000. Early consumer worries about privacy are easing.

Online shopping has just begun to focus on healthcare as a broad consumer niche. Health-related products and services likely to be sold widely on the web include: prescription drug refills; over-the-counter drugs; medical supplies for the chronically ill, such as diabetics; durable medical equipment; vitamins and homeopathic medicines; and home fitness equipment.

Shopping on the web offers convenience, speed, comparability, and price. It is just like opening an electronic catalog, but with an almost limitless range of products and services. Internet shopping combines *Consumer Reports* information with discount outlet prices. Smart shoppers like the detailed product descriptions available from web-based emporiums, and cost-conscious consumers have the ability to purchase name brands online, often at substantial savings.

5. Internet Pharmacy

Pharmaceutical refills have been identified as a high-volume, high-dollar niche that may be just right for the Internet. Mail-order pharmacies may rapidly become obsolete in the face of Internet competitors. Firms such as drugstore.com are just getting started. Selling pharmaceuticals requires state licenses, which has slowed the arrival of online access to drug refills. Prices will be competitive with the deepest discounts available, but with the convenience of next-day home delivery. The nation's most active health web site, drkoop.com, offers pharmaceutical refills and bundles a free "drug checker" software screen for drug compatibility.

6. Health Insurance Sales

Health insurers and HMOs are targeting the web as a future channel for consumer registration, eligibility verification, and transaction processing. Internet-savvy health insurance customers in the future may shop for a health plan from discount Internet brokers, a web-enabled market already widely used for online purchase of automobiles, life insurance, and airplane tickets. Consumers like the price savings of "disintermediation" (cutting out the middleman).

Health insurance sold on the web could become a national business, leapfrogging state and local markets. The biggest health plans and HMOs, which are already licensed in multiple states, could jump most quickly to national marketing. Companies such as United Healthcare, Aetna U.S. Healthcare, CIGNA, and the Blue Cross-Blue Shield Associations have the multimarket presence and local networks to service customers on a national basis. National health plans have moved quickly to adopt the Internet as an integral component in their sales and marketing plan.

At the same time, these big health plans may be vulnerable to new web-based "virtual insurers" with low overhead that would contract at wholesale prices with local provider networks and revolutionize the health insurance market. Medicare HMOs and PPOs could be sold online to a national market of the "wired retired," the estimated 40 percent of seniors who now have online access. These national Medicare HMOs could become licensed by Health Care Financing Administration (HCFA) in every state. Medicare PPOs are authorized by the Balanced Budget Act of 1997, but have not yet been implemented by HCFA.

7. Electronic Medical Records

Predictions for the proliferation of electronic medical records (EMRs) are being realized. No paperless hospitals exist in the United States today, but the Mayo Clinic's new Scottsdale hospital hopes to become virtually paperless within five years. Internet connectivity offers a low-cost architecture of "intranets" and "extranets" that link internal and external provider sites, including physician offices, nursing homes, and in-home electronic monitoring equipment for the chronically ill.

Medical information will be universally accessible to participating providers in "data warehouses" with huge electronic storage capacities. Patient information can be accessed on a real-time basis for diagnosis and treatment. Health plans and provider-sponsored integrated delivery networks can "mine" their databases to assess and predict risks, as well as to measure their own medical care against clinical and economic benchmarks.

Internet-based patient records can allow consumers to "own" their electronic medical records. Internet health information providers such as drkoop.com encourage consumers to register their health history, and to build a record of their own health status over time. Universal patient identifiers such as Social Security numbers can provide an Internet address for future medical data from providers to be electronically compiled. The goal is to have informed consumers who are empowered to monitor and manage their health improvements.

8. Online Health Advice and Telemedicine

With little regulation in place yet, some healthcare consumers and providers are venturing into new territory by dispensing health advice online, and even prescribing pharmaceuticals for a fee. The practice is frowned upon by professional organizations, and the source of frustration for state-based regulators who are concerned about health professionals doing business across state boundaries without state licenses. Although prescribing drugs over the Internet is controversial, online consultations for patients seeking Viagra are already available, through web sites such as viagra purchase.com, with 48-hour delivery of the pharmaceuticals.

Internet-based telemedicine may become widely used in the coming decade as a cost-effective method for remote diagnosis, patient information, case management and monitoring, and remote medical consultation.

9. Customer Service

The Internet will be widely used by health plans, hospitals, and large medical groups to provide customer service, including:

- verification of health plan eligibility;
- explanation of health plan benefits;
- search for a plan-approved provider;
- off-hours questions from patients or enrollees;
- requests for referral information, such as long-term care;
- online registration of new enrollees; and
- notification of changes in status, such as a new address.

Internet access for patient self-scheduling is likely to be a popular service enhancement. This allows patients to scan their doctors' calendars and then self-schedule an appointment. Such a system can also provide patients with Internet reminders of appointment times and dates.

Looking Forward: Reinventing Medicine on the Net

Internet connections and high-speed telecommunications will not just speed up medicine—they may revolutionize it. In other fields, e-mail and the Internet have created an "X-factor" that has stimulated the U.S. economy through increased productivity and efficiency, observes Andrew Grove, Chairman of Intel (Ukens 1998). Now it is time for an X-factor to be applied to healthcare, where Internet technology can be used to keep costs in check, while deepening patient-provider relationships through increased communication and care.

References

Brock, K. 1998. "Website Offers Long-Term Care Information." *Business Journal—Portland* 15 (27): 6.

Howgill, M. W. 1998. "Health Care Consumerism, the Information Explosion, and Branding: Why 'Tis Better to Be the Cowboy Than the Cow." *Managed Care Quarterly* 6 (4): 33–43.

Reuthe, E., and V. Allee. 1999. "Knowledge Management: Moving the Care Model from a Snapshot to a Story." *Healthcare Forum Journal* 42 (3): 26–28.

Santiago, R. 1998. "Supply and Demand Increase for Internet Health Resources." *Crain's Cleveland Business* Dec. 7: 18.

Schaich, R. L. 1999. "Internet Commerce and Managed Care." *Health Management Technology* 19 (7): 43–47.

Ukens, C. 1998. "Internet Access Transforming Health Care, Says Koop." *Drug Topics* 142 (22): 80.

Weber, D, 1999. "Web Sites of Tomorrow: How the Internet Will Transform Healthcare." *Healthcare Forum Journal* 42 (3): 40–45.

Discussion Questions

1. This chapter outlines strategies for bringing health care onto the web. What are some of the positive and negative outcomes of these strategies?
2. How would a move toward e-health affect consumers who do not have Internet access?
3. Should having health-care business information online reduce the responsibility of health-care providers to distribute information in traditional formats (i.e., in person, over the phone, through postal mail services)? ✦

Chapter 4 Illness Narratives and the Social Construction of Health

Barbara F. Sharf and Marsha L. Vanderford

Chapter 4 completes the framework of Part I by focusing on the socially constructed reality that shapes all of our notions of health, illness, sickness, well-being, and the various concepts that are part of looking at the role of communication in health care. Our social constructions create the walls that define our boundaries, as well as forge the doors through which it is possible to go outside those walls. Health communication has traditionally been researched from a biomedical, social-scientific perspective. As you read this chapter, consider the argument that there are many benefits to viewing health communication as socially constructed and that there are specific benefits to focusing on illness narratives. Using a variety of different studies, as well as a narrative of one woman's experience living with a neurological disease, this chapter suggests that health communication could be fruitfully explored by placing a greater emphasis on patients' own experiences of health and illness.

Related Topics: culture, health-care behaviors, history, patient-centered communication, patients' perspectives, role of the patient, social support

From "Illness Narratives and the Social Construction of Health," Barbara F. Sharf and Marsha L. Vanderford, 2003, *Handbook of Health Communication,* edited by A. M. Dorsey, K. I. Miller, R. Parrott, T. L. Thompson, pp. 9–34.

Rose, a 20-year-old college sophomore, was the designated driver for a group of friends coming home from a party one evening in the suburbs of Charleston, South Carolina. The group lost their way, and while searching for a familiar landmark, Rose failed to stop for a blinking red light. After a police vehicle tailed her car for a few miles, she was signaled to pull over to the side of the road. The police officer shined a flashlight on the three occupants of the car, asked to see Rose's driver license, directed her to get out of the car, then queried, "What's the matter with your eyes?" Though Rose explained that, because of a neuromuscular problem, her eyelid muscles sag when she is tired (a condition called ptosis*), the officer accused Rose of driving while under the influence of alcohol or drugs, an allegation that Rose vehemently denied.*

The officer replied that she could see the effect of alcohol in Rose's eyes. Rose explained that she suffered from a neurological disease called myasthenia gravis*, in her case a congenital condition. Myasthenia gravis is caused by inadequate connections between the nervous system and the muscles, resulting in generalized muscle weakness and periods of extreme fatigue. Medications help to keep the symptoms from being overpowering and to slow degeneration but do not eliminate all the problems.*

Although Rose showed the officer a disability parking permit, the officer did not buy this explanation. Instead, she insisted that Rose walk a straight line, but being stressed and tired, the young woman had trouble with this task. Rose asked to be given a breath[a]lizer test twice, but her requests were denied. In the end, the officer ticketed her for driving under the influence of alcohol (DUI), took her bail bond card, and gave her a date for a court appearance. Rose followed the advice of a disabilities lawyer, who arranged to have Rose's DUI charges dropped in exchange for her having to take a test for a special driver's license that permanently categorizes her as a person with a neuromuscular ailment and that requires an annual retest.

Rose's story is an excellent illustration of how matters of health and illness are socially constructed; that is, how bodily and psychological states of being are perceived and imbued with social and cultural meaning. In this chapter, we start with a brief overview of the social construction perspective, its bases in rhetorical and communication theory, and its application to communication referencing matters of health and illness. Following this introduction, we center our attention on socially shared health-related narratives, among the most common and powerful forms of symbolic construction. Although we refer to a widely diverse scholarly literature, we have not tried to present an exhaustive survey of the field. Instead, we refer to exemplary studies, including some of our own, that we find particularly instructive for understanding the health narrative approach. We then identify, discuss, and illustrate five functions of health narratives: sense-making, asserting control, transforming identity, warranting decisions, and building community. We conclude with several points to consider as the narrative perspective becomes increasingly incorporated into health communication scholarship. Throughout this chapter, we use Rose's narrative to illuminate our conceptual explanations.

Evolution of the Social Construction Approach

Sociologists Peter Berger and Thomas Luckmann (1966) defined the social construction of reality as a dialectic between social reality and individual existence—in other words, a symbolically based tension between commonly accepted knowledge and personal understanding. Social constructions of reality are mediated through linguistic expression articulated among people and communities, shaped and recorded as history.

The philosophical roots of the symbolic representation of reality are clearly evident in historical and contemporary rhetorical and communication theories. Ever since Plato in the *Gorgias* ridiculed the sophistic practice of teaching rhetoric as a vehicle of appearance rather than of truth, scholars have debated the role and purpose of communication. Two opposing positions have characterized the controversy: (1) communication ought to *represent,* to the extent possible, the material world and its truths and (2) language *creates* the world and its meanings. Two thousand years ago, the Sophists were vilified for holding a relative view of truth and teaching rhetorical skills designed to create appearances and influence public perception. The early Christian Church fathers looked with suspicion on later sophistic rhetoricians, believing that possession of religious truth was inherently persuasive without interpretation or elaboration.

This controversy has endured up until the present. Thirty-five years ago, rhetorician Robert L. Scott (1967) argued that rhetoric is epistemic, a way of knowing. His argument presumes that truth is not immutable, able to be conveyed from one person to another, but rather a "set of generally accepted social norms, experience or matters of faith that serve as reference points in working out [human] contingencies" (p. 12) and that are "the result of a process of interaction at a given moment" (p. 13). In short, truth is created through the process of communication. Scott's position has prompted a variety of responses, resulting in a debate between contrasting stances. One group of disputants claims that rhetoric is an inadequate vehicle for truth (e.g., Croasman & Cherwitz, 1982), whereas another group holds that all knowledge, even our understanding of physical objects, is created through language and intersubjective consensus (Brummett, 1976, 1982). A middle ground was laid out by Railsback (1983), who proposed that material reality is separate from language but not meaningful without symbolic interpretation. Her outlook provides a framework for examining the tension between material reality and the symbolic representation of health, illness, and disease. In a recent review of communication theories, Robert Craig (1999) reiterated the dialectic of acquiring and communicating knowledge of reality in slightly variant terms. Craig differentiated between a *transmission* concept that posits communication as the transfer of information in the form of messages "from one mind to another" (p. 125) and a *constitutive* approach that conceptualizes communication as a "process that produces and reproduces shared meaning" (p. 125). Elaborating upon this basic distinction, he made a case for using the constitutive or social construction perspective as a "metamodel" encompassing all the various particular theories that attempt to explain how communication works.

In the context of health, illness, and medical care, the application of the constitutive model of communication reveals the complexities of moderating between scientific truth derived from the physicality of organic disease and the materiality of bodies, and the meanings of human suffering experienced by patients, their loved ones, and the health professionals who care for them. The social construction approach to health communication has primarily emerged as a reaction to the biomedical perspective, long dominant in the health care arena. Similar to the ancient and contemporary schisms in communication theory we have described, the medical community has historically divided communication about health into two kinds of discourse. The first kind uses *objective* language to present traditional,[1] biomedical information about organic, verifiable, measurable signs of disease conveyed in the authoritative voices of physicians and other health providers, evidenced by clinical signs, laboratory tests, imaging, and other technologies. The second kind uses *subjective* language to talk about the internal, nonverifiable experience of illness, of being in disease. People undergoing health problems and their families develop their own understandings about physical symptoms, revealing health beliefs, augmented with personal and cultural significance, that transcend the material signs relied upon by clinicians. In medical contexts, the scientific detachment and empiricism of practitioners is valorized, whereas the subjective experiences of patients, reflecting moral, spiritual, and social elements of illness, "inevitably connote insubstantiality, something 'existing only in the mind' " (Donnelly & Brauner, 1992, p. 481). Patients whose accounts stray from physical symptoms, the review of bodily systems, and the medical chronology are characterized as "poor historians" (Brody, 1987) who distort reality with subjective perception and tangential interpretation.

However, over the past 25 years, many participants in the health care system, including clinicians, health educators, social scientists, medical humanists, and patients, have challenged biomedicine's hierarchical epistemological claims, asserting that the "scientific method is only one of several routes to knowledge" (McWhinney, 1989, p. 38). Social psychologist Elliot G. Mishler (1981) laid the foundation for seeing the implications of social construction theory in the context of clinical care. Starting with the proposition that "the world as a *meaningful* reality is constructed through human interpretative activity, " Mishler explained that "whether or not a particular behavior or experience is viewed . . . as a sign or symptom of illness depends on cultural values, social norms, and culturally shared rules of interpretation" (p. 141). Thus, observation of the same biological phenomenon, such as Rose's heavy-lidded eyes and inability to walk a straight line, is imbued with quite a different meaning for the police officer, for Rose's friends, and for Rose herself.

Furthermore, Mishler (1984) helps us to understand that within a clinical encounter, although the practitioner and the patient are ostensibly discussing the same physiological symptoms and reported history, there is nearly always a contrast, and often outright conflict, between what he calls "the voice of medicine" and "the voice of the lifeworld." Rose has enjoyed a positive relationship with Dr. Harvey, her neurologist, for several years. Nonetheless, there are inevitably significant differences between how the doctor understands the manifestation of myasthenias gravis in his patient as an organic process and Rose's experience of the impact of the disease on her intellectual, social, and emotional life. For instance, as the voice of medicine, Dr. Harvey is concerned with quantitatively assessing changes in the degree of muscle weakness in her eye. For Rose, the voice of the lifeworld, her concern with optical fatigue is focused on how it will impact her working on a computer screen under stress and thereby affect her performance on the Graduate Record Exam.

From a social construction perspective, the work of health communication scholarship is to unpack the sociocultural sources of symbolic usage in health care, for people often accept it as natural and inevitable without considering how meanings emerge from contextual and political sources in ways that mold health beliefs and behaviors, clinical judgments, and organizational routines.[2] Two influential works exemplify how the voices of medicine and of the lifeworld have become commingled within everyday discourses. Social critic and cancer survivor Susan Sontag's (1978, 1988) astute comparative analyses of tuberculosis in the 19th century and cancer and AIDS in the 20th century demonstrate the pervasiveness of disease-related connotations in many nonmedical spheres of life as well as how language shapes the identities of people suffering with those diseases, often in negative, problematic ways. For example, over the past 30 years, cancer metaphors have been used to describe the Watergate coverup of the Nixon administration, the scandalous personal behaviors that propelled the impeachment of Bill Clinton, and, most recently, rhetoric from the Bush Administration concerning terrorism in the United States (e.g., expressions of commitment to keep terrorist cells from growing). Sontag claimed convincingly that such insidious verbal comparisons contribute considerably to the suffering of people with cancer.

Pushing the direction of Sontag's work further, cultural studies scholar David Morris (1998) indicated the limits of the biomedical model of health and disease in his discussion of *postmodern illness*—"situated at the crossroads of biology and culture" (p. 71). In his view, postmodern illness is characterized by ambiguity of existence, is reflective of lifestyle and politics, and is fragmentary and interdisciplinary. Morris cites such biocultural manifestations of postmodern illness as medically mysterious diagnoses like chronic fatigue syndrome, depression, and attention deficit disorder, as well as equally mysterious modes of therapy like pain clinics and modes of complementary healing (mysterious insofar as they resist verification through empirical techniques).[3]

Cross-cultural scholarship has been particularly useful in revealing the misunderstandings that arise from conflicting cultural constructions. The work of Arthur Kleinman (1988; Kleinman, Eisenberg, & Good, 1978), a psychiatrist and medical anthropologist, has been pivotal in illustrating how illnesses are understood, explained, and acted on through ethnocultural lenses, which he calls explanatory models. His examples show how differences in explanatory models in clinical settings often increase patients' suffering and sometimes have life-threatening results. An especially striking application of Kleinman's conceptualization of cultural constructions in conflict is journalist Anne Fadiman's (1997) tragic ethnographic description of a young girl caught between the American medical system's approach to epilepsy and her immigrant family's comprehension of the condition they called "the spirit catches you and you fall down." Even modern Western societies that ostensibly share the tenets of biomedicine interpret the practice of medicine in culturally distinct ways, resulting in strikingly different clinical discourses and modes of care (Payer, 1988).

To better understand the confluence of the biomedical and sociocultural, the material and the symbolic, let's briefly consider the multiple and changing ways in which the concept of health is discussed and applied in everyday contexts by various agents. One of the most common definitions of health is in terms of its opposite: Health is the absence of disease. But health is not necessarily such an absolute state. On the popular television drama *The West Wing,* the fictional President Bartlett, an ostensibly astute, ethical, and tough-skinned chief executive, suffers from multiple sclerosis, a degenerative disease that threatens his physical and mental stamina. The public revelation of this illness raises questions that have been asked of politicians in real life as well. Is the president sufficiently healthy to continue his role as a national and international leader? What reasons might have justified the president's not disclosing his health status from the beginning? In fact, we often speak of being healthy in relative terms. We might say someone is healthy who has a chronic illness or permanent disability but is able to carry out key functions of daily living and enjoy mental well-being despite the presence of pain and physical limitations. Conceptualizing health in this way makes explicit that there are psychological and spiritual components of health integrated with the physical components.

In another common usage, the term *healthy* is used to characterize what is found in nature. Although manufactured pharmaceuticals have been increasingly relied upon to protect against or clear up infections and allergic reactions, decrease pain, and even rejuvenate bones and other body tissues, their undesired side-effects have led to the widespread popularity of herbal remedies, accompanied by an ideology that equates what is "natural" with what is healthy, even if substances found in nature also have unintended, unpleasant consequences.

This usage of the term contrasts with the way health care is increasingly viewed as an economic commodity. Consumers purchase it, providers supply it, third-party payers and health care organizations manage it, and primary care practitioners coordinate and guard entry to more specialized modes of treatment. Individuals "shop" for doctors (often from a list of those who are "preferred" financially), and physicians find ways to "fire" problematic patients. A variety of practitioners provide care that is considered alternative (or, more recently, complementary) to what is known as traditional or regular medicine, even if the alternative treatments have existed for centuries, predating modern biomedicine. When the concept of health is applied to populations or communities instead of individuals, other indices may come to the surface (e.g., safety from violence, adequate nutrition and shelter, and availability of meaningful employment). At times, the health concerns of the "public" may conflict with the rights of individuals, as in the case of vaccinations or the segregation of infectious citizens.

The several ways in which the concept of health has been situationally applied at a symbolic level clearly have serious material consequences—financial, physical, and social—for an array of stakeholders, including patients, caregivers, insurers, clinical scientists, policymakers, and guardians of public health. In short, materiality and meaning are commingled in the social construction work of health communication scholars.

Narrative Approaches to Health Communication Scholarship

As we have indicated, the social construction approach to health communication can serve as a conceptualization and method of analysis for a wide variety of issues and purposes. In this chapter, we focus primarily on a particular type of social construction, the application of the narrative perspective to health contexts, especially in the form of illness narratives. Our objective is to explain and illustrate how viewing narration as the defining paradigm of human communication (Fisher, 1987) illuminates common health-related discourses. Although we might have used this perspective to concentrate on clinical interactions, drug advertisements, the policies and practices of managed care, or other facets of health communication, much of our own previous work has investigated discourses reflecting the experience of illness, both at a personal level and as it is represented in popular media, and so we have chosen this kind of discourse as our exemplar.[4]

Following rhetorician Walter Fisher's argument that humans are *homo narrans,* the species distinguished by its ability and predisposition to tell stories, it is our assertion that the most common way of communicating our personally constructed ideas of the realities we experience is through the social sharing of narratives—stories about our lives. Narratives not only reflect individual views of the world but also provide explanations for why things happen in certain ways. They help us to recount people and events of significance, account for motives, causes, and reasons (Fisher, 1987), and are the primary means for involving others in our own world view (Bruner, 1986). Such stories regularly occur in many kinds of contexts. Some are carefully crafted accounts conveyed in public settings and mass media, others are informal tales incorporated into ordinary conversations. As a form of interaction, the illness narrative implies a reciprocal role for listeners, namely, to witness—through attentive listening, acknowledgment, understanding, and perhaps empathy—the suffering of others (Kleinman, 1988).

Attention to personal narratives began to emerge in health communication scholarship concurrently with the development of a conceptual distinction between disease, defined as organic malfunctions and pathological processes whose signs and symptoms typically can be observed and quantitatively assessed; and *illness*, the patient's experience of disease or ill health (Kleinman, et al, 1978). Ahmed, Kolker, and Coelho (1979), among others, posited a third concept, *sickness*, to talk about the labels, roles, and societal expectations projected onto diagnosed individuals. Illness is the phenomenon studied by health communication scholars who are interested in the ways that individuals, and sometimes groups, portray their experiences of ill health in specific, individualized contexts. Narrative-based investigations extend the discussion of health and disease beyond the biomedical to encompass the meaning that patients ascribe to their illnesses as they affect roles, relationships, and identities, as well as levels of meaning that reflect social, organizational, ethnocultural, and familial assumptions and influences (Sharf & Kahler, 1996).

Clinical medicine has also been shown to employ narrative in its most fundamental activities, including clinical rounds and case reports (Good, 1994; Hunter, 1993; Poirier & Brauner, 1988) and chart notations (Poirier & Brauner, 1990; Poirier et al, 1992), but notably without representation of the patient's voice (Donnelly, 1988). Patients' accounts of their illnesses, Mishler's "voice of the lifeworld," are proving to be significant alternate "routes to knowledge," serving as a means to comprehend the storytellers' construction of their illness experience. As increasingly depicted through ethnographies, patients' writings, and media portrayals, such stories give legitimacy to the often unacknowledged expertise of patients, help to establish identity (both of individual patients and groups who share a common health concern), and provide unrivaled insight into the experience of illness (Vanderford, Jenks, & Sharf, 1997). Video representations of patients' voices are starting to have a significant impact on the education of physicians (Makoul, 1999; VIA Website).

Like other types of stories, *illness narratives* are implicitly appealing and comprehensible because they make use of familiar elements with which we have learned to shape our perceptions of the world. Such elements include characters, the people who enact the events of the story (for example, heroes, villains, victims, and innocent bystanders)[5]; scenes, the settings in which key events occur (e.g., a clinic or hospital, home, the workplace); motives, the thoughts, emotions, and circumstances that impel characters to take certain actions (for example, fear, concern, anger, accommodation); chronologies or time frames (which emphasize past, present, or future); plots or dramas, the meaning that emerges from how key events and characters' actions are configured in relation to one another (Charon, et al, 1996; for example, battling disease, accepting one's fate, or being empowered to make choices and take action); and narrator's voice or point of view (for instance, a story is always told from someone's perspective, thus necessarily not representing other perspectives). Finally, as important as the story elements that constitute a narrative is the *telling* of the story—the process and style of communicating the narrative.

Implicit in the way stories of sickness are told are underlying values, such as the desire for information, personal control, recognition of individuality, or enjoyable quality of life. Lack of congruence between the explicit or implicit values within the stories of practitioners and patients is often the source of significant problems in clinical care (Geist & Gates, 1996; Vanderford, Smith, & Harris, 1992). Patient accounts compensate for the partiality and objectification of medical records, creating a more complete picture of illness, health, and disease. Health communication scholars have approached illness narratives as psychosocial maps, revealing the storytellers' emotional and cognitive journeys. These narratives challenge the voice of medicine as the primary means of understanding health and disease. To interweave both the voice of medicine and the voice of the life-world into a consistent, mutually agreed upon story that functions as the basis for clinical care and decision-making is a primary communicative goal, albeit one that is often difficult to achieve (Geist & Dreyer, 1993; Sharf, 1990).

Sociologist Kathy Charmaz's (1999) discussion of her research on patients' accounts of suffering due to chronic disease illustrates the range of communicative experiences of interest to narrative scholars. "[Suffering] is of the self and it is social. As suffering spreads out, it shapes social relations and limits social worlds" (p. 365). It changes the interaction that sufferers have with others and the roles they can play. As a result, the patient's very identity is affected. "Although meanings of suffering may begin with the body, they include emotions, accompany losses, and thus, can arise through social as well as corporeal existence" (p. 366).

Patients' changing relationships, interactions, roles, identities, emotions, losses, and growth are the elements of dramatic stories, naturally drawing the attention of narrative scholars (Vanderford et al., 1997). In defining how the application of narrative thought has changed the practice of health care ethics, Jones (1996) pointed to the importance of the particular circumstances and situational details that form the basis for inductive analysis; the acceptance of complicated human emotions, behavior, and connections; and the nonhierarchical recognition and support of people's capacities "to construct their own life stories and make their own decisions" (p. 268).

In their analysis of narratives that unfolded during a support group for epileptic patients, Arntson and Droge (1987) identified four functions of health-related storytelling, that have since been identified in subsequent studies of individuals' illness accounts. Illness narratives help patients (a) make sense of health and disease, (b) assert control in the midst of physical and psychological losses, (c) transform their identities and social roles as a result of altered health and disease, and (d) make decisions about their health. As illness narratives increasingly move beyond clinical and interpersonal levels of communication and are shared in broader, more public venues, they serve a fifth function: to solidify health-based communities with common visions and social agendas. These five socially constructive functions of health-related storytelling provide the organizational structure for the remainder of this chapter.

In summary, the narrative approach to health communication highlight the meaning of the illness experience, primarily to the individual or group with a particular health problem and secondarily to others who witness or read those personal accounts. All who participate in the telling or hearing of an illness narrative help in creating its significance and act as its interpreters.

Narrative as Sense-Making

In the incident described at the beginning of this chapter, the young woman appears to have been unfairly treated. But had the same events been narrated from the police officer's perspective, that is, from the viewpoint of an individual charged with looking out for reckless drivers, the meaning of the anecdote would almost certainly be very different. After all, Rose's ailment is, for practical purposes, a largely invisible disability (Matthews & Harrington, 2000) and therefore easy to misinterpret. Unlike paralyzed people confined to wheelchairs or blind people who walk with white canes or guide dogs, Rose appears "able-bodied." Heavy-lidded eyes due to muscle fatigue constitute a visible but rather subtle sign that the officer noted and interpreted as evidence of alcohol or drug intake. As an alternate narrator, the officer would provide a strikingly different interpretation of this same physical symptom.

Most narrative research focuses on the sense-making function of stories—the ability of narratives to create meaning of random events, people, and action. Organizational theorist Karl Weick (1995; see also Miller, 2001; Miller, Joseph, & Apker, 2000) has developed a conceptualization of the process of sense-making that emphasizes the pivotal role of communication and includes attributes particularly relevant to the creation of narratives that enable us to cope with chaotic or confusing conditions often encountered in our everyday lives. According to Weick, sense-making is, among other things, retrospective (is affected by our past experiences); emergent (needs to take into account new experiences); interactive (is influenced by social relations and information gained from others); and driven by plausibility (focuses on "what can account for sensory experience, but what is also interesting, attractive, emotionally appealing, and goal relevant" [Fiske, 1992, p. 879]). Weick also points to the strong reciprocal connection between situational sense-making and one's notions of personal identity; this link will be explored below as one of the key functions of narrative. Considering these characteristics, much of the development of social and personal meaning is inherent in the creation of good stories.

Fisher (1985) asserted that narratives are focused on "words and/or deeds—that have sequence and meaning for those who live, create or interpret them" (p. 2). Individuals are believed to make sense of unexpected, random events as they construct accounts of what they experienced, connecting people and events to create some understandable pattern (Churchill & Churchill, 1982). Critical to this sense-making activity is the distance in time between the actions in the story and the "telling" of it in retrospect. Recalling the events in hindsight, the storyteller can "assume a reflective, observant posture toward those events in a way that was impossible when the events were in progress." (Brody, 1987, p. 14).[6] Storytellers can interpret events, ascribe meanings, justify actions, and make links in retrospect that are less likely to be discerned when the narrator experiences events in real time. Although the sense-making role of storytelling is apparent in accounts in which illness does not occur, this function is especially significant for patients whose lives have been altered by the suffering that results from severe chronic or acute disease or disability. While the details of individual illness narratives are personal and context-specific, scholars who study patients' stories as a discursive genre have derived general categories of meta-narratives based on how the storytellers make sense of the illness experience. Literary analyst Anne Hunsaker Hawkins (1993) calls this genre *pathography,* which she asserted has spawned four major types of myths or stories: those of rebirth and the promise of cure, those of battle and journey, those of dying, and those of health beyond medicine (i.e., health through alternative modes of healing). Similarly, sociologist Arthur Frank (1995), himself a survivor of heart disease and prostate cancer, argued that "wounded storytellers" create stories of restitution or recovery, stories of chaos or illness with no hope of recovery, and stories of quest or journey in which the suffering engendered by illness leads to larger purposes or understandings. Whatever the category, narrative scholars agree that the very voicing of an illness experience in story form is itself an act of healing and agency. By virtue of providing a reason for the person's illness experience, a narrative has the potential to diminish suffering (Brody, 1987) and to allow the person to assume accountability for him- or herself and perhaps others in similar circumstances (Frank, 1995).

Naturally, not only people diagnosed with a disease but their family and friends are affected by the illness experience. As caretakers, providers of social support, and fellow sufferers, people in a patient's extended network create their own explanations of events and experiences. Although narrative scholarship has not sufficiently explored the comparative accounts of patients and their loved ones, a few excellent examples exist, such as two remarkable, intertwined narratives in which a surviving life partner and a partner dying of breast cancer recorded concurrent impressions of shared events over a 2-year period from diagnosis through death (Butler & Rosenblum, 1991). Writes Sandy, the surviving partner:

> Last night I wrote, "I am excused. I excuse myself. Cancer is what I do now." Cancer is my work. Barbara's mood swings, doctor's appointments, medicines. My feelings. Our writing together. All of it has become my central activity. Cancer swallows up the air of my life

> and insinuates its presence everywhere. Nothing remains untouched. Inviolate. (p. 48)

Sense-making may also differ among people with seemingly similar illness experiences. A striking example of the power of narrative to help make sense of illness is found in contradictory accounts of women with breast implants (Vanderford & Smith, 1996). In an extended study of patients', physicians', and popular press accounts of the breast implant controversy, the stories of women who blamed subsequent illnesses on their implants are compared with the stories of those who also had undergone synthetic breast surgery but did not hold their implants responsible for health problems. The latter group did not blame their problems on implants because their health issues fit within a larger narrative concerning the imperfection of medicine. In one account, a woman tells a story that integrates her understanding of general medical risks with her personal experience:

> They told me in '77, "This [implant] is going to last forever." I didn't question it any further. It didn't dawn on me to question it further, but I do remember them saying that, because I had a good rapport with the doctor. The doctor that I had was the head of plastic surgery at Duke at that time. Dr. X, you know, he just laughed about it. And I said, "You mean when I die they are still going to be there? " And he said, "You are going to be laid out, they are still going to be up there. " I mean, that was their attitude at that time. And of course they were mistaken. But I don't have any, I don't know. It was an error, nothing in our bodies last. A hip replacement is silicone, it doesn't last. (p. 82)

This storyteller integrates the rupture of her implants into the natural evolution of knowledge about medical devices and health risks. In this account, the physician is not a villain; his knowledge was just incomplete, albeit the best possible at the time. For the narrator, the risk of a rupture is to be expected as the natural consequence of the deterioration of medical devices.

In contrast, women who blamed their implants for a host of illnesses generated stories in which no reason other than their implants could account for their health problems. The chronological relationships developed in the accounts pointed the blame directly on the implants (and indirectly at the plastic surgeons who implanted them), as in the following excerpt:

> I started having problems a few weeks after that with the implants. . . . The implants were placed directly in, and then three weeks after that I had an infection in where the skin turned real black . . . I mean problem after problem . . . I kept getting infections . . . and there was a bunch of lymph nodes . . . they just kept swelling up . . . swelling of the joints and dryness in your eyes, your mouth . . . I've had a rash that would come upon my hands and my feet . . . my dermatologist didn't know where it was coming from. . . . Since all this started with the implants, I get colds easier and infections, like these little skin cancers they've been freezing off . . . nothing heals, I mean every time I turn around they have to put me on antibiotics to get anything to heal. . . . My menstrual cycle . . . has been irregular for a little over a year now. (Vanderford & Smith, 1996, p. 32)

This woman's story highlights the implant procedure as the point at which never-before experienced symptoms and health problems begin to occur.

As these excerpts illustrate, narrative sense-making frequently involves assigning responsibility and sometimes blame, a process of attribution that occurs both at the level of personal reasoning about illness as well as at more public levels, such as a health campaign. As rhetoricians William G. Kirkwood and Dan Brown (1995) point out in their study of a variety of nontechnical public communications about cancer, heart disease, drug addiction, and so on, questions of responsibility interwoven into particular health-related narratives (Is being overweight an issue of heredity or lifestyle? Is cancer prevention a matter of individual surveillance or environmental regulation?) are as much rhetorical as scientific. These messages are constructed to vary with the audiences to whom they are addressed. Their objectives include fostering healthy behaviors among the undiagnosed public, easing feelings of guilt among and empowering those who have been diagnosed with a disease, and motivating favorable or unfavorable treatment of the sick (e.g., people with AIDS or smokers). In effect, how causative factors of disease are accounted for provides scenarios of innocent and culpable victims, careless perpetrators, or factors of nature or chance beyond human management. Yet, even in the midst of unavoidable disease or disability, the very act of generating a story allows the narrator a certain degree of agency.

Narrative as Asserting Control

In recalling her childhood experiences of growing up with myasthenias gravis, Rose has vivid, painful memories of being teased by schoolmates because she had a difficult time with many ordinary physical activities. As a way of responding to this situation, Rose chose to give a fifth-grade oral report on this disease in which she described what the problem is and how it affects people who have it without specifically mentioning that she herself suffered from it. She remembers this experience with a sense of satisfaction, because she felt she had managed to educate her peers and reduce the teasing without directly sacrificing her privacy. In short, she had discovered her own way to exert control over a hurtful situation through a form of narration that she had chosen. However, 2 years later she experienced the opposite effect. When her medication dosage suddenly failed to manage her symptoms, she became very ill and needed to be hospitalized for nearly 6 weeks, a very difficult episode for a seventh grader. Although she asked the school not to disclose to her classmates why she was in the hospital, her science teacher did exactly that, disregarding her request. In this instance, the suffering from being physically sick was increased by a loss of control of personal information—what she came to regard as a usurping of her personal narrative.

The relationship of storytelling to increased perceptions of control is especially important in illness accounts. The experience of severe and/or chronic illness strips away multiple sources of an individual's perception of control within the realm of his or her own life. A sense of suffering can be exacerbated by varying degrees and kinds of lost autonomy. Some forms of loss are physiological but also have emotional repercussions, such as shame, embarrassment, and frustration. For instance, prostate cancer survivors frequently experience loss of control over their bladders and sometimes their bowel functions. Women who have undergone a mastectomy, in addition to the more obvious change in appearance, may experience a loss of range of arm motion, a loss of strength, and a permanent severe swollenness of the affected arm (a condition called *lymphedema*). People with epilepsy experience unpredictable seizure activity, losing control of their entire bodies and mental concentration. Those with myasthenias gravis, like Rose, are subject to debilitating bouts of fatigue and weakness. Severe and chronic illness frequently is accompanied by physical restrictions which, in turn, leads to the diminishment of social relationships. Patients may no longer be able to work, socialize, or participate in as wide a range of activities as they did previous to the onset of disease. Further contributors to suffering often include a reduction in financial resources, a loss of personal energy, and the need to forgo other pursuits in order to focus primarily on pain relief or rehabilitation.

Compounding these losses is an increased dependency on family caregivers, medications, and health care providers. The patient role has traditionally been passive, requiring that individuals seek medical help and comply with their physicians' recommendations (Brody, 1980; Smith & Pettegrew, 1986). Medical diagnosis and categorization has the potential to stigmatize patients as well as restrict their opportunities for recovery, development, and empowerment (Arntson & Droge, 1987). All these sorts of deficits may combine to create a "loss of certainty . . . loss of certainty means losing the collective myth of a 'taken for granted' future as well as the personal belief in sustained health" (Charmaz, 1999, p. 366).

Assuming that authorship allows individuals with health problems to reassert some control in the midst of multiple losses, Frank (1995) explained that "seriously ill people are wounded not just in body but in voice. They need to become storytellers in order to recover the voices that illness and its treatment often take away" (p. xii). Turning one's experiences into a narrative creates order by placing previously unexplainable events into relationships. The act of ordering and predicting the future is an act of control (Churchill & Churchill, 1982), as is recounting the history of previous occurrences. Rose's remembrances of childhood illness narratives illustrate the importance of constructivist issues including: Whose voice is narrating the story? What information is selected for inclusion or exclusion and for which audiences? An additional significant aspect of authorial control is sequencing. A narrator imposes order on experience by creating, a chronology of events:

> [She] is required to sequence the events of the story temporally: "A" happens, then "B," then "C." These temporal associations may then well turn into cause-effect relationships. The story's "illusion of sequence" can impose order on a chaotic, if not random set of events. [For example,] scientifically there may be no explanation for [the occurrence of symptoms or side effects from medication]. By placing these events within a narrative, they may longer be so unpredictable for the narrator. (Arntson & Droge, 1987, p. 161)

By creating order and attributing causes for symptoms and disease, patients may regain a measure of control, denying the dominance of disorder and unpredictability.

Importantly, illness narratives sometimes serve as vehicles for patients to project control into a future in which, as the disease or disability accelerates, they might no longer be able to express their choices to physicians and family members. Such stories told to family members or health care practitioners can serve as an advanced directive in place of institutionalized documents. Although for some, dying of an illness is characterized as losing a hard-fought struggle for life, for others, being able to plan how death occurs (i.e., enabling a "good death") is one of the ultimate measures of asserting control. A man diagnosed as HIV positive explained: "If you are talking to your doctor and you tell him that you don't want to be saved by any kind of machine that would help you breathe or whatever, the doctor ought to be able to put that in the chart and he ought to be able to respect your wishes on that point . . . if my heart gives out, don't start it again" (Vanderford et al., 1992, p. 132).

Sullivan's (1997) analysis of women coping with living with breast cancer also described patient narratives in which women asserted control in the midst of terminal illness. Like the man with HIV, these women described themselves acting in ways that projected their wills into situations in which they would later lack agency. For example, they told the interviewer how they had planned and arranged their own funerals, written their personal obituaries, and even arranged care for their pets for after their own deaths. As characters taking action in their own life stories, these women featured themselves as agents in control, despite the impending loss of life itself.

In short, narrative form puts the "I" back into a person's understanding of his or her life. Rather than silently comply with the initiatives and orders of others, the patient narrator asserts him- or herself as agent: "The actual narration of a story, saying the words in the appropriate form, makes a place in the world for [the] narrator" (Churchill & Churchill, 1982, p. 77). Creating a story also allows the narrator to emphasize certain aspects of who that agent is, and how illness has influenced that persona.

Narrative as Transforming Identity

How does Rose make sense of her illness in telling her own story? Would she define herself as disabled? Depending on whom she's speaking with, she might describe how she faces moderate restrictions in physical exertion and makes regular adaptations in various aspects of her life, such as the kind of work she does or how much rest she needs. Yet her mom told her a long time ago that everyone is born with or develops some kind of imperfection, so she doesn't consider herself particularly special and feels only occasionally inconvenienced. Although obviously aware that she suffers from a chronic disease, she doesn't label herself as "sick," nor does she feel impeded from living her life in ways that she chooses; hers would likely be a narrative about a busy psychology major, nursery school instructor, and fun-loving young adult.

Of course, there have been times in her life when the official diagnosis of her disease, sanctioned by a neurologist, has been a necessity, creating a different version of her narrative. For instance, in the large high school she attended, a special designation of disability was needed to excuse her from certain physical education requirements and to ensure a schedule that limited the distance she would need to walk between classes. Her handicapped parking permit allows her to park her car near the buildings where she needs to go for university classes or business. Because of her ailment, she receives tuition assistance from the state of South Carolina. In these cases, an account that labels her as a disabled individual is necessary and welcomed. On the other hand, she would much prefer to focus on stories that do not categorize her primarily as a person with myasthenia gravis in her social and professional identities.

Narratives not only serve as a means to assert agency for persons whose control has been diminished but also provide "wounded" storytellers with a means to reshape their identities, either in functional, enabling ways or, alternatively, with an emphasis on loss, trauma, or impairment. Churchill and Churchill (1982) describe the act of storytelling as an approach to self-knowledge: "Storytelling . . . is a mode of coming to know ourselves. . . . [s]tories are devices which shape agents and events into some intelligible pattern. They weld actors to their actions and doers to their deeds" (p. 74). Chronic illness often disrupts a person's previously established self-image (Corbin & Strauss, 1988). As individuals experience dramatic changes in their health and "realize the crisis has lasting consequences for their lives" (Charmaz, 1994, p. 269), they also face "identity dilemmas," including changes in roles, relationships, social circles, and activities. Physician Howard Brody (1987) explains that illness threatens a person's "continuity of memory " or narrative coherency when the individual's confidence in his or her ability to carry out a "rational life plan" is shaken. When severe and/or chronic illness disrupts one's life plan, "getting better" may not be possible through physical cure but instead requires the creation of a revised life story with a modified identity; "healing involves moving beyond thoughts of recovery and survival to the creation of a self that can 'thrive' " (Sullivan, 1997, p. 50) despite impairment, pain, or a more uncertain future. A familiar example of a transformative story that underscores identity issues is Christopher Reeve's (1998) first-hand account of his physical and existential journey from movie star and Superman persona to quadriplegic patient and survivor to national health activist for spinal cord injuries. Despite such radical transformations, he claim[ed] to be "still me," a pun referring both to his paralysis and to the preservation of a consistent inner core of self-identity.[7]

Stories that reflect transformation of identity make use of key narrative features that may include identification of critical, life-changing incidents; the revelation of character through multiple perspectives; and the integration of personal expertise and adaptation to illness. The intersection of chronology with critical incident is frequently told in a before-and-after format, in which the narrator's sense of self alters at a moment of changed health status (Vanderford & Smith, 1996). Inevitably, the narrative turns to challenges brought on by disease or disability, revealing which circumstances, symptoms, and interactions are normal and which abnormal for the narrator. Usually disease and the resulting sickness contribute to changes in bodily appearance and function that may require difficult and radical changes in self-image and ways of living. Comparing his experience of enduring a heart attack with a later bout of prostate cancer, Frank (1991) observed, "During my heart problems I could no longer participate in certain activities; during cancer I felt I had no right to be among others. . . . Heart attacks are invisible on the body's surface. To myself and to others, I looked no different. One wears cancer. My own visible stigmas were hair loss and my intravenous line" (p. 92).

Another kind of challenge revealed through narrative analysis is the way in which illness alters relationships, an inherent dimension of identity. While renegotiation of relationship roles tends to be gradual, the impact can still be quite dramatic. In a study of men's accounts of prostate cancer, Arrington (2000), focused on "sex talk"—stories men told in support groups about changes in their relationships with their wives that fundamentally challenged their role as sexual beings and intimate partners.[8] In one example, a participant described the tension between him and his wife that his illness had caused: "He complained that the messages presented through the media suggested that sex goes on for one's entire life, and he lamented that such was not always the case. He expressed frustration that women saw those messages and consequently expected a full lifetime of sex."

Based on research interviews with individuals suffering from a variety of chronic diseases, Charmaz (1995) described the process of adaptation to bodily limits and other illness-related losses as gradual accommodation and acceptance, "flow[ing] with the experience" (p. 657), although other possible reactions include ignoring, minimizing, resisting, reconciling, and embracing. Adaptation in this sense involves a close reexamination of one's goals, expectations, and terms of self-acceptance. Therefore, illness narratives may convey personal identity both through repetitive patterns and changes in actions and choices involving struggle, surrender, and accommodation to alterations in one's capacities. Indeed, the self revealed during a serious illness may prove to be a complex mix of continuity and transformation. Not surprisingly, the storytelling process allows for various facets of one's identity to be expressed. As Holstein and Gubrium (2000) pointed out, "narrative editing" allows the storyteller to shift perspectives, both as a way of incorporating complex adaptations and as a strategy for taking various listeners into account: "The storyteller, in effect, is an editor who constantly monitors, modifies, and revises themes and storylines . . . to attend to perspective and to the ways they expect their accounts to be heard" (p. 113). In Rose's case, we can see two versions of identity, one emphasizing the healthy self and the other focused on the disabled self. Both versions are ways of coping with her varied needs and circumstances; her chosen anecdotes reflect a lifetime of having to accommodate to an ongoing health condition.

Charmaz (1995) pointed out that some surgical procedures and medical regimens can result in "upward changes" (p. 668), including improvements in appearance, stamina, and possibly prognosis. Even positive changes in health inspire stories in which patients must redefine themselves. Brashers et al.'s (1999) study of HIV patients focused on the accounts of individuals who had experienced restored hope after protease inhibitor drugs had rescued them from a terminal prognosis. "Revival" required each HIV patient to change their identities to "a person living with a chronic illness rather than a person dying from a terminal illness." Having already accepted their impending deaths, the narrators' new circumstances included a change of social status and expectations, hence a need to renegotiate roles and identities. Just as they had earlier adjusted to the "sick role," revival led the patients to resume seeing themselves as "workers" and to place a positive value on independence, self-sufficiency, responsibility and stability.

Some of the best-told and most insightful illness narratives not only prove helpful in strengthening the teller's capacity for dealing with illness-related problems but also awaken listeners or readers to issues that they may not have been aware of or that they are attempting to deal with in their own lives. One influential and long-enduring example is poet Audre Lorde's journal (1980) following treatment for breast cancer. In one entry, she pondered the silence surrounding the experience of mastectomy that kept women from sharing their wisdom and fears with one another. Significantly, the crucible of a life-threatening illness experience can change people's identities in ways they never would have imagined. For instance, Sullivan's

(1997) interviews with breast cancer patients helped transform these women into advocates for the health of future generations, turning their disease into a mission. Reflecting their discussions, the researcher described their

> collective and personal efforts to increase awareness and educate others about breast cancer. These women were concerned about future generations of women, especially their own daughters. They strongly advocated breast self-examination as a vital way to save lives. Other "ways to spread the word" included donating books to resource centers, participating in fundraising activities, and acting as local resource persons. Nora helped conduct a survey to determine possible causes for the high incidence of breast cancer in the area. . . . Two other women began their own health related businesses. (p. 47)

A final interesting aspect of narrative identity construction we wish to underscore is the ability of many narrators to apply essential personal resources and expertise to the illness experience in order to derive perceptive insights. For instance, sociologist Robert Murphy (1987) analyzed how others reacted to his degenerative paralysis as he labored to maintain his social and professional identities, and writer Reynolds Price (1994) incorporated original poetry into his account of learning to deal with the intense pain of a spinal cord tumor. Particularly refreshing is comedian Julia Sweeney's account (1997) of living with her brother Mike, who was being treated for a terminal brain tumor, while she was simultaneously diagnosed with cervical cancer, turning her Hollywood bungalow into the "International House of Cancer." And here is how she describes an evening in which Mike was extremely ill and nauseated:

> We got to the emergency room and they could see that Mike was really dehydrated. They wanted to get a saline solution into him right away, but the veins in his arms were all exhausted and so they were trying to get a needle in up over his ear. And he was continuing to throw up and I was standing in the doorway looking in on this. And, to just show you what a wonderfully dark sense of humor Mike had, in even the most horrific of circumstances, he turned to me and said, "I guess it's not so funny now that you have cancer too, huh?" And I said, "Yeah, Mike. 'Cause normally I'd be laughing my ass off." (p. 121)

In the words of Kathy Charmaz (1995), "Adaptation to impairment takes people with serious chronic illness on an odyssey of self" (p. 675). The same is true for people undergoing other forms of suffering, and the process of narrating an illness experience can reveal a person's essential character through the struggles to adapt, persist, and thrive.

Narrative as Warranting Decisions

As mentioned previously, Rose does not consider her illness the defining characteristic of her life. This is not to say that having lived with myasthenias gravis hasn't deeply affected certain life choices. In fact, Rose has decided to continue with graduate education that will lead to a career as a counseling psychologist, working specifically with children with disabilities and their families. In this very important matter, her illness has shaped her future life story in a direction that she feels is positive—both personally rewarding and of social value. "I want to advocate for others so they won't have to deal with the same problems I've had."

Still, she routinely makes choices about health-related disclosures, deciding what is necessary to say to friends, professors, and people she dates and when it is appropriate to raise these issues. One decision that has been especially significant for her is selecting situations in which she will use a wheelchair. Because she often needs to lean on a friend or family member due to sudden feelings of weakness, she has frequently been mistaken for being drunk. Dr. Harvey dissuaded her from using a wheelchair during high school even though school officials had wanted her to do so. Thus far she has chosen to use a motorized cart on three visits to the Disney World theme park, where her close friend works. Although she is used to being attuned to sudden bouts of fatigue and weakness that necessitate rest and changes in medication, she real-

ized on her first visit that she would not be able to cope in her usual ways with the immense distances and dense crowds in the park. The motorized cart enabled her to maneuver and truly enjoy Disney World. During a visit to New York City, however, she elected not to use a wheelchair. She found herself having to stop and rest constantly, reduced to being a burden to the friends she was visiting and treated like a nonperson by people who didn't know her well. In the end, she concluded she would have been better off in a wheelchair despite the social stigma it bestows.

Nonetheless, making use of a wheelchair changes the nature of her hidden disability; her identity suddenly becomes one of a publicly acknowledged disabled person. This is a difficult shift, and because she doesn't define herself as part of the "disabled community," she says she has the feeling of being an "imposter" when she makes use of a motorized chair. Perhaps this feeling is increased by the reactions and assumptions made by others about people who use wheelchairs (Cahill & Eggleston, 1995). The complexities and contradictions of integrating the use of a wheelchair into her life are still in the process of being developed and understood within her ongoing story of experiencing illness.

Narratives reveal the storyteller's values or reasons for actions, including routine activities as well as those involved in medical decision making (Vanderford & Smith, 1996). Charmaz (1999) calls stories of suffering "moral parables of right and wrong, of moral virtue and moral flow, of reason and rationalization" (p. 367; see also Bochner, 1998). The inherently moral function that she refers to includes making judgments about desirable and undesirable behaviors, describing appropriate and inappropriate relationships and roles, and implying desired transformations. In telling about their experiences of sickness, narrators are able to position themselves so as to portray character and actions taken within the plotline. Narrative chronology may place the locus of one's decision making on past events, current demands, or future consequences. The retrospective stance of the narrator allows for ethical reflection; "the temporal gap between one's actions and the telling allows the narrator to assume a distance about his or her actions as narrated in the story, which creates a space for recognizing actions as 'good' or 'bad,' 'better' or 'worse.' This space provides the reflective ground for change " (Churchill & Churchill, 1982, p. 74). In this example taken from a discussion within a prostate cancer support group, one participant reveals the motives behind his treatment decision: "That is what my physician told me [that radiation had fewer side effects]. So I opted on the radiation, uh, because, uh, it seemed like that would have less effect upon, uh, the sex life, uh, than an operation, which, uh, I had heard anyway, that the changes that, of losing your ability to have sex was much greater than just by radiation. So l went through the radiation starting in October of 1995." (Arlington, 2000)

Accounts of chronic illness and suffering describe conflicts and explain problems, including the difference between the way things were in the story and the way the storyteller desired them to be. They disclose a storyteller's attitudes and judgments about events, actions, people, motives, types of relationships, and goals. As a result, stories reveal (implicitly or explicitly) the way the teller thinks the world ought to operate. One HIV patient 's conclusion to a story about his treatment in a V.A. hospital provides a clear example: "I won't ever come back here. I won't come back here because I'm not an animal and I don't behave like an animal. . . . They . . . did nothing to build and boost my esteem and help me deal with the problem of being HIV positive" (Vanderford et al., 1992, p. 134). Just below the surface of complaint, the patient's emphasis on the values of human dignity and compassion is easy to see.

One person's story frequently has a salutary impact on another's decision. In a study (Sharf, 1997) of people participating in an online breast cancer listserv, the husband of a woman with early-stage breast cancer asked about the advisability of her becoming pregnant.[9] Several women replied with stories revealing their own struggles with this perplexing question, including this response, which detailed the narrator's attempt to weigh pros and cons (unfortunately, after finally deciding to become pregnant, she miscarried):

> I'm posting to the list in hopes my personal experience is helpful. This is an issue I have been struggling with since I was diagnosed 7 yrs ago. . . . After the miscarriage I worried a lot about whether I'd increased my risk of new breast cancer—those worries have subsided at this point. . . . My best wishes to you and your wife, whatever you decide, (p. 75)

When more than one person is involved in the health care decision-making process, then the issue of co-constructing or overlapping stories frequently comes to the fore. Earlier we referred to the dichotomy that often arises between the voice of medicine and the voice of the lifeworld. Thus, in medical consultations, a negotiated story that interweaves elements of both the patient's and the practitioner's distinct narratives is sometimes needed in order to arrive at a care management plan acceptable to both parties (Sharf, 1990). In a different context, sociologist Carolyn Ellis (1995) tells the painful story of her becoming the primary caretaker of Gene, her life partner, who was dying from emphysema. Over several years' duration, their versions of Gene's course of illness variously melded and differed as to severity, burdens and responsibilities, and ways of coping. Toward the end of Gene's life, Carolyn's story was colored by thoughts of what it would mean to be a survivor, while Gene struggled with impending death. Through very open conversations, both had to come to agreement on whether to use a respirator as a treatment of last resort, since Carolyn would almost surely be the surrogate decision-maker for Gene when the disease prevented him from thinking and speaking coherently. This process of co-constructing a narrative among family members that incorporates a person's advance directive in the event of life-threatening illness is perhaps one of our most difficult communication challenges.

Ultimately, "decisions about health are based on the meaning patients give to symptoms and experiences with disease and their physicians. Narratives function to justify decisions already made and determine future decisions" (Vanderford & Smith, 1996, p. 23, citing Fisher, 1985). Understanding a patient's story is key to understanding his or her decisions.

Narrative for Building Community

Rose doesn't particularly identify with the disabilities activists in her community. From her perspective, they seem to make their disabilities the centerpiece of their lives, something she has tried not to do. She'd prefer not to be "lumped into a group." Her sense of community will be fulfilled from the counseling work with disabled children she has chosen to do. It's not likely that she will see much public attention given to her particular disability-related problems since myasthenias gravis affects a relatively small number of people, nor are there any mass media images with which she identifies directly. In her youth, the television show that made the biggest impression upon her was Life Goes On, *a program that featured a family whose members included a young man with Down's syndrome played by an actor with Down's syndrome. Both the fictional character and the real actor proved themselves to be attractive people with capabilities that surprised and pleased the viewing audience. Rose feels that the more the public is exposed to non-stereotypical depictions of illness and disability, the better the chance of acceptance and understanding.*

So far, we have discussed illness narratives primarily as individual stories of sickness that serve multiple functions for the teller and sometimes have the power to influence others as well. We have also alluded to the co-construction of illness narratives as an important aspect of the interaction between patients and clinicians. Communication theorist Ernest Bormann (1985) conceptualized the interactional ways in which multiple individuals or organized groups are attracted to and build upon stories (what he calls *fantasy themes*), leading to the development of rhetorical visions that provide common histories, coherent depictions of current reality, and desires for the way the world should be. He calls this process—in which stories cohere and build upon each other—*symbolic convergence*. Applying the theory of symbolic convergence to health-related situations, we assert that narratives serve a communal function in at least three ways: by helping disparate individuals with common maladies provide support to one another, by raising public awareness about specific issues inherent in experiences of illness, and by serving as highly recognizable discourses for advocacy. In this section, we discuss these three aspects of how stories told in group and public formats help to solidify health-based communities.

Illness-defined organizations such as face-to-face support groups and online chat groups and listservs share a socially constructed reality shaped by commonly expressed interests, rules of operation, and vocabulary. Communities like these serve the communicative and social functions of enabling members to access a wider range of information than one person is apt to have; giving attention to socioemotional needs and coping skills; and empowering participants to participate in medical decision making, political activist events, and related matters (Sharf, 1997). This occurs largely through discussion generated by the sharing of individuals' stories of experience. The aforementioned analysis of a support group for individuals diagnosed with epilepsy illustrates how this kind of group discourse changed the way members viewed themselves and their disease. Participants encouraged one another to tell stories in which their disease did not stigmatize them:

> The narrative mode of communication can provide an opportunity for self-help members to develop a functional language for talking about themselves. . . . Many members described themselves in stigmatizing and helpless words: epileptic, out of control, an embarrassment, depressed, unattractive, and so on. The Chicago self-help group that we observed and taped did not allow members to describe themselves as being epileptic. Victim narratives were also not well received after a while. (Arntson & Droge, 1987, p. 162)

Adelman and Frey's (1997) ethnographic analysis of Bonaventure House, a residential facility for people with AIDS, is a richly detailed case study of an illness-based community. Because of the particular necessities inherent in this living situation, modes of storytelling evolved that helped to initiate incoming members and to prepare established residents for the deaths of others; create private boundaries and cooperation within a limited physical space; and balance a sense of normalcy with ongoing loss and crisis. Of particular interest are the symbolic strategies used to positively reframe grief and fear with celebration and continuity. These rely heavily on rituals, tokens, and stories of departed residents that help to sustain, both spiritually and materially, those currently coping with the problems of the disease.

The sense of community emanating from ongoing support groups and residential organizations is focused on participants who choose to identify with the goals and activities of those groups. Community building may also be assisted through popular dramatizations that serve as outreach to people who might otherwise never perceive themselves as identified with a common set of health concerns. There are any number of excellent examples of media portrayals that raise public consciousness about the difficulties of living with serious and/or chronic disease. Singhal and Roger's (1999) analyses of "entertainment-education" focused on how health prevention topics such as safe sex, family planning, and other lifestyle behaviors are dealt with on soap operas and other types of televised entertainment programs. In fact, entertainment television can be seen as an important element of planned health promotion campaigns. Less scholarly attention has been given to television dramas (and occasionally comedies) and films featuring problematic narratives of illness, such as a young mother's lengthy struggle to remain connected with her husband, children, and friends as she coped with life-threatening ovarian cancer on *thirty something* (Sharf & Freimuth, 1993); actor Tom Hank's portrayal of a lawyer with AIDS battling job discrimination in *Philadelphia; NYPD Blue* detective Andy Sipowicz's fear of submitting to treatment for prostate cancer (Arlington, 2000); and professor Morrie Schwartz's lessons on coming to grips with terminal illness and the orchestration of a good death.[10]

Although entertainment-education about health issues is generally treated as the province of the electronic mass media, ethnographer and performance studies scholar Dwight Conquergood (1988) provides an example of using live performance for similar purposes. While serving as a public health officer in a Hmong refugee camp in Thailand, Conquergood organized a theatrical presentation using the refugees' mythologies and cultural stories, along with newly-developed characters, to convey messages about how to maintain sanitary conditions in the crowded campground, so different from the environment these people had lived in previously. Entertainment-educational efforts include teaching audiences about diagnoses, symptoms, and treatments about which they may not have been aware; considering good and poor role-modeling behaviors in approaching problems related to illness; and initiating talk among family and friends on previously ignored or repressed topics (Sharf, Freimuth, Greenspon, & Plotnick, 1996). In a sense, the engaged audience becomes a community of learners, hopefully better prepared to think about and act upon similar episodes in their own lives.

A third way in which narratives help to form the foundation of an illness-related community is in the service of various forms of advocacy, especially to raise funds and change policy (Sharf, 2001). Personal stories of lived experiences of illness told by admired celebrities have helped to rivet public and political attention to an unprecedented degree. Notable examples include actor Christopher Reeve's speech at the 1996 Democratic presidential convention and his appearances in front of other audiences on behalf of spinal cord injury research and Michael J. Fox's testimony to Congress in support of funding for Parkinson's disease research. Equally effective are strategies to bring the narratives of suffering and courage of ordinary people to our attention. One of the best-known and affecting works of this kind is the AIDS quilt, whose immense expanse of personally-dedicated patchwork pieces poignantly reminds spectators of the human toll of this health problem.[11] The National Breast Cancer Coalition has widely disseminated its "Faces of Breast Cancer" exhibit in a variety of venues, including museums, shopping malls, and scientific conferences. The exhibit comprises photographs of women from each of the 50 states who have died from breast cancer, along with brief narratives describing their contributions to family and community. Participants in the various versions of the Race for the Cure participate and wear T-shirts in memory of loved ones who did not survive their fight with this disease. In each of the examples, the accumulation of personal stories serves a similar purpose—to illustrate the extent and proximity of the problem in a way that generalized statistics cannot.

Social Construction of Health Scholarship: To Be Continued

This review of the social construction perspective in health communication scholarship has highlighted the rhetorical origins of the tension between the physical world and symbolic representation, and the application of this approach to communication issues related to health and illness. Although narrative inquiry is only one of many ways of approaching health communication research, its benefits lie in the application of knowledge related to the meanings that individuals like Rose and others that we have quoted, paraphrased, and described here create out of health and illness. The voice of the patient, so often absent in clinical research, is now heard more often because of the emphasis that health communication as a field of inquiry has given to it. The construction of personal stories of suffering is useful to the individual dealing with serious and/or chronic sickness by allowing the individual to make sense of a situation that may at first seem to have no discernible explanation; assert control over what feels like a chaotic set of circumstances; document the transformations in identity spawned by the illness experience; and identify reasons for making decisions related to treatment, adaptation, and coping. The sharing of illness narratives contributes to the formation of community, be it for purposes of public education, social support, or political advocacy.

Although we cannot forecast in what directions health communication studies using a social construction approach will develop, clearly this kind of scholarship, once rare, is now accumulating with increasing frequency. We would like to conclude with a few guidelines that we think can help maximize the utility and influence of the social construction approach:

- *Contextualize discourse.* Whether it be historical, social and/or cultural, the context in which the discourse under investigation emerges and is articulated is critical to interpreting its meaning. Social construction emphasizes the connectedness of context and significance.
- *Identify contrasting perspectives.* When there is more than one account of reality among key participants in the situation being studied, key points of divergence and commonality should be identified and explored.
- *Incorporate cultural sensitivity.* Our understanding of cultural differences as they are manifested in narrative content and styles of story telling is limited. Awareness of actual distinctions is increasingly important in both clinical and public health contexts as populations continue to diversify and cross-cultural communication becomes at once more prevalent and more problematic.
- *Reveal what is rhetorical.* Social construction analysis should be concerned with how language and other forms of symbolization both shape and reflect people's shared perceptions of reality. In health communication research, the Health promotion messages (along with the public's response to these) and health policy are particularly important to explore from a rhetorical vantage point.[12]
- *Be alert to the clinical implications of personal narrative.* Social construction analysis should strive to clarify how patient narratives are understood by and responded to by clinicians; how the communication of narratives (by or about patients) affects the quality of clinical care; and how sharing of illness-related narratives impacts patient empowerment, participation, and decision making.
- *Recognize the tension between emancipation and appropriation of voice.* It has been argued that scholarship that helps to break the silence about experiences labeled as vulnerable or shameful are acts of social justice, insofar as the telling of stories enables self-knowledge, promotes healing, and encourages societal change (Varallo, Ray, & Ellis, 1998).[13] Still, the liberating effects of providing a platform for the public telling of powerful personal stories must be tempered with the realization that the same process of scholarship is necessarily one that edits and punctuates those narratives so that they become supporting evidence for the researcher's own arguments and point of view. The use of others' stories in the service of one's own research leads anthropologist Susan Estroff (1995) to ask, "Whose story is it anyway?"

Finally, we will conclude by underscoring the insight of communication scholar Arthur Bochner (1998), who reminds us that narrative inquiry is at its core a *moral* activity, one that is purposely and self-consciously entwined with the values of narrator and characters and is always *personal,* whether it be a matter of telling our own stories or "thinking with" (p. 349), resonating with, another's story, inevitably from the framework of our own lives. As we "listen" to Rose's story, her voiced struggle to make moral choices throughout her young life seems palpable. Though the situations impelled by her particular illness may seem rare, her ongoing quest to manage her identity with a sense of empowerment in the face of physical and social adversities is one with which many of us can identify.

> Even though I need the assistance of others sometimes, I don't like to be treated as fragile. . . . Control is a big issue for me. I conserve my energies and know my

limits. And I like doing things that help others; it helps my sense of self-esteem. . . . My illness has given me good things. It's made me really self-aware—things I like and don't like about myself. It helps me to empathize with others.
—Rose, at age 22

Acknowledgment

The authors wish to thank "Rose" for agreeing to share her narrative through a series of interviews conducted for purposes of this chapter.

Notes

1. Labeling biomedicine as "traditional" is itself an act of social construction. Many of the healing or treatment modalities referred to as "alternative" or "complementary" long predate regular medicine.
2. While a wide variety of methodological approaches have been used in social construction work, depending on the nature of the questions asked, there has been particular emphasis on qualitative, naturalistic methods, including archival explorations, discourse analysis, depth interviewing, autoethnography, and participant observation.
3. No wonder, then, that popular fictional media icon, Mob boss Tony Soprano, is afflicted with psychosomatic anxiety attacks, necessitating weekly appointments with a psychiatrist.
4. It will be evident from the range of references cited that we do not claim the health-related narrative as the sole province of health communication. To the contrary, this research on this topic is quite interdisciplinary. Nonetheless, we strongly believe that health communication scholars have made significant contributions to its study.
5. Stories of sickness sometimes treat the body or body parts as characters independent of the person to whom they belong (Cassell, 1985).
6. In some renditions, the narrator is not only relaying past events, but is looking to the future as well. In cases where death appears to be imminent, the reduction of distance in time and psyche between the narrator and the yet-to-be experienced resolution often adds to the power and poignancy of the narrative. See, for instance, Christina Middlebrook's account (1996) of coping with metastatic breast cancer.
7. For an in-depth analysis of Reeve's transformative illness narrative see Geist-Martin, Ray, & Sharf (2002), pp. 23–31.
8. Although Arrington does not label his method as "narrative," characterizing it instead as grounded theory, the cancer patients accounts reveal their construction of themselves and their relationships with their wives by focusing on characters, actions, and motives.
9. Clinical studies are not consistent as to whether the increased estrogen levels that accompany pregnancy encourages growth of malignant tumors, and if so, under what conditions. Many women with breast cancer have successfully given birth without tumor recurrence.
10. *Tuesdays with Morrie* eventually appeared as a best-selling book (Albom, 1997), a series of interviews with Ted Koppel on *Nightline*, and a televised, feature-length movie.
11. The availability of effective new generations of drugs to combat HIV in the United States have quickly changed the social construction of AIDS from a certain killer to a problematic but chronic disease. In the meantime, the devastation of lives from AIDS in the resource-poor African continent continues at an alarming rate, largely out of view from the American public. Perhaps an international version of the quilt needs to be produced and exhibited.
12. For example, see Kimberly Kline's rhetorical analysis (1999) of breast self-examination campaigns, which in part supports the criticism of women's health activists that these messages detract from perceptions of agency and efficacy in the early detection of breast cancer. Rather than simply dismiss these campaigns, she suggests specific ways in which they can be improved so that women audiences feel empowered and health promotional behavior is encouraged at the same time.
13. The assertion of narrative-based research as social justice stems from the authors' interviews with incest survivors.

References

Adelman, M. B., & Frey, L. R. (1997). *The fragile community: Living together with AIDS.* Mahwah, NJ: Lawrence Erlbaum Associates.

Ahmed, P. L, Kolker, A., & Coelho, G. V. (1979). Toward a new definition of health: An overview. In R I. Ahmed & G. V. Coelho (Eds.), *To-*

ward a new definition of health: Psychosocial dimensions (pp. 7–22). NY: Plenum.

Albom, M. (1997). *Tuesdays with Morrie: An old man, a young man, and life's greatest lesson.* New York: Doubleday.

Arntson, P., & Droge, D. (1987). Social support in self-help groups: The role of communication in enabling perceptions of control. In T. Albrecht & M. Adelman (Eds.), *Communicating social support.* Sage.

Arrington, M. (2000). Sexuality, society, and senior citizens: An analysis of sex talk among prostate cancer support group members. *Sexuality and Culture, 4,* 151–158.

Berger, P. L., & Luckmann, T. (1966). *The social construction of reality: A treatise in the sociology of knowledge.* Garden City, NY: Doubleday.

Bochner, A. P. (1994). Perspectives on inquiry II: Theories and stories. In M. Knapp & G. R. Miller (Eds.), *Handbook of interpersonal communication* (pp. 21–41). Beverly Hills, CA: Sage.

Bochner, A. P. (1998). Storied lives: Recovering the moral importance of social theory. In J. S. Trent (Ed.), *Communication: Views from the helm for the 21st century.* Boston: Allyn & Bacon.

Bormann, E. (1985). Symbolic convergence theory: A communication formulation. *Journal of Communication, 35*(6), 128–138.

Brashers, D. E., Neidig, J. L., Cardillo, L. W., Dobbs, L. K., Russell, J. A., & Haas, S. M. (1999). 'In an important way, I did die': uncertainty and revival in persons living with HIV or AIDS. *AIDS Care, 11,* 201–219.

Brody, H. (1980). The patient's role in clinical decision-making, *Annals of Internal Medicine, 93,* 718–722.

Brody, H. (1987). *Stories of sickness.* New Haven, CT: Yale University Press.

Brummett, B. (1976). Some implications of "process" or "intersubjectivity": Postmodern rhetoric. *Philosophy and Rhetoric, 9,* 21–54.

Brummett, B. (1982). On to rhetorical relativism. *Quarterly Journal of Speech, 68,* 425–430.

Bruner, J. (1986). *Actual minds, possible worlds.* Cambridge, MA: Harvard University Press.

Butler, S., & Rosenblum, B. (1991). *Cancer in two voices.* San Francisco: Spinsters Ink.

Cahill, S. E., & Eggleston, R. (1995). Reconsidering the stigma of physical disability: Wheelchair use and public kindness. *Sociological Quarterly, 36,* 681–698.

Cassell, E. J. (1985). Talking with patients: Vol. 2. *Clinical technique.* Cambridge, MA: MIT.

Charmaz, K. (1994). Identity dilemmas of chronically ill men. *Sociological Quarterly, 35,* 269–288.

Charmaz, K. (1995). The body, identity, and the self: Adapting to impairment. *Sociological Quarterly, 36,* 657–680.

Charmaz, K. (1999). Stories of suffering: Subjective tales and research narratives. *Qualitative Health Research, 9,* 362–382.

Charon, R., Brody, H., Clark, M. W., Davis, D., Martinez, R., & Nelson, R. M. (1996). Literature and ethical medicine: Five cases from common practice. *Journal of Medicine and Philosophy, 21,* 243–265.

Churchill, L. R., & Churchill, S. W. (1982). Storytelling in medical arenas: The art of self-determination. *Literature and Medicine, 1,* 73–79.

Conquergood, D. (1988). Health theatre in a Hmong refugee camp: Performance, communication, and culture. *TDR: Journal of Performance Studies, 32,* 174–208.

Corbin, J., & Strauss, A. (1988). *Unending work and care: Managing chronic illness at home.* San Francisco: Jossey-Bass.

Craig, R. T. (1999). Communication theory as a field. *Communication Theory, 9,* 119–161.

Croasman, E., & Cherwitz, R. A. (1982). Beyond rhetorical relativism. *Quarterly Journal of Speech, 68,* 1–14.

Donnelly, W. J. (1988). Righting the medical record: Transforming chronicle into story. *Journal of the American Medical Association, 260,* 823–825.

Donnelly, W. J., & Brauner, D. J. (1992). Why SOAP is bad for the medical record. *Annals of Internal Medicine, 152,* 481–484.

Ellis, C. (1995). *Final negotiations: A story of love, loss, and chronic illness.* Philadelphia: Temple University Press.

Estroff, S. (1995). Whose story is it anyway? Authority, voice, and responsibility in narratives of chronic illness. In S. K. Toombs, D. Barnard, & R. A. Carson (Eds.), *Chronic illness: From experience to policy* (pp. 76–102). Bloomington, IN: Indiana University Press.

Fadiman, A. (1997). *The spirit catches you and you fall down: A Hmong child, her American doctors, and the collision of two cultures.* New York: Farrar, Straus & Giroux.

Fisher, W. R. (1985). The narrative paradigm: In the beginning. *Journal of Communication, 35*(4), 74–89.

Fisher, W. R. (1987). *Human communication as narration: Toward a philosophy of reason, value, and action.* Columbiasc: University of South Carolina Press.

Fiske, S. (1992). Thinking is for doing: Portraits of social cognition from daguenrotype to laserphoto. *Journal of Personality and Social Psychology, 63,* 877–889.

Frank, A. W. (1991). *At the will of the body: Reflections on illness.* Boston: Houghton Mifflin.

Frank, A. W. (1995). *The wounded storyteller: Body, illness, and ethics.* Chicago: University of Chicago Press.

Geist, P., & Dreyer, J. (1993). Juxtapositioning accounts: Different versions of different stories in the health care context. In S. Herndon & G. Kreps (Eds.), *Qualitative research: Applications in organizational communication* (SCA Applied Communication Series, pp. 79–105). Cresskill, NJ: Hampton Press.

Geist, P., & Gates, L. (1996). The poetics and politics of recovering identities in health communication. *Communication Studies, 47,* 218–228.

Geist-Martin, P., Ray, E. B., & Sharf, B. F (2002). *Communicating health: Personal, political, and cultural complexities.* Belmont, CA: Wadsworth.

Gergen, K. J., & Gergen, M. M. (1983). Narratives of the selves. In T R. Sarbin & K. E. Scheibe (Eds.), *Studies in social identity* (pp. 254–273). New York: Praeger.

Good, B. J. (1994). *Medicine, rationality, and experience: An anthropological perspective.* Cambridge, England: Cambridge University Press.

Hawkins, A. H. (1993). *Reconstructing illness: Studies in pathography.* West Lafayette, IN: Purdue University Press.

Holstein, J. A., & Gubrium, J. F. (2000). *The self we live by: Narrative identity in a postmodern world.* New York: Oxford University Press.

Hunter, K. M. (1993). *Doctors' stories: The narrative structure of medical knowledge.* Princeton, NJ: Princeton University Press.

Jones, A. H. (1996). Darren's case: Narrative ethics in Perri Klass's Other Women's Children. *Journal of Medicine and Philosophy, 21,* 267–286.

Kirkwood, W. G., & Brown, D. (1995). Public communication about the causes of disease: The rhetoric of responsibility. *Journal of Communication, 45,* 55–76.

Kleinman, A. (1988). *The illness narratives: Suffering, healing and the human condition.* New York: Basic Books.

Kleinman, A., Eisenberg, L., & Good, B. (1978). Culture, illness, and care: Clinical lessons from anthropologic and cross-cultural research. *Annals of Internal Medicine, 88,* 251–258.

Kline, K. N. (1999). Reading and reforming breast self-examination discourse: Claiming missed opportunities for empowerment. *Journal of Health Communication, 4,* 119–141.

Lorde, A. (1980). *The cancer journals.* Argyle, NY: Spinsters Ink.

Makoul, G. (1999). Using patient narrative videos for understanding better the illness experience. *Academic Medicine, 74,* 580–581.

Matthews, C. K, & Harrington, N. G. (2000). Invisible disability. In D. G. Braithwaite & T. L. Thompson (Eds.), *Handbook of communication and people with disabilities: Research and application* (pp. 405–421). Mahwah, NJ: Lawrence Erlbaum Associates.

McAdams, D. P. (1993). *The stories we live by: Personal myths and the making of the self* New York: Morrow.

McWhinney, I. (1989). The need for a transformed clinical method. In M. Stewart & D. Roter (Eds.), *Communicating with medical patients* (pp. 25–40). Newbury Park, CA: Sage.

Middlebrook, C. (1996). *Seeing the crab: A memoir of dying before I do.* New York: Anchor.

Miller, K. (2001). *Communication theories: Perspectives, processes, and contexts.* Boston: McGraw-Hill.

Miller, K., Joseph, L., & Apker, J. (2000). Strategic ambiguity in the role development process. *Journal of Applied Communication Research,28,* 193–214.

Mishler, E. G. (1981). The social construction of illness. In E. G. Mishler, L. R. Amarasingham, S. D. Osherson, S. T. Hauser, N. E. Waxier, & R. Liem (Eds.), *Social contexts of health, illness and patient care* (pp. 141–168). Cambridge, England: Cambridge University Press.

Mishler, E. G. (1984). *The discourse of medicine.* Norwood, NJ: Ablex.

Morris, D. B. (1998). *Illness and culture in the postmodern age.* Berkeley: University of California Press.

Murphy, R. F. (1987). *The body silent.* New York: Henry Holt & Co.

Payer, L. (1988). *Medicine and culture: Varieties of treatment in the United States, England, West Germany, and France.* New York: Henry Holt & Co.

Plato. (1998). *Gorgias* (J. H. Nichols, Jr., Trans.). Ithaca, NY: Cornell University Press.

Poirier, S., & Brauner, D. (1988). Ethics, language, and the daily discourse of clinical medicine. *Hastings Center Report, 18,* 5–9.

Poirier, S. & Brauner, D. (1990). The voices of the medical record. *Theoretical Medicine, 11,* 29–39.

Poirier, S., Rosenblum, L., Ayres, L., Brauner, D. J., Sharf, B. F., & Stanford, A. F. (1992). Charting the chart: An exercise in interpretation(s). *Literature and Medicine, 11,* 1–22.

Price, R. (1994). *A whole new life: An illness and a healing.* New York: Scribners.

Railsback, C. C. (1983). Beyond rhetorical relativism: A structural-material model of truth and objective reality. *Quarterly Journal of Speech, 69,* 351–363.

Reeve, C. (1998). *Still me.* New York: Ballantine.

Scott, R. L. (1967). On viewing rhetoric as episternic. *Central States Speech Journal, 18,* 9–17.

Sharf, B. F. (1990). Physician-patient communication as interpersonal rhetoric: A narrative approach. *Health Communication, 2,* 217–231.

Sharf, B. F. (1997). Communicating breast cancer on-line: Support and empowerment on the Internet. *Women and Health, 26,* 63–82.

Sharf, B. F. (2001). Out of the closet and into the legislature: The impact of communicating breast cancer narratives on health policy. *Health Affairs, 20,* 213–218.

Sharf, B. F., & Freimuth, V. S. (1993). The construction of illness on entertainment television: Coping with cancer on thirty something. *Health Communication, 5,* 141–160.

Sharf, B. F., Freimuth, V. S., Greenspon, P., & Plotnick, C. (1996). Confronting cancer on thirty something: Audience response to health content on entertainment TV. *Journal of Health Communication, 1,* 157–172.

Sharf, B. F., & Kahler, J. (1996). Victims of the franchise: A culturally sensitive model for teaching patient-physician communication in the inner city. In E. B. Ray (Ed.), *Communication and the disenfranchised: Social health issues and implications* (pp. 95–115). Mahwah, NJ: Lawrence Erlbaum Associates.

Singhal, A., & Rogers, E. M. (1999). *Education-entertainment: A communication strategy for social change.* Mahwah, NJ: Lawrence Erlbaum Associates.

Smith D. H., &. Pettegrew, L. S. (1986). Mutual persuasion as a model for doctor-patient communication. *Theoretical Medicine, 7,* 127–146.

Sontag, S. (1978). *Illness as metaphor.* New York: Farrar, Straus & Giroux.

Sontag, S. (1988). *AIDS and its metaphors.* New York: Farrar, Straus & Giroux.

Sullivan, C. F. (1997, Spring) Women's ways of coping with breast cancer. *Women's Studies in Communication, 20,* 31–53.

Sweeney, J. (1997). *God said "Hal": A memoir.* New York: Bantam.

Vanderford, M. L., Jenks, E. B., & Sharf, B. F. (1997). Exploring patients' experiences as a primary source of meaning. *Health Communication, 9,* 13–26.

Vanderford, M. L., & Smith, D. H. (1996). *The silicone breast implant story: Communication and uncertainty.* Mahwah, NJ: Lawrence Erlbaum Associates.

Vanderford, M. L., Smith, D. H., & Harris, W. S. (1992). Value identification in narrative discourse: Evaluation of an HIV education demonstration project. *Journal of Applied Communication Research, 20,* 123–161.

Vanderford, M. L., Stein, T., Sheeler, R., & Skochelak, S. (2001). Communication challenges for experienced clinicians: Topics for an advanced communication curriculum. *Health Communication, 13,* 261–284.

Varallo, S. M., Ray, E. B., & Ellis, B. H. (1998). Speaking of incest: The research interview as social justice. *Journal of Applied Communication Research, 26,* 254–271.

VIA (Video Intervention/Prevention Assessment) Website. Learning from patients about the illness experience. Downloaded on October 14, 2002 from http:www.viaproject.org.

Weick, K. (1995). *Sensemaking in organizations.* Thousand Oaks, CA: Sage.

Discussion Questions

1. What is an illness narrative? How is it related to the social constructivist perspective? Based on this article, do you think that there is a need for more health communication scholarship done from this perspective?

2. What does it mean to be "healthy"? How are our definitions of health influenced by illness narratives?

3. Sharf and Vanderford discuss the many roles and functions of illness narratives. What are your own narratives of health/illness? What influences do they have on your life? ✦

Part II

PATIENT-PROVIDER COMMUNICATION

Chapter 5
'But Basically You're Feeling Well, Are You?'
Tag Questions in Medical Consultations

Annette Harres

Part II of this anthology addresses patient-provider communication, one of the two most studied areas of health communication, the other being health promotion campaigns (see Parts VI and VII). The six chapters in this part of the reader discuss a variety of topics that provide a sense of the issues that present themselves as patients seek the care of health-care professionals. This section will address the complexity of communication between providers and patients and the ways in which communication scholars reach outside the academic world into the everyday practices of health care and its provision.

In Chapter 5, Annette Harres uses conversation analysis techniques to look at the impact of the way doctors ask questions following up on the responses they get. She focuses primarily on tag questions, questions that follow a statement, and analyzes their use in the health-care provider interaction with the patient. Tag questions in medical consultations may be used for a number of reasons that are in opposition to how this communication style has been traditionally viewed. Understanding the tag question as a valuable tool or strategy in these interactions allows for greater insight into the doctor-patient relationship.

From " 'But Basically You're Feeling Well, Are You?': Tag Questions in Medical Consultations," Annette Harres, 1998, *Health Communication*, Vol. 10:2 pp. 111–123.

Related Topics: culture, patient-provider communication, qualitative methods

Tag questions represent an interesting analytical focus for the study of doctor-patient communication because they have been described by various researchers as conducive or leading (Thomas, 1989), as preemptory or closed (Algeo, 1988), and as facilitative or open (Cameron, McAlinden, & O'Leary, 1988). They also constitute one of the most quoted strategies in terms of indirect or nonassertive speech and are thus theoretically at odds with authoritative linguistic strategies. This article explores the use of tag questions by 3 Australian female doctors working in general practice. In particular, I show how tag questions function to establish rapport between doctor and patient yet also to maintain control of the interaction. The insights gained from such a linguistic analysis allow some conclusions with regard to the communicative processes involved in doctor–patient interaction and can contribute to more efficient clinician communication. After a brief discussion of the form and functions of tag questions in general, I review aspects of the use of tag questions in health communication before presenting some excerpts from consultations in Australia.

Form and Function of Tag Questions

The term *tag question* refers to the combination of a clause and an auxiliary verb + pronoun + interrogative. The auxiliary is either the primary auxiliary *be, have,* or *do* or a modal auxiliary. The negation used in the tag is either *n't* or *not,* however, the latter is uncommon in Australian and American English. The following sentences are examples of tag questions:

1. You aren't in pain, are you?
2. You can bend your knee, can't you?

When the clause is declarative or interrogative and includes an auxiliary, this auxiliary remains constant in the tag. When the clause is declarative or interrogative and has no auxiliary, the verb of the clause is replaced by *do* in the tag, as in

3. You know her well, do you?

There are two types of polarity among tag questions: *constant polarity* in which both phrases are positive, illustrated in Example 4, and *reverse polarity* in which one phrase is positive and the other negative, illustrated in Example 5.

4. You've survived the weaning, have you?
5. You've survived the weaning, haven't you?

Nässlin (1984) stated that in constant polarity tag questions, the speaker expresses no personal opinion about the truth of the proposition, whereas in reverse polarity tag questions, the speaker believes the proposition to be true.

Bublitz (1979) termed tag questions *reduced questions* and argued that the functions fulfilled by tag questions in the process of communication were specific to discourse occasions and depended also on prosodic factors, such as intonation. Allan (1986) argued that rising intonation clearly showed the speaker's orientation toward the hearer and was used when speakers were not speaking with finality or certainty. Thus, tag questions in which speakers indicate that they are checking the proposition with the hearer have a rise or fall–rise tone. Tags by which speakers indicate that they expect the hearer to agree with them have a fall or a rise–fall tone. As Allan commented, a rising intonation contour is associated with politeness and deference as well as hesitancy, uncertainty, and a lack of confidence. It represents a cooperative strategy by the speaker to ascertain that the hearer is comprehending.

Thus, a falling intonation contour invites agreement from the hearer and tends to constitute a closure of the discourse, whereas a rising intonation contour is more open to disagreement. The rising intonation contour is essentially hearer-oriented and generally associated with deference and uncertainty. By contrast, the falling intonation is typical of assertion and command. Leading questions will be more likely to possess a falling intonation contour because the speaker presumes that the hearer agrees with the proposition.

Types of Tag Questions

Holmes (1990, 1995) summarized tag question usage according to four categories, depicted in Table 5.1. Tags were either *content oriented (modal),* that is, they were used predominantly to satisfy the information needs of the speaker, or *hearer oriented (affective).* A modal tag has a confirmatory or informative function, for example

1. Doctor to patient: "You've been here before, haven't you?"

An affective tag can be facilitative (Example 2), challenging (Example 3), or softening (Example 4); for instance,

2. Doctor to patient, who has talked about marital problems: "That's the last straw, isn't it?"
3. Magistrate to defendant: "You hit her, didn't you?"
4. Teacher to pupil: "That's not very tidy, is it?"

Tag questions used for their facilitative function are a cooperative strategy aimed at reducing social distance and expressing solidarity or support. As part of their coercive or challenging function, tag questions force addressees to respond to and agree with the speaker (conducive tag questions). Acknowledging the ambiguity of some tag questions, Holmes nevertheless maintained that although tags may serve more than one function, it was generally possible to allocate a primary meaning and assign tags to one of the categories mentioned for the purpose of data analysis.

How does all this relate to doctor–patient communication? First, modal tag questions are clearly an effective means of eliciting information from the patient. Second, affective tag questions provide doctors with a valuable tool to establish rapport with patients and to facilitate involvement. Prosodic features, such as intonation and stress, help to fine-tune the utterance—for instance, to diminish the force of a negative comment. At the same time, tag questions

Table 5.1
Categories and Functions of Tag Questions

Category	Function
Modal meaning (content-oriented)	To express uncertainty
Affective meaning (hearer-oriented)	To express positive politeness
Facilitative	To invite addressee to participate in conversation
Softening	To express negative politeness
	To reduce force of criticism and or directive
Challenging	To intensify force of negative speech act
	To force addressee to contribute to conversation

give patients a chance to participate in the exchange, to monitor whether the doctor's assessment represents their own, and to correct any misconceptions. Whether these opportunities are actually realized by patients is a different matter: It has been suggested that patients are reluctant to take the floor and ask questions (Ten Have, 1991).

Tag Questions and Health Communication

In asymmetrical discourse in which the participants in verbal interaction do not have equal status, tag questions are an important strategy to manipulate interactional involvement. Cameron et al. (1988) investigated the use of tag questions in three different asymmetrical settings: in a classroom, in a TV talk show, and during a phone-in between a doctor and a patient. They found that powerless speakers never used facilitative tags but used modal tags almost twice as often as powerful speakers. Hence, affective tags seemed associated with powerful discourse rather than inferiority, as Lakoff (1975) claimed. For both symmetrical and asymmetrical discourse, the person in the role of conversational facilitator (i.e., who was responsible for eliciting contributions from other speakers) in the study by Cameron et al. (1988) seemed to favor the use of affective tags. Similarly, Holmes (1987) found that participants responsible for the flow and success of an interaction ("leaders") used more tags.

Winefield, Chandler, and Bassett (1989) investigated the use of tag questions during a course of psychotherapy. They found that the female patient used more tag questions as therapy progressed and she gained in self-confidence. According to Winefield et al., the patient's tags remained predominantly speaker centered (i.e., modal rather than affective) throughout the course of therapy, indicating that the basic asymmetry between doctor and patient had not been disturbed. In addition, they argued that tags following opinions functioned to express the patient's growing assertiveness and confidence. The authors found that the patient's tags did not function to yield the floor to the therapist but were used to check the therapist's response to her views and functioned therefore as appeals to solidarity.

In their study the patient used four times as many utterances as the therapist during the course of therapy. Sequential analysis revealed that the patient's tag questions resulted in advice and help from the therapist, who was less likely to merely acknowledge her communication after she included tags in her utterance. In later sessions, tags were occasionally used for their affective function by the patient, especially sentence-medial tag questions, for example, "It is difficult, isn't it, to understand how it works." In these instances the patient appealed to shared information between herself and the therapist.

Given that therapeutic discourse often involves self-monitoring of speech on the part of the therapist, the male therapist involved in the study by Winefield et al. (1989) explained that he resisted being drawn into doing most of the work in the early stages of therapy. As far as the tag use of the therapist is concerned, he did not use more tags towards the end of the course of therapy than at the beginning, mainly due to his tendency for speech monitoring. This fact would also explain why, given that tag questions can be hearer oriented and function to elicit contributions from them, the therapist in this study did not use many tags in the early stages of therapy, during which he was most reliant on patient contributions.

According to Cameron et al. (1988), the results of their study support the claim that affective tags are the domain of the powerful speaker, used to elicit lengthy responses from the addressee. By contrast, modal tags were used by less powerful speakers to request reassurance and by powerful speakers to gain information. In particular, they found that during the phone-in, doctors used modal tags to establish or summarize the facts of a case and to cut off the caller's narrative. Although tag questions have been classified as indirect, they are obviously very effective in expressing assertiveness. The significance of tag questions for understanding the process of doctor–patient communication becomes clear when we analyze how doctors actually employ these linguistic strategies.

Method

For this study, 29 tape-recorded consultations between 3 female general practitioners and their patients were analyzed with regard to the functions of tag questions. The consultations took place in the doctors' practices in the Australian state of Victoria and included 11 interactions for Dr. Alice Durham (age 50), 8 interactions for Dr. Belinda Forbes (age 36), and 10 interactions for Dr. Carol Lang (age 42). The consultations were transcribed[1] and coded, using encounter codes allocated by the Community Medicine Program at the Monash Medical Centre, Monash University.

Holmes' (1990) classification of tag questions according to modal and affective function was used for the analysis. As mentioned previously, coding of tag questions can be ambiguous, so to ensure reliability the tag questions were coded independently by three researchers. Multiple functions of tag questions appeared in only two cases overall, but it was then possible to allocate a primary function to those tag questions.

Analysis

Overall, the doctors used 98 tag questions, of which 43% had modal meaning, and 55% had affective meaning. Table 5.2 shows the distribution of tag questions among the three doctors. (It must be noted that the relative paucity of tag questions in the corpus does not allow any statistically significant conclusions.)

All doctors used both modal and affective tags in all major stages of the consultation, and the following linguistic analysis investigates how tag questions shaped the verbal interactions between doctors and patients.

Modal Tag Questions

Doctors used modal tag questions mainly to elicit information from their patients about aspects of their medical condition or to summarize medical facts, as in the following excerpts (D = Doctor, P = Patient):

EC31:73F349DT1
D: .although,
. . . (13.1)uhm,
. . . (5.7) you were ^on *Aprinox* at one stage,
[^weren't you↓]
P: [Ye=s I was].

In this example, the doctor, Alice, uses a modal tag with falling intonation and reverse polarity: the clause is positive, but the tag is negative. These features render the tag question less interrogative: The doctor is summarizing information she believes to be correct and about which she is reasonably certain. Her tag question is a request for confirmation from the 73-year-old female patient, whose response overlaps with the doctor's. She has not anticipated the doctor's tag and is ready to answer the question. By contrast, Alice is less certain about her

Table 5.2
Distribution of Tag Questions by Function

	Doctor					
	Alice		Belinda		Carol	
Function	%	n	%	n	%	n
Modal	55	17	37	10	40	16
Affective	45	14	63	17	60	24
Total	100	31	100	27	100	40

proposition in the following exchange with a 30-year-old male patient:

EC29:30M349DT2
D: .But ^when did you get him?
At the ^weekend,
→was it↑
P: Uhm yeah,
this ^weekend.

Alice wants to know on which day her male patient had access to his son, who had arrived from Sydney. After a direct WH-question ("When did you get him?"), she uses the rising intonation tag to elicit information that she genuinely does not possess. The tag shows constant polarity in that both the clause and the tag are positive sentence types. However, her tag serves to direct her patient's reply as a cue towards the answer that she assumes is correct and so has a more conducive effect. The combination of the two questions has a "cluster" quality and thus conveys a sense of impatience on the doctor's part. Paradoxically, the tag also softens the impact of the question. The interrogative nature of the tag is emphasized by the rising intonation contour, which carries with it a strong appeal to the patient to respond. Alice's patient replies to her question, prefacing his response with a hesitation marker.

Similarly, the second doctor, Belinda, used modal tag questions to confirm information pertaining to the patient's medical condition:

EC25:53M394DT3
D: Alright,
a=nd.. ^I'm just wondering,
you've still got your ^machine at home,
→^haven't you ↓
P: Yeah.
D: (0) For your ^blood pressure?
P: Mhm.

The function of the modal tag with its reverse polarity and falling intonation contour is to satisfy the speaker's information needs and it elicits the desired response from the patient. Again, the doctor is reasonably certain about her proposition, as signaled by the falling intonation contour. Although the patient confirms her assumption, she follows up quickly with a clarification of her tag question.

The third doctor, Carol, used the modal tag effectively to provide her patients with a chance to talk about any additional medical or psychological concerns. A typical example is given here:

EC1754M429DT2
D: @,
. . . so=,
, but ^basically you've been feeling well,
→<R. have you ↑ R>
P: (0) <H Oh yeah H>.
. . I don't feel ^any . . measurable . . pain.
. . . (1.7) Happy ^enough I think.
D: <P Good P>.

Here the modal tag question serves to elicit information from the patient and gives him the opportunity to mention any concerns about his health. The rising intonation contour reinforces the interrogative nature of the utterance. At the same time, Carol seeks confirmation that the patient feels fine overall. In fact, Carol uses this particular type of tag question several times with other patients, usually prefacing it with *but*. The pragmatic particle points forward in this case, away from previously raised health issues to direct talk to other relevant business. The brief hesitation that precedes the tag highlights the elicitative function of the modal tag question in this case.

The constant polarity feature gives the patient the possibility to disagree with the doctor's assumption, which is stated in the clause preceding the tag. Constant polarity, like rising terminal intonation, emphasizes the interrogative aspect of the utterance, especially when it contains a rising intonation contour. Although it can be argued that Carol is leading the patient to reply in the affirmative, the constant polarity tag opens up the exchange for disagreement. The less categorical nature of the clause is also expressed by the adverbial hedge basically. However, rather than expressing uncertainty, the modal tag here provides an opportunity for the doctor to elicit necessary information from the patient. By using the modal tag in this way, the doctor reduces social distance and provides patients with an opening to contribute to the discussion about their health.

Affective Tag Questions

The doctors frequently used affective tags in their facilitative function to express empathy and alignment with their patients. At a later stage in the same consultation while examining the patient's stitched hand, Alice comments on the condition of the wound:

EC27:65M349DT2
D: Now that's looking ^good,
→^isn't it↓
P: I—
I—
I yes,
it doesn't—
you know the couple of times I've ^seen it,
it ^looked quite—
. . . even ^despite the fact that I hadn't been,
taking me medication as regular as I ^should,
not because I ^didn't ^intend to,
D: (0) That's the te-
tenth,
^wasn't it↓

She empathizes with the patient about how well the hand is healing, the implication being that the patient is looking after it well. The tag functions here as an instance of positive politeness and by implication as praise for the patient. He in turn replies hesitatingly, with several false starts, and the reason for this is revealed when he confesses that he has not always taken his medicine. Alice seems to ignore this completely, because she proceeds to ask him for the date when his injury occurred, phrased as a modal tag question. She does not refer back to what her patient has said; instead she introduces a new topic immediately after he has finished his turn ("latching"). The falling intonation contour on the tag indicates that here the use of the tag question is predominantly phatic, with the doctor not expecting agreement from the addressee.

Alice also uses the affective tag in a preemptory way as a means to ward off pressure from the mother of a 2-year-old girl who is visiting the practice for the first time. The child has been vomiting for the last few days and is very weak, and the mother is very upset. When the doctor fails to make an outright diagnosis and refers the child to a pediatrician, the mother continues to press for information:

EC26:02F349DT3
M: [It's just not] ^normal,
to vomit every few ^days.
D: No.
M: And she just seems to be ^getting worse,
I mean—
. . . (10.1) ((UNINTELLIGIBLE DUE TO TRAFFIC NOISE))
If the ^other one gets it—
D: Well.
. . we'll have a better ^idea,
↓won't we↓
M: Yeah.

At this stage the patient's mother is very concerned about her daughter's condition. Alice is in the process of writing the referral letter as the mother continues to talk about her concerns. The doctor's affective tag accomplishes several things at once: First, it serves to cut off the mother's list of worries without being openly impolite; second, it excludes her from the decision-making process through the personal pronoun we as the doctor draws on the authority of the medical community; and third, it forces the mother to agree with the doctor. The falling intonation contour of the tag question emphasizes the categorical closure of the sequence and makes the reading of the personal pronoun as a marker of solidarity unlikely. Here, the affective tag is not so much a device for the doctor to align herself with the patient, but for the patient to be aligned with the doctor. The doctor is no longer interested in discussing the issue and uses the tag question to close the topic, but the mother continues to pressure her for a diagnosis even though it is clear that Alice does not know what is wrong with the girl. The mother's continued remarks constitute a potential challenge to the doctor's authority. By using the affective tag, Alice cuts off any further challenges from the mother.

Belinda used not only affective tags to express solidarity with her patients but also self-disclosure, as in the following excerpt from a consultation with a 31-year-old female patient:

EC19:31F394DT4
P: . . My ^father has . osteoporitis [sic],
. my mother had rheumatoid ^arthritis,
D: and ^cancer,
. . uhm . . no,
apart from ^arthritis,
no @ @
D: I've got that in ^my family too.
P: Oh.
D: It's an ^awful thing,
→^isn't it↓
P: It doesn't ^help,
no.

Asked whether there are any severe illnesses in her family, the patient lists a number of conditions and the doctor discloses that one of them—arthritis—also runs in her family. The patient acknowledges the information with an information management marker (*oh*), indicating that the information is news to her, and Belinda continues with an affective tag question, expressing empathy and eliciting agreement from her patient. The tag question shows a falling intonation contour that reduces its interrogative character and signals that the speaker is appealing to shared knowledge. Self-disclosure by the dominant speaker does not occur often in institutional discourse. Coates (1993) described self-disclosure as characteristic of talk between women friends, in which it signals intimacy and solidarity. In this particular case, it reduces the distance between doctor and patient. It can, of course, be used as a powerful strategy to encourage patients to disclose issues in return.

Finally, Carol's use of affective tag questions demonstrates how they can provide feedback and signal attentiveness by the doctor and thus encourage patients to continue with their turn. In the following example, Carol is talking to a 25-year-old female patient, who has finally become pregnant:

EC1925F429DT1
P: . I'm really ^rapt Carol,
D: . . Yes,
<H it's ^good,
→^isn't it H>↓
P: . Uhm,
I'm a different person now,
I'll—
D: Yeah.
P: compared to two ^years ago.

In this example, the affective tag shows a falling intonation contour as well as increased pitch. The doctor is providing positive feedback, sharing the patient's joy at her pregnancy. The patient recognizes it as phatic and continues her train of thought, rather than treating it as a genuine request for information. The affective tag question signals to the patient that the doctor is not just interested in her medical but also her psychological well-being.

Although this study is concerned with doctors' use of tag questions, it makes sense to discuss briefly the use of patients' tag questions. Most importantly, perhaps, is the observation that the patients who participated in this study used almost no affective tag questions, which confirms findings reported in the literature. It appears that the asymmetrical relationship between doctors and patients and the ritualized nature of their encounters means that affective tag questions are the domain of the doctor. It is not up to the patient to demonstrate solidarity, express empathy, or reduce social distance: These moves are initiated by the more powerful speaker.

Conclusion

This study shows how women doctors used tag questions on one hand to maintain control of the consultations and on the other hand to align themselves with patients. They used tag questions as linguistic strategies that served as means to an end: the diagnosis of conditions and their treatment or management. In other words, they were a discourse strategy that helped them realize themselves as competent professionals within the framework of the medical consultation. Given that the medical consultation has clearly defined parameters that both doctors and patients are aware of, the expectations brought to the encounter by both parties will affect their discourse structure. Tag questions played an important part in how interactional control and involvement, respectively, were realized in face-to-face interaction. In this manner, doctors were able to decrease social distance in an attempt to present themselves as active and sympathetic listeners, and patients responded by volunteering information.

Modal tag questions provided doctors with a valuable linguistic tool to summarize medical information and to elicit confirmation of information from their patients. In addition to serving the information needs of the doctor, it also provided patients with an idea as to how their doctors saw and thought about their condition. By giving patients the chance to respond, doctors also opened up the discourse to them, offering them an opportunity to either talk about additional problems or to correct the doctor's version of their condition. It must be kept in mind that these initiatives came from the doctors, which means that the essentially asymmetrical character of the consultations was not challenged.

Affective tag questions were a very effective way of showing that the doctor was genuinely concerned about the patient's physical and psychological well-being. All three doctors used these types of tag questions to express empathy, acknowledge their patients' experiences, appeal to shared knowledge, and even show solidarity. When necessary, however, doctors also used affective tags to close off the interaction and direct it towards a new topic. They can obviously function as a powerful linguistic strategy, especially in combination with the personal pronoun *we,* which is still used by practitioners when they perceive the need to refer to the authority of the institution of medicine. Clearly, doctors as well as patients need to protect face, but the use of tag questions as a means to cut off patients' questions, comments, or even challenges can easily be interpreted as patronizing.

Practitioners who are aware of the role that tag questions can play in eliciting information from patients or in establishing rapport with them have at their disposal a valuable linguistic tool. Tag questions are not necessarily leading questions: They can indicate to patients that their concerns are taken seriously. In the linguistics literature, tag questions used to be associated with nonassertive talk. This study indicates that tag questions are much more versatile than that, and future research should focus on the use of different types of tag questions by male practitioners to determine whether gender makes a difference.

Note

1. Transcription conventions: [is overlapping speech; = is lengthened segment; ^ is primary stress; @ is laughter; . . . (n) is timed pause; . . is short pause; ((words)) is comments; ↑ is direction of intonation contour; <F F> forte is increased loudness; <H H> high is raised pitch; <R R> rapid is increased speed; <P P> piano is decreased loudness; (0) is latching, no pause; —is truncated intonation unit.

References

Algeo, J. (1988). The tag question in British English: It's different, isn't it? *English World-Wide, 9,* 171–191.

Allan, K. (1986). *Linguistic meaning* (Vol. 2). London: Routledge & Kegan Paul.

Bublitz, W. (1979). Tag questions, transformational grammar and pragmatics. *Papers and Studies in Contrastive Linguistics, 9,* 5–22.

Cameron, D., McAlinden, F., & O'Leary, K. (1988). Lakoff in context: The social and linguistic functions of tag questions. In J. Coates & D. Cameron (Eds.), *Women in their speech communities: New perspectives on language and sex* (pp. 74–93). London: Longman.

Coates, J. (1993). *Women, men and language* (Rev. ed.). London: Longman.

Holmes, J. (1987). Hedging, fencing and other conversational gambits: An analysis of gender differences in New Zealand speech. In A. Pauwels (Ed.), *Women and Language in Australian and New Zealand Society* (pp. 59–79). Sydney, Australia: Australian Professional Publications.

Holmes, J. (1990). Hedges and boosters in women's and men's speech. *Language and Communication, 10,* 185–205.

Holmes, J. (1995). *Women, men and politeness.* London: Longman.

Lakoff, R. (1975). *Language and women's place.* New York: Harper & Row.

Nässlin, S. (1984). The English tag question: A study of sentences containing tags of the type isn't it? is it? Stockholm: University of Stockholm.

Ten Have, P. (1991). Talk and institution: A reconsideration of the "asymmetry" of doctor-patient interaction. In D. Boden & D.

Zimmerman (Eds.), *Talk and social structure: Studies in ethnomethodology and conversation analysis* (pp. 138–163). Cambridge, England: Polity.

Thomas, J. (1989). Discourse control in confrontational interaction. In L. Hickey (Ed.), *The pragmatics of style* (pp. 133–156). London: Routledge.

Winefield, H., Chandler, M., & Bassett, D. (1989). Tag questions and powerfullness: Quantitative and qualitative analyses of a course of psychotherapy. *Language in Society, 18,* 77–86.

Discussion Questions

1. Do you think tag-questions serve similar functions and are perceived similarly in different cultures?

2. The author of this chapter mentions that future research should look into possible gender differences in the use of tag questions. Do you think there would be a difference if the research had included males? Explain your answer.

3. Do the power differences between providers and patients play a role in the effectiveness of tag questions? ✦

Chapter 6
Blood, Vomit, and Communication

The Days and Nights of an Intern on Call

Krista Hirschmann

Chapter 6 uses a different qualitative research approach, participant observation, to follow first-year residents as they deal with patients. By following and observing residents in their rounds, Krista Hirschmann provides insights into the practice of medicine and interactions with patients. Training to be a physician is an arduous process, involving many years of school followed by several years of training, or residency, in hospitals. Through a narrative of her experience observing interns (first-year residents) over two, 24-hour shifts, Hirschmann observes some of the barriers to developing good communication skills among new doctors. Through offering a first-hand account of her own experiences "shadowing" interns, she also offers insight into the direct emotional experiences that residents and health-care workers encounter.

Related Topics: culture, groups, organizations, patient-provider communication, qualitative methods

Health care is a messy field. Not only are the daily menial tasks filled with indelicate odors and sights, but the context of shifting power from physicians to managed care has created administrative, financial, and legal tensions among health care professionals that must be negotiated regularly. In addition, new technology has led to ethical dilemmas that in earlier times did not exist. What it means to be a physician, the role one must play, and skills one needs to perfect are, in some instances, drastically different in today's health care climate. However, despite these dynamic changes, physicians-in-training, otherwise known as residents, continue to be initiated in much the same tradition as were their predecessors—by being overworked, overstressed, and underappreciated. This situation is particularly true of the first year of training, internship year, which is often the hardest due to an intern's amount of work and lack of experience. Yet, health communication researchers often fail to consider this context as a site of study. Also, health communication research (much like Western medicine) tends to focus on remedying problems by teaching "old docs new tricks," rather than by preventing problems by examining the system from which they emerge.

This research provides an evocative account of the internship context based on a series of observations in the hospital setting. Specifically, I shadowed an intern, Kevin, during 2 nights on call to describe the fragmented, chaotic, and exhausting experiences of an intern. It is not intended to be a generalizable account of all hospitals, residents, or even of Kevin's typical work day, especially because the number of people he admitted easily quadrupled as his training progressed. Instead, this article is a reminder, or perhaps an introduction, for health care researchers whose theories, particularly critical ones, neglect the mess.

Through Sickness and in Health Care . . .

The flames of the citronella candles scattered about a small screened-in porch flicker as a soft October breeze passes through. While reaching for another piece of pan pizza from the open box between us, I turn to my partner, Kevin, and for the fifth time that week ask, "Are you sure you don't mind me shadowing you during your on-call night at the hospital?"

"No, I don't mind at all," he responds. "It'll be fun to have some company for a change."

From "Blood, Vomit, and Communication: The Days and Nights of an Intern on Call," Krista Hirschmann, 1999, *Health Communication*, 11:1, pp. 35–57.

"Are you sure I won't distract you or make you nervous?" I ask, thinking back to an incident the month before when another intern on call prescribed a medication to which the patient was allergic.

"No, you'll be just like another medical student following me around."

"You know what intimidates me most about doing this project?" I muse.

"The thought of working for 24 hours?" Kevin guesses.

"Yeah," I nod.

"Just think of it as staying up until 2 in the morning. And then you only have 5 more hours."

Internship, the first year of a medical residency, is considered by most in the field to be the hardest, because an intern is required to do the most work based on the least amount of knowledge. By title, interns are doctors and have a medical school diploma along with lots of happy graduation pictures to prove it. However, in the hierarchy of medicine, interns are the dirt on which the ladder stands. Consequently, personal descriptions of this first year of postgraduate education vary in their degree of melancholy (Harrison, 1982; Marion, 1991; Peschel & Peschel, 1986; Shem, 1978), with most lamenting long hours, hard work, and lack of power. . . . Despite the menial status of interns and residents, the system for educating them has caused quite a stir in recent years. In particular, the long sleepless hours faced by those on call, that is, those having to stay in the hospital overnight and through the next day resulting in 36-hour shifts, is argued to be unhealthy for both the residents and their patients. Consequently, mistakes resulting from both fatigue and lack of supervision are inevitable and potentially deadly. One highly publicized case is that of Libby Zion, an 18-year-old woman who died in a New York hospital for reasons that are contested to this day. Yet, despite the ambiguity surrounding her death, investigations revealed a series of medical errors, partially attributable to overworked residents. Consequently, on July 1,1989, as a result of a grand jury investigation and recommendation, "The Bell Regulations went into effect in New York State [and] forbid residency programs . . . to work their residents more than an average of eighty hours a week, or more than twenty-four hours in a single shift" (Duncan, 1996, p. 118). Though pertaining only to New York State, reactions within the medical community to such measures are divided. Those physicians supporting medical education reform believe that the reduced hours are not only more reasonable but also result in fewer mistakes, which in the long run is beneficial both to the patients and the hospital. Others argue that the longer hours provide continuity of care for the patients as well as teach the residents how to function under demanding situations (Duncan, 1996). Fox (1990) briefly reviewed the history of this discussion, noting that both the *Journal of the American Medical Association* in 1981 and the American Medical Association in 1987 sought to address the grueling schedules of interns and residents. In both instances, adamant rebuttals argued that "such rites-of-passage challenges have indispensable value in preparing young initiates into the medical profession" (Fox, 1990, p. 206).

In the past, such long shifts were less problematic because there was simply less to do, including paper work. Residents often slept through a night on call, or waited by the side of a dying patient knowing that lifesaving procedures or drugs were unavailable. However, as medicine evolves, so do the technological and pharmacological procedures residents need to know how to perform. For instance, an estimated 10,000 new drugs have been introduced since 1973, with an additional 500 coming out each year (Blumgart, 1991). Also, hospital patients today are sicker, with more complicated illnesses (Duncan, 1996, p. 70) that ultimately result in more tests and procedures to complete, more work for the interns, and less time and energy to communicate with the patients. In addition to the pressures of the hospital context, the focus on "serious teaching" by senior or attending physicians has consistently declined since World War II, largely due to a shift toward research (Fox, 1990, pp. 207–208). Such an absence of mentoring leaves residents without adequate role models or guidance on how best to manage their stressful responsibilities and potentially life-or-death decisions.

Literature Review

"Do you remember our first conversation on the steps of the library?" I ask playfully.

"Yeah," Kevin grins.

"Do you remember the part where you disagreed when I said 'patients' should be called 'clients'?"

"Uh, no, I don't remember that specifically," he admits.

"Well, I remember arguing that without changing the language and making it more consumeristic, and empowering the patient to take more responsibility for asking questions and demanding answers, patients will continue to passively receive medical care like a child taking orders [Beisecker & Beisecker, 1993]. And you thought . . ."

"I thought," Kevin recalls, "that calling patients 'clients' is a result of the influence of managed care, and that managed care contributes to a breakdown in the relationships between doctors and patients."

"Has your attitude towards any of that changed?"

"No, I think physicians still attempt to treat patients like they always have. But the way they view patients outside the office has changed a lot, and most of that change has to do with insurance companies and health care in the 90s. Just completely running an office more and more like a business every day and every week."

"Hmm. What about communication? Do you think I'm wasting my time studying the health care context?"

"No!"

"Why not?"

"Everything I do in the hospital," he begins, "revolves around communication with someone, whether it's another physician, another intern, a nurse, a patient, or a patient's family. And when problems arise, it's mostly because of communication breakdown between whoever is on the hospital staff. Also, I think it's easier to point problems out than it is to solve them, especially for those people who may not recognize that they have a problem communicating. And that's the biggest hurdle—when physicians think they're masters at communicating, when actually they're the poorest communicators in the entire hospital. So people's perceptions of how well they communicate are often skewed."

Malpractice attorneys would probably agree with Kevin's assessment. When asked the most frequent cause for malpractice suits, they responded that 80% of their cases were attributable to "communication issues," such as "physician attitudes" and "failure in communication" (Levinson, 1994, p. 1619). Yet, a review of communication literature reveals a glaring absence of research dedicated to positing theories and promoting skills that consider the reality of a physician's, particularly a resident's, high stress, sleep-deprived, caffeine-enhanced lifestyle. Sharf (1993) agreed that such research accounting for "professional, institutional, political, and sociocultural contexts . . . has been minimal, with doctor-patient dyads treated as generic and interchangeable across assorted circumstances" (p. 36). In addition to this need for contextualization, research needs to address how support systems, such as marriages, often crumble as the demands of work overshadow relational commitments and a social life outside of work. Furthermore, drug and alcohol use among physicians is a recognized problem, as are higher-than-average suicide rates (Duncan, 1996, pp. 108–109). With all this in mind, who am I to say, as the literature does, that if physicians responded better to indirect questions (Weijts, Widdershoven, Kok, & Tomlow, 1993) and used expertise in compliance-gaining strategies (Burgoon, Parrott, Burgoon, Birk et al., 1990), but made these strategies nonaggressive (Burgoon, Parrott, Burgoon, Coker, et al., 1990) that their patients would comply more readily? Furthermore, how can I tell them that if they interpreted patients' cues better (Geist & Hardesty, 1990), if they stopped making one-up statements when talking to their patients (O'Hair, 1989), and if they shared more sociodemographic similarities with their patients (Beisecker, 1990), they would be perceived as better communicators, and hence better doctors? Who am I, as a well-rested, professionally mentored graduate student, to say, "You know, forget that your decision making might kill somebody, what you should really concentrate on are you nonverbals." Who am I to say anything?

Ethnography? What's That?

7:05 A.M.: Looking around the physicians' dining room, I see an ample array of breakfast food and beverages. I am standing with Greg, Kevin's roommate, another intern whom I will be shadowing during the day. Greg is tall and slim, with looks that reflect his Middle-Eastern heritage. He has a broad smile and polite manners, both of which many women find attractive. His father, late brother, sister, and brother-in-law are all doctors, a network of privilege that creates both beneficial support and the pressures of high expectations. Playing the role of tour guide, Greg introduces me to another intern, a red-headed man, carrying a plateful of scrambled eggs and bacon.

After a brief exchange of credentials, the redhead backtracks to an earlier comment. "You mentioned something about doing an ethnography," he inquires. "I'm not familiar with that word. What is that exactly?" (Later another intern was to ask, "Ethnography? What is that? Some kind of Ph.D. word?") I pause for a moment to form a response. Van Maanen (1988) would argue that doing ethnography involves bridging fieldwork with culture (p. 4). That is, ethnographies are a written means of representing a culture by describing and understanding localized practices, particularly communicative practices (Bantz, 1995, p. 107). Ethnography as a method was largely popularized by Goffman (1989), who once said that to do ethnography, participant observation in particular,

> You must [subject] yourself, your own body, and your own personality, and your own social situation, to the set of contingencies that play upon a set of individuals, so that you can physically and ecologically penetrate their circle of response to their social situation, or their work situation, or their ethnic situation . . . so that you are close to them while they are responding to what life does to them. (p. 125)

Although ethnography can be a wonderful means of gathering vivid descriptions, it is also "politically mediated, because the power of one group to represent another is always involved" (Van Maanen, 1988, p. 5). Consequently, the current politics of both the researcher and his or her discipline impact the nature of the description (Van Maanen, 1988, p. 5). Essential to ethnography, then, is the understanding that the cultures under examination are portrayed in relation to a particular intersubjective experience, which is "always subject to multiple interpretations" (Van Mannen, 1988, p. 35).

This dynamic context reflects the characteristics of the "fifth moment," or the current tensions that exist in qualitative research (Lincoln & Denzin, 1994). This tension includes the representation of multiple voices, and the interdisciplinary nature of qualitative research, including ethnography (Lincoln & Denzin, 1994). One form of writing emerging in response to these tensions is the narrative account. The narrative account encourages researchers to engage in experimental writing that is both evocative and multivocal (Richardson, 1994). Furthermore, narrative writing brings the researcher into the account in a way that is both meaningful and self-reflexive. For instance, Ellis (1991) and Kleinman and Copp (1993) discussed the role of emotions when doing field work. They argued that researchers can experience multiple, simultaneous emotions (Ellis, 1991), and that exploring these emotions in writing can contribute to understanding both the successes and failures of a project (Kleinman & Copp, 1993, pp. 16–17). (Van Maanen, 1988, called such accounts "confessional tales" and gave them consideration equal to the more traditional "realist tales.") Thus, for the researcher, ethnography includes observing both the participants and one's self to construct a meaningful account of how understandings emerge during interaction.

"Well," I begin, "what it means is that instead of watching you in a lab or just handing you surveys, I actually observe you in your natural environment so that I can get a better idea of the whole picture."

"Oh, okay," he replies with an understanding smile. I wonder how many nuances are lost as people continue to translate medical jargon for me.

Description

Morning (Yawn) Report

7:10 A.M.: One thing particularly odd about the Sun Coast Area Hospital is that it doesn't have that usual overwhelming hospital smell of disinfectant. So moving from the low-ceilinged hallway, past the office of medical education into the small carpeted lecture room/hospital library is not the olfactory relief it might otherwise have been. Instead, the scent of aftershave, subtly detectable on most individuals, is compounded to produce an effect slightly less dramatic than the anticipated disinfectant. And no wonder. The room is filled with 13 young, white-coated, close-shaven men. Looking like an older version of the *Dead Poets' Society* with an Asian flair, the mix of interns and medical students wear Docker pants and comfortable shoes. Their hair is cut short, and slicked in place with moderate amounts of gel. Although there is one female intern, and frequently female students who rotate through the hospital, today I am the only woman present. I feel slightly uncomfortable and rather conspicuous because of this gender discrepancy, and shift quietly in my seat to observe the room. Stethoscopes are draped over shoulders, around necks, and stuffed into the large pockets of lab coats. Stressing pocket seams still further is the bulging weight of pharmacological references and other mini-sized but essential resources. I was later told that you can determine a physician's experience and level of confidence by how many resources he or she carries. Consequently, the most experienced doctors, who seldom carry reference books, often don't even wear their lab coats.

During the next 2 minutes, the front line of the hospital filters in carrying various plates of breakfast food—eggs, bacon, Danishes, doughnuts, bagels, juice, and, of course, coffee. And I presume it is coffee that fills the large purple, plastic, lidded mug in front of the attending physician, who himself sits in the front of the room facing his audience. Short of stature, with a full middle-aged build, he has dark hair, bushy eyebrows, and an accent suggesting New England roots. As he begins the morning report, his probing questions, though asked dryly, reveal a solid understanding of his trade.

"I want to see more history to give me a better picture of this person. Note what questions you can't get answers to. This way at least the attendings know that you were smart enough to ask them even if you don't have answers." Turning to Dr. Wong, the intern who just finished his night on call, and who is responsible for updating everyone at morning report, the attending says "I appreciate you presenting this patient, but if at all possible I would like the admitting physician to present the case." His demand for better history and physical taking skills continues. "Try to relive the admission—what you saw and felt. . . . That is a good history and physical for morning report. Now," he drones on, "if a patient with known IV drug abuse . . . has hepatitis B, what should that clue you in on?" There is no answer. "Has anybody ever heard of hepatitis D? *D* as in David?" he asks, slightly exasperated.

7:30 A.M.: Twenty minutes into morning report, people are starting to wake up. With increasing frequency, responses are called out, and whispered conversations in the back of the room begin to punctuate the answers. As they drift from case to case, I realize that even though I cannot follow all of the dialogue, with the necessary training I could. Like any other jargon, the coded language of medicine is used to define group membership and participation. Of course, if the pedagogy before me serves as an index of quality, I would happily forego such training. To me, the outsider, both the attending's presentation and teaching skills leave a lot to be desired. He appears unenthusiastic, aggressive, and demanding, but not necessarily demeaning. Noting the interns' reluctant responses, I wonder if this direct style of inquisition would encourage them to develop shells of confidence and cores of fear and insecurity. That is, I sense that during these question-and-answer sessions, the interns learn to hide their uncertainties and replace them with a facade of authority and decisiveness. Fox (1990) names this experience "training for uncertainty" (p. 205).

Shattered Assumptions

8:12 A.M.: Later, in the hallway, Greg confides, "That was really an atypical morning report." I nod with sympathetic understanding. "It was really good," he continues. "There was a lot of learning going on in there." In an instant, my assumptions are shattered. Like any researcher who enters a foreign culture, I too must not expect local customs and standards to match my own. I should not accept the belief that our educated, middle-class, professional similarities override the differences of our lived experiences, philosophies, and training. Yet, as Riessman (1993) discovered in her analysis of divorce narratives, "Contrasting assumptions [and] trouble in interaction provided a fruitful beginning point" (p. 58). As I was soon to discover, sexual appropriateness was another site of difference.

Although Greg is house officer this month, meaning he is responsible for all new admissions during the day, the morning is a leisurely one, mostly spent getting coffee, chatting with the staff, and roaming the hospital. Because the hospital only sponsors a general internship program of six people, and no residents, the interns have more responsibility than usual. Not only do they complete 1-month rotations of various specialties (sometimes outside the hospital), they also cover the entire hospital every fourth to sixth night on call. Therefore, slower mornings like this are savored. Using my presence as an excuse to avoid other duties in radiology, Greg leads me on a tour of the single-story, 100-bed hospital. The hospital is owned by a large national health care organization, which has a reputation with insiders for its cost-cutting measures. Despite its relatively small size, I am disoriented by the sameness of the hallways that radiate out from a central nursing station. On the medical floor, pale blue cabinets line the hallways. Like the name tags and nurses' lights outside the patients' rooms, there is one cabinet for every bed. Pulling open the cabinet creates a small surface on which staff can write notes in a binder-styled chart that is stored, along with medical dictionaries and some medicines, in the cabinet. Moving through the rest of the hospital, I note that, despite its nondescript smell, the hospital is clean and fairly modern. The pale blue of the cabinets repeatedly appears as the coordinating hue for signs, floor tiles, wallpaper, carpets, and furniture. The blue contrasts with the white walls and floors tinged yellow by fluorescent lights. Touches of peach round out the passive color scheme that thankfully is enlivened by colorful smocks worn by some of the nurses. Occasional posters promoting home care or (ironically) patient confidentiality decorate the maze of hallways.

During the tour, the staff is politely inquisitive as to my interests, with a common response of, "Well, you should find a lot to study here." The usual pleasantries, however, are disrupted when a male emergency room (ER) nurse, Sam, grows adamant about informing me of Greg's reputation as a ladies' man. Sam assures me that there are many stories that he could tell me about Greg's conquests. Greg shifts uncomfortably during the razzing, while I wonder what prompts this man to make sexual references in a professional environment. During my observations, this nurse was not the only person to do so, but certainly the most explicit and least apologetic. Because I know Greg and his dating patterns relatively well, and have heard about the hospital's penchant for gossip, I readily dismiss the comments. Greg later assures me that the nurse is an alcoholic who drinks a 12-pack a night. When I consider the nurse's responsibilities, Greg's assurance does not relieve my dismay.

Unfortunately, we bump into Sam again later that morning. This time Greg is giving a tour to a fourth-year medical student applying for an internship spot for the following fall. She happens to be a tall, poised woman with an enviable figure and long, wavy auburn hair. She is wearing little makeup and a form-fitting but professional green dress. She presents herself as a serious student in search of a potential job. She asks and answers questions efficiently, barely letting a smile emerge. Her controlled self-presentation does not, however, prevent Sam from making a comment as we pass him a second time, with me a few feet behind Greg and the student.

"Ah, wow, must be Greg's lucky day. It looks like Greg and the Gregettes." This was the lowest point of my day, and I doubt that the medical student felt much better about it. At the time, I laughed more out of bewilderment than amusement, but realized again that the increasingly politically sensitive context of academics had lowered my resistance against the comments of differently educated people. Although feminists have consistently pointed out the patriarchal nature of medicine (Hicks, 1994; Riessman, 1987; Treichler, 1989), I still found myself somewhat stunned with the experience of being blatantly objectified. Although this situation might be sexist in its own right, the earlier trivializing of Greg illustrates that because sexism involves issues of power, men also are subject to sexual inappropriateness within the hospital. With this distinction in mind, I grew increasingly aware that "punitive consequences" do not exist for those staff members engaging in various forms of sexual banter (Butler, 1990, p. 273). However, that is not to say that mutual banter can't also serve as a release from stress. The tour ends soon after this incident, and we part ways with the student.

Discipline and Punish

11:45 A.M.: "So maybe you want me to spread eagle for you too? How would you like that?" The question comes from a woman, probably in her late 50s, who currently is in wrist restraints because earlier that morning she tried to set her hair on fire. Greg grabs the bed rails and looks away. Considering the woman's scrawny frame, weather-beaten appearance, and admission for alcoholism, I don't think Greg would like it at all.

"Now, Rhonda," reprimands her husband, "you're actin' crazy talking like that. These people are trying to help you. They're professionals."

"I feel like some kind of farm critter tied up like this," she laments, lifting her hands.

Funny, that's exactly what I thought of you when I walked into your room.

Greg has little patience at this point, but does his best to reason with her. "But we need to keep you here so that you can get better. You need to keep the restraints on so you don't hurt yourself."

You need to keep the restraints on so you don't cause us problems.

"But I'm so bored," she argues. "I want to go home." Greg makes the mistake of asking her what she can do at home that she can't do in the hospital. "I want to go dancing, take a bubble bath, work on my crafts," she answers.

I don't blame you lady, you can only watch so much TV. Affirm her Greg. Tell her that you understand how frustrated she must be just lying there.

"Well, there are some things you can't do here. But you need to stay here so we can take care of you," Greg reasons once again. Rhonda's husband finally agrees to bring back her knitting if she settles down. As Greg and I leave the room, he comments, "Now see, that's the stuff I can't stand." In the hallway two attendings and another intern affirm Greg's annoyance by referring to the patient as a "schizo" and a "lunatic." As I wonder what the exact symptoms of these diagnoses are, I begin to recognize how easily a patient gets labeled in terms of behavior. Even more startling, Hafferty and Franks (1994) argued:

> What students learn about the core values of medicine . . . takes place not so much in the content of formal lectures . . . and . . . not so much at the bedside . . . but via its more insidious and evil twin, "the corridor." It is time medicine started claiming ownership of both realms. . . . (p. 869)

The Conversation

4:05 P.M.: "How long does it take to become cynical?" I ask the three interns with whom I am sitting in the physicians' dining room. The day is unbelievably slow and the afternoon hours are dragging by.

"About a week," responds Kevin. He is shifting restlessly and starting to get antsy about being on call soon. "I always get this sick feeling in the pit of my stomach right before it starts," he admits.

"About a day," corrects Dr. Wong, the intern who presented at morning report. He appears giddy that his 34-hour shift is almost over.

"You see," Greg continues, trying to explain his intolerance with Rhonda, "some people are just dirtballs. They're scumbags and money or race or age has nothing to with it. It's what they do to themselves as alcoholics."

"What about people who die because of lung cancer? They did that to themselves from smoking," I argue.

"That's different," corrects Greg. "Smokers aren't belligerent to the staff and their families—the people who are trying to help them." At that moment, Geist and Hardesty's (1990) distinction between good and bad patients pops into my head. They wrote:

> Physicians evaluate patients' attitudes to form impressions of them being either "problem patients" or "good patients" (Lorber, 1981). Good patients have cooperative attitudes, do not complain, are pleasant, do not disagree, make staff aware of their medical needs, are not too passive, appear to understand, accept medical instructions, offer little resistance to the regimen prescribed, and do not make trouble (Fisher & Groce, 1985; Lorber, 1981; Speedling & Rose, 1985). Problem patients are quite the opposite. (p. 72)

Later, Kevin expands on Greg's perspective. "You see, alcoholics will be admitted, and usually they'll go through what are called delirium tremens (DTs). Because of this they can be really abusive to the staff and their families—even violent. And these families have usually been through so much with this person already. These DTs can last a couple of days, and they're really painful because the body is going through withdrawal, so we put the person on pain killers. So we have to care for them while they're acting irresponsibly, and after the DTs are over they don't remember what they went through, or what they put other people through. And a lot of times," Kevin continues, "they're back in the hospital the next week with liver failure or some other complication, and they have to go through it all over again. I know it's a disease, but when you see the families, especially the children, it's very hard to be sympathetic towards the alcoholic when you know they won't remember it, and will probably keep doing until they kill themselves." The literature (Mizrahi, 1986) notes that such disgust by medical personnel is common. As Hafferty and Franks (1994) explained it:

> Patients . . . are cast concurrently as victims of disease, objects for learning, and subjects for research. . . . They can be transformed into objects of work and sources of frustration and antagonism—evocatively recast as "hits," "gorners," "geeks," and "dirtballs." They become "the enemy," with students feeling justified in their use of negative labels and corresponding behaviors. (p. 865)

Covering the Floor

5:16 P.M.: With Kevin and I both changed from dress clothes into scrubs, and most of the other doctors and students gone for the day, I feel more relaxed. However, I can't say the same about Kevin, especially because his beeper just went off.

"Okay, I'll be right down," he says. Hanging up the phone, he turns to me and says, "It's someone on the floor," We leave the intern lounge and find the patient's room. Kevin checks the chart before entering the softly lit room. I am excited to finally see him work with patients one-on-one.

"I heard you had some diarrhea," Kevin says loudly and clearly as he approaches an older woman with shiny gray hair.

"Yeah, I'd like to get it fixed," she responds.

"Well, when did it start?" Kevin inquires.

"Oh, about 10 years ago," she informs him. The nurse and I look at each other and smile as I try to suppress a laugh.

"When did it start this time?" Kevin asks specifically.

"It never left."

Kevin tries a different approach. "Why are you in the hospital?"

"Oh, you'll have to ask my doctor."

So much for communication theory.

5:55 P.M.: Kevin is waiting at the end of the medical floor hallway to help move a patient. I am at a cabinet writing up my notes when a woman approaches me to ask if her father, who is sick to his stomach, can have a 7-Up®. I admit that I don't work here but she explains her reason anyway: "Oh well, he's sick to his stomach and I hate to bother the doctor because he looks busy, but I still wanted to ask just in case." She disappears into the room. I look at Kevin, who is standing at the end of the hall chatting with a nurse about something inconsequential. I continue writing, and the woman reappears from the room. I am half tempted to give her permission myself—I mean, it's only a 7-Up®—but I decide against it, partially because of the legal consequences, and partially because I think ginger ale is better for an upset stomach.

"Do you still want to ask?"

"Yes."

"Kevin," I command, "this woman has a question for you." He stops his conversation and comes to the patient's door. Kevin checks the chart, asks a question, and then gives permission for the carbonated beverage. At first I am amused by the woman's intimidation, but then I grow dismayed when I recognize myself in her. I think of different visits to doctors' offices where I felt guilty for taking their time by asking questions. I even have apologized to Kevin for discussing some health concern during his time off. Even though neither my physician nor Kevin has ever belittled me for my concerns, I wonder how the aura or myths surrounding doctors and deeming them unapproachable become constructed.

6:35 P.M.: "What seems to be the problem?" Kevin asks.

"This is not my stomach," answers a woman who had a ruptured ovarian cyst removed yesterday. Kevin discreetly pulls back the covers and lifts the woman's gown to listen to her heart and intestines.

"This is not my stomach," the woman repeats. "My stomach is flat." Her belly looks a bit distended, the lower part covered by a huge white bandage. "Nobody has been in to check on me or told me what's going on. This is not my stomach." Kevin asks a few questions about the surgery and her surgeon. He begins to explain that everything sounds normal, and that she probably has some gas, which usually takes about a day after the surgery to relieve. The woman doesn't buy his explanation. "But I had the surgery last night and this isn't my stomach."

"Well, sometimes it takes 2 days," Kevin revises. He pauses for a moment and then takes out a notebook on which he begins to crudely sketch the stomach and intestines. Meanwhile, he explains the intestines' garden hose-like structure and their natural response to shut down after surgery while still accumulating air. The woman's tense face begins to soften as she finally gets her questions answered and receives reassurance that her flat stomach eventually will return.

"I wish I could just let out a big old fart," she laments. "That would make me feel better."

"Well, essentially that's what. . . ." Kevin drifts off, not sure how to respond. Outside her room, I compliment Kevin for taking the time to answer her questions.

"She's going to keep me up all night," he disagrees.

"Why do you say that?"

"Because the discomfort will get worse and she'll want something for the pain."

"No, she won't. Didn't you see how grateful she was that somebody took the time to explain things? She won't bother you for the rest of the night because now she knows what's going on, and what to expect. I'll bet you a backrub," I challenge.

"Okay," Kevin agrees. I won.

The Code

7:40 P.M.: BEEEEP! Kevin looks at his beeper and reaches over to dial the phone in the intern lounge. "I'll be right there." Click. He grabs his lab coat and quickly explains he has to go to the Intensive Care Unit (ICU) for a code. He takes long leaping strides down the hallway as I jog behind him.

"CODE BLUE ICU! CODE BLUE ICU!" blares a woman over the intercom. We pick up our pace. The scene unfolds as we reach the ICU.

The ICU has seven beds, all within a few steps of the nurses' station. The most seriously ill patients, many of whom are older, are in the ICU, where the ratio of nurses to patients is 1:2. For convenience, the rooms contain only one bed, and four rooms have no door, but rather a doorway about 8 feet wide, with a purple curtain that can be drawn for privacy. At the moment, the curtain of Room 2 is pushed aside, allowing me a full view of the code blue—a response to a full respiratory arrest. Apparently, during the process of being moved from the ER to the ICU, the patient had gone into seizures and begun *arrhythmia,* or irregular heartbeats. In addition, he had a severe gastrointestinal bleed that is decreasing his oxygen circulation, called *hypoxemia,* and possibly damaging his heart.

Kevin is the first doctor to enter the room. The attending is still on his way to the hospital, and the ER doctor is not there yet. Because the patient has just arrived in the ICU, neither the nurses nor Kevin know what is going on. For the first minute Kevin must run the code until, finally, the ER doctor enters the room, followed shortly by the attending. These two senior doctors stand at the foot of the bed giving orders, which Kevin and the nurses carry out. Twelve people in all crowd around the patient, a 76-year-old man named Sumner. Through the crowd, I can see him stretched out, completely naked except for his black nylon socks. By now he is in both hand and foot restraints, as several nurses simultaneously prod him with six different needles, two IVs to deliver medicine, one saline solution, one delivering blood, one to draw blood for a blood gas, and a sixth located in his fem[o]ral artery at the top of his thigh to measure his blood pressure. About every 2 seconds, Sumner lets out a loud groan, "UHH! . . . UHH! . . . UHH!" Ignoring his outburst, the staff continues to work efficiently. One of the nurses motions to me to shut the doors to the ICU. Another tells me to hand him a pillow from the stretcher in the hallway. Sumner still is groaning.

During the first minute, Kevin had intubated him, or put a tube into his lungs to deliver oxygen more efficiently. Early in the code the ER doctor moved from the foot of the bed to remove it, possibly believing that Kevin had placed the tube incorrectly. Now, Sumner, despite his restrained body, tries to sit up as he repeatedly moans, "I can't . . . I can't . . . I can't . . . I can't . . ." *He can't breathe,* I advocate silently. Meanwhile, the nurses are rotating turns doing chest compressions, or manually pumping his heart by pushing on his chest. The work is tiring and one nurse jokes to the other, "Good thing you've been working out!" The other nurse laughs.

I stand in the hallway silently watching. The doors to the ICU open and a man pops his head in, motioning to me that he wants to see his mother in Room three. Seeing the man in the doorway, the attending asks me what he wants, and I tell him. He tells me to wave the son in, and I do. The man walks quickly past the commotion in front of me to which I redirect my attention. Within minutes, the room has grown into a jungle of IVs and wires leading ambiguously from beeping machines and plastic bags to Sumner's chest, arms, groin, and penis, which lies limp among tufts of gray pubic hair. *Who is this man? A father? A brother? A lover? When he pictured his death as all mortals do, is this what he imagined? Lying naked in front of strangers who torture him with heroics as they banter with one another?*

"I can't . . . I can't . . . I can't . . . I can't," Sumner continues to gasp. *He can't breathe,* "I can't move," he finally wheezes out. *Oh, he can't move.*

"But, Sumner," replies a nurse, "we don't want you to move. Try to relax. Stay calm. We're trying to help you." She repeats the instructions several times while another nurse continues to pump on his chest. *What if that were me? How would it feel to die so vulnerable, surrounded by people who are unimpressed by the finality of death.* I begin to fabricate his life. Sumner has a wife, whom he sent daily love letters to while they were separated by war; he has three children for whom he played Santa every year until they had children of their own; five grandchildren who now are in college but still receive cards from him containing crisp 20s. He worked hard and saved his money to retire to a little house in Florida. A house that his wife will now think about selling due to her beloved loss and perpetual loneliness. I fade back to the reality before me and realize that Sumner's pleas have ceased. The execution of orders is now deliberately delayed, perhaps to encourage the inevitable.

"Okay, I'm calling it. Time of death is 8:03," announces the attending. With the staff clearing the room, I look at Sumner's lifeless body in full view. Dried blood crusts around the needles' holes. His mouth sits slightly agape. A nurse closes his eyes. Then she turns off the machines and disconnects the wires. I try to remember Sumner's last words, but in light of the past several minutes I can only wonder, *My God, my God, why have you forsaken him?*

I'm Not a Doctor on TV But I Play One in Real Life

10:20 P.M.: "I'm so glad that we finally got to spend a day together," I admit as I snuggle closer to Kevin over a month later, during my second observation. Sitting in front of the TV on Thanksgiving night, we decide a rerun of NBC's *ER* is our best option, particularly because it's one of our favorite shows.

"Me, too," Kevin sighs as we watch Dr. Ross swim into a sewer tunnel to save a young boy's life.

"Wow, do you think we'll get to do that tonight?" I ask, poking his ribs.

BEEEEP! Kevin looks at his beeper. "It's the ER." We both groan as we reach for our shoes, leaving the irony of the situation unspoken.

Reflecting back on the day's activities, I note the steady business. This is particularly true of the ICU, where people, who are trying their best to die, are miraculously saved with a shot of this here and a slight adjustment of the ventilator there. Of course, it's not always the hospital's "fault" that these people live. Sometimes it is the family who, divided over a parent's or grandparent's fate, agonize as to whether living permanently attached to a machine is a quality life. Take, for instance, Patient 4, a 78-year-old man who was extubated this morning, in the hopes of weaning him off the machine that was breathing for him. As his breathing started to fail in the early afternoon, the ICU staff—nurses, Kevin, and respiratory therapists—spent the remainder of the day trying to contact the attending to get permission to put Patient 4 back on the ventilator. The attending took over 2 hours to return the calls, while the staff juggled the legal implications of what they could do. Finally, just as the staff was ready to make the decision on their own and face the consequences, the attending called to order the unconscious patient placed back on the ventilator.

5:00 P.M.: In walks the attending on-call, his pungent cologne preceding him. I had met him previously on the night of Sumner's death, and my second impression remains consistent with my first. "Are you children having fun yet?" he condescendingly asks of those clustered about the ICU nursing station. Already pissed off by his earlier response (or lack thereof), they become visibly agitated with his obnoxious demeanor. He checks on Patient 4, then leaves to speak with the family who has been camping in the waiting room for several hours. The attending returns within a few minutes to the nurses' station. "The problem here is a lack of communication," he announces. Knowing that he is aware of my background, I sense that he is putting on this show for me. "They think that he is going to get better," he continues. "There's been no communication with the family practitioner. Their doctor has kept them in the dark about the seriousness of his condition, and they won't make a decision to DNR [do not resuscitate] until they speak with him. And he's one of those guys who believes in taking whatever measures you can just to keep someone alive." Kevin nods in agreement. "This is hogwash," the attending raves. "You don't do this to people. When they're like this you make them comfortable and let them go in peace." For a second, the stink of his cologne almost disappears.

A Holiday Special

7:20 P.M.: Arriving in the ER for the first time that night, we find another variation of postponed death. An 86-year-old woman, Mrs. Rempe, arrived by ambulance from the nursing home where she lives. After she passed out earlier in the evening, the nursing home staff resuscitated her, intubated her, and transferred her to the hospital, where she currently is stable but unconscious. She needs to be admitted, and Kevin must write the orders as soon as the nurse finishes talking with the woman's physician.

"Really," the nurse says. She listens for a minute. "Uh huh, okay." She hangs up the phone. "Get this," she says turning to us. 'This woman was just discharged from another hospital yesterday with orders to DNR. But her doctor forgot to write them up and send them to the nursing home, so when she coded tonight they resuscitated her." We turn and look at the woman who should really be dead. "But we can't extubate her now, so we need to admit her," she finishes. Kevin begins writing up the chart and orders when an emergency medical technician (EMT) breaks through on the radio that they are a minute away with a 68-year-old woman who's having trouble breathing. Kevin continues writing until she arrives.

True to their word, within a minute the ambulance arrives. "She coded in the parking lot!" an EMT shouts as he comes rushing through the automatic doors. Behind him on a stretcher is a large woman whose big round belly and white dimpled skin remind me of a stuffed turkey ready for the oven. They take her to Room 3 for round one of her medical care. As usual, the staff begins poking and prodding.

Meanwhile, an EMT is sent to get scissors from the ambulance so they can cut off her dress, which has been shoved up to her neck. The staff "bags her," or puts over her face a mask attached to a bag that they squeeze to help her breathe. Chest compressions begin, and the IVs are set up. The nurse finally gets the scissors and cuts away the woman's white underwear, only to discover a large sanitary napkin between her legs. At the other end, the woman begins to throw up her recent Thanksgiving dinner, causing foul-smelling odors to drift into the hallway where I stand. "Get some wet towels," a nurse shouts. The chunks of food are apparently too big, thick, and plentiful to be suctioned out, and the meal starts to pool in her mouth like a boat of gravy. The ER doctor tries to intubate her, but can't see anything due to the vomit. They roll her on her side to clear her mouth and try again. Meanwhile, two nurses work to spread the woman's legs to insert the catheter into her urinary tract. However, the rolls of fat along her inner thigh swallow the nurses' gloved hands, making the job more difficult than usual. It is 15 minutes into the code.

Come on lady, just get it over with and die. For a moment, I think about Sumner and my reaction to his violent passing from this world. I look at "Turkey Woman," whose situation is now not so very different. My reaction is less personal this time. The day has been full of dealing with unconscious bodies, whose identities are distinguished more by room numbers and medications than their given names. It is exhausting work to remind myself of their human potential, and much easier to believe that none exists. *Come on lady, don't survive to be a vegetable. Make it easy on yourself (and me, and the staff) and go now.* Kevin is somewhere in the midst of the shuffle, though safely distanced from the puke. (Kevin hates the heaves and stale smell that accompany vomit.) He seems to be playing with his stethoscope a lot, listening for breathing, heartbeats, and pulses. I begin to chat with the EMTs, who are discussing exactly which tools they should carry with them at all times, as well as the woman's last words, which apparently were, "I don't think I'm going to make it."

"I've got a pulse," shouts the ER doc 20 minutes into the code. The eight people crowded in the small exam room simultaneously stop and stare at him, as if waiting for the punch line.

"Yeah, there's a pulse," someone else confirms.

10:20 P.M.: Now, having switched from the TV version to the real thing, we are back in the ER for the second time that evening to help transfer Turkey Woman to the ICU, where Kevin needs to place his first A-line (artery) to measure her blood pressure. She is still a mess, with yellow and brown leftovers smeared across her face. An impressive display of teamwork among the ER and ICU nurses allows them to physically transfer Turkey Woman to an ICU bed. A nurse sets up an A-line kit along with sterile gloves and gauzes. Having gloved, Kevin opens the contents of the kit, which resembles a small tackle box. He lifts a folded piece of paper out of the kit and opens it. "Ah, the directions. Better save these," he says as he lays them on the bed. Over 1 hour, two kits, and three nurses later, the line is placed in her left wrist. Kevin originally aimed for the artery leading to her right thigh; however, the needle was too short to go through all her fat and stay in place. Apparently people who are obese are not considered part of the medical model. Kevin sighs in relief as her blood pressure appears on the monitor, and an ICU nurse finally begins cleaning her up.

1:30 A.M.: Kevin goes to speak with Turkey Woman's adult children, who have been waiting for several hours. "She's holding her own," he reports to the brother and sister, after selectively explaining why it took so long.

"We went through this with our dad a couple of years ago," the woman explains. "We know that she has a lot of health problems. But what we need to know is what will she be like after this? I know she wasn't breathing for awhile and that can't be good. Do we need to think about nursing care, or will she be able to live on her own?" Obviously their time in the waiting room was spent sorting through the possibilities.

"It's hard to say," Kevin responds. "She coded in the parking lot, so we were quickly able to start her breathing artificially. But the first 24 hours are the most crucial. We'll know a lot better in the morning what her chances are." I miss part of the conversation because the patient's ICU nurse has pulled me aside to give me directions to pass along to Kevin. I realize in that moment that I have been temporarily integrated into their culture. Somewhere between disposing of sharp instruments, finding their pens, and staying out of their way, I had gained enough trust from the nurses to become an intermediary. "So you can go see her now," Kevin finishes. I relay the message. Walking back to the intern lounge, Kevin explains why he was so ambiguous with the children. "I just didn't feel that that they were ready to make a decision tonight about anything. And that's just based on my own judgment," he adds. "Besides, you never know, I've seen people gradually improve. It happens."

Duty and the Sleep

1:45 A.M.: We crash in the lounge, having been up almost 20 hours. Kevin's beeper goes off at 2:04, 3:11, 3:45, 4:32, and 5:28. Each time I wake with him, but he tells me to go back to sleep, that he just needs to check on something and will be right back, and he usually is. Cursing ethnography under my breath, I agree. Finally rolling awake at 6:00, I realize that I just slept through the gist of my project, while Kevin caught a total of about an hour of sleep. Apparently everyone is still breathing this morning, but now we need to do an admit for a surgical patient. With only an hour to go (thankfully there is no morning report, and he has the rest of the day off), I follow Kevin to pre-op, where a woman is about to undergo a biopsy on her right breast. Walking into the room, I am startled to see an alert, responsive person after my night of observing the near-dead. Suddenly, I feel self-conscious and unpracticed as to how I should interact with this young woman, who must be close in age to my own 24 years. This similarity is disturbing, especially when I hear that she already had a lump removed from her left breast. Past experience may explain her remarkable calmness, as Bing Crosby sings "White Christmas" in the background. Kevin runs through the standard list of questions from memory and wishes her luck. It is 6:40 A.M. as we leave the operating room and Kevin muses, "I wonder what happened to that chest pain last night?" The night is a blur, and without my watch and notes I would have no idea as to when anything happened. I struggle to recall the chest pain, but it alludes my memory. My body is in a scummy daze as we wait for the next shift to arrive. Dressed in a shirt and tie, Greg is the first to walk into the lounge.

"Hey, how was it?" he asks, wondering what he should expect this morning.

"Busy," Kevin replies. "But doable. Very doable."

Hi Honey, How Was Work Today? (Last Night? Yesterday?)

As a partner, visiting the stage myself allows me to picture Kevin's daily drama more clearly, and digest his fragmented narratives without expecting either a coherent plot or resolution. However, in response to Kleinman and Copp's (1993) discussion of confessional tales (p. 17), I readily admit that my observations were not necessarily successful and are certainly open to multiple interpretations. Specifically, I am disappointed to have missed the series of early morning calls through which I so restfully slept. In addition, my trip to the field has only raised more questions and concerns for me regarding the education of physicians, particularly in terms of healthy communication. For instance, based on the literature (Sharf, 1993), this research, and my many conversations with Kevin, it appears that current communication theory regarding physician-patient or client interaction focuses on specific constructs that emerge in clinical settings such as nonverbals, domineeringness, and interviewing skills. Although these constructs are also relevant to the hospital setting, the frequent context of emergency care, unconsciousness, and disorientation on behalf of the patient (and sometimes the intern) alters possible expectations of healthy or effective communication. Consequently, a physician's first experience with communicating as a professional is filled with fragmented interactions and questionable role models (Fox, 1990). It is easy to imagine, then, how the deemphasized role of communication in these situations leads to deemphasis in other interactions. In sum, the chaotic nature of interaction during residency is not conducive to developing healthy communication skills, which are essential to a physician's clinical career.

Although part of the reason a deemphasis on communication occurs is due to the context of interaction, including the intern's own physical state, another reason is found in the culture of medicine and its socialization of residents (Fox, 1990; Hafferty & Franks, 1994; Mizrahi, 1986). Despite medicine's reflection of larger cultural practices (Fox, 1990; Sharf, 1993) it is also a culture that, as described, is potentially very different, both in terms of experiences and norms, from the assumptions and practices of those outside the field. Part of the culture of medicine is the heightened awareness of the body as a site of potential struggle and transformation in the physical, legal, and moral sense. Therefore, although I do not condone being objectified, it is understandable why the young, healthy, well-dressed, and well-rested body—the unstruggling body, that is—is cause for attention and comment. Furthermore, in many of the scenarios, objectifying the body is arguably a defense mechanism to remain humane rather than an inherent lack of humanity. To constantly consider the implication of one's actions is perhaps as exhausting as the work itself. Inflicting pain in the name of healing, being the bearer of hope, the messenger of death, are potentially emotional roles when consciously embraced. Consequently, disassociating the physical body from its humanness is one form of coping. As Kevin explained to me:

> It's only rough when I'm pronouncing somebody dead whom I've worked on. So I've seen them in their last hours, and I've seen how families can react. I try to be sympathetic towards the family, but I try not to get overly involved, because it can be taxing. As hard as it is, as soon as I leave that situation, I have to force myself to say, "Okay, that's over. It's behind you. Next."

Thus, the challenge for communication researchers lies with focusing on specific skills within specific contexts. Our theories must not gravitate only toward the convenience of clinical observations, but also to the trenches and training grounds where young physicians live the formative parts of their careers. As Sharf (1993) argued, "Taking account of contextual variability will sharpen the utility of our work and clarify which findings transcend these distinctions" (p. 37). In addition, such theory building should consider not only the formal interactions with patients and other staff, but should also attend to a physician's personal growth and development, which is undoubtedly impacted by her or his career and training (Mizrahi, 1986). Admittedly, such a proposal appears overwhelming at first glance. However, it is not nearly as overwhelming as the need to encourage competent and compassionate communication skills that enhance the quality of life for all involved.

Yet, reflecting on my own experiences, I realize the difficulty behind this need. My own 2-day transformation from an idealistic (annoying?), distanced communication researcher to a subdued participant observer was startling. The ethical concerns I had about patient confidentiality vanished with my discomfort of looking at nakedness and the revealing silhouettes visible through flimsy hospital gowns. That is not to say that my concerns were resolved appropriately. Rather, as seen during my own objectification of Turkey Woman, I adopted the same justification of convenience that medical professionals grant themselves when organizing the hospital culture. Oddly enough, I can still split my feelings between Turkey Woman and Sumner. The best I can explain such a stark emotional division lies with having heard Sumner's repeated pleas for help, and watching him struggle against the medical treatment. In short, I saw him as a person. Unlike Sumner, Turkey Woman was passive; she did not have a voice, or a half-dozen family members waiting in the lounge to compose an identity for her. To me, she was human only in form. Considering my education, it scares me to feel this way, but helps me to understand why health care professionals sneer at overeager and idealistic attempts to make them more compassionate and humane. Does the current system really allow them to do any better?

Finally, I realize that, like the labeling of patients, both good and bad doctors exist, and often they are the same person at different times or to different people. Consequently, traditional dichotomous assumptions do not offer adequate or accurate guidance with theory construction and practice. Instead, as health communication researchers, we must use our naturally dynamic context as a prototype for more systemic theory construction. Although praxis has undoubtedly contributed valuable understandings to our literature, we also must work to return our borrowed theories as more complex and useful tools. In this way, "We gain significant insights that will enhance the quality of health care while increasing understanding about the nature of human communication" (Sharf, 1993, p. 35). Likewise, medicine must continue to seek and utilize social science research that offers alternative paradigms for quality care, work life, and education. With the joint effort of social scientists and the medical community to explore the messy field called health care, we heighten the potential of offering contextualized advice so that physicians can begin to heal themselves.

Acknowledgments

I thank both Carolyn Ellis for her many careful readings of this text and Kevin for sharing his story.

References

Bantz, C. (1995). Ethnographic analysis of organizational cultures. In S. L. Herndon & G. L. Kreps (Eds.), *Qualitative research: Application in organizational communication* (pp. 107–119). Cresskill, NJ: Hampton.

Beisecker, A. (1990). Patient power in doctor-patient communication: What do we know? *Health Communication, 2,* 105–122.

Beisecker, A. E., & Beisecker, T. D. (1993). Using metaphors to characterize doctor-patient relationships: Paternalism versus consumerism. *Health Communication, 5,* 41–58.

Blumgart, H. (1991). Medicine: The art and the science. In R. Reynolds & J. Stone (Eds.), *On doctoring* (pp. 105–118). New York: Simon & Schuster.

Burgoon, M., Parrott, R., Burgoon, J. K., Birk, T., Pfau, M., & Cocker, R. (1990). Primary care physicians' selection of verbal compliance-gaining strategies. *Health Communication, 2,* 13–27.

Burgoon, M., Parrott, R., Burgoon, J. K., Cocker, R., Pfau, M., & Birk, T. (1990). Patients' severity of illness, noncompliance, and locus of control and physicians' compliance-gaining messages. *Health Communication, 2,* 29–46.

Butler, J. (1990). Performative acts and gender constitution: An essay in phenomenology and feminist theory. In S. Case (Ed.), *Performing feminisms* (pp. 270–282). Baltimore: Johns Hopkins University Press.

Duncan, D. E. (1996). *Residents: The perils and promise of educating young doctors.* New York: Scribner's.

Ellis, C. (1991). Sociological introspection and emotional experience. *Symbolic Interaction, 14*(1), 23–50.

Fox, R. (1990). Training in caring competence. In H. C. Hendrie & C. Lloyd (Eds.), *Educating competent and humane physicians* (pp. 199–216), Bloomington: Indiana University Press.

Geist, P., & Hardesty, M. (1990). Reliable, silent, hysterical, or assured: Physicians assess patient cues in their medical decision making. *Health Communication, 2,* 69–90.

Goffman, E. (1989, July). On field work. *Journal of Contemporary Ethnography, 17,* 123–132.

Hafferty, F. W., & Franks, R. (1994). The hidden curriculum, ethics teaching and the structure of medical education. *Academic Medicine, 69,* 861–871.

Harrision, M. (1982). *A woman in residence.* New York: Random House.

Hicks, K. M. (Ed.). (1994). *Misdiagnosis: Women as a disease.* Allentown, PA: People's Medical Society.

Kleinman, S., & Copp, M. A. (1993). *Emotions and fieldwork.* Newbury Park, CA: Sage.

Levinson, W. (1994). Physician-patient communication: A key to malpractice prevention. *Journal of the American Medical Association, 272,* 1619–1620.

Lincoln, Y. S., & Denzin, N. K. (1994). The fifth moment. In N. K. Denzin & Y. S. Lincoln (Eds.), *Handbook of qualitative research* (pp. 575–586). Thousand Oaks, CA: Sage.

Marion, R. (1991). *Learning to play God: The coming of age of a young doctor.* Reading, MA: Addison-Wesley.

Mizrahi, T. (1986). *Getting rid of patients.* New Brunswick, NJ: Rutgers University Press.

O'Hair, D. (1989). Dimensions of relational communication and control during physician-patient interactions. *Health Communication, 1,* 97–115.

Peschel, R., & Peschel, E. R. (1986). *When a doctor hates a patient and other chapters in a young physician's life.* Berkeley: University of California Press.

Richardson, L. (1994). Writing: A method of inquiry. In N. K. Denzin & Y. S. Lincoln (Eds.), *Handbook of qualitative research* (pp. 516–529). Thousand Oaks, CA: Sage.

Riessman, C. K. (1987). Women and medicalization: A new perspective. In H. D. Schwartz (Ed.), *Dominant issues in medical sociology* (pp. 101–121). New York: Random House.

Riessman, C. K, (1993). *Narrative analysis.* Newbury Park, CA: Sage.

Sacco, J. (1989). *Morphine, ice cream, and tears: Tales of a city hospital.* New York: Morrow.

Sharf, B. (1993). Reading the vital signs: Research in health care communication. *Communication Monographs, 60,* 35–41.

Shem, S. (1978). *The House of God.* New York: Richard Marek.

Treichler, P. A. (1989). What definitions do: Childbirth, cultural crisis, and the challenge to medical discourse. In B. Dervin, L. Grossberg, B. J. O'Keefe, & E. Wartella (Eds.), *Rethinking communication* (Vol. 2, pp. 424–453). Newbury Park, CA: Sage.

Van Maanen, J. (1988). *Tales of the field.* Chicago: University of Chicago Press.

Weijts, W., Widdershoven, G., Kok, G., & Tomlow, P. (1993). Patients' information-seeking actions and physicians' responses in gynecological consultations. *Qualitative Health Research, 3,* 398–429.

Discussion Questions

1. This article is what ethnographers call a "confessional tale," detailing the researcher's personal experience at the research site. Does this style of writing help or hinder your understanding of the study that was done? In what ways?

2. Considering the communication constraints among health providers, what are some ways that health communication in hospital settings can still be improved?

3. Cynicism among health-care providers is evident in several areas of this account, most notably with the "turkey woman." What function does depersonalization serve in medicine? Is it necessary, or should we strive to overcome it? ✦

Chapter 7 Components of Patients' and Doctors' Perceptions of Communication Competence During a Primary Care Medical Interview

Donald J. Cegala, Deborah Socha McGee, and Kelly S. McNeilis

In another approach to studying patient-provider interactions, Donald J. Cegala, Deborah Socha McGee, and Kelly S. McNeilis present some of the differing elements that can affect perceptions of doctor competence during medical interviews. Taken together with the earlier chapters in this section, it becomes increasingly clear that many variables are at play in determining the ways in which patients and their health-care providers communicate. Communication competence of both doctors and patients can be a significant component of a medical interaction. The authors present research that provides insight into the elements affecting perceived communication competence for both patients and doctors during a medical interview. This information becomes valuable in understanding the doctor-patient relationship, especially when considering effective communication in a health setting.

Related Topics: media, patient-provider communication, patients' perspectives, qualitative methods, quantitative methods, role of the patient

From "Components of Patients' and Doctors' Perceptions of Communication Competence During a Primary Care Medical Interview," Donald J. Cegala and Deborah Socha McGee, with Kelly S. McNeilis, 1996, *Health Communication*, 8, 1–28.

Over the last decade, several researchers have focused attention on the concept of interpersonal communication competence (e.g., Bostrom, 1984; Cegala & Waldron, 1992; O'Keefe & Delia, 1982; Spitzberg & Cupach, 1984; Wiemann, 1977). Recently, some health communication scholars have suggested that the concept of competence may serve as a useful theoretical framework for future research into provider-patient communication (e.g., Kasch, 1984; Kreps & Query, 1990; Morse & Piland, 1981).

The purpose of this research is to take initial steps in developing a theoretical and operational connection between interpersonal communication competence and doctor–patient communication. In particular, our purpose is to identify and define components of doctors' and patients' communicative competence in the primary care medical interview.

Critique of Competence Literature

There are several available summaries of the competence literature (e.g., Rubin, 1990; Spitzberg, 1986; Spitzberg & Cupach, 1984; Wiemann & Backlund, 1980). Our intent here is not to provide a detailed analysis and assessment of that literature, but, rather, to isolate key problematic characteristics that most of the current approaches to communication competence have in common. We then use this critique as a foundation for articulating an alternative approach to competence (also see Cegala & Waldron, 1992).

Despite extensive research, there is little

agreement on what interpersonal communication competence is or how to assess it. Most research on competence appears to be driven by the desire to develop a general theory of communication. Although this is laudable, we believe that the desire for a general theory of communication has prompted scholars to search for and develop broad transsituational constructs that have abstract theoretical appeal but weak operational specificity and predictive power. Thus, for example, we have competence models that include such factors as knowledge, motivation, and skills (Spitzberg & Cupach, 1984) but do not clearly specify how these constructs relate to one another or how they are measured. One of the results of this sort of approach is that it de-emphasizes the need to examine actual behavioral manifestations of competence (especially language-in-use), and it all but ignores the role of context. As an alternative, we propose an approach to research on competence that is grounded in communicative behavior and, as such, is inherently context-bound (see Cegala & Waldron, 1992). Our approach is by no means adverse to striving toward a general theory of communication, but it assumes that such a theory is likely to evolve from deep understanding of what competence is within several different contexts.[1]

Thus, our approach assumes that communication competence is best defined in terms of participants' language-in-use and that such usage is largely bound by the limitations and resources available within the immediate social setting in which communication takes place. Accordingly, definitions and assessments of competence are assumed to be grounded in participants' understanding of what they are trying to achieve communicatively and the extent to which they are able to perceive and appropriately accommodate and align each other's intentions and communicative moves.[2]

Such an approach to competence demands a process-oriented research model that allows for the monitoring of emergent meanings and corresponding communicative moves during the course of interaction. Unfortunately, current methods in the social sciences are rather limited in their ability to provide content-level information about online cognitive and affective processes involved in virtually any aspect of meaning (see Waldron & Cegala, 1992). Conversational moves, however, often can be made available for observation and analysis. Thus, our approach to the definition and assessment of communication competence begins with an analysis of the actual communicative behavior of participants. This analysis is enhanced to the extent that the observer (i.e., researcher) is reasonably knowledgeable about participants' goals and their perceptions of each other's goals. Communicative moves that effectively advance a participant's goals and, at the same time, reflect understanding and appropriate[3] accommodation of the other's goals are defined as competent.

Application of the Competence Model to the Medical Interview

Similar to McFall (1982), our approach to competence requires a task analysis of the communicative context within which interaction occurs. The purpose of such an analysis is to determine what likely goals are relevant to communicators.[4] Our assessment of the doctor–patient communication literature reveals that the medical interview is characterized by two primary communicative tasks: information exchange and relational development.

Information Exchange in the Medical Interview

Although physicians and patients may have other goals during the medical interview, it appears that effective information exchange is the primary task (see Guttman, 1993; Roter, 1989; Roter, Hall, & Katz, 1988; Street, 1991a). Thus, competent doctor–patient communication, in part, entails exchanging information that facilitates such matters as obtaining an accurate medical history, describing and understanding the medical problem, providing information about diagnosis and prescribed treatment, and understanding prescribed procedures and their rationale. Perhaps not surprisingly, differing perceptions about information exchange appear to be a major source of misunderstanding between doctors and patients. For example, research shows that though a majority of patients indicate they are interested in obtaining as much information as possible, physicians often do not perceive patients' information needs accurately, and physicians often overestimate how much information they provide patients (e.g., Beisecker, 1990; Beisecker & Beisecker, 1990; Waitzkin, 1984, 1985).

Although the concept of information exchange has been central to considerable research into doctor-patient communication, relatively little is actually known about the dynamics of how doctors and patients seek and provide information during the medical interview. One major reason for this is that researchers typically have used rather gross categories to measure information exchange, such as *asks questions* and *provides information* (see Roter, 1989), and have ignored subtle, yet important, aspects of information exchange (e.g., Frankel, 1990; Todd, 1984; Tuckett & Williams, 1984). Another reason for the lack of knowledge about how doctors and patients exchange information is that little attention has been given to defining exactly what information means from the perspective of doctors and patients. It may be expected that what constitutes informative messages about such matters as diagnosis and treatment options is very different from the perspectives of patients and doctors. Clearly, baseline knowledge differences between doctors and patients with respect to such topics could affect how they define informative messages.

Overall, then, information exchange is a significant communicative component of the medical interview and should be central to a definition and assessment of doctors' and patients' communication competence. Yet, the current state of knowledge about information exchange during the medical interview does not provide adequate input into conceptual or operational definitions of competence. One objective of this research is to provide needed information along these lines.

Relational Dimension

Research suggests that there are other important functions, besides information exchange, served by communication during the medical interview. The patient-centered model of medical communication emphasizes the relational (sometimes called affective) dimension of doctor–patient interaction (Ben-Sira, 1980; Smith & Hoppe, 1991). For the most part, research demonstrates a significant correlation between physicians' expression of care and concern for the patient as a person and patients' satisfaction with the medical encounter, and, to a lesser extent, patients' compliance with recommended treatment (e.g., Hauck, Zyzanski, Alemagno, & Medalie, 1990; Kreps, 1988; Thompson, 1994).

Among the factors that lead to patients' dissatisfaction with relational aspects of health care delivery are the lack of feedback, insensitivity to and misinterpretations of relational needs, failure to express empathy, and disregard for the other's input in decision-making (see Kreps, 1988). For the most part, research has focused on doctors' communication and has concluded that, typically, physicians are not relational enough in their interactions with patients. The usual interpretation of these findings is that the manner in which doctors relationally communicate with patients has implications for matters such as trust, respect, and loyalty, as well as general satisfaction with health care.

Although research suggests that the relational component of medical communication is important, little is actually known about how doctors convey relational messages or exactly how these messages impact outcomes (see Stiles, 1993). In addition, very little attention has been given to doctors' relational satisfaction, especially with respect to their perceptions and assessments of patients' communication (Suchman, Roter, Green, Lipkin, & The Collaborative Study Group of the American Academy on Physician and Patient, 1993). Similar to the research on information exchange in the medical interview, there is little in the literature on relational communication to provide a clear direction for conceptual or operational definitions of doctors' and patients' communication competence. A second purpose of this research is to provide information with respect to these concerns.

Despite the lack of specific data on communicative competence in the medical interview, previous research into doctor–patient communication suggests that information exchange and relational development should be important aspects of doctors' and patients' communicative competence. However, very little work in doctor–patient communication provides clear direction for how communication competence may be defined along the lines of information exchange and relational communication. Thus, research is needed to facilitate such connections. With this objective in mind, we pose the following research questions:

> *Research Question 1:* What specific components of information exchange and relational communication are perceived by doctors and patients as comprising competent communication during the medical interview?

> *Research Question 2:* To what extent will doctors and patients agree on the components of information exchange and relational communication with respect to their perceptions of self- and other-communication competence?

Although the literature on doctor–patient communication has emphasized the communicative functions of information exchange and relational development, surprisingly little attention has been given to the relation between these functions. Recently, however, Roter offered a hypothesis about how these functions relate to each other through their connection to various outcomes (Roter, 1989; Roter & Hall, 1991). For example, she argued that patients evaluate doctors on both technical and relational competence, but that doctors' messages achieve positive therapeutic effects (i.e., patient compliance) through both explicit content (i.e., sharing of technical information) and an implied message of interest and caring. In other words, an informative physician may also be perceived as concerned and caring and positively affect compliance, but a physician who is merely nice or caring without providing information does not provide the evidence patients need to encourage adherence to a therapeutic regimen. Thus, Roter suggested that the information component of doctors' messages carries more weight in influencing patients' compliance (also see Buller & Street, 1991). Street (1991b) reported results that extend this hypothesis to effects on patients' satisfaction. He found that 34% of the variance in patients' satisfaction was accounted for by the informativeness (i.e., technical relevance) of physicians' communication, whereas only 17% of the variance in patients' satisfaction was accounted for by physicians' interpersonal sensitivity. Overall, then, there is some support for expecting the information exchange component of patients' perceptions of communicative competence to carry more weight in a medical interview than the relational component. Although we are not aware of any research addressing how doctors weigh these components, one might assume that information exchange is especially important for doctors, as it is a primary means by which they arrive at a diagnosis and determine appropriate treatment regimens. Thus, we hypothesize that:

> *Hypothesis 1:* Information exchange behaviors will account for more of doctors' and patients' perceptions of communicative competence than will relational behaviors.

Method

Participants

The primary participants for this study were 27 patients and 15 family practice residents at an outpatient clinic associated with a large, Midwestern university medical school and hospital. The patients' average age was 37 (range 20 to 64). Of the 27 patients, 8 were men, 16 were White, and 11 were Black. Eighteen patients were new to the doctor and 9 were return patients.

The average age of residents was 32. Ten of the residents were men. Four of the residents were in their first year of residency in the Family Practice Department, 5 were in their second year, and 6 were in their third year. Six of the residents were White, 5 were Hispanic, 3 were of East Indian origin, and 1 was of Far Eastern origin. The initial plan was to videotape each resident twice.[5] This was successful for all but three residents.

Thus, the data reported here are based on 27 interviews.

In addition to the main participants, six faculty physicians in the Department of Family Medicine at the same university hospital clinic also provided data for the study. Three were men. Five were White and one was of Far Eastern origin. On average, they were 12 years past residency and members of the faculty for 6.5 years.

Design and Procedures

Patients were telephoned prior to their appointment with a doctor and asked if they would participate in a study of doctor–patient communication. They were told that their visit with the doctor would be videotaped and that after the interview they would complete a brief questionnaire and then view the tape of the interview. If the patient agreed to participate (most did so), he or she was paid $20.00. Once a patient agreed to participate in the study, the appropriate physician was contacted and permission was secured to videotape the appointment. Prior to videotaping, both the patient and physician were again briefed about the procedures and asked to sign consent forms.

Two examination rooms were equipped with video cameras and a microphone (though all the taping was actually conducted in the same examination room). The cameras were suspended from the ceiling in a corner of the room, and the microphone was placed on a small desk where history-taking and treatment discussions were conducted. The entire interview was videotaped, but the examination table was intentionally placed out of camera range to ensure the patients' privacy during physical exams. The video and audio equipment was connected to recording equipment and monitors in a central control room down the hall from the examination rooms.

Taping began when the physician arrived in the examination room and continued until the end of the appointment. Immediately after the appointment, the physician and patient were taken to separate rooms. There they completed a postinterview questionnaire. After completing the postinterview questionnaire, patients engaged in a stimulated recall procedure as they viewed the videotape of their appointment. The stimulated recall data are not relevant to this article. Subsequent to completing the postinterview questionnaire, residents were engaged in a brief interview. The purpose of the interview after the first taping session was to elicit information about how residents defined information exchange during a medical interview. This information is not relevant to this article. The purpose of the interview after the second taping was to elicit information about residents' views of doctors' and patients' communication competence during a medical interview.

Data Sets

Three data sets served as information for analysis of doctors' views of communication competence. Residents provided two data sets; faculty physicians provided the remaining data set. Residents provided data relevant to (a) a specific interview via responses to a postinterview questionnaire and (b) medical interviews in general via responses to an interview with the senior author. Faculty physicians provided data relevant to medical interviews in general via responses to a questionnaire that paralleled the interview questions given to residents. A fourth data set was provided by patients who saw the residents for a scheduled visit. The patients' views of communication competence were based on their perceptions of the communication occurring during this scheduled visit.

Postinterview questionnaire data. Doctors and patients completed parallel questionnaires consisting of 16 items (each on a 5-point, Likert-type scale) designed to assess perceptions of doctors' information exchange and relational communication during the interview. Most of these data are not directly relevant to this article. However, included on the postinterview questionnaire were two Likert-type items designed to assess perceptions of self- and other-communication competence during the interview (i.e., "I was a competent communicator during the visit" and "The patient [doctor] was a competent communicator during the visit"). Following each item, was an open-ended question asking the respondent to indicate "What specific aspects of your [the other's] behavior during the interview led you to form this judgment?" Thus, both doctors and patients judged self- and other-competence and provided information about the basis upon which these judgments were formed. The relevant data for this study consist of the responses to the two open-ended questions. The two Likert-type scales (i.e., for self- and other-competence assessment) were used to verify the positive or negative connotation of the open-ended statements.

Interview data. Only data from the second posttaping interview with residents are relevant to this study. These data consist of responses to the following questions:

1. How important do you think a doctor's communication skills are to the quality of health care patients receive? (Responses were recorded on a 5-point, Likert-type scale.)
2. What are the most important communication skills for a doctor to have?
3. How important do you think a patient's communication skills are to the quality of health care he or she receives from doctors? (Responses were recorded on a 5-point, Likert-type scale).
4. What are the most important communication skills for a patient to have?

The data elicited by Questions 2 and 4 were examined for each respondent and redundancies with responses to the open-ended, postinterview questionnaire items were eliminated when they occurred. Thus, residents in the sample provided information about specific competence assessments relevant to a particular interview or interviews and information about competence in medical interviews in general.

Faculty physician questionnaire. The six faculty physicians completed a questionnaire with the same items that residents were asked in the interview (i.e., Questions 1–4). These data provided information about what faculty physicians considered to be important communication skills for doctors and patients to have in general.

Development of the Content Coding Scheme

All of the handwritten competence descriptions provided by residents, faculty physicians, and patients were transcribed to a typewritten document. Participants provided 257 behavior statements in all. There was no need to compute unitizing reliability for the statements because they appeared clearly as natural units (i.e., complete sentences, single words, or phrases). Occasionally, a participant wrote a complex sentence containing more than one behavior. When this happened, participants used commas or some other form of punctuation to clearly separate the behaviors, thus making unitizing of data straightforward even in instances of complex sentences.

After the behavior statements were typed, Donald J. Cegala developed a content category scheme for each of four data sets (i.e., doctors' self-competence, patients' self-competence, doctors' and patients' judgments of the other's competence). The constructs of information exchange and relational communication served as the conceptual framework for examining the behavior statements. Information exchange was defined as communication involving the giving, seeking, or processing of information (see Cegala, McNeilis, Socha McGee, & Jonas, 1995). *Relational communication* was defined as communication showing care and concern for another, establishing rapport, displaying emotional support and, in general, conveying confirmation and support for another as a person.

Specific categories under these general constructs were allowed to emerge from the raw data in a manner similar to analytic induction (Baxter, 1991). Thus, for each data set, the behavior statements were initially examined for general concerns about either information exchange or relational matters. Then the data were examined again in an effort to search for meaningful categories within the two broad labels of information exchange and relational communication. On the basis of this examination, an initial set of category labels was used to classify the behavior statements.

After about 1 week, the category labels were used to classify all of the behavior statements again. Adjustments were made in category labels and definitions when needed. Part of the data and category schemes were then given to a person unfamiliar with this study. The individual classified the behavior statements using the provided categories. The coding results were examined to identify problems in interpretation of category labels and definitions. When such problems were noted, adjustments were made.

Final category schemes. The final four category schemes are reported in Table 7.1. These category schemes were given to three graduate students in communication who were not involved in any other way with this project. The three students independently coded the data and each of their results were compared to Donald J. Cegala's coding for each category scheme using Holsti's (1969) method.

Of the 13 categories (excluding Other) in Table 7.1 describing doctors' self-competence, five are oriented to information exchange and four reflect relational communication. The remaining four categories do not clearly indicate a focus on information exchange or relational matters, although the Be Open and Honest category could be construed as concerned with information exchange. However, because it is less clearly reflective of information exchange as defined here (perhaps reflecting both information exchange and relational concerns), it is not included as part of the information exchange category.

Next in Table 7.1 are the data relevant to doctors' judgments of patients' competence. The first five categories clearly indicate a concern about information exchange, whereas the remaining two categories do not appear to be directly reflective of either information exchange or relational communication. The third data set reported in Table 7.1 displays the categories associated with patients' perceptions of their own competence. The first three categories are clearly concerned with information exchange. No behavior statements reflect concerns about relational communication. As already suggested, the remaining category (Be Open and Honest) may reflect both information exchange and relational communication, and thus does not appear to be purely one category or the other. The last data set reported in Table 7.1 consists of categories describing patients' judgments of doctors' competence. The first four categories reflect information exchange concerns, whereas the remaining three categories are concerned with relational communication.

Results and Discussion

Research Question 1 asked: What specific components of information exchange and relational communication are perceived by doctors and patients as comprising competent communication during the medical interview?

Physicians' Perceptions of Competence

Doctors' perceptions of self. In Table 7.1, doctors' perceptions of their own competence in information exchange (i.e., the first five categories) focused on concerns about the extent to which they (a) provided explanations to patients, particularly with respect to such matters as diagnosis, treatment options, and prognosis; (b) verified that patients understood explanations; (c) were able to explain technical information in understandable terms; (d) encouraged patients to share or seek information; and (e) sought relevant information from patients. Doctors' perceptions of competent relational communication included the extent to which they (a) were able to establish a warm, friendly, trusting environment; (b) conveyed care, interest and concern for the patient; (c) demonstrated affective support, such as sympathy and empathy; and (d) were responsive to the patient's needs and concerns.

Doctors' perceptions of patients. Doctors' judgments of patients' competence in information exchange were based on the extent to which the patient (a) was informative about the medical problem, such as communicating symptoms and other potentially useful diagnostic information; (b) actively sought information by asking questions; (c) was able to provide clear, thorough answers to questions; (d) presented an organized, accurate medical history; and (e) stayed on topic without going off on tangents. None of the behavior statements reflected relational communication concerns.

Patients' Perceptions of Competence

Patients' perceptions of self. Patients' self-judgments of their own competence in information exchange were a function of the extent to which they (a) provided thorough descriptions of their medical problems; (b) sought information by asking questions; and (c) provided answers to doctors' questions. None of the patients' self-judged, competent behaviors reflected relational matters.

Patients' perceptions of doctors. The specific components of information exchange relevant to patients' judgments of doctors' competence were a function of the extent to which doctors: (a) were informative about the medical problem, such as conveying information about test results and treatment procedures; (b) verified that patients understood what they were told; (c) explained medical terms in language patients could understand; and (d) appeared to be knowledgeable about the patients' medical history and problems. The components of relational communication indicated that patients' judgments of doctors' competence were a function of doctors (a) communicating in an open, friendly manner; (b) showing care, interest, and concern for the patients' problems; and (c) displaying emotional support and confirmation.

In summary for Research Question 1, perceptions of competent information exchange were primarily accounted for by categories concerned with providing or seeking information about the patient's medical problem, including concerns about diagnosis, treatment, history, and test results. Also relevant, but less dominant in participants' judgments, were categories concerned with information processing, particularly with respect to verification of understanding and message clarity. Perceptions of competent relational communication were accounted for by behavior that conveyed a friendly, trusting atmosphere; affective support, especially in the form of sympathy and empathy; and care, interest, and concern about the other.

The second Research Question asked: To what extent will doctors and patients agree on the components of information exchange and relational communication with respect to their perceptions of self and other communication competence? Tables 7.2 and 7.3 provide a comparison of the categories relevant to doctors' and patients' behavior statements.

Perceptions of Physicians' Competence

Turning to Table 7.2, doctors' self-competence and patients' judgments of doctors' competence agree on the relevance of three information exchange categories: Explain/Inform, Assess/Enhance Fidelity, and Use Plain Language. Thus, both doctors and patients agreed that doctors' competence in information exchange was, in part, a function of their ability to: adequately explain aspects of the medical problem, such as diagnosis and treatment options; verify that patients have understood information given to them; and explain technical information in terms patients can understand. The apparent relative weight,[6] in terms of percentage figures that doctors and patients gave to information processing concerns (i.e., fidelity enhancement and use of plain language) were also quite comparable (8.1% and 7.1%; 13.1% and 11.9%, respectively). However, patients as a group placed nearly three times as much weight on obtaining information about their medical problem as doctors placed on providing such information (28.6% vs. 10.1 %). This result supports previous research that suggests that patients place more value and importance on being informed about their medical problems than doctors generally recognize (e.g., Waitzkin, 1984, 1985).

Table 7.2 also reveals similarities between doctors' self-judgments of relational competence and patients' judgments of doctors' relational communication. Both doctors and patients viewed doctors' relational competence in terms of their ability to establish a friendly, trusting atmosphere; express care, concern, and interest; and display affective support. However, patients placed about twice as much emphasis on doctors' competence in establishing a friendly, trusting atmosphere (16.7% vs. 8.1%) and somewhat more emphasis on doctors showing care, in-

Table 7.1
Content Category Schemes For Doctors' and Patients' Data

Data Set	Category	Definition	Sample Items*
Doctors' self-competence			
	Information exchange:		
	Explain/inform about medical problems	References to explaining or informing another about such matters as symptoms, medications, medical problems, causes, treatment, test results, diagnosis, prognosis (or failure to do so).	I explained possible causes of her problem and treatment options. I conveyed how to use the medication and possible side effects. I explained his medical problems and long-term consequences.
	Assess/enhance fidelity of communication	References to reviewing or repeating information, or in some way evaluating reception of information, to determine if the other understood what has been conveyed (or failure to do so).	I asked if she understood what I just explained. I tried to evaluate if the patient understood my explanations. Rephrasing to assess if correctly understood.
	Use plain language	References to the use of lay person terms, or simple terms or understandable or appropriate terms in place of medical terminology (or failure to do so).	Use simple, nonmedical language. I explained in layperson terms. Use language the patient understands.
	Encourage information sharing/seeking	References to permitting or urging another to ask questions or provide detailed information about something (or failure to do so).	I allowed the patient to elaborate on the details of his condition. I allowed the patient to speak and express his concerns. Encouraged the patient to feel free about asking more.
	Seek relevant information	References to asking types of questions (i.e., open, closed) or asking questions without specific indication of question content (or failure to do so).	I used open questions. I asked the patient questions. Ask the right questions.
	Relational communication:		
	Create a friendly/trusting atmosphere	References to establishing a positive relationship with another (e.g., being friendly, warm) or, in general, establishing rapport and trust (or failure to do so).	I was warm and friendly. Create a warm environment. Establish rapport with patients.
	Show care, concern, and interest in the patient	References to showing that patients are cared for or that there is interest in or concern about them or their medical problems (or failure to do so).	Communicate in a caring manner. Show you care about the patient. Show you are really interested in the patient getting better.
	Convey affective support	References to sympathizing, empathizing, understanding, or, in general, supporting another (or failure to do so).	I tried to sympathize with the patient. Empathy/sympathy. I listened to his concerns with understanding and empathy.

Data Set	*Category*	*Definition*	*Sample Items**
	Responsive to the patient's needs/concerns	References to in some way addressing the patient's reasons for the visit (or failure to do so).	Address the patient's needs and concerns. I answered her questions and the reason why she came in today. Be sensitive to the patient's needs.
	Other:		
	Be a good listener	References to listening well or just listening (or failure to do so).	I listened to the patient. Be a good listener Listening to major problems.
	Use of appropriate nonverbals	References to using any sort of nonverbal communication (or failure to do so).	I used good eye contact. Gesturing. Nonverbal aspects.
	Set goals/expectations	References to explaining or in some way communicating about goals or expectations (or failure to do so).	Discussed the patient's expectations. I explained my expectations for the patient. I communicated the direction I wanted her to take.
	Be open and honest	References to straightforward, open, and frank communication (or failure to do so).	Direct, open, and frank communication. Honesty. Straightforward dealing with the patient.
	Other	Any reference that does not clearly fit one of the above categories.	Wise use of time allotted for the visit. Use humor. Show confidence.
Doctors' evaluations of patients' competence			
	Information exchange:		
	Explain/inform about medical problems	Same as above.	Related wishes for treatment. Told me his problems/symptoms. Able to tell me necessary information for a good diagnosis.
	Seek information about medical problems	References to the other asking questions (or failure to do so).	Not afraid to ask questions if they don't know. Asked me questions about her problem. Knew what she wanted and asked for it.
	Responsive to questions	References to the other answering questions or evaluations of how the other answered questions (or references indicating a failure/reluctance to answer questions).	Able to respond to questions, answered them appropriately. Did not feel threatened by the questions I asked. She didn't answer questions very clearly.
	Provide accurate, organized, detailed history	References to providing historical information in a chronological, organized form or assessments of accuracy/amount of medical history provided (or failure to do so).	Be knowledgeable and organized in presenting a history. Put symptoms, signs, and co-occurrences in chronological order. Provide an accurate history.

(Continued)

Table 7.1 *(Continued)*

Data Set	Category	Definition	Sample Items*
	Stay focused	References to staying focused on topic when relaying information, and being specific/detailed, as opposed to going off on tangents or listing numerous problems (or failure to do so).	Be specific. Don't wander. Patient didn't go into tangents, but stayed focused on the reason for being there.
	Other:		
	Be open and honest	Same as above.	No concealment of any aspect of their health care. Open about personal life. Honest when asked questions about compliance.
	Expression of concern about one's health	References to or assessments of the patient's interest/concern about his or her own health (or failure to do so).	She doesn't seem to bother too much about her health problems. Patient is motivated and shows serious consideration for his problems. The patient should show concern and interest for his or her problems.
	Other	Same as above.	Be receptive to doctor's advice. Willing to hear criticism. State expectations.
Patients' self-competence			
	Information exchange:		
	Explain/inform about medical problems	Same as above.	I was thorough in my descriptions. I informed the doctor of my medical concerns. I talked about my problems thoroughly.
	Seek information about medical problems	References to self asking questions of the other (or failure to do so).	I felt comfortable asking questions. I asked what I needed to know. I got the answers I wanted.
	Responsive to questions	References to self answering questions or evaluations of how self answered questions (or references indicating a failure/reluctance to answer questions).	I answered all questions thoroughly. I wasn't too shy to answer. I answered all his questions.
	Other:		
	Be open and honest	Same as above.	I was open and honest. I was able to speak openly and freely about my concerns. I admitted to not following up.
	Other	Same as above.	None.

Data Set	*Category*	*Definition*	*Sample Items**
Patients' evaluations of doctors' competence			
	Information exchange:		
	Explain/inform about medical problems	Same as above.	Let me know what my medical situation was. Told me what to expect from the tests. Explained what treatment I had to do.
	Assess/enhance fidelity of communication	Same as above.	She explains everything and makes sure I understand. Asked me over and over if I had any questions. If I showed reason not to understand, he would rephrase/explain.
	Use plain language	Same as above.	Explained in terms I could understand. Some words I don't understand, so I stop him and he breaks them down. Didn't use a lot of medical terminology that I didn't understand.
	Display medical/historical knowledge	References to the extent of medical knowledge or extent of knowledge/understanding of medical history, including information accessed from written records (or the lack thereof).	Seemed knowledgeable. Had a good understanding and knowledge of my history. Displayed her knowledge.
	Relational communication:		
	Create a friendly/trusting atmosphere	Same as above.	Made me feel comfortable. Friendly and nice. He was open and honest.
	Show care, concern and interest in the patient	Same as above.	He was very concerned. Interested in my diabetes and other problems. Concerned.
	Convey affective support	Same as above.	Related my problems with his or her own feelings. Wanted me to know the seriousness of my condition without scaring me. She didn't make me feel like I was important.
	Other:		
	Other	Same as above.	He kept cutting me off. He rushed the appointment. Way he carried on the conversation.

*Relatively few ($n = 26$, 10%) behavior statements were negative (i.e., implying the absence or failure to do something), consequently, most of the sample items are positive in nature. Except for three sample items, all were independently classified the same by all four coders.

Table 7.2
Frequencies and Percentages of Content Categories: Doctors' Self- and Patients' Other Judgments

Doctors' Self-Competence[a]			*Patients' Judgments of Doctors' Competence*[b]		
Category	*Frequency*	*%*[c]	*Category*	*Frequency*	*%*[c]
Explain/inform	10	10.1	Explain/inform	12	28.6
Assess/enhance fidelity	8	8.1	Assess/enhance fidelity	3	7.1
Plain language	13	13.1	Plain language	5	11.9
Encourage information seeking/sharing	5	5.1	Display medical knowledge	8	19.1
Seek relevant information	8	8.1			
Friendly/trusting	8	8.1	Friendly/trusting	7	16.7
Show care, concern, interest	6	6.1	Show care, concern, interest	4	9.5
Convey affective support	12	12.1	Convey affective support	3	7.1
Responsive to needs/concerns	6	6.1			
Be a good listener	10	10.1			
Appropriate nonverbals	6	6.1			
Set goals/expectations	4	4.0			
Be open/honest	3	3.0			
Other	12	10.8	Other	6	12.5

[a] *n* = 111.
[b] *n* = 48.
[c] For all but the Other category, percentages are based on the total, excluding the Other frequency. Percentages for the Other category represent percentage of the total with Other frequency included.

terest, and concern (9.5% vs. 6.1%), whereas doctors placed somewhat more emphasis on their competence in displaying affective support (12.1% vs. 7.1%). These results suggest that patients' concerns about doctors' relational behavior are most focused on the doctor's ability to create a trusting atmosphere in which the patient feels comfortable and secure in being open about the patient's problems. In this sense, the data provide some indirect support for the general notion that patients may blend informational and relational aspects of communication in the medical interview (e.g., Roter & Hall, 1991). Given the foreign and sometimes threatening context in which patients seek medical attention (see Bochner, 1983; B. R. Rubin, 1990, p. 52), it may be especially important for them to feel assured and comfortable with the doctor to engage freely in the seeking and giving of information that is important to the effective accomplishment of their, and the doctors', goals with respect to information exchange.

Although there is considerable overlap between behaviors doctors view as competent on their part and behaviors patients consider competent on the doctor's part, there is also evidence of mismatching. Doctors associated a much broader range of competent behaviors with their own communication than patients associated with doctors' communication. In particular, doctors had two additional information exchange categories (Encourage Information-seeking/Sharing, Seek Relevant Information) that together accounted for 13.2% of the self-competent behaviors they identified. Additionally, doctors had one more relational category (Responsive to Needs/Concerns) and four more categories that did not clearly fit under information exchange or relational communication. Together, the behaviors in these categories accounted for approximately 29.3% of the behaviors doctors identified. Thus, 42.5% of the behaviors identified by doctors did not fall under comparable categories for patients. On the other hand, all of the behaviors patients associated with doctors' competence (with the exception of Display Medical Knowledge) overlapped with behaviors that doctors identified as relevant to themselves. Each of these overlapping categories fell under information exchange or relational communication. Overall, the most useful results in

Table 7.3
Frequencies and Percentages of Content Categories: Patients' Self- and Doctors' Other Judgments

Patients' Self-Competence[a]			*Doctors' Judgments of Patients' Competence*[b]		
Category	*Frequency*	*%*[c]	*Category*	*Frequency*	*%*[c]
Explain/inform	12	36.4	Explain/inform	11	19.0
Seek information	11	33.3	Seek information	8	13.8
Responsive to question	4	12.1	Responsive to questions	6	10.3
			Provide accurate history	9	15.5
			Stay focused	7	12.1
Be open/honest	6	18.2	Be open/honest	13	22.4
			Expression of concern about one's health	4	6.9
Other	0	0	Other	7	10.8

[a]*n* = 33.
[b]*n* = 65.
[c]For all but the Other category, percentages are based on the total, excluding the Other frequency. Percentages for the Other category represent percentage of the total with Other frequency included.

terms of Research Question 2 indicate considerable agreement between doctors and patients on the components of doctors' competence in information exchange and relational communication. This has important implications for the development of language categories and self-report measures that can be used to assess doctors' and patients' actual communication and their perceptions of the communication that occurs in primary care medical interviews.

Perceptions of Patients' Competence

Reported in Table 7.3 are comparison data for patients' self-judged competence and doctors' judgments of patients' competence. In terms of Research Question 2, patients and doctors agreed on three information exchange categories—Explain/Inform, Seek Information, and Responsiveness to Questions. Thus, both patients and doctors agree that patients' competence in information exchange is, in part, a function of their ability to explain the medical problem (e.g., symptoms), seek information by asking questions, and be responsive and thorough in answering the doctor's questions. Patients and doctors placed about the same emphasis on being responsive to questions (12.1% vs. 10.3%), but patients placed considerably more emphasis on providing explanations of their medical problem (36.4% vs. 19.0%) and seeking information about it (33.3% vs. 13.8%) than did doctors.

The apparent discrepancy between patients' and doctors' emphasis on the Explain/Inform category is accounted for by the fourth category in Table 7.3—Provide an Accurate History. From a doctor's perspective, providing an accurate history is integral to explaining one's medical problem. When the history and explain categories are combined, the total is comparable to the patients' percentage of Explain/Inform behaviors (i.e., patients, 36.4%; doctors, 34.5%). Thus, patients and doctors actually were in agreement on the emphasis they placed on the Explain/Inform category. The discrepancy concerning information-seeking supports the notion that patients place more value on asking doctors questions and, in general, becoming informed about their medical situation than doctors do. This is consistent with previous research that shows that doctors think they provide more information to patients than patients believe they do (e.g., Guttman, 1993; Waitzkin, 1984, 1985).

The Stay Focused category is the only information exchange behavior that is not shared by patients and doctors. It is clear why doctors would view staying on task as important to patients' competence, as it implies more concise, to-the-point information sharing and, thus, more efficient use of time. However, given that staying focused did not appear among patients' behaviors of self-competence, there is the implication that patient education in communication skills should include attention to ways of avoiding rambling, off-task messages. The only remaining category in Table 7.3 is Be Open and Honest, which both patients and doctors identify with patients' competence and with somewhat comparable emphasis (18.2% vs. 22.4%).

Overall, there was considerable agreement between patients and doctors on the components of patients' competent information exchange. Both groups agreed that competent patients should provide thorough descriptions of their medical problem (including history, for doctors), seek information, and be responsive to questions. It is interesting that neither patients nor doctors included relational communication behaviors as part of their competence judgments of patients. Thus, they seem to agree that the onus of relational work in the medical interview should fall on the doctors' shoulders. This is further supported by the data relevant to our hypothesis.

Our hypothesis predicted that information exchange behaviors would account for more of doctors' and patients' perceptions of communicative competence than relational behaviors. Turning first to Table 7.2, the sums of the percentages of doctors' self-competence categories in information exchange and relational communication are 44.5% and 32.4%, respectively. Comparable data for patients' judgments of doctors' information and relational competence are 66.7% and 33.3%, respectively. In Table 7.3, the sums of patients' self-competence categories in information exchange and relational communication are 81.8% and 0%, respectively. Comparable data for doctors' judgments of patients' competence in these categories are 70.7% and 0%. Thus, in both data sets, the percentage of behaviors comprising information exchange is greater than the percentage of behaviors comprising relational communication.

However, there are some clear differences between these data sets. Both patients and doctors identified far more information exchange behaviors with patients' competence than they identified with doctors' competence (doctor mean, 55.6%; patient mean, 76.2%). As might be expected, most of these patient behaviors involved categories of information-giving (patients' self, 48.5%; doctors' other, 56.9%). However, patients also identified one third of their information exchange competence behaviors as information-seeking, whereas doctors placed relatively little emphasis on patients' competence in information-seeking. This suggests that patients place more value on their competence in obtaining information from doctors than doctors place on such skills. Examination of the data in Table 7.2 provides insight into perceptions of behaviors that compliment these skills.

The sum of doctors' self-competence behavior percentages in information-giving categories is 23.2%, whereas comparable data for patients' judgments of doctors' competence in information-giving is 59.6%. Thus, patients placed more emphasis on doctors' competence in information-giving than doctors placed on their own competence in this category. Together, these results suggest that patients are more concerned about their ability to access, and doctors' ability to provide, information during medical interviews than doctors are concerned with these behaviors. Thus, the results provide clear direction for training doctors in communication skills. They suggest that attention should be given to matters such as perceiving and being sensitive to patients' information needs and providing appropriate information to meet those needs.

Overall, then, although doctors and patients agree that information exchange behaviors are especially important to self- and other-competence, patients appear to place more emphasis on their own competence in obtaining information and the doctor's competence in providing information than doctors place on comparable behaviors relevant to self- or other-competence. Also, consistent with results pertinent to Research Question 2, there is a clear indication that both doctors and patients agree that relational behaviors are identified with doctors' competence but that such behaviors are not viewed as part of patients' competence. Though perhaps not surprising, this is an interesting result that merits further examination. From our research experiences over the last 2 years, it is quite clear that doctors do have concerns about patients' relational communication. For example, it is not at all difficult to get doctors to discuss their views of "difficult" patients, and our results relevant to doctors' thoughts and feelings during medical interviews indicate that they develop very clear positive or negative attitudes toward patients (Cegala et al., 1995). Given this, it is curious that relational communication did not show up in at least doctors' views of patients' competence.

To our knowledge, this study provides unique insight into the components of doctors' and patients' perceived communication competence during a medical interview. The results provide direction for future research regarding the particular behavioral components that comprise the constructs of information exchange and relational communication. We are currently engaged in two follow-up projects based on the data reported here. One project is focused on the development of language categories for assessing doctors' and patients' actual information exchange and relational communication during the course of an interview. Another project involves the development of a competence scale that may be used to record doctors' and patients' judgments of self- and other-communication competence during a medical interview. These and related projects are part of an ongoing program of research on doctor-patient communication that is directed to the development and implementation of a communication skills training program for family practice residents and their patients.

Notes

1. Of course, the term *context* itself lacks clear specificity, as it can reasonably include everything from individuals' perceptions of a situation to collective cultural definitions of a communicative setting. Indeed, the breadth of the potential meanings of context, in part, explains the difficulty scholars have experienced in addressing the term conceptually or operationally. Our context-bound approach to communication competence does not claim to address all of the potentially relevant dimensions of context that may relate to individuals' communicative competence. However, we believe that our approach to competence seriously incorporates the construct of context and, in at least this regard, is ultimately a more useful approach than most of the existing alternatives.
2. The term *moves* here is a general reference to a view of communication based on an analogy to games. The particular view of this analogy subscribed to here is best reflected in the work of scholars such as Jacobs and Jackson (1983).
3. The term *appropriate* is used here to avoid the connotation that competent communication necessarily entails communicative moves that are accommodating to another's desires. Although we expect that many, or even most, competent communicative moves at least minimally accommodate another's goals, we also recognize that there are instances in which the most competent move may be to block or in some way ignore another's goal (e.g., in denying a con artist a desired objective). Thus, what is appropriate in a given instance is defined by the participants' goals and the circumstances of the particular interaction.
4. A limitation of our approach to competence is that some communicative settings may not reveal enough information about participants' communicative goals to allow for an accurate initial determination of the criteria needed for defining and assessing communicative moves.
5. The plan was to videotape each resident once with a patient we had trained in communication skills and once with an untrained patient. The results of the training are topics for another research paper and are not examined here.
6. The term *weight* is used throughout this article in reference to frequencies only. This is a restricted use of the concept of weight, as participants may place different value, utility, or some other form of emphasis on various components of information exchange and relational communication. The restricted use of the term weight in this article is a potential limitation in interpreting results. Future research should be directed toward assessing the emphasis doctors and patients place on various aspects of communication competence in ways other than frequency of response.

References

Baxter, L. (1991). Content analysis. In B. Montgomery & S. Duck (Eds.). *Studying interper-*

sonal interaction (pp. 239–254). New York: Guilford.

Beisecker, A. E. (1990). Patient power in doctor–patient communication: What do we know? *Health Communication, 2,* 105–122.

Beisecker, A. E., & Beisecker, T. D. (1990). Patient information-seeking behaviors when communicating with doctors. *Medical Care, 28,* 19–28.

Ben-Sira, Z. (1980). Affective and instrumental components in the physician-patient relationship. *Journal of Health and Social Science Behavior, 21,* 170–180.

Bochner, S. (1983). Doctors, patients and their cultures. In D. A. Pendleton & J. C. Hasler (Eds.), *Doctor patient communication* (pp. 127–138). London: Academic.

Bostrom, R. N. (Ed.). (1984). *Competence in communication: A multidisciplinary approach.* Beverly Hills, CA: Sage.

Buller, D. B., & Street, R. L., Jr. (1991). The role of perceived affect and information in patients' evaluations of health care and compliance decisions. *Southern Communication Journal, 56,* 230–237.

Cegala, D. J., McNeilis, K. S., Socha McGee, D., & Jonas, A. P. (1995). A study of doctors' and patients' perceptions of information processing and communication competence during the medical interview. *Health Communication, 7,* 179–203.

Cegala, D. J., & Waldron, V. R. (1992). A study of the relationship between communicative performance and conversation participants' thoughts. *Communication Studies, 43,* 105–123.

Frankel, R. (1990). Talking in interviews: A dispreference for patient-initiated questions in physician-patient encounters. In G. Psathas (Ed.), *Interaction competence* (pp. 231–262). Washington, DC: International Institute for Ethnomethodology and Conversation Analysis and University Press of America.

Guttman, N. (1993). Information exchange in medical encounters: Problems and problems. In B. D. Ruben & N. Guttman (Eds.), *Caregiver patient communications* (pp. 151–168). Dubuque, IA: Kendall/Hunt.

Hauck, F. R., Zyzanski, S. J., Alemagno, S. A., & Medalie, J. H. (1990). Patient perceptions of humanism in physicians: Effects on positive health behaviors. *Family Medicine, 22,* 447–452.

Holsti, O. R. (1969). *Content analysis for the social sciences and humanities.* Reading, MA: Addison-Wesley.

Jacobs, S., & Jackson, S. (1983). Speech act structure in conversation: Rational aspects of pragmatic coherence. In R. T. Craig & K. Tracy (Eds.), *Conversational coherence* (pp. 47–66). Beverly Hills, CA: Sage.

Kasch, C. R. (1984). Interpersonal competence and communication in the delivery of nursing care. *Advances in Nursing Science, 6,* 71–88.

Kreps, G. L. (1988). Relational communication in health care. *Southern Speech Communication Journal, 53,* 344–359.

Kreps, G. L., & Query, J. L. (1990). Health communication and interpersonal competence. In G. M. Phillips & J. T. Wood (Eds.), *Speech communication essays to commemorate the 75th anniversary of the Speech Communication Association* (pp. 293–323). Carbondale: Southern Illinois University Press.

McFall, R. M. (1982). A review and reformulation of the concept of social skills. *Behavioral Assessment, 4,* 1–33.

Morse, B. W., & Piland, R. N. (1981). An assessment of communication competencies needed by intermediate-level health care providers: A study of nurse-patient, nurse-doctor, nurse-nurse communication relationships. *Journal of Applied Communication Research, 9,* 30–41.

O'Keefe, B. J., & Delia, J. G. (1982). Impression formation and message production. In M. E. Roloff & C. R. Berger (Eds.), *Social cognition and communication* (pp. 33–72), Beverly Hills, CA: Sage.

Roter, D. L. (1989). Which facets of communication have strong effects on outcome—A meta analysis. In M. Stewart & D. Roter (Eds.), *Communicating with medical patients* (pp. 183–196). Newbury Park, CA: Sage.

Roter, D. L., & Hall, J. A. (1991). Health education theory: An application to the process of patient-provider communication. *Health Education Research, 6,* 188–193.

Roter, D. L., Hall, J. A., & Katz, N. R. (1988). Patient-physician communication: A descriptive summary of the literature. *Patient Education and Counseling, 12,* 99–119.

Rubin, B. R. (1990). The health caregiver-patient relationship: Pathology, etiology, treatment. In E. B. Ray & L. Donohew (Eds.), *Communication and health: Systems and applications* (pp. 51–68). Hillsdale, NJ: Lawrence Erlbaum Associates, Inc.

Rubin, R. B. (1990). Communication competence. In G. M. Phillips & J. T. Woods (Eds.), *Speech communication essays to commemorate the 75th anniversary of the Speech Communication Association* (pp. 94–129). Carbondale: Southern Illinois University Press.

Smith, R. C, & Hoppe, R. B. (1991). The patient's story: Integrating the patient- and physician-centered approaches to interviewing. *Annals of Internal Medicine, 115,* 470–477.

Spitzberg, B. H. (1986). Issues in the study of communicative competence. In B. Dervin & M. J. Voight (Eds.), *Progress in communication sciences: Vol. 8* (pp. 1–46). Norwood, NJ: Ablex.

Spitzberg, B. H., & Cupach, W. R. (1984). *Interpersonal communication competence.* Beverly Hills, CA: Sage.

Stiles, W. B. (1993). The process-outcome correlation problem and the uses of verbal interaction process coding. *Southern Communication Journal, 58,* 91–102.

Street, R. L., Jr. (1991a). Information-giving in medical consultations: The influence of parents' communicative styles and personal characteristics. *Social Science and Medicine, 32,* 541–548.

Street, R. L., Jr. (1991b). Physicians' communication and parents' evaluation of pediatric consultations. *Medical Care, 29,* 1146–1152.

Suchman, A. L., Roter, D. L., Green, M., Lipkin, M., Jr., & The Collaborative Study Group of the American Academy on Physician and Patient. (1993). Physician satisfaction with primary care office visits. *Medical Care, 31,* 1083–1092.

Thompson, T. L. (1994). Interpersonal communication and health care. In M. L. Knapp & G. R. Miller (Eds.), *Handbook of interpersonal communication* (2nd ed., pp. 696–725). Newbury Park, CA: Sage.

Todd, A. D. (1984). The prescription of contraception: Negotiations between doctors and patients. *Discourse Processes, 7,* 171–200.

Tuckett, D., & Williams, A. (1984). Approaches to the measurement of explanation and information in medical consultations: A review of empirical studies. *Social Science and Medicine, 18,* 571–580.

Waitzkin, H. (1984). Doctor-patient communication: Clinical implications of social scientific research. *Journal of the American Medical Association, 252,* 2441–2446.

Waitzkin, H. (1985). Information giving in medical care. *Journal of Health and Social Behavior, 26,* 81–101.

Waldron, V. R., & Cegala, D. J. (1992). Assessing conversational cognition: Levels of cognitive theory and associated methodological requirements. *Human Communication Research, 18,* 599–622.

Wiemann, J. M. (1977). A model of communicative competence. *Human Communication Research, 3,* 195–213.

Wiemann, J. M., & Backlund, P. (1980). Current theory and research in communication competence. *Review of Educational Research, 50,* 185–199.

Discussion Questions

1. In what ways could health communication scholars or medical scholars use the information from this chapter to improve patient-provider communication?
2. Does the information in this chapter coincide with your experiences in medical interactions? Explain.
3. Reflect on your own experiences and knowledge. Do you agree with the categories of competence for doctors and patients as they are discussed in this chapter? Why? Would you add or delete any of the categories? Why? ✦

Chapter 8
Virtually He@lthy
The Impact of Internet Use on Disease Experience and the Doctor-Patient Relationship

Alex Broom

Chapter 8 looks at the Internet and its role in health care as a source of information that may be at once empowering and an alternative source of medical information. The Internet can take a person outside the walls that once separated health-care institutions, and the information found therein, from immediate access to patients and interested others. The Internet often has effects on how people experience health and disease and on the relationship between doctors and patients. In this chapter, Alex Broom investigates a group of Australian men and how their use of the Internet affected their experiences of prostate cancer, including control over their disease and limiting inhibitions. Internet-informed patients and their relationships with their doctors are also discussed. The Internet has a role as a source of information that can empower, as an aid in decision-making, and as a power-balancing tool that can improve communication and satisfaction.

Related Topics: cancer, e-health, Internet, media, patient-provider communication, qualitative methods, role of the patient, social support

There has been considerable discussion of the Internet's potential to contest and disrupt belief systems by breaking down geographical and political boundaries, and to challenge understandings of gender (Cole, Conlon, Jackson, & Welch, 1994; Spender, 1995), community (N. Fox & Roberts, 1999), and intimacy (Collins, 1999). However, little has been published on the consequences of Internet usage for health care consumers and providers. People are "surfing" the Internet for information about their health (Ahmann, 2000; Diaz et al., 2002; Hardey, 1999; Nettleton & Burrows, 2003; Pemberton & Goldblatt, 1998), with the Internet playing an increasingly important role in self-health education. For example, in 2002 a national survey by the Pew Internet and American Life Project (S. Fox & Rainie, 2002) found that 73 million American adults have gone online searching for health information. This study found that a significant proportion of people rely on the Internet to make critical health decisions, often bringing information retrieved from the Internet into medical consultations as an aid to decision making (see also Anderson, Rainey, & Eysenbach, 2003; Berland et al., 2001; Friedewald, 2000; Pemberton & Goldblatt, 1998). In S. Fox and Rainie's (2002) study, 61% said the Internet had improved the way they take care of their health. Brotherton, Clarke, and Quine (2002) have completed the only Australian study hitherto into the impact of the Internet, surveying oncology patients (n = 142) from two teaching hospitals with a 2-year follow-up. Although, given the small sample and the nature of the setting, their results should be treated with caution, of the patients surveyed in 2001, 46% used the Internet, a 13% rise from 1999. Substantial research is needed in this area, but it seems likely that, as is the case in the United States, a significant proportion of Australian consumers use the Internet for health-related information and support.

In addition to the informative potential of the Internet for individuals, it is clear that online communities are developing around particular health problems, with people "chatting" with others about their health problems, treatment programs, and encounters with medical professionals (Hardey, 1999; Lamberg, 1997; Sharf, 1997). According to Rainie and Fox (2001), 84% of American Internet users have used the Internet to access online groups. Moreover, 28% of their respondents had used an on-

From "Virtually He@lthy: The Impact of Internet Use on Disease Experience and the Doctor-Patient Relationship," Alex Broom, 2005, *Qualitative Health Research*, Vol. 15:3, pp. 325–345.

line support group for a medical condition or personal problem. Despite this, little is known about the effects of actively seeking information and support about health on the Internet on patients' disease experiences.

Moreover, the consequences of the Internet-informed patient for patient–clinician encounters remain underresearched. Diaz et al. (2002) found that 59% of Internet users did not discuss with their doctor the information they had retrieved (n = 512). It has also been reported that clinicians can feel threatened by patients' seeking information and react negatively in the consultation (Anderson et al., 2003; Crocco, Villasis-Keever, & Jadad, 2002; S. Fox & Rainie, 2002; Henwood, Wyatt, Hart, & Smith, 2003).

There are many important questions that remain unanswered: Are online support groups, mailing lists, and informative Web sites changing the way in which patients think about their health? What is the role of the Internet in health self-education? Is the Internet empowering patients to question biomedical knowledge and thus medical decision-making processes? Are doctor-patient dynamics changing as a result of patients' Internet usage, and, if so, how are doctors coping with these changes?

Although there is considerable social commentary on the effects of the new social spaces and interpersonal dynamics arising from online interaction (see Morley & Robins, 1995; Nunes, 1995; Rheingold, 1993; Sadar, 1996), few researchers (e.g., Anderson et al., 2003; Diaz et al., 2002; Hardey, 1999; Sharf, 1997) have attempted to address how this new medium influences patients' perceptions of disease, treatment decisions, and encounters with medical professionals.

Drawing on 33 interviews with Australian men who have prostate cancer, I argue in this article that by providing patients with knowledge and support, the Internet has the potential to empower patients and increase their sense of control over their disease. However, this study also illustrates a number of the problems associated with the Internet as a source of information and support, focusing on the reactions of some medical specialists to Internet-informed patients, timing of access and retrieval of information, and patients' perceptions of "risk" in relation to misinformation and deception online.

Background

The effects of the Internet within health care has seen increasing attention from social commentators in the past 5 years (see Anderson et al., 2003; Hardey, 1999; Kassirer, 2000; Lindberg & Humphreys, 1998; McLellan, 1998; Pemberton & Goldblatt, 1998; Sharf, 1997). There has been debate concerning the potential of the Internet to provide patients with a source of empowerment (Sharf, 1997) and increase their sense control over their disease (Hardey, 1999). Buckland and Gann (1997) have suggested that the Internet is particularly powerful, in that it challenges previous hierarchical models of information giving by freeing patients from the passive reception of information and empowering them to seek answers actively. Light (2001) has expanded on this argument, suggesting that the Internet has the potential to foster democratic discourse and participation, assisting in the production of "decentralised and participatory decision-making structures" within health care (p. 1179). Prior to the emergence of the Internet, clinicians were the only readily accessible source of information for most patients (Hellawell, Turner, LeMonnier, & Brewster, 2000). Health self-education involved considerable time and effort for most patients, resulting in their inevitable reliance on clinicians for advice and support, thus reinforcing the authority and power of the clinician in the medical encounter. Although other sources of information were available to patients, such as books, magazine and newspaper articles, pamphlets, journal articles, and so on, seeking information from written sources was considerably time consuming and inevitably too difficult for most patients (Anderson et al., 2003, p. 69). Added to this, it often involved travel and thus mobility and was often difficult to understand because of medical jargon, and much of the material available was out of date by the time it was published.

In this article, I argue that the Internet can empower patients and increase their sense of control over their disease. However, exactly what do I mean by empowerment? K. Roberts (1999) has used the term *patient empowerment* to identify a new patient role in which the distribution of power between patient and physician has altered such that patients are more in control of their health and their encounters with health care professionals (p. 82). Gibson (1991) suggested that empowerment is best understood as the absence or decrease of powerlessness, helplessness, hopelessness, alienation, victimization, subordination, oppression, paternalism, loss of a sense of control over one's life, and dependency. Sharf (1997) suggested that empowerment (as seen in her study of women with breast cancer who use the Internet) is how people perceive online information and support as providing them with the knowledge, skills, attitudes, and self-awareness necessary to make more informed decisions, to improve the quality of their lives, and to take actions they might not have otherwise (p. 74).

In the current study, I viewed empowerment as how it was experienced and articulated by the patient. It can involve the elements identified by the authors above for certain individuals, but for others, it might constitute something very different. It is thus a very slippery concept, in that there is no concrete, identifiable "empowered" state. Empowerment is unique to the individual patient rather than primarily a set of abstractions or behaviors (i.e., knowledge level, activeness, or emotional composure). Thus, in this article, I am concerned with these men's subjective perceptions of their disease experience and their accounts of empowerment (or lack of thereof) resulting from the Internet usage.

The importance of empowerment can be seen in studies that have shown that patient empowerment is associated with better treatment outcomes and significantly higher levels of patient satisfaction. Greenfield, Kaplan, and Ware (1985) evaluated the impact of a health education intervention, with patients in the experimental group given individualized information about their disease and encouraged to ask questions when they met with their physicians. Results showed that patients in the experimental group talked more during consultations than patients in the control group did and also were better able to elicit information from their physicians. Greenfield and colleagues concluded that a more active role relates to a greater sense of control over disease and, therefore, better health outcomes. These results are consistent with other studies that have shown a positive relationship between sense of control and enhanced coping ability (Kiecolt-Glaser & Glaser, 1995). In the context of the current study, such evidence leads to the question of whether the use of the Internet contributes to patient empowerment: Is the Internet reducing feelings of powerlessness, helplessness, hopelessness, loss of a sense of control over one's life, and dependency?

I argue in this article that patient empowerment and the impact of the Internet are inextricably tied to the doctor–patient relationship. Moreover, discussion of the effects of the Internet must involve consideration of the responses of medical professionals to the Internet-informed patient within the context of the medical consultation. There has been considerable discussion concerning the changing role of the medical professional over the past few decades and implications for how patients are interacting with doctors (see Charavel, Bremond, Moumjid-Ferdjaoui, Mignotte, & Carrere, 2001; Freedman, 2002; Ishikawa, Takayama, Yamazaki, Seki, & Katsumata, 2002; Lang, 2000; Lupton, 1997; Zadoroznyj, 2001). In recent years, researchers have speculated about the impact of Internet-informed patients in the medical encounter and the challenge they pose to traditional medical authority (see Anderson et al., 2003; Friedewald, 2000; Hardey, 1999; Pemberton & Goldblatt, 1998). Some commentators have suggested (although little evidence has thus far been presented) that the Internet is changing doctor–patient dynamics (Anderson et al., 2003) and breaking down traditional power imbalances based on previous exclusive access to expert medical knowledge (see Hardey, 1999). Hardey has suggested that by breaking down hierarchical models of information giving (i.e., doctor to patient), the Internet has contributed to clinicians' loss of control over medical knowledge or deprofessionalization, contributing to a decline in awe of and trust in doctors (p. 832). Some clinicians might also feel threatened by patients' seeking information and react negatively in the consultation (Anderson et al., 2003; Crocco et al., 2002; S. Fox & Rainie, 2002). In their study of American Internet users, S. Fox and Rainie found that 13% of respondents had "got the cold shoulder" when presenting Internet material to their doctor (p. 7). Although effects vary between individual patients and individual doctors, there seems to be an increase in concern from doctors that neither they nor the patient can cope with the amount of information patients are bringing into the medical consultation (McLellan, 1998).

The doctor–patient relationship is a vitally important facet of medical care, as, in the large part, it determines the quality of care a patient receives within the medical system. More specifically, effective doctor–patient communication is related to patient satisfaction with medical care, favorable attitudes toward physicians, recall and understanding of information, improved emotional state, and overall health status (see Bennett & Alison, 1996; Frederickson, 1995; Ong, De Haes, & Lammes, 1995; C. Roberts, Cox, Reintgen, Baile, & Gibertini, 1994). With the amount of information now available to patients on the Internet, some might feel they know as much about a certain condition as a doctor does (Anderson et al., 2003; Dudley, Falvo, Podell, & Renner, 1996). This, according to some commentators, poses a new and real challenge to the medical profession (Dudley et al., 1996). Patients are able to become informed about their disease but also to evaluate the performance of their medical specialist as compared to those that other patients talk about online.

I argue in this article that the potential of the Internet to empower patients is, in part, dependent on the responses of the medical professional to changes in the way patients approach decision-making processes and, in particular, the medical consultation. This is not to suggest that doctors are the barrier to the Internet's empowerment of patients. On the contrary, this study illustrates important reasons, unrelated to their clinicians, why men do not access the Internet or find it problematic and unhelpful for making treatment decisions. Conflicting narratives concerning the effects of the Internet illustrate that although it can be empowering for many patients, in other cases it has little or no impact on patients' disease experience. I argue that retaining the complexity and contradictory nature of the effects of the Internet is important to avoid romanticizing its impact on disease experience (i.e., as purely a source of power and liberation) and, second, to provide indications of how to improve it as a source of information and support for patients.

Prostate Cancer

The lifetime risk of being diagnosed with prostate cancer in Australia is about 1 in 10, with the lifetime probability of dying of prostate cancer approximately one in 68 (Australian Institute of Health and Welfare, 1999). Despite the high prevalence of prostate cancer, except in cases of advanced disease, there is little agreement about effective treatment (Garnick, 1993). The causes of prostate cancer are unclear, although studies have shown that it is likely that both genetic and environmental factors play a role (Starr, 1998). Every year, about 10,000 Australian men are diagnosed with the disease, and more than 2,500 die of it (Frydenberg, 1998), making prostate cancer the second largest cause of male cancer deaths, after lung cancer. The old adage "most men die with, not of, prostate cancer" is certainly not true today (Prostate Foundation of Australia, 2003). Men are living longer, giving the cancer more time to spread beyond the prostate, with potentially fatal consequences. Younger men are now developing prostate cancer, and many die of the disease and not with it (Frydenberg, 1998). Earlier onset, combined with greater male life expectancy, means those cancers have more-than-adequate time to spread and become life threatening unless diagnosed and treated (Prostate Foundation of Australia, 2003). Despite high rates of morbidity and mortality of prostate cancer in Australia, however, public awareness and support services lag behind those for comparable diseases such as breast cancer (Prostate Foundation of Australia, 2003). The Internet is an increasingly important source of information and support for men with prostate cancer. Research to assess both its effects for those men currently using it and its potential for those who are not is essential if we are to reap the full benefits of this new technology.

Masculinity and 'Risk'

A central concern in this article is the multiple logics of "risk" (Lupton & Tulloch, 2002) constructed by men in relation to the Internet, and how these logics, for some men, are tied into the pressure felt in face-to-face situations to conform to stereotypical constructions of masculinity. There has been significant discussion about how constructions of masculinity, exacerbated by media images of the "bullet-proof," hard man (Saunders, 2000), create an environment in which men are generally less able than women to recognize physical and emotional distress and to seek help (Reddin & Sonn, 2003). For most illnesses, men are less likely than women to consult their general practitioners, yet their hospital admission rates for diseases such as coronary heart disease and stroke are higher (Bradlow, Coulter, & Brooks, 1992; Cameron & Bernardes, 1998). A recent American survey found that 41% of men would wait at least a week to seek care for a serious medical problem, and 34% would not seek immediate help if they experienced severe chest pain or shortness of breath (Walsh, 2000). Australian men have higher death rates than women for all major causes of death. Furthermore, their use of health services is 40% lower than that of Australian women (MANNET, 2002). Men are said to be less aware of potential risks to their health, and this seems to be true in the case of the prostate. Although research needs to be done in the Australian context, a British survey (N = 2,000) found that when asked to identify the prostate gland on a diagram of the body, 16% of women got it right, compared to only 11% of men (Court, 1995, p. 759). Moreover, only 50% of the men surveyed knew that prostate cancer affects only men.

The reluctance of men to consult medical professionals and seek social support is amplified for prostate cancer sufferers, who at various stages in the course of the illness and its treatment might experience problems with sexual performance and continence (Hines, 1999), resulting in a fear of humiliation. This is compounded by the fact that the majority of men with prostate cancer are over 60 years of age, an age group not as accustomed as other groups to taking an active role in their health or treatment decisions (Beisecker & Beisecker, 1990; Nathanson, 1975). Furthermore, according to Walsh (2000), physicians often do not deal well with the "male mentality" and tend to be "uninformed and uncomfortable with male problems" (p. 42). As a result, men are often unaware of where to turn for health information and support.

The lack of research into the Internet as a source of information and support within health care, and the tendency of men to be less active in seeking information and getting involved in decision making, prompted the development of the current study. In their study of American Internet users, S. Fox and Rainie (2002) found that men were more likely than women to have used the Internet to find information about sensitive health topics that they found difficult to talk about (38% of male and 29% of female respondents). A central concern in the current study was the potential of the Internet as a source of "safe" information and support for men with prostate cancer. Hardey (1999) suggested that the anonymity experienced by users of online communities promotes trust by allowing patients to "open up" and disclose sensitive information in a safe environment. In this article, I examine the Internet as both a source of risk and a tool for minimizing risk for men with prostate cancer.

There has been considerable sociological commentary of the prominence of risk in modern society (Beck, 1992) and the ways in which people make sense of and respond to specific risks (Lupton & Tulloch, 2002). In this article, I examine multiple logics of risk and the ways in which these men engage in risk management (Elliott, 2002, p. 293) in relation to the Internet and online communities. The Internet might provide a haven for some men by minimizing the risk of embarrassment or humiliation that they might feel when sharing their experiences and emotions in face-to-face settings (see also Anderson et al., 2003; Hardey, 1999; Sharf, 1997). Furthermore, access to both lay and expert narratives of illness through the Internet and online forums, and the enhanced ability to self educate, minimizes the risk of reliance on the medical expert. However, I found in this study that some men employ different risk logics, actively avoiding the Internet and/or online forums because of the risk of misinformation or deception.

Method

The Sample

After reviewing the literature and obtaining ethics approval, I arranged meetings with local support group organizers to explain the study, and, with their support, I sent information letters to group members, asking them to participate in the study. Eventually, 25 men were recruited from three face-to-face support groups operating in Victoria, Australia. Overall, 37% (25 of 68) of those approached through the support groups agreed to take part after follow-up and reminder letters. The remaining 8 responded to an article written about the current study in a personal computer magazine, in which I requested that readers with prostate cancer interested in participating in the study contact me. The description of the study in the information letter, outlining the focus on men's Internet usage, meant that the majority of the men who responded (28 of 33) were current Internet users. To provide some comparison with the Internet users, I interviewed 5 men who had never used the Internet. The sample was not designed to be representative of all men prostate cancer; rather, the purpose was to get a sample that would allow an investigation into the effects of Internet usage on disease experiences. In total, 33 men were recruited. Interviews continued until the sample included men of varying ages, with a range of prognoses, and who had been through a range of treatments. All the men were fluent English speakers.

The Interviews

All the respondents were subsequently interviewed in their homes for between 1 and 2 hours. In two cases, the men's wives were present during the interview. The interviews were relatively unstructured, exploring the impact of the Internet on their coping and decision-making ability, and the implications of becoming Internet informed for interactions with medical specialists. Empowerment, enhanced sense of control, and risk emerged as important themes, with many men talking spontaneously about the benefits of the Internet in terms of empowerment and heightened sense of control, and others about their fears concerning the accuracy of information and the authenticity of relationships on the Internet. It is these three themes, empowerment, control, and risk, that I examine in this article.

The Analysis

The method for this project draws on the interpretive traditions within qualitative research, in which the researcher seeks an in-depth understanding of the experiences of the respondents and, in particular, how they made sense of the role of the Internet within their experiences of disease. I took an in-depth exploratory approach to data collection, aimed at documenting the subjective and complex experiences of the respondents rather than merely reflecting on such things as frequency of Internet usage, sources of information, and the type of information retrieved. I maintained a focus on unpacking the complex ways in which the Internet has affected the lives of the respondents, building theory from their narratives rather than imposing it on them (see Charmaz, 1990, p. 1162).

The process of analysis began during data collection. This provided an opportunity to establish initial themes and then to look for deviant or negative cases, complicating my initial observations and retaining the complexity of the data. I approached the analysis initially by systematically reading through each transcript several times, writing notes, discussing ideas with colleagues, and noting emerging patterns within the data collected. Within this process, I continually sought to retain the complexity of the respondents' experiences, documenting atypical cases, conflicts, and contradictions within the data.

Following this initial analysis, I looked back through these notes in the margins of the interviews to establish themes emerging across the interviews. Within this process, once I had identified a theme, I would search through the interviews for other related comments, employing constant comparison to develop or complicate these themes further. This process meant that events that I initially viewed as unrelated could be grouped together as their interconnectedness became apparent. The final step involved revisiting the literature and seeking out conceptual tools that I could use to make sense of the patterns that had emerged from the data.

Results

It is important to emphasize at this point that there is no one archetypal effect of the Internet on disease experience. Experiences and attitudes differed for each patient and were influenced by many factors, such as disease stage, age, literacy level, socioeconomic status, and social support networks. However, although embracing the complexity of effects and perspectives within such a heterogeneous group of men, one is able to identify certain themes within their narratives that provide an idea of the effects the Internet can have on patients' experiences of disease.

The Internet and Control

The role of the Internet in enhancing these respondents' power and control over their disease and decision making processes were prominent themes within the interviews. One respondent talked about this in relation to an online community:

> I found [the online community] extremely useful. I'm one of these people who has a high need for information and knowledge. Knowledge is power. I like to be in control of my situation and the way I want to do that is by knowing what is going to happen . . . That need for knowledge or need for control means I really need that information to feel ok. There are some people who are really quite happy just to not have that information. I'm not one of those. (Internet user, 6 months posttreatment, organ-confined disease)

Another patient recalled his experience of using the Internet:

> In terms of the actual outcome it [the Internet] probably doesn't make any difference. In terms of people's need to feel that they are in control of the situation . . . if people have confidence in their treatment they're more likely to have a positive outcome. I wasn't stressed out by the information I gained, I just thought I was in greater control . . . that's what I thought. (Internet user, 1 year posttreatment, organ-confined disease)

Several of the men who had used the Internet stated that online information sources (and, in some cases, online communities) provided an invaluable method of seeking knowledge and thus control over their treatment process. As the above respondent notes, the information provided by online forums provided clarity in terms of treatments options and, as a result, diminished his reliance on his specialists, allowing him to "take control of my treatment instead of having to rely on my specialist." Although several of the respondents reported that their Internet usage did not necessarily influence the decisions made, and certainly not the physiological outcome of treatment, it was seen as greatly improving the decision-making process by reducing the uncertainties involved in making a treatment decision.

Some members of the medical community have suggested that the Internet is problematic, or even harmful, because of its tendency to either sway patients away from conventional cancer treatments or mislead them in relation to their efficacy (Kiley, 2002; Whiting, 2000). Moreover, fear of increased consumer access to alternative knowledges has contributed to the labeling of Internet usage as an activity that represents dissatisfaction with conventional medicine. Three respondents talked about alternative treatments and the Internet:

> I fairly quickly decided that I didn't want to take these alternative treatments so I didn't really search for them. It was better to get rid of cancer, particularly if it was contained. (Internet user, 3 years posttreatment, organ-confined disease)

> Well, if you went into a site that was telling you to eat green peas six days a week and that will help you [laughs], I wouldn't be eating green peas six days a week. I've made a decision, I've had the operation, so, I look for a particular type of information now and I don't think alternative medicine was much of an option. (Internet user, 1 year posttreatment, organ-confined disease)

> [The Internet] is quite good for people who might be trying alternative treatments who say, no, I don't want the knife. I didn't go down that path. I was happy that my urologist had advised me correctly and that I had made the right decision too so I wasn't really seeking alternative information. I had made up my mind that I wanted to have surgery and then it was a matter of concentrating on achieving fitness to be able to have it happen. So I wasn't really looking around on the Internet for information other than stuff on surgery. (Internet user, 1¼ years posttreatment, organ-confined disease)

Contrary to the fears of the medical community, for the majority of the men interviewed here, accessing support and information online did not increase their negativity or skepticism toward biomedical cancer treatments. Rather, the result was clarification of the subtleties involved in particular biomedical treatments, enabling a significant proportion of the respondents to experience a heightened sense of control and therefore enter into a comprehensive negotiation with their specialist and make what they perceived to be an informed choice. This ability of patients to negotiate with specialists once informed by the Internet was also observed by Hardey (1999, p. 829).

The reaction of medical specialists to Internet-informed patients was of particular interest in this study. One respondent's response to the question of what effect information seeking had on his encounters with medical professionals was

> A lot of the medical community basically see it as loss of control. The standard advice is if you want information about your condition ask your doctor. They don't like it when you seek information from other sources . . . it [is] the standard, well, you're not medically trained, you're not competent to understand this, we will interpret it for you. This is back to we have exclusive control over this area of knowledge-type mind-set. I felt that particularly in contact with the urologist I saw. (Internet user, 6 months posttreatment, organ-confined disease)

Like this respondent, the majority of the men who had used the Internet felt that their information seeking was effective and that they were competent to decipher the "good" from the "bad." Despite this, they were acutely aware that their specialists might view this as outside the patient's role, or, as the above respondent suggests, as a challenge to his or her authority. This same respondent states later in the interview, "I don't feel completely comfortable sharing the information that I have found with my specialist," reflecting a pattern in the men interviewed here of being disapproved of in terms of his Internet usage and information seeking. Another respondent explained his specialist's reaction when he disclosed his use of the Internet in the consultation:

> I asked him questions and he answered them and I said, "Well, listen, I was on the Internet last night and I've got all these questions for you." And he goes, "Oh, look you've got to be careful when you go on the Internet," and he's telling me, "Keep away, steer away, because information overload is just no good for you." And I thought to myself, hmm, that's thick, for me, and I like the Internet, I like reading, I'm right into it and this bloke is telling me to keep away from it. "That means I leave it up to you and I rely totally on you for information"—he goes, "yes." And I said, "Well, how do I know what to ask you?" He said, "Oh, you just do." I said, "Hmmm." . . . And he didn't like that. (Internet user, pretreatment, organ-confined disease)

This perception of feeling disapproved of is

a significant barrier to patient–clinician communication that inevitably results in higher levels of anxiety, confusion, and frustration. As Beisecker (1990) has suggested, the behaviors of specialists might discourage patients from asking questions and entering into an open dialogue with them about their treatment preferences and concerns. The reaction of some specialists to the apparent threat of a disruption to the lay–expert divide within the consultation is to create a relationship dynamic whereby the patient feels "bad" for attempting to understand or question the information being provided by the specialist. This produces a complex process of contesting, redefining, and, in some cases, reinforcing the dominance of the passive patient role in the treatment process.

As was the case for several of the respondents, there is clearly a discrepancy between what the above respondent viewed as his role in the treatment process and his specialist's expectations of the patient's role. Thus, increased access to information and support online does not necessarily result in better doctor–patient communication. Being well informed, and attempting to engage in a comprehensive dialogue in treatment decisions might, in fact, result in hostility, irritation, and a less satisfactory level of care. This has the effect of reducing patient control and power in decision making, thus complicating claims of the liberating nature and positive effect of the Internet on disease experience. The narratives of several of the respondents reveal that patients might feel their level of knowledge seeking creates a barrier to receiving effective care from their specialist. Control or power, then, cannot be seen as confined to any one particular facet of a patient's experience, as feelings of power and control are, in part, determined by the reception of patients' Internet usage by medical specialists.

The Internet and Empowerment

In the current study, I asked respondents how their Internet usage affected their decision-making ability. One man talked about his and his wife's use of the Internet:

> The information available on the Internet was a revelation. It was a real revelation to us. We were reading reports and information about different treatments right up to the minute—material that just wasn't available anywhere else. We picked the bones out of each particular subject. We could log on to brachytherapy and a new world opened up to us. We were able to then sort out statistical information about cure rates, and define centres of excellence. We finally felt as if we had some control over things. (Internet user, midtreatment, extracapsular disease)

The Internet allowed this respondent to "do something" rather than just being "told what to do by our specialist." It provided him with a sense of purpose and control, having a profound effect on his ability to deal with his cancer. Being a very active person, this respondent strove to be able to "throw my energy into getting better," and the Internet, he suggested, provided a vehicle for him to feel as though there was something he could do. Furthermore, it provided him with the resources to help other men with prostate cancer by explaining to them what was happening to them based on the information he retrieved from the Internet. The Internet gave him the knowledge and skills to counsel his friends and take a leadership role in the face-to-face support group he attends, dramatically improving the quality of his life. As he put it, "It made me feel like I had some power over this disease, I could understand it, so I could fight it."

Despite the powerful and liberating effect of the Internet for several of the respondents, findings from the current study indicate that for others, it was a case of too much information too late. Although several of the men found important information on the Internet, by the time they began searching and became computer literate enough to find useful information, they had either already begun a particular treatment regimen or had already gone through surgery. As a result, for several of the respondents, searching the Internet became more a matter of discovering information they felt they should have known before making a treatment decision. Several expressed regret regarding how much more useful the Internet would have been if they had been exposed to it immediately after diagnosis and, in particular, before making a treatment decision:

> The Internet wasn't really very useful in helping to make the decision but it certainly made a tremendous difference in your background information for either accepting what was decided or regretting the decision. I think that that it was extremely useful in reassuring me that that had been the right decision. . . . I suppose decisions have to be made in real life before you get all the information. (Internet user, midtreatment, extracapsular disease)

This excerpt captures one of the many the practical limitations of the Internet for patients. Often, the testing, diagnosis, and treatment takes place over a number of weeks or just a couple of months, leaving little time for research, let alone learning to use communication technologies such as the Internet. Moreover, for several of these respondents, there was considerable self-imposed and, sometimes, clinician encouraged pressure to make a quick decision to "get the cancer out" as soon as possible, even in the case of low-grade, nonaggressive tumors that are relatively slow growing. As a result, searching the Internet was about making sense of the treatment process they had been through or exploring alternatives if treatment had been unsuccessful. In particular, they often sought information about side effects and how successful their surgery and/or radiation treatment was compared with others (whether their situation was typical or whether something "went wrong").

The Internet and the Patient's Role

As Hardey (1999) has argued, the Internet is, to a certain degree, generating new dynamics between doctors and patients by providing patients with the information and support necessary to understand and, at times, question medical decisions. In the following excerpt, a respondent talks about specialists' attitudes toward patients' seeking information from the Internet and other sources:

> I more than think, I know what their attitude is. We extensively searched the Internet [and] at one urologist's office I was asking about certain information and this went on for some time. I went back to his secretary and we are paying the bill. He was talking into a dictaphone and he was making the referral to somebody else and he said, "[patient's name] is somewhat difficult and over-informed" . . . The first urologist that I went to said, "have an operation," he didn't even discuss other forms of treatment. No, they definitely don't really like well-informed people. (Internet user, 1 year posttreatment, organ-confined disease)

As this respondent experienced firsthand, the Internet tests the limits of the "conventional" doctor–patient relationship, having a leveling effect (but not necessarily making them level) in a relationship historically marked by an imbalance of power (McLellan, 1998). However, this can result in specialists' adopting various strategies to discourage this leveling, such as giving patients the impression that they are disapproved of or treating men who ask questions as "problem" patients. Another respondent responds to the question of why specialists are resistant to questioning and informed patients:

> *Participant*: Well, they are probably that busy or whatever that it's all dollars and cents to them. The thing that really disheartened me was that I went away rather shocked like anyone is when they are told they have got cancer and I made a list of things to ask him in the next consultation. I had two foolscap sheets of questions . . . I said to him "Could you please tell me what my Gleason score[1] is." He said, "Oh, you've got some questions, have you," and I said yes and he said, "oh, show them to me," and I gave him the two pieces of paper and he just grabbed them like that [shows me] and went [ticking motion] yes, no, yes, no . . . not applicable, yes, no, and handed them back to me.
>
> *AB:* Why do you think your urologist reacted like that?
>
> *Participant:* Why . . . when you park your car, one parking officer won't even speak and will write out the ticket, but the other bloke will give you a bit of a warning. It's attitudes . . . that happens in all

> professions I guess. (Internet user, 4 years posttreatment, organ-confined disease)

The reaction of this specialist is an example of a strategy to avoid dialogue and reclaim the consultation model whereby it becomes merely a process of, at best, one-way information provision. His response of "yes, no, no" and ticking the questions listed by the respondent disempowers the respondent by not allowing him to initiate a dialogue to work through his concerns. This specialist ignores the respondent's request for his Gleason score, reacting, according to the respondent, as if it was inappropriate and "suspicious for me to want this type of information." This is one example of the various strategies employed by some of the respondents' specialists to limit the successfulness of their attempts to understand and question medical decisions and initiate a dialogue within the consultation.

It is tempting to romanticize the effects of the Internet and the empowering nature of information. However, as a number of the respondents suggested, the empowering nature of the information they retrieved from the Internet and other sources depended on how receptive providers and specialists were to their desire to take part in decision-making processes. Financial constraints combined with a desire to "deal quickly" with their disease meant that several respondents felt that they could not afford to spend a lot of time "shopping around" for sympathetic specialists. One respondent explains the limits to the potential of the Internet:

> You can be empowered to be happier with decisions that are made for you and you also can participate more to a degree in the decision but it's still dependent on finding a consultant or even the hospital which is reactive to this situation or sympathetic. That seems to me to be the difficulty in that, in my case, or in the individual case, you can't go to 4 or 5 specialists. Sooner or later you have to make a choice. (Internet user, midtreatment, suspected extracapsular disease)

The benefits of information are constrained by a number of factors, including an individual's skill in accessing and comprehending it, the amount of time (both perceived by them and prescribed by the specialist) that they have to make a treatment decision, and their access to receptive medical professionals. Several of the men interviewed could not afford to get a second opinion or to choose a specialist. Even though they had access to a substantial amount of information, they either could not afford to see other specialists or opt for limited, costly treatments such as high dose rate (HDR) brachytherapy. Furthermore, their resistance to getting a second opinion was amplified by the fact that they thought it would "slow down" their progress and mean their cancer would be worse when they were eventually treated. The view seemed to be that it would "irritate" their specialists if they sought a second opinion or presented them with information that questioned their advice and possibly result in their receiving less effective care. Thus, information was only one variable in determining whether the respondents were empowered to make an informed decision, with other structural constraints severely limiting their ability to negotiate satisfactory treatment processes.

Trust and Uncertainty

A number of the respondents, particularly the nonusers, were suspicious of the Internet and talked consistently about their reliance on the expertise and advice of their medical specialists. In the following excerpts, two respondents talk about whether patients should seek information and be "active" in making treatment decisions:

> Even now I ask myself: these people, they sit in front of their computers and they search the Internet and they read this but for what reason? Maybe they are chasing something that's not there . . . I figure if you go to a specialist and you don't follow his advice it's bordering on stupidity—he's the expert and I trust his judgment. (Non-Internet user, 6 years postdiagnosis, hormone treatment for secondary disease)

> I don't think that's my job. I sort of believe you've got to judge your surgeon. I know he goes overseas to conferences. I think you've sort of got to assume that

> they're up with the latest, um, you've got to hope that they have got a steady hand [laughs] and just go from there. I would be wary of designing me own treatment. (Non-Internet user, 3 years posttreatment, organ-confined disease)

The latter respondent articulates a common feeling of a lack of ability to judge information and a heavy reliance on the expertise of the specialist. This same respondent is then asked why he did not seek information or support from the Internet. He responds, in relation not to the Internet explicitly but, rather, to the futility, in his view, of trying to take control of his treatment process:

> Even though I had been diagnosed with cancer, which is a word everybody fears, I guess I'm fairly accepting of the situation. If I've got little or no control over it . . . When I went into hospital for this they said, you know, do you want to be a public or a private patient. If you're a private patient you have a doctor of your own choice. Well, I mean, who am I going to pick, I've never had that operation before, obviously, or I wouldn't have a prostate. Am I going to say, well, gee, bring us in the yellow pages and I'll pick one out. So, at the end of the day you sort of go with something but you've got the stress . . . I mean you've got the stress of your own situation and your family is under stress, you're exploring this information and you have got to make good judgments and you can't actually necessarily judge the source. (Non-Internet user, 3 years posttreatment, organ-confined disease)

This respondent vividly articulates the sense of loss of control that a significant proportion of the respondents (not just the nonusers) experienced attempting to make treatment decisions. The provision of options, such as public versus private, gives a perception of choice, whereas clearly this choice almost constricts the previous respondent in the sense that information is not provided for him to make the choice. There are no performance criteria for particular doctors provided. The choice, from the perspective of this respondent, is meaningless, because he has no knowledge and, in his mind, has no way of gaining the knowledge to make a decision that would produce the better outcome.

Three of the non-Internet users considered reliance on their specialist not a negative thing but, rather, the intelligent option. As suggested in one of the earlier excerpts, they considered it "stupid to try and learn what they [specialists] already know." Reliance was viewed as the "safe" option, and using the Internet, as one respondent put it, "is a stupid thing to do. I think they [other men] are probably grasping at straws anyway. Why bother? My specialist knows his stuff." These narratives illustrate the complex needs of men with prostate cancer and the importance of not assuming that all men want to self-educate or develop a sophisticated understanding of the treatment options available.

Masculinity and Risk Management

A theme that emerged from the interviews was the potential of online communities to allow men to "open up" and reduce the risk they might feel in sharing their experiences in face-to-face situations. One respondent spoke about his experience of using an online community, reflecting on the benefits of this new medium in terms of an effective forum for him and other men, to talk about the more sensitive aspects of their disease experience:

> One of the things you find is an amazing openness and frankness about these sort of matters that I'm sure men if they were meeting face to face would not talk about. I mean it's amazing stuff when you actually look at it that if they were sitting around a table in a room I'm fairly positive they would not be talking about such intimate details because it's a community out there . . . we're doing it through this medium and we can be a lot more frank. We could discuss things that if we knew each other face-to-face, we wouldn't have been quite as frank and open. There's the anonymity, there's the disembodiment which is slightly different than anonymity. Anonymous is, your not known and you have all these people who . . . you're able to project in a way that isn't having any comeback on you . . . in terms of your not having to deal with the face-to-face reactions or anything like that. It is disembodying from

> you, from what you're putting there. It's away from me. It's out there. (Internet user, 6 months posttreatment, organ-confined disease)

This respondent's comment reinforces Hardey's (1999) argument that the Internet provides a haven for patients (in this case men) to talk about the more sensitive aspects of their disease experiences, discussions that, according to this respondent (and several others interviewed), would not occur in a face-to-face situation. Sharf (1997), who participated in an online breast cancer support group, also observed the potential of this medium to encourage "a more uninhibited outpouring of feelings, without consciousness of tears, disfigurement or other physical barriers" (p. 74). The Internet presented a number of these men with a method for managing the risk of sharing sensitive information with other men. The risk of attempting such a dialogue in face-to-face situations is precisely that of not being able to share their experiences at all.

Several of the respondents suggested that the Internet distanced them from their disease and their symptoms. They found it much easier to share their experiences, if only at first, if they perceived them to be dislocated from their body. Seen in the previous excerpt, there is a differentiation between being anonymous, which this respondent sees as negative, and being disembodied, which he views as a positive state with regard to feeling able to share his experiences. The separation of the embodied self from the disembodied-but-diseased self allows some of these men to open up to other men and seek information and support, an opening up that might not have occurred in a face-to-face situation. This perceived disembodiment allows a controlled transition toward intimacy and mutual support.

For several of the men interviewed, the protection felt online helped them extend themselves, allowing different types of interactions and personal growth (see also Myers, 1987). This perception of anonymity or disembodiment in online forums might lead people to reveal more about themselves than they do face-to-face (Joinson, 2001). As suggested by the following respondent, the risk of expression might be amplified in the case of prostate cancer, as societal perceptions of manliness and the nature of the disease and treatment (incontinence, sexual dysfunction, etc.) make open, face-to-face discussion problematic for men:

> Some men don't want to be face-to-face. Maybe they're frightened of it, maybe they don't want to travel the distances. Maybe they're scared of being ridiculed or something . . . all sorts of reasons like that. Maybe they're a bit anxious about having the problem and not wanting to share it with other people. I think that's men for you. Some will find it easier to talk online. (Internet user, 3 years posttreatment, organ-confined disease)

The ability to "lurk" online and not necessarily post messages was also viewed as a significant advantage of online communities. In particular, men could participate without feeling the pressure to share their specific experience, as might be felt in face-to-face situations. One respondent discussed different levels of participation in his online support group and the benefits of lurking for patients attempting to find information and support:

> In terms of people being active there's a hard core, whose names you will see just about everyday, of about 10 or 12. There's a much wider group of about 50 who constantly . . . every couple of months they will bounce up. So they are obviously sitting there monitoring it, they will respond to something that interests them. And then there is a lot more who are lurking, who occasionally . . . someone will come on and say, "Well, I've been lurking on this site for three or four months, now I have a specific question to ask." But there are also people that are obviously just monitoring it and not actually contributing anything . . . maybe they'll make the occasional contribution. It suits some people to post messages but not others. (Internet user, 2 years posttreatment, metastatic disease)

For this respondent, lurking is an invaluable characteristic of this community, allowing participants who do not feel able to ask questions to benefit from the interactions of the more active participants. Although they were not looking specifically at health-oriented online communities, Rainie and Fox (2001) found in their study that 60% of members of online communities post messages, leaving 40% who merely observe the postings of other members (p. 11). The respondents who used online communities reported going through stages of needing more or less information and support, with periods during which they would post more than once a day and times when they would not post at all for months. The point of making a decision about treatment and the period immediately following treatment were, according to several of the respondents, the times that they posted the most messages. There was a collective understanding of the dynamic nature of the need for information and support during the patient's "career" (Gustafson, 1972). The acceptability of both varying and low levels of involvement within such groups was appealing for a number of the respondents.

There was a clear division among the respondents as to the context in which they were willing to share their experiences and their perceptions of what constituted risk. The respondents who used online support networks emphasized the importance of being able to get information and support from a "safe" distance and the value of a forum that was separate from their "everyday life." However, several of the respondents who attended face-to-face support groups, particularly those who had never used the Internet, were adamant about their suspicion of communication that was not face-to-face and the importance of being able to "see who I am talking to." These reflect two different ways of managing risk within this particular group of men. The risk for those using the online support groups was having to share their experiences in a public situation—to be exposed to the "public" gaze and reveal themselves to other men face-to-face. Online support groups presented a way of negotiating this risk and a safe way of sharing, receiving, and providing emotional support and information. However, for others, online support groups presented a serious risk in terms of authenticity of relationships ("who am I talking to") and information ("they could tell me anything"). As is shown in the following discussion, for these respondents, not searching the Internet or being involved in online support groups was considered a method of reducing risk. One respondent talks about the risk of online communities:

> *Participant:* I would be very wary of [online communities]. For the same reason as the Americans are finding out when they are interrogating these Afghans. They are getting fed wrong information, sometimes deliberately, and they're going out and bombing innocent people on the basis of information extracted out of these people.
>
> *AB:* How does that relate to prostate cancer?
>
> *Participant:* Well, if I talk to you I can gauge that you are a fine young man and so on and so forth. If it's an anonymous person on the Internet and I was talking about sexual things, I wouldn't know if it was a female who's getting some sort of kicks out of it. Also, it's a pretty asocial sort of activity, isn't it[?] If I sit in there on my computer and my wife's in there watching the TV. If I, this was not a cause of friction, but, it's not very . . . she's a sort of widow sitting in there on her own. If I get the Internet and I'm on there every night doing things she could be wondering, oh, is he talking to some girl in America—that's what the next-door neighbour did. She was talking to some bloke in America. As a consequence her marriage has gone. (Non-Internet user, 3 years posttreatment, organ-confined disease)

For this respondent, the concept of communicating via a computer is bizarre and devious. He could not think of sharing any personal details unless he could see the person face-to-face. Furthermore, his social group had demonized the Internet as a corrupting force in light of what happened to the next-door neighbor's marriage. Justification for not using the Internet and/or online support groups generally ranged from concerns regarding the stigma of being "on the Internet" (i.e., being viewed as promiscuous or unfaithful) to the perceived risk of being "fed the wrong information." These concerns represent the flip side of the benefits described by the men who had used online support groups, who viewed anonymity and secrecy as conditions allowing greater personal disclosure and considered the multiplicity of views offered in chat rooms not as potential sources of misinformation or deception but, rather, as opportunities to hear descriptions and perspectives other than those provided by their medical specialists.

Discussion

This study showed considerable support for the potential of the Internet to provide patients with a sense of empowerment and greater control of their disease. The results indicate that accessing information and/or support online can have a profound effect on men's experiences of prostate cancer. For a number of the respondents, the Internet was an essential coping strategy and, in particular, a method of taking some control over their disease. The immense value of the Internet lies in its role as a source of information that empowers men in decision making, providing some balance to traditional imbalances in knowledge and power in doctor–patient encounters, thereby improving communication and satisfaction with treatment processes. Regardless of whether their Internet usage changed the actual decisions made, the majority of the men viewed it as greatly improving their ability to reduce the uncertainties involved in making a treatment decision.

However, this study highlights the limitations of the Internet for patients, particularly in terms of the responses of medical specialists. The narratives of these men illustrate the impact of specialists' responses to Internet usage in terms of patients' feeling respected, competent, and able to engage in decision-making processes. The evidence presented suggests that increased access to information and support online does not necessarily result in better doctor–patient communication. Being well informed and attempting to engage actively in decision-making processes can result in hostility and irritation within the medical consultation. Specialists might react by employing strategies that implicitly or explicitly discredit the ability of patients to become informed via the Internet, presenting serious barriers to shared decision making and to the acceptance of the importance of information seeking for their disease experiences. It is clear that for some medical specialists, Internet-informed patients challenge their power within the medical encounter, resulting in the employment of strategies to reinforce paternalistic dynamics and alienate patients who use the Internet. This has the effect of reducing patient control and power in decision making, thus complicating the potentially positive influence of the Internet on disease experience. This backlash against Internet-informed patients presents a considerable barrier to reaping the benefits of the Internet as a source of information and support, with serious implications for doctor–patient communication and thus quality of care. Medical specialists must provide encouragement, guidance, and support to patients in relation to their Internet usage to achieve the maximum benefits from this potentially empowering and liberating source of information and support.

This study also illustrates the potential of online support groups to provide men with a unique and potentially liberating source of support and information, limiting inhibitions felt in face-to-face encounters, thereby fostering increased expression of emotion and intimacy. The potential benefit of online support groups lies in their ability to allow some men to transcend cultural expectations of masculinity (non-emotive, strong, well, tough, inexpressive, etc.) and share personal experiences that they would not in a face-to-face situation. For several respondents, the risk of expression was reduced with the anonymity of the Internet and the perceived safety of "doing it at home." However, for the men who chose not to use online forums, risk consisted of the potential for deception and misinformation. It is argued that understanding different forms of risk management is essential if we are to understand the multiple and complex informational and support needs of men with prostate cancer.

Note

1. The Gleason system evaluates how effectively the cells of any particular cancer are able to structure themselves into glands resembling those of the normal prostate. The ability of a tumor to mimic normal gland architecture is called its differentiation, and a tumor whose structure is nearly normal (well differentiated) will probably have a biological behavior that is not very aggressively malignant (see the Prostate Cancer Info Link Web Site, www.phoenix5.org/Infolink/).

References

Ahmann, E. (2000). Supporting families' savvy use of the Internet for health research. *Pediatric Nursing, 26*(4), 419–423.

Anderson, J., Rainey, M., & Eysenbach, G. (2003). The impact of cyberhealthcare on the physician–patient relationship. *Journal of Medical Systems, 27*(1), 67–84.

Australian Institute of Health and Welfare. (1999). *Cancer in Australia 1996: Incidence and mortality data for 1996 and selected data for 1997 and 1998.* Canberra, Australia: Author.

Beck, U. (1992). *Risk society: Towards a new modernity.* London: Sage.

Beisecker, A. (1990). Patient power in doctor–patient communication: What do we know? *Health Communication, 2*(2), 105–122.

Beisecker, A., & Beisecker, T. (1990). Patient information-seeking behaviours when communicating with doctors. *Medical Care, 28,* 19–28.

Bennett, M., & Alison, D. (1996). Discussing the diagnosis and prognosis with cancer patients. *Postgraduate Medical Journal, 72,* 25–29.

Berland, G., Elliot, M., Morales, L., Algazy, J., Kravitz, R., Broder, M. et al. (2001). Health information of the Internet: Accessibility, quality and readability in English and Spanish. *Journal of the American Medical Association, 285*(20), 2612–2621.

Bradlow, A., Coulter, A., & Brooks, P. (1992). *Patterns of referral.* Oxford, UK: Health Services Research Unit.

Brotherton, J., Clarke, S., & Quine, S. (2002). Internet use by oncology patients: Its effect on the doctor–patient relationship. *Medical Journal of Australia, 177,* 395.

Buckland, S., & Gann, B. (1997). *Disseminating treatment outcomes information to consumers: Evaluation of five pilot projects.* London: King's Fund Publishing.

Cameron, E., & Bernardes, J. (1998). Gender and disadvantage in health: Men's health for a change. *Sociology of Health & Illness, 20*(5), 673–693.

Charavel, M., Bremond, A., Moumjid-Ferdjaoui, N., Mignotte, H., & Carrere, M. (2001). Shared decision-making in question. *Psychooncology, 10,*93–102.

Charmaz, K. (1990). "Discovering" chronic illness: Using grounded theory. *Social Science & Medicine, 30*(11), 1161–1172.

Cole, A., Conlon, T., Jackson, S., & Welch, D. (1994). Information technology and gender: Problems and proposals. *Gender and Education, 6*(1), 77–84.

Collins, L. (1999). Emotional adultery: Cybersex and commitment. *Social Theory and Practice, 25*(2), 243–270.

Court, C. (1995). Survey reveals men's ignorance about health. *British Medical Journal, 310* 759.

Crocco, A., Villasis-Keever, M., & Jadad, A. (2002). Analysis of cases of harm associated with use of health information on the Internet. *Journal of the American Medical Association, 287*(21), 2869–2872.

Diaz, J., Griffith, R., Ng, J., Reinert, S., Friedmann, R., & Moulton, A. (2002). Patients' use of the Internet for medical information, *Journal of General Internal Medicine, 17,*180–185.

Dudley, T., Falvo, D., Podell, R., & Renner, J. (1996). The informed patient poses a different challenge. *Patient Care, 30*(19), 128–138.

Elliott, A. (2002). Beck's sociology of risk: a critical assessment. *Sociology of Health and Illness, 36*(2), 293–316.

Fox, N., & Roberts, C. (1999). GP's in cyberspace: The sociology of the virtual community. *Sociological Review, 47*(4), 643–671.

Fox, S., & Rainie, L. (2002). *Vital decisions: How Internet users decide what information to trust when they or their loved ones are sick.* Washington, DC: Pew Internet & American Life Project.

Frederickson, L. (1995). Exploring information-exchange in consultation: The patients' view of performance and outcomes. *Patient Education and Counselling, 25,* 237–246.

Freedman, T. (2002). "The doctor knows best" revisited: Physician perspectives. *Psychooncology, 11,* 327–335.

Friedewald, V. (2000). The Internet's influence on the doctor–patient relationship. *Health Management Technology, 21*(11), 7980.

Frydenberg, M. (1998). Management of localised prostate cancer: State of the art. *Medical Journal of Australia, 169,* 11–12.

Garnick, M. (1993). Prostate cancer: Screening,

diagnosis and management. *Annals of Internal Medicine, 118,* 804–818.

Gibson, C. (1991). A concept analysis of empowerment. *Journal of Advanced Nursing, 16,* 354–361.

Greenfield, S., Kaplan, S., & Ware, J. (1985). Expanding patient involvement in health care: Effects on patient outcomes. *Annals of Internal Medicine, 102,* 520–528.

Gustafson, E. (1972). Dying: The career of the nursing home patient. *Journal of Health and Social Behaviour, 13,* 226–235.

Hardey, M. (1999). Doctor in the house: The Internet as a source of health knowledge and a challenge to expertise. *Sociology of Health and Illness, 21*(6), 820–835.

Hellawell, G., Turner, K., Le Monnier, K., & Brewster, S. (2000). Urology and the Internet: An evaluation of Internet use by urology patients and of information available on urological topics. *British Journal of Urology, 86,* 191–194.

Henwood, R., Wyatt, S., Hart, A., & Smith, J. (2003). Ignorance is bliss sometimes: Constraints on the emergence of the "informed patient" in the changing landscapes of health information. *Sociology of Health and Illness, 25*(6), 589–607.

Hines, S. (1999). Treating early prostate cancer: Difficult decisions abound. *Patient Care, 33* (16), 82–91.

Ishikawa, H., Takayama, T., Yamazaki, Y., Seki, Y., & Katsumata, N. (2002). Physician-patient communication and patient satisfaction in Japanese cancer consultations. *Social Science & Medicine, 55,* 301–311.

Joinson, A. (2001). Self-disclosure in computer-mediated communication: The role of self-awareness and visual anonymity. *European Journal of Social Psychology, 31,* 177–192.

Kassirer, J. (2000). Patients, physicians, and the Internet. *Health Affairs, 19*(6), 115–123.

Kiecolt-Glaser, J., & Glaser, R. (1995). Psychoneuroimmunology and health consequences: Data and shared mechanisms. *Psychosomatic Medicine, 57,* 269–274.

Kiley, R. (2002). Does the Internet harm health? *British Medical Journal, 324,* 238.

Lamberg, L. (1997). Online support group helps patients live with, learn more about the rare skin cancer CTCL-ML. *Journal of the American Medical Association, 277*(18), 1422–1424.

Lang, F. (2000). The evolving roles of patient and physician. *Archives of Family Medicine, 9,* 65–67.

Light, D. (2001). Managed competition, governmentality, and institutional response in the United Kingdom. *Social Science & Medicine, 52,* 1167–1181.

Lindberg, D., & Humphreys, B. (1998). Medicine and health on the Internet: The good, the bad, and the ugly. *Journal of the American Medical Association, 250*(15), 1301–1302.

Lupton, D. (1997). Consumerism, reflexivity and the medical encounter. *Social Science & Medicine, 45*(3), 373–381.

Lupton, D., & Tulloch, J. (2002). "Risk is part of your life": Risk epistemologies among a group of Australians. *Sociology, 36*(2), 317–335.

MANNET (Men's Awareness Network). (2002). Aussie health. Retrieved October 10, 2002, from http:// www.mannet.com.au

McLellan, F. (1998). Like hunger like thirst: Patients, journals and the Internet. *The Lancet, 352,* (2 Suppl. 3), el2.

Morley, D., & Robins, K. (1995). *Spaces of identity: Global media, electronic landscapes, and cultural boundaries.* London: Routledge.

Myers, D. (1987). Anonymity is part of the magic: Individual manipulation of computer-mediated-communication contexts. *Qualitative Sociology, 10,* 251–266.

Nathanson, C. A. (1975). Illness and the feminine role: A theoretical review. *Social Science & Medicine, 9* 57–62.

Nettleton, S., & Burrows, R. (2003). Escaped medicine?: Information, reflexivity and health. *Critical Social Policy, 23*(2), 165–185.

Nunes, M. (1995). Jean Baudrillard in cyberspace: Internet, virtuality and postmodernity. *Style, 29*(2), 314–318.

Ong, L., De Haes, J., & Lammes, F. (1995). Doctor–patient communication: A review of the literature. *Social Science & Medicine, 40,* 903–918.

Pemberton, P., & Goldblatt, J. (1998). The Internet and the changing roles of doctors, patients and families. *Medical Journal of Australia, 169,* 594–595.

Prostate Foundation of Australia. (2003). *Prostate cancer: What is it?* Lane Cove, Australia: Author. Retrieved February 20, 2004, from http://www.prostate.org.au

Rainie, L., & Fox, S. (2001). *Online communities: Networks that nurture long-distance relationships and local ties.* Washington, DC: Pew Internet & American Life Project.

Reddin, J., & Sonn, C. (2003). Masculinity, social support, and sense of community: The men's group experience in Western Australia. *Journal of Men's Studies, 11*(2), 207–224.

Rheingold, H. (1993). *The virtual community: Homesteading on the electronic frontier.* Reading, MA: Addison-Wesley.

Roberts, C., Cox, C., Reintgen, D., Baile, W., &

Gibertini, M. (1994). Influence of physician communication on newly diagnosed breast cancer patients' psychological adjustment and decision-making. *Cancer, 74,* 336–341.

Roberts, K. (1999). Patient empowerment in the United States: A critical commentary. *Health Expectations, 2,* 82–92.

Sadar, Z. (1996). alt.civilisations.faq: Cyberspace as the darker side of the West. In Z. Sadar & J. Ravetz (Eds.), *Cyberfutures: Culture and politics on the information superhighway* (pp. 14–41). London: Pluto.

Saunders, C. (2000). Where are all the men? *Patient Care, 34*(11), 10.

Sharf, B. (1997). Communicating breast cancer on-line: Support and empowerment on the Internet. *Women and Health, 26*(1), 65–84.

Spender, D. (1995). *Nattering on the net: Women, power and cyberspace.* North Melbourne, Australia: Spinifex.

Starr, C. (1998). Prostate cancer: Who's at high risk? *Patient Care, 32* (16), 150.

Walsh, N. (2000). Men are out of touch with the health care system. *Family Practice News, 30* (20), 42.

Whiting, R. (2000, December 11). A healthy way to learn: The medical community assesses online healthcare. *Information Week,* p. 60. Retrieved October 19, 2004, from http://www.informationweek.com/816/kin4.htm

Zadoroznyj, M. (2001). Birth and the "reflexive consumer": Trust, risk and medical dominance in obstetric encounters. *Journal of Sociology, 37*(2), 117–141.

Discussion Questions

1. The author of this chapter presents research that suggests that increasing support and access to information online does not always result in better communication between the doctor and patient. How can patients be both well-informed and engage actively in decision-making while avoiding irritation and hostility in the medical consultation?

2. When using online support groups or obtaining information from the Internet, how can people safeguard themselves from misinformation?

3. Do you feel it is essential for patients to share their experiences of online support groups and information obtained from the Internet with their physicians? ✦

Chapter 9 Promoting Communication With Older Adults

Protocols for Resolving Interpersonal Conflict and for Enhancing Interactions With Doctors

Patricia Flynn Weitzman and Eban A. Weitzman

Chapter 9 addresses aging and the unique challenges present in the patient-provider interaction with elderly patients. Effective communication is important at all ages, but it may become more complicated as we age and have new experiences. This chapter presents several ideas for effective communication training and for targeting older adults in interpersonal conflict and medical contexts. Contextual factors play a role in these communicative experiences.

Related Topics: aging, culture, media, patient-centered communication, patient-provider communication, role of the patient

1. Introduction

Some of the concerns that can plague adults as they age have to do with maintaining health and functional abilities, managing household hassles, and dealing with trying situations with social network members (Backer, 1995; Clarke, Preston, Raksin, & Bengston, 1999; Weitzman, Dunigan, Hawkins, Weitzman, & Levkoff, in press). Ways to address concerns around personal health and household hassles, while not always agreeable, are at least often straightforward. Addressing issues involving relationships, however, can feel less straightforward to older adults (Clarke et al., 1999; Weitzman & Weitzman, 2000).

One of the reasons for this may be that many members of the current generation of older adults, particularly women, believe that the way to preserve relationships with social network members and to minimize social stress is by avoiding conflict and suppressing anger when conflicts do arise (Minick & Gueldner, 1995; Weitzman, Dunigan, et al., in press; Weitzman & Weitzman, 2000). Unfortunately, habitual conflict avoidance can increase stress over time rather than decrease it (Pearlin, Mullan, Semple, & Skaff, 1990). Yet, it can be difficult for some older adults to accept the notion that replacing avoidant behaviors with those that involve communicating openly and honestly about a difficult interpersonal issue is actually better for their relationships and for their health (Sandy, Boardman, & Deutsch, 2000; Steptoe, Fieldman, Evans, & Perry, 1996; Steptoe, Moses, & Edwards, 1990; Weitzman & Weitzman, 2000).

Since experiments show increased cardiovascular reactivity to psychosocial stressors in older compared to younger adults (e.g., Jennings et al., 1997; Uchino, Uno, Holt-Lunstad, & Flinders, 1999), and since the avoidant coping behaviors that many in the current generation of older adults may use can exacerbate stress (Pearlin et al., 1990), this group may be at increased risk for stress-related illness due to poorly resolved conflicts. Furthermore, for people of all ages, effective interpersonal conflict resolution skills often do not come naturally (Opotow, 1991). Rather, the skills need to be learned and practiced.

Unfortunately, a surprising lack of programmatic attention has been paid to promoting constructive and effective interpersonal communication for older adults

From "Promoting Communication With Older Adults: Protocols for Resolving Interpersonal Conflict and for Enhancing Interactions With Doctors," Patricia Flynn Weitzman and Eban A. Weitzman, 2003, *Clinical Psychology Review*, Vol. 23:4, pp. 523–535.

(National Eldercare Institute, 1996). We are unaware of any training programs in interpersonal conflict resolution developed specifically for older adults. While printed literature is available to help older patients communicate better with their doctors, we do not know of any training programs that allow older adults to directly practice such techniques. The National Institute on Aging has developed educational materials to help physicians maximize communication with older patients, which are based on research on emotional and cognitive factors that may affect the processing of medical information in older patients (see Gastel, 1994; Park, Morrell, & Shifren, 1999). These considerations include recognizing that older patients may experience increased emotional discomfort when visiting doctors, may have age-related memory deficits that interfere with the reporting of symptoms, and may be suffering from increased anxiety in general, which they are reluctant to discuss (Gastel, 1994; Hocking & Koenig, 1995). Our training protocol for older patients likewise draws from this literature, and represents the translation of these research insights into practical skills for older patients. It also draws from literature showing that older patients can be reluctant to ask questions of doctors, which has particular ramifications in the managed care context. We present an overview of this protocol, along with one in constructive interpersonal conflict resolution that we have developed and begun to use. These protocols can serve as a starting point for others to refine for use with specific older adult groups.

2. Theoretical Concepts and Skills

Our understanding of interpersonal communication draws from Roger Brown's and from Morton Deutsch's theoretical work on intergroup processes. Brown (1965) emphasizes that all successful communications require that the point of view of the other person be realistically understood. While this may seem obvious, significant research shows that it is a task difficult for most people to achieve during the heat of an argument or other stressful social interaction (see Deutsch, 2000). Both Brown and Deutsch have pointed out that mastering the ability to understand the other person's perspective, however, is worth the effort in that it can lead to more open and trusting communication. According to Deutsch's (1973, 2000) *Crude Law of Social Relations,* open and trusting communication on one person's part can, in turn, induce similar communication from the other person.

With regard to older adults' communication with doctors, we have also drawn from Levkoff, Levy, and Weitzman's (1999) theoretical model of elderly helpseeking during illness. This model emphasizes that many older adults feel reluctant to seek help during illness, and may require support to do so. Once helpseeking is initiated, the older person who perceives a successful communicative interaction with a doctor or provider will be more apt to return to the doctor at the worsening of symptoms, than the person who has felt dismissed or not listened to by his/her doctor. Thus, the process operates like a feedback loop, with the success or failure of each communicative encounter affecting all subsequent encounters, and by extension health outcomes. Levkoff et al. point out that training for older adults on how to communicate effectively with doctors can help reduce the likelihood that health regimens will be followed incorrectly or abandoned altogether, as can often happen with older adults (Boyd & Bywaters, 1999; Levkoff, Cleary, Wetle, & Besdine, 1988).

3. Definition of Skills

Turning to the skills that promote good communication and aid in the constructive resolution of conflict, a review of some of the empirical literature on interpersonal communication and conflict shows a concurrence that the following are important: self-disclosure, explaining, active listening, perspective taking, refraining, and brainstorming, among others (Cahn, 1994; Deutsch, 1994, 2000; Hartley, 1993; Hayes, 1991; McCann & Higgins, 1984). The empirical efforts that have tested these skills, particularly active listening and perspective taking, reinforce both Brown's and

Deutsch's focus on the mutual benefit that can be derived when at least one person in a conflict makes an attempt to listen fully and understand the point of the view of the other person (Burggraf & Sillars, 1987; Deutsch, 2000; Sillars, Wilmot, & Hocker, 1993). Definitions of these skills (presented in language that can be incorporated directly into trainings) might be as follows.

3.1. Self-Disclosure

When you self-disclose, you reveal to the listener some aspect of how you are feeling, especially that which you might have heretofore been trying to conceal. You also share with the listener what it is that you really need, without engaging in bargaining ploys to manipulate the listener.

3.2. Explaining

When you explain, you provide the listener with information about the aspects of the situation about which you are most concerned. To facilitate communication, both self-disclosure and explaining must be done without the use of language that is blaming or disrespectful to the other person.

3.3. Active Listening

When you actively listen, you turn your full attention to the overall message of the speaker, as well as the details, rather than focusing on your own concerns or on counterarguments. You also provide feedback to the speaker in order to ensure that you understood the message. The feedback can involve paraphrasing what you think the speaker said, and asking questions to clarify. It should not include an evaluation of, or a counterargument to, what the other person said; rather, it should be an attempt to understand the other person's needs and concerns as he/she sees them.

3.4. Perspective Taking

Perspective taking is largely an internal process in which you try to understand how it might feel to be the other person in the situation. It is fostered by active listening. In other words, perspective taking is trying to understand the other person's needs, concerns, difficulties, and pain in this situation. It is often referred to as "putting yourself in the other person's shoes." Perspective taking and active listening can help move the situation from an adversarial one in which your needs are pitted against the other person's, to a collaborative one in which you are working with the other person to satisfy both sets of needs.

3.5. Reframing

Reframing proceeds from active listening and involves moving further away from an adversarial "me against you" situation toward seeing the situation as a mutual problem to be solved collaboratively. It can be initiated by such statements as "what can we do so that you get what you need which is [fill in the blank] and I get what I need which is [fill in the blank]?"

3.6. Brainstorming

Brainstorming comes after active listening and reframing, and involves coming up with as many solutions as possible for the problem, without critiquing them at first, and then narrowing them down to come up with the solution or set of solutions that best fits everyone's needs. Generating many solutions, quickly and without evaluation, can help with creativity, and lead to unexpected solutions.

4. Interpersonal Conflicts and Older Adults

Before discussing how these skills might be applied in work with older adults, it seems important to also consider contextual factors that may be associated with older adults' experiences of interpersonal conflict. Understanding contextual factors can help finetune a training, making it more relevant which, in turn, can help make older adults who are resistant to training more open to it. One of the contextual factors relevant to older adults' conflicts, namely beliefs about the health benefits of conflict avoidance, has already been discussed. From our own work with older women, we have found that older European-American women report conflicts with neighbors, adult children, and community service providers as particularly stressful and challenging to resolve (Weitzman & Weitzman, 2000). Older African-American women report conflicts with adult children, peers, and grandchildren as particularly difficult to resolve (Weitzman, Weitzman, & Levkoff, 2002). A survey of nursing home administrators revealed that many older women residing in nursing care experience conflicts with roommates (Weitzman et al., 2002).

Research has also shown that older adults living in multigenerational households may often be in conflict with their adult children over financial matters and lifestyle issues (Halpern, 1994). In fact, conflict between older adults and their adult children, may be common. In a large study with older adults by Clarke et al. (1999), two-thirds of older parents reported frequent conflict with adult children. Both older parents and their adult children frequently described communication with each other as strained or nonexistent, and/or characterized by yelling.

5. The Older Patient

In understanding the context of older adults' interactions with doctors, one must start with the fact that such interactions tend to increase with age (National Center for Health Statistics, 1995). Studies show that middle-aged and older women often feel dissatisfied with the quality of their communications with doctors (Adler, McGraw, & McKinlay, 1998; Beisecker, 1996). Yet, somewhat paradoxically, research with older breast cancer patients shows that some older women believe that not questioning doctors is necessary for good healthcare. Asking "too many" questions seems to be perceived by some as potentially antagonistic to doctors, which then might lead doctors to provide the patient with poorer care (Adler et al., 1998). Older adults also recognize that in today's managed care climate, doctors have less time to spend with patients, and while this fact is unpleasant, many believe that the appropriate response is to limit questions (Greene & Adelman, 1996). Yet, we know that patients who do ask questions and insist on courtesy, respect, and responsiveness from providers are more likely to report satisfaction with healthcare experiences (Herzlinger, 1997); may experience less severe treatment side effects (Shapiro et al., 1997); may be more likely to keep appointments (Roter, 1977); and may be more likely to follow recommended health routines (Kaplan, Greenfield, & Ware, 1989).

This problem of holding back on questions can be compounded by the fact that, despite the greater frequency of doctor visits compared to younger adults, many older adults put off going to the doctor and suffer a worsening of symptoms because of it (Levkoff et al., 1988). Older adults may arrive at the doctor's office in an extreme state of psychological and physical stress, with the psychological stress stemming from not having been "successful" at steering clear of the doctor, and the physical stress from the fact that their symptoms are now at an acute stage. Furthermore, up to 20% of older patients with chronic, treatable illnesses experience clinically significant anxiety (Hocking & Koenig, 1995). Higher levels of anxiety can make it harder to communicate with doctors; harder to remember questions to ask; and harder to retain treatment information (Hocking & Koenig, 1995).

Another critical concern with regard to older adults in the healthcare interaction is that up to 60% does not know what medications they are supposed to take, what the correct dosages are, and the reasons for which their doctors prescribed particular medications (Ruscin & Semla, 1996). Lack of communication with doctors is a primary cause of medication mismanagement in older adults. Statistics show that about 50% of all prescriptions are not taken properly, and account for an estimated 125,000 deaths in America per year (Johns Hopkins Medical, 1996). Some estimates show that adverse drug reactions due to medication mismanagement affect older adults three times as often as the general population (cf. Haber, 1999). Providing older patients with a framework for maximizing communication with doctors may help overcome anxiety-related communication problems, and improve their adherence to and understanding of medication regimens.

6. Constructive Conflict Resolution Training With Older Adults

We have applied the concepts and contextual information outlined above to our training efforts with older adult women in constructive conflict resolution. In preliminary work, we translated concepts into three basic skills: active listening, reframing, and brainstorming, which are defined above (see Weitzman, Hardaway, Smakowski, Weitzman, & Levkoff, in press). We have limited our training approach with older adults to three skills, not only because the cognitive psychology literature shows that conceptual triads are easier to remember than dyads or larger groupings (Baddeley, 1986), but also because we believe that in working with older adults, especially the physically frail, it can be important to limit the training session to about 1.5–2 h. In our experience, this amount of time is adequate for introducing three skills. Limiting the training group size to 6–12 is also useful in keeping the training to about 1.5 h.

6.1. Format

To facilitate trainees' thinking about conflict, it can be helpful to open the training with a discussion in which trainees are asked to describe interpersonal situations from their everyday lives that are challenging, and how they have responded to them. These situations can then be integrated into the training, which helps ensure that it is more accessible, relevant, and useful. The discussion group also allows trainers to identify and incorporate the language of the participants for describing their conflict experiences into the training, e.g., situations that "get on my nerves," which can help make the training more culturally appropriate. The real-life examples gathered in one training session can then also be used in future trainings with similar groups, particularly to encourage participants who seem reluctant to talk about their conflicts. At the opening of a training with older adults, for example, it can be pointed out that in past trainings, some older adults have said that they are often distressed about conflicts occurring with neighbors. This can help current trainees identify and talk about similar situations from their own lives.

After the discussion to raise trainees' awareness of their own responses to conflicts, the trainer(s) can then introduce the three skills by first role-playing the skills themselves, and then aiding the trainees in role-playing the skills using their own and their fellow trainees' conflict situations. Trainees can be divided into groups of two to role-play the skills. The trainer(s) can circulate around the room to provide assistance as needed. After each role-play session, the group can come back together to discuss the process and be introduced to the next skill to be worked on. After each skill has been discussed and role-played, additional time can be allotted for trainees to practice using the skills for specific conflicts in their lives with which they are struggling. We have found this simple format to be effective for improving trainees' understanding of and facility with the skills for constructive conflict resolution (Weitzman, Dunigan, et al., in press; Weitzman, Hardaway, et al., in press).

6.2. Incorporating Contextual Factors

We have already discussed some aspects of context that may be relevant to older adults. For example, trainings with nursing home residents may be best focused on roommate conflicts or conflicts with family members over healthcare issues, and include a discussion of the various ways that such conflicts are handled by administrators, and whether or not these administrative measures are helpful. Further adaptations that consider context may also be helpful. For example, because of the belief held by some older adults that conflict avoidance is health protective, it can be emphasized at the beginning of the training that the medical research shows the opposite to be true. It can also be useful to ask trainees if conflict avoidance actually leads them to feel better. Most likely, the answer will be no. Second, by eliciting conflict examples from their own lives, the training can then be focused on those areas. For example, in the opening discussions of our trainings with older African-American women, many have cited examples of challenging situations with their grandchildren and the trainings were focused on such situations. The benefits of this approach have been twofold: it provides social support from peers around real-life stressful situations, and it provides numerous examples that can be focused on by trainers to make the training most relevant.

Because conflicts with adult children may be common across older adult groups, trainers might want to explore this issue as well. The uniqueness and complexity of parent–adult child relationships are widely recognized (see Henwood, 1995), and beyond the scope of this discussion. What may be most relevant for training, however, is the fact that these conflicts can center on practical issues such as money and household management or around lifestyle choices and religious, moral, or political beliefs (Clarke et al., 1999; Halpern, 1994). Research indicates that conflicts over limited, concrete, and/or practical issues are easier to resolve than those that have to do with lifestyle issues or moral, religious, or personal values (Coleman, 2000; Deutsch, 1973). It may be important to spend some time discussing this with trainees, and talking about the different course that conflict can take depending upon the issue of conflict, i.e., practical or value-related. Trainees should understand what kinds of resolutions are realistic for a given conflict. If the issue is value-based, the goal of resolution may not be getting the other persons to change their behavior (e.g., sexual preference), but rather to come to a place of mutual understanding with the other persons.

A final point to emphasize with any group being trained in constructive conflict resolution skills is that even though the other person(s) with whom one experiences conflict may not have gone through such training, the use of the skills by one person, particularly active listening, typically helps to deescalate the conflict and make it easier to resolve constructively (Burggraf & Sillars, 1987; Deutsch, 2000; Sillars et al, 1993). The reason for this is that once the other person in the conflict feels really listened to, he/she will likely start to feel calmer, and is going to be more likely and able to, in turn, listen to your needs and concerns, which paves the way for a satisfactory resolution.

7. Protocol for Effective Patient Communication

The same general format outlined above, i.e., awareness-raising discussion that elicits real-life examples, introduction to three basic skills using role-plays, and keeping to a roughly 1.5 h session, can be used for training in communication with doctors. Stating one's needs clearly is the central focus of the training. Doing so along with asking questions appears central to good communicative encounters with doctors, resulting in more information being provided about diagnosis, medical procedures, and treatment options (Herzlinger, 1997; Street, 1991). Such self-expression, however, may feel particularly difficult for older adults (Adler et al., 1998; Beisecker, 1996; Levkoff et al., 1988). Because of this, the three skills we describe for promoting good communication with doctors center on stating needs and asking questions (see Deutsch, 1973, 1994; Gordon, 1997; Karp, 1994). We will define these skills in language that can be incorporated directly into trainings.

"I" statements involve expressing your needs and concerns clearly to the doctor. It is critical to focus on what *you* need or what *you* are concerned about, and not extraneous issues. One of the best ways to do this is to state clearly what your medical concerns are (symptoms, problems, etc.). Examples of "I" statements are "I am having pain in my foot" or "I don't like the side effects of my medication" (rather than "you made me sick with that medicine"). "I" statements in which you clearly state your medical concerns are usually easy.

Another type of "I" statement that is very important during doctor's visits is stating when you do not understand something your doctor has said, e.g., saying "I don't understand what you said about the cause of my back pain," which can be more effective then a more challenging statement such as "you're not making sense" or a more general comment such as "I don't understand." It is also very important to use "I" statements when you feel the doctor has not really listened to your concerns by saying, e.g., "I don't feel you understood what I said about how I felt," and then explaining your concerns again.

Although "I" statements may seem simple, many of us are uncomfortable telling doctors when we do not understand something he/she said. We also may feel uncomfortable telling doctors when we do not feel that he/she understood what we said. Focusing on your own concerns can help you to avoid sounding like you are blaming the doctor if you think he/she has not fully understood or listened to you, and thus make the conversation more comfortable for both you and the doctor. The more a person practices both types of "I" statements, the more comfortable he/she will be at using them during doctor's visits.

Active listening in the doctor–patient interaction is mainly listening carefully to what your doctor has said to you about your condition, so that you gain all the information that you need to make treatment decisions. One of the best ways to do this is by asking as many questions as you need, and then summarizing the doctor's responses by repeating back what you think the doctor has said. This ensures that you really understand what he/she is saying, and are not confused. Asking questions is key to active listening during visits with the doctor. Do not be afraid to "bother" your doctor with questions. In order to be well, you need to understand your condition and how it can be treated.

Brainstorming is working collaboratively with your doctor to come up with a treatment plan that is satisfactory to both you and the doctor. You can do this by asking the doctor what your treatment options are, asking him/her what the pros and cons are of different treatments, and proposing ideas yourself about how to proceed with treatment. You and your doctor can then decide *together* what treatment plan is the most appropriate for you. Again, asking questions is essential to making good decisions about treatments.

8. Incorporating Contextual Factors

Since asking questions may feel particularly difficult for the older patient but is key to successfully patient–doctor communication, each of the skills emphasizes the use of questions. Understanding the importance of asking questions and *practicing doing so* may help older patients overcome inhibitions about question asking. Another step that addresses the issues of anxiety and age-related memory deficits that might impede the older patient's ability to obtain adequate information from doctors involves using written notes before and after the visit. The sequence of the training, then, might be as follows: (1) notes—discussing the importance of writing down one or two main symptoms/questions to discuss with the doctor. The use of a prepared list of questions has been shown to reduce anxiety in older cancer patients (Brown, Butow, Dunn, & Tattersall, 2001); (2) training and practice in "I" statements, active listening, and brainstorming; and (3) notes—coming back to the subject of note taking, and now discussing the importance of writing down at the end of the visit new medication names, dosages, and reasons for usage.

Incorporating into the discussion other helpful strategies to minimize anxiety and enhance retention of information can be helpful. These include bringing along a friend or family member to assist in asking questions, to help in remembering treatment advice, and to possibly help with taking notes. Another helpful strategy is encouraging the older patient to make follow-up phone calls to the doctor to get further information or clarify issues.

9. Summary

In presenting these approaches to training older adults in effective communication during interpersonal conflict and during doctor visits, we have emphasized the contextual factors that may shape older adults' communicative experiences in both domains. It is our belief that context, including the social context in which such communicative encounters occur, can exert a powerful influence on the course of communication (Deutsch, 1994; Krauss & Morsella, 2000). In most social situations, individuals carry an implicit set of norms for appropriate behavior. It can be important in developing a communication skills training program for a particular group to identify the social norms that may be influencing behavior in different settings. For example, one's beliefs about the social acceptability of questioning an authority figure, such as a doctor, may influence one's behavior in that situation (Adler et al., 1998). Examining with a target group what the perceived norms are for a given situation, how malleable they may be, and how to achieve one's own communicative goals within that particular setting can make it more likely that the skills taught are the appropriate ones, and are going to be used in real life.

Further qualitative research on older adults' communications with doctors is needed. Very little applied work from the point of view of older adults has been done. In particular, there is little research that explores how cultural background and/or health condition, e.g., chronic or terminal, can shape communications of older adults with doctors. Also, because hearing and vision losses can contribute greatly to communication problems late in life, it seems important to consider ways to not only teach new concepts to older adults, but also to encourage them to maintain communicative abilities as visual and hearing impairments increase (see Worrall, Hickson, Barnett, & Yiu, 1998 for a program to address communicative disorders in older adults).

On a final note, it is well recognized in the field of aging research that certain types of cognition may decline with age, such as solving of abstract relations problems, memory tasks, or novel problems, and that certain types of cognition may remain stable or improve with age (Salthouse, 1998). As for the latter, these tend to pertain to tasks that are social in nature and/or in a domain that is so often used that competence is more a function of knowledge than of ability to solve novel problems (Salthouse, 1998; Sinnott, 1989). Combining this information with what we know about older adults' poorer outcomes due to ineffective communication suggests that older adults may actually be better able to integrate new skills for use in conflict and doctor–patient situations than their younger counterparts. Our evaluation research on the constructive conflict resolution protocol suggests, at a minimum, that older adults may be readily able to absorb such skills and related concepts (Weitzman, Hardaway, et al., in press). Further development and evaluation of programs in these areas can help determine more about the actual transfer of skills to real-life situations, and possibly about cognition in old age.

References

Adler, S., McGraw, S., & McKinlay, J. (1998). Patient assertiveness in ethnically diverse older women with breast cancer: Challenging stereotypes of the elderly. *Journal of Aging Studies, 12,* 331–350.

Backer, J. (1995). Perceived stressors of financially secure, community-residing older women. *Geriatric Nursing, 16,* 155–159.

Baddeley, A. (1986). *Working memory.* New York: Oxford University Press.

Beisecker, A. (1996). Older persons' medical encounters and their outcomes. *Research on Aging, 18,* 9–31.

Boyd, M., & Bywaters, P. (1999). Towards understanding women's decisions to cease HRT. *Journal of Advanced Nursing, 29,* 852–858.

Brown, R. (1965). *Social psychology.* New York: Free Press.

Brown, R., Butow, P., Dunn, S., & Tattersall, M. (2001). Promoting patient participation and shortening cancer consultation. *British Journal of Cancer, 85,* 1273–1279.

Burggraf, C., & Sillars, A. (1987). A critical examination of sex differences in marital communication. *Communication Monographs, 54,* 276–294.

Cahn, D. (Ed.) (1994). *Conflict in intimate relationships.* Hillsdale, NJ: Erlbaum.

Clarke, E. J., Preston, J., Raskin, J., & Bengston, V. (1999). Types of conflicts and tensions between older parents and adult children. *Gerontologist, 39,* 261–270.

Coleman, P. T. (2000). Intractable conflict. In M. Deutsch & P. Coleman (Eds.), *The handbook of conflict resolution* (pp. 428–449). San Francisco: Jossey-Bass.

Deutsch, M. (1973). *The resolution of conflict:*

constructive and destructive processes. New Haven: Yale University Press.

Deutsch, M. (1994). Constructive conflict resolution: principles, training, and research. *Journal of Social Issues, 50*(1), 13–32.

Deutsch, M. (2000). Cooperation and conflict. In M. Deutsch & P. Coleman (Eds.), *The handbook of conflict resolution* (pp. 21–40). San Francisco: Jossey-Bass.

Gastel, B. (1994). *Working with your older patient: A clinician's handbook.* Bethesda, MD: National Institute on Aging.

Gordon, T. (1997). *Leader effectiveness training.* New York: Bantam.

Greene, M. G., & Adelman, R. D. (1996). Psychosocial factors in older patients' medical encounters. *Research on Aging, 18,* 84–102.

Haber, D. (1999). *Health promotion and aging: Implications for health professionals.* New York: Springer.

Halpern, J. (1994). The sandwich generation: Conflicts between adult children and their aging parents. In D. Cahn (Ed.), *Conflict in personal relationships* (pp. 143–162). Hillsdale, NJ: Erlbaum.

Hartley, P. (1993). *Interpersonal communication.* London: Routledge.

Hayes, J. (1991). *Interpersonal skills.* New York: Harper Collins.

Henwood, K. L. (1995). Adult parent-child relationships: A view from feminist and discursive social psychology. In J. Nussbaum & J. Coupland (Eds.), *Handbook of communication and aging research* (pp. 167–184). Mahwah, NJ: Erlbaum.

Herzlinger, R. (1997). *Market driven health care.* New York: Addison-Wesley.

Hocking, L., & Koenig, H. (1995). Anxiety in medically ill older patients: A review and update. *International Journal of Psychiatry in Medicine, 25,* 221–238.

Jennings, J., Kamarck, T., Manuck, S., Everson, S., Kaplan, G., & Salonen, J. (1997). Aging or disease? Cardiovascular reactivity in Finnish men over the middle years. *Psychology and Aging, 12,* 225–238.

Johns Hopkins Medical (1996, January). *Johns Hopkins Medical letter: Health after 50. Protecting yourself against prescription errors.* Baltimore, MD: Johns Hopkins Medical.

Kaplan, S., Greenfield, S., & Ware, J. E. (1989). Assessing the effects of physician-patient interactions on the outcomes of chronic disease. *Medical Care, 27,* sll0–sl27.

Karp, F. (Ed.) (1994). *Talking with your doctor: A guide for older people.* Bethesda, MD: NIH.

Krauss, R., & Morsella, E. (2000). Communication and conflict. In M. Deutsch & P. Coleman (Eds.), *The handbook of conflict resolution* (pp. 131–143). San Francisco: Jossey-Bass.

Levkoff, S., Cleary, P., Wetle, T., & Besdine, R. (1988). Illness behavior in the aged. *Journal of the American Geriatrics Society, 36,* 622–629.

Levkoff, S., Levy, B., & Weitzman, P. F. (1999). The role of ethnicity and religion in the help seeking of family caregivers to dementia-affected elders. *Journal of Cross-Cultural Gerontology, 14,* 335–356.

McCann, C. D., & Higgins, E. T. (1984). Individual differences in communication. In H. Sypher & J. Applegate(Eds.), *Communication by children and adults* (pp. 172–210). Beverly Hills: Sage Publications.

Minick, P., & Gueldner, S. H. (1995). Patterns of conflict and anger in women sixty years and older. *Journal of Women and Aging, 7,* 71–84.

National Center for Health Statistics (1995). Current estimates from the National Health Interview Survey: US 1994. *Vital and health statistics, series 10,* no. 193.

National Eldercare Institute (1996). *Senior centers in America.* Washington, DC: National Eldercare Institute.

Opotow, S. (1991). Adolescent peer conflicts: duplications for students and for schools. *Education and Urban Society, 23*(4), 416–441.

Park, D., Morrell, R., & Shifren, K. (1999). *Processing medical information in aging patients: Cognitive and human factors perspectives.* Mahwah, NJ: Erlbaum.

Pearlin, L. I., Mullan, J., Semple, S., & Skaff, M. (1990). Caregiving and the stress process: An overview of concepts and their measures. *Gerontologist, 30,* 583–594.

Roter, D. (1977). Patient participation in the patient–provider interaction: The effects of patient question asking on the quality of interaction, satisfaction, and compliance. *Health Education Monographs, 5,* 288–311.

Ruscin, J., & Semla, T. (1996). Assessment of medication management skills in older outpatients. *Annals of Pharmacotherapy, 30,* 1083–1088.

Salthouse, T. A. (1998). Cognitive and information-processing perspectives on aging. In I. Nordhus, G. VandenBos, S. Berg, & P. Fromholt (Eds.), *Clinical geropsychology* (pp. 49–59). Washington, DC: APA.

Sandy, S., Boardman, S., & Deutsch, M. (2000). Personality and conflict. In M. Deutsch & P. Coleman (Eds.), *The handbook of conflict resolution* (pp. 289–315). San Francisco: Jossey-Bass.

Shapiro, D., Boggs, S., Rodrigue, J., Urry, H., Algina, J., Hellman, R., & Ewen, F. (1997). Stage II breast cancer: Differences between 4 coping patterns in side effects during adjuvant chemotherapy. *Journal of Psychosomatic Research, 43,* 143–157.

Sillars, A. L., Wilmot, W., & Hocker, J. C. (1993). Communicating strategically in conflict and mediation. In J. Wiemann & J. Daly (Eds.), *Communicating strategically* (pp. 24–32). Hillsdale, NJ: Erlbaum.

Sinnott, J. (1989). *Everyday problem solving: theory and applications.* New York: Praeger.

Steptoe, A., Moses, J., & Edwards, S. (1990). Age-related differences in cardiovascular reactions to mental stress tests in women. *Health Psychology, 9,* 18–34.

Steptoe, A., Fieldman, G., Evans, O., & Perry, L. (1996). Cardiovascular risk and responsivity to mental stress: The influence of age, gender, and risk factors. *Journal of Cardiovascular Risk, 3,* 83–93.

Street, R. (1991). Information-giving in medical consultations: The influence of patients' communicative styles and personal characteristics. *Social Science and Medicine, 32,* 541–548.

Uchino, B., Uno, D., Holt-Lunstad, J., & Flinders, J. (1999). Age-related differences in cardiovascular reactivity during acute psychological stress in men and women. *Journal of Gerontology: Psychological Sciences, 54B,* 339–346.

Weitzman, P. F., Dunigan, R., Hawkins, R., Weitzman, E., & Levkoff, S. (in press). Everyday sources of conflict and stress among older African American women. *Journal of Ethnic and Cultural Diversity in Social Work.*

Weitzman, P. F., Hardaway, C, Smakowski, P., Weitzman, E., & Levkoff, S. (in press). A constructive conflict resolution training protocol for older African American women. *Gerontology and Geriatrics Education.*

Weitzman, P. F., & Weitzman, E. (2000). Interpersonal negotiation strategies in a sample of older women. *Journal of Clinical Geropsychology, 6,* 41–51.

Weitzman, P. F., Weitzman, E., & Levkoff, S. E. (2002). Interpersonal conflicts of women in nursing homes: An administrative perspective. *Journal of Clinical Geropsychology, 8,* 139–147.

Worrall, L., Hickson, L., Barnett, H., & Yiu, E. (1998). An evaluation of the Keep on Talking Program for maintaining communication skills in old age. *Educational Gerontology, 2,* 129–140.

Discussion Questions

1. How is the information presented in this chapter useful to students studying health communication?
2. Is it ethical to encourage patients to deviate from their cultural experiences or the behavior they believe is appropriate so that the patient may more effectively communicate in medical interactions? Explain your answer.
3. Do you believe it is necessary to provide the training described in this chapter to older adults? Explain. If so, who should be held responsible for providing this training? ✦

Chapter 10
Listening to Women's Narratives of Breast Cancer Treatment

A Feminist Approach to Patient Satisfaction With Physician-Patient Communication

Laura L. Ellingson and Patrice M. Buzzanell

Chapter 10 looks at the ways in which patients write of their experiences with cancer. Physician-patient communication is perhaps one of the most studied areas of health communication. However, it remains somewhat problematic. In this chapter, Laura Ellingson and Patrice Buzzanell examine women's stories of their breast cancer treatment and how they view satisfaction. This offers us not only a different perspective on what "good" physician-patient communication is, but also a new way of understanding what leads to patient satisfaction. This chapter bridges to the next part of the reader in which the focus of the patient-provider interactions shifts to the patient and the ways in which patients are changing the roles they take in relation to their providers.

Related Topics: cancer, culture, groups, health-care behaviors, media, patient-centered communication, patient-provider communication, patients' perspectives, qualitative methods, role of the patient, social support

Physician–patient communication has usually focused on interactions within a single episode, has been quantitative, has been studied using primarily medical students or residents in primary care practice, and has utilized a biomedical standpoint that privileges the experiences, perceptions, and power of the physician (Bennett & Irwin, 1997; Borges & Waitzkin, 1995; Gabbard-Alley, 1995; Mishler, 1984, 1986; Sharf, 1993; Vanderford, Jenks, & Sharf, 1997). In addition, research on physician–patient communication rarely has used biological sex or psychological gender as a central variable (Gabbard-Alley, 1995).

Our goal was to give voice to the experience of women breast cancer survivors, with the intention of modifying traditional concepts of patient satisfaction with physician–patient communication. K. A. Foss and Foss (1994) contended that "the information gathered about women's perceptions, meanings, and experiences cannot be understood within constructs and theories that were developed without a consideration of women's perspectives" (p. 39). As such, in order to rethink satisfaction, our study addressed gender by focusing on female breast cancer patients' experiences with female and male physicians. Our approach is not only consistent with feminist research principles (e.g., Cook & Fonow, 1990; K. A. Foss, 1989; Nielsen, 1990; Reinharz, 1992) but is also aligned with current health care trends toward "patient-centered" health communication research (Bennett & Irwin, 1997; Vanderford et al., 1997). Patient-centered approaches position the patient as an active part of the health care team rather than as a complex problem to be solved by those with knowledge and power. To study patients' experiences in their own words, we asked breast cancer patients to tell stories about

From "Listening to Women's Narratives of Breast Cancer Treatment: A Feminist Approach to Patient Satisfaction With Physician-Patient Communication," Laura L. Ellingson and Patrice M. Buzzanell, 1999, *Health Communication*, Vol. 11:2, pp. 153–183. Copyright © 1999 by Lawrence Erlbaum Associates, Inc. Reprinted by permission.

their interactions with health care providers and to describe satisfaction with physician–patient communication (North, 1996; Sandelowski, 1991).

Literature Review

There are numerous reasons why we would want to improve our understanding of physician–patient communication. More effective communication can be an end unto itself. Yet it can also be used to (a) elicit patient concerns, particularly on sensitive issues that patients find uncomfortable or difficult to discuss; (b) maximize patient satisfaction; (c) improve preventative medicine; (d) produce more accurate diagnoses; (e) increase patient compliance; (f) decrease malpractice suits; (g) enlist political support from patients in shaping federal medical policy decisions; and (h) create more professionally rewarding medical practices (Mann, 1998; Wyatt, 1991). An additional reason is to better understand women's perceptions, feelings, and beliefs about what they need in their physician–patient communication.

To enhance our understanding of women's medical experiences, we briefly summarize research on physician-patient communication, including patient satisfaction, and offer a critique of this research. Next, we describe the gendered nature of health communication, particularly as it affects female patients. We discuss how gender relations, or the ways in which women and men "do gender" that preserves asymmetrical power, can offer possibilities for creating more equitable interactions and expectations about patients' and physicians' identities and needs (see West & Zimmerman, 1987).

Physician–Patient Communication

Patient satisfaction, as a specific aspect of physician–patient communication, is of central concern to health communication researchers. Sharf (1993) stated that in medical encounter studies patient satisfaction had been researched more than other outcomes. Zastowny, Roghmann, and Hengst (1983) argued that "the prominence of concern with satisfaction has its roots in the premise that it is meaningfully and functionally related to specific health behaviors and other health attributes" (p. 296). Consistent with this premise, researchers have correlated patient satisfaction with: physicians' affiliative communicative style (Buller & Buller, 1987); compliance (Burgoon et al., 1987); interpersonal involvement of the physician and expressiveness (DiMatteo, Hays, & Prince, 1986; DiMatteo, Taranta, Friedman, & Prince, 1980; Hall, Roter, & Katz, 1988; Heath, 1984; Street & Wiemann, 1987); less control dominance by the physician (Cecil, 1998); information giving (Hall et al., 1988); perception of physicians' technical competence (Hall et al., 1988); partnership building (Hall et al., 1988); communication skills training for medical students (Evans, Stanley, & Burrows, 1992); and age of chronically ill patients (Linn & Greenfield, 1982).

Yet patient satisfaction can be difficult to study. It has been operationally defined in many different ways (Schneider & Tucker, 1992). Researchers often have proposed dimensions or aspects of satisfaction with the physician–patient interaction that then are assessed using scales in survey research. Some of these dimensions include affective, cognitive, and behavioral components (Burgoon et al., 1987; Cardello, Ray, & Pettey, 1995; Schneider & Tucker, 1992); physician's communicative style, affective tone, technical competence, and expressed interest (DiMatteo & Hays, 1980); art of care, technical quality, and efficacy (Linn & Greenfield, 1982); expressive and instrumental dimensions (Korsch & Alley, 1973; Korsch, Gozzi, & Francis, 1968); personal qualities, professional qualities, and competence of the physician and cost and convenience of services (Hulka, Zysanski, Cassel, & Thompson, 1971); access to care, continuity of care, availability of services, and physician conduct (Ware & Synder, 1975); general satisfaction via assessment of physicians and medical care and specific satisfaction via assessment of past experiences with regular source of care (Roghmann, Hengst, & Zastowny, 1979); and overall assessment of the medical visit, technical and interpersonal qualities of the doctor, completeness of services, and the length of office waiting time (Ware & Hays, 1988). As can be seen, the variety of components is broad, but a listing of dimensions does not present a core understanding of what patients mean by *communication satisfaction* as it emerges over time.

Specifically, most research has sought to measure rather than define satisfaction. Scales developed by various researchers for the physician–patient communication context or adapted from other contexts for this use usually include different variables of satisfaction based on two to four primary dimensions of satisfaction. Then researchers attempt to correlate the dimensions with each other and with other factors such as patient compliance or return visits.[1]

These quantitative measures offer a valuable but limited view of a complex interaction (Borges & Waitzkin, 1995; Gabbard-Alley, 1995; Sharf, 1993). Rather than being able to address relationships over time between patients and providers, studies have centered primarily on interactions within a single episode (Sharf, 1993), with the concepts of effective communication and of patient satisfaction with physician–patient communication being intertwined. At present, most studies have not distinguished between communication that patients find effective and communication that patients find satisfying. *Effective* connotes a more pragmatic assessment, but the studies that focus on effective communication and its relation to patient satisfaction examine most of the same variables and use similar methods as those studies that examine satisfaction with communication (e.g., Burgoon et al., 1987; Street & Wiemann, 1987). Finally, most studies measure satisfaction with the medical visit in general rather than satisfaction with the communication experience between patient and physician. In this way, communication is positioned as just one dimension within an overall measure of satisfaction.

To understand how patients experience physician–patient communication, we asked the following research question (RQ):

> RQ1: How do patients conceptualize satisfaction with their physician–patient communication?

Gender and Physician–Patient Communication

In physician–patient communication, gender may shape the ways in which (a) both parties share personal information, (b) power dynamics favoring physicians are played out during interactions, and (c) bodily integrity is questioned and perhaps violated by disease or injury and subsequent treatment.[2] Bodily integrity is important in breast cancer treatment not only because breast cancer is central to women's sexuality and identity (Montini, 1996) but also because 70% of the risk in contracting this disease is related only to being a woman (Nechas & Foley, 1994).

Little research to date has emphasized the professional, social, institutional, and sociocultural contexts of physician–patient interaction; physician–patient interactions have been treated as generic and interchangeable across a wide assortment of circumstances (Borges & Waitzkin, 1995; S. Fisher, 1984; Gabbard-Alley, 1995; Sharf, 1993). Yet contextual matters are critical to understanding encounters between physicians and female patients. Gabbard-Alley's (1995) review of gender in health communication stressed the need to consider historical, social, and personal aspects of both physician and patient (e.g., economic level, race, education, gender).

In physician–patient communication we see the gendered politics of everyday life. Social control occurs as a subtle feature of the discourse between female patients and their doctors (Borges & Waitzkin, 1995). The physician "reflects, helps to sustain and reproduces the status quo and as such is political" (S. Fisher, 1984, p. 5). Because physicians rarely address gender roles and contexts, they have the effect of reinforcing them: "The patient–doctor encounter thus seldom elicits a critical analysis of troubling social patterns that affect women . . . Lacking a critical thrust, the ideologic impact of medical discourse helps reinforce women's gender roles as they are" (Borges & Waitzkin, 1995, p. 50). The power of the physician to make decisions and exercise authority over patients is part of this generally uncontested gendered construct. An asymmetrical relationship places the physician as the holder of knowledge, authority, activity, and dominance, whereas the patient is passive (Boston Women's Health Book Collective, 1984; S. Fisher, 1984, 1986; Todd, 1989). This power dynamic is exacerbated further when the doctor is a man and the patient is a woman, due to gender roles that ascribe a subordinate position to women in our society (Borges & Waitzkin, 1995; S. Fisher, 1984, 1986; Gabbard-Alley, 1995; Wood, 1997). Given the gendered nature of physician–patient communication, we ask:

RQ2: How might patients' conceptualizations of satisfaction with physician–patient communication be gendered?

Method

Research Participants

All research participants (*N* = 14) were diagnosed with breast cancer from 9 months to 7 years before this research project. Although all of the women had completed breast cancer treatment, they saw physicians, oncologists, radiologists, or surgeons between two and four times per year. Many took Tamoxifen (a drug designed to decrease chances of recurrence) or received long-term treatment, regular testing, or both.

Participants' ages ranged from 33 to 70 years. All were White and lower middle to middle middle class.[3] With one exception, all the women lived in a suburban or rural area in the midwestern United States. Twelve of the women currently were married, and 2 were divorced. Among research participants, four had finished high school and had some college level courses, two had completed a bachelor's degree, four had taken some master's level courses, three had taken some doctoral-level courses, and one had a Ph.D.

Procedures

First, we discuss the ways in which we gathered the data, including protocol development and research participant recruitment techniques. Next, we describe our data analytic techniques, including transcription procedures and narrative and thematic analyses.

There were two forms of data collection: interviews using a moderately structured interview protocol (see Stewart & Cash, 1991) and surveys requesting background information. The protocol consisted of four primary questions with probes. The first question requested a description of the physician, how he or she was selected, and the research participant's positive and negative feelings about the physician. The next three questions asked the participant to tell positive and negative stories and an imagined retelling of the negative stories. On completion of each interview, we administered a brief written questionnaire requesting demographic characteristics and any details that participants thought were important for data analyses. We refined our question wording in the protocol and survey after interviewing a female breast cancer survivor.

Next, the first author recruited research participants for this study by attending support groups for breast cancer survivors located throughout area hospitals and the American Cancer Society and by using a snowball approach (Reinharz, 1992; Vanderford et al., 1997). Six participants were recruited through support groups, and seven women were contacted through acquaintances. The final participant heard about our study through a mutual acquaintance and asked to participate. The first author conducted 13 interviews face-to-face in settings selected by participants and 1 interview over the phone for logistical reasons.

All interviews were audiorecorded for transcription, following participants' permission. Interviews lasted between 17 and 55 min, with an average interview time of about 30 min. In total, we collected 7 hr of audio tape that translated into 350 double-spaced pages using transcription guidelines developed by Waitzkin (1990). The Waitzkin system encourages researchers to represent sounds accurately (rather than correcting for grammar or clarity), which DeVault (1990) argued is essential in giving voice to women (see also Reinharz, 1992). The first author and two assistants transcribed interviews, then checked random selections of transcriptions against audiotapes for accuracy. Before data analyses, the first author compared all recordings with transcripts and failed to locate differences.

To analyze data, we employed both narrative and thematic analytic techniques. Narrative analyses allowed for "systematic study of personal experience and meaning: how events have been constructed by active subjects" (Riessman, 1993, p. 70; see also Sandelowski, 1991). We independently read transcripts for content and for narrative structure, including how the story was organized and how it fit within the participant's overall discussion through symbolic actions or meanings, sequences, character, and storytelling processes (Bertgen & Costermans, 1994; W. R. Fisher, 1987; M. M. Gergen, 1992; Riessman, 1993; Sandelowski, 1991).

Next, we independently isolated themes or common semantic issues, concerns, and phrases that emerged within and across participants' interviews. We conducted inductive analyses (Janesick, 1994) using Owen's (1984) three criteria for assessing themes: *recurrence* (same meaning, different wording), *repetition* (same wording), and *forcefulness* (nonverbal cues that stress or subordinate words or phrases). We discussed our preliminary findings and derived our results collaboratively. We enhanced accuracy and trustworthiness by audio-recording data, incorporating different researchers' interpretations, and utilizing interdisciplinary triangulation to broaden our understanding of patient communication satisfaction (see Janesick, 1994; Lincoln & Guba, 1985). We utilized Fitch's (1994) criteria for evaluating qualitative data and findings.

Results and Interpretations

This section is organized according to our two interrelated RQs: (a) How do patients conceptualize satisfaction with physician–patient communication? and (b) How are these conceptualizations of satisfaction with physician–patient communication gendered? In general, we found that women see patient satisfaction with physician–patient communication as a dynamic process designed to negotiate tensions and to serve specific communication functions. Three themes emerged: respect, caring, and reassurance of expertise. Two *root themes,* or underlying interactive processes, described the dynamics of patient satisfaction with physician–patient communication: dialogic of power and control and context of women's lives.[4] On examination of communication satisfaction themes and root themes, we found that two gendered processes—women's ways of knowing and feminine communication styles—form a backdrop for how themes, root themes, and interactions are negotiated into viable physician–patient relationships. Finally, women showed how they integrated these themes, root themes, and gendered communication patterns through storytelling.

Patients' Satisfaction With Physician–Patient Communication

This study focused on patient satisfaction with physician–patient communication specifically, rather than considering communication as one part of a larger context of patient satisfaction with health care. In contrast to traditional literature, our research participants did not express satisfaction with physician–patient communication as a list of specific behaviors, dimensions, or attitudes. Instead, they described satisfaction as a negotiated dialectical process of both needing to be cared for and of needing to be active participants in their treatment. Satisfaction emerged as an ongoing dynamic process through which the self and the physician–patient relationship were revised continuously. To address RQ1, three themes emerged as prominent over the course of physician-patient interactions: (a) respecting the patient as an intelligent and autonomous being, (b) caring about and for the patient as an individual, and (c) reassuring the patient of the physicians' expertise (see Table 10.1). However, describing these themes is insufficient for understanding patient satisfaction with physician–patient communication. Therefore, after we present the themes, we explore two root themes, or underlying dynamics, that enable patients (and physicians) to participate in and construct patient satisfaction with physician–patient communication: dialogic of power and control and contextualization.

Respect. Respecting the patient as an intelligent and autonomous human being means that patients perceive their physi-

Table 10.1
Themes in Conceptualization of Patient Satisfaction With Physician-Patient Communication

Theme	Description	Functions
Respect	Patient wants respect as an intelligent being who is capable of processing information and decision making.	To process information and to establish and maintain relationship.
Caring	Patient wants to be cared about as an individual, with specific needs and issues.	To establish and maintain relationship.
Reassurance of expertise	Patient wants physicians to be knowledgeable about the latest, "cutting-edge" research and to be exhaustive and thorough in use of tests and preventative measures.	To establish and maintain trust and to differentiate roles and tasks.

cians as (a) talking in a straightforward manner, (b) answering questions and providing information, and (c) displaying consideration of the patient's time (see Table 10.1). Almost all of the women commented that their physicians were straightforward, "up front," or both when giving information about patient diagnosis, prognosis, and treatment options. Participant F remarked that straightforwardness is comforting and even empowering: "she was just so calm and straightforward that . . . I felt like we can do this." Although straightforwardness implies the unadulterated truth, being "plainly stated" does not mean without a degree of hope. Participant D said that she wanted the "information" message but also wanted to have the alternative reading of the message reinforced when she explained that her physician "still gives you the truth . . . [but she says] so if 90 percent of the people have this happen, who's to say you're not in the 10 that's not." When alternative readings, optimistic messages, and possibilities are missing, patients notice and object to these omissions.

Straightforwardness should not be confused with extreme bluntness. Participant B felt that this straight talk could go too far, not only because possibilities and hope were missing but also because she felt that the physician should have anticipated how upsetting certain kinds of news, such as impending hair loss, would be to her. She wanted her physician to give her information that would help her to cope with the issue at hand. Some patients recognized that straightforwardness is negotiated and includes their right to tell the physician how much straight talk they want to receive at different points in their treatment. Participant C noted that it would be unfair to expect a physician to guess how much information she wanted and exactly how she would like the information presented. So she instructed her physician to only tell her positive news at first, but she then wanted her physician to not "sugar-coat" anything later in treatment.

Participants also noted that patient communication satisfaction includes a desire to have their questions answered with detailed information and to have written documents made available to them. When details are not given verbally, the effects are devastating. Participant D described the physical pain she experienced after her physician failed to offer (and she did not request) information about a specific treatment issue. After the needle biopsy, "he totally wrapped my breast in surgical tape. . . . And gave me no instructions . . . it really hurt . . . I took the tape off as soon as I could and ended up terribly, terribly bruised." For whatever reason, her physician did not check to make sure she had the necessary information. Miscommunication not only produced painful results for the patient but also was so detrimental to establishing a trusting relationship that she left this physician soon after she received her biopsy results. Besides oral messages, written information is considered "a sign that your physician thinks you're intelligent enough to be able to read" and be proactive in your own treatment (Participant E).

Besides straightforward talk and adequate information provision, a third aspect of respecting the patient is the recognition that the patient's time is valuable. Participants expressed the desire that if the physician's time was considered valuable, so should the patient's time be treated as equally valuable. Almost all the women commented either that they really appreciated not having to wait or that they felt prolonged waiting was very disrespectful. In other words, patients wanted acknowledgment that their lives outside of their cancer treatment were important.

To summarize, respecting the patient as an intelligent and autonomous human being is displayed through physicians' straightforward talk, responses to questions and information needs (without being asked), and consideration of the patient's time. Participants framed respecting as a negotiated, continually evolving process. The theme of respect was mentioned very often in all of the interviews, and participants stated their feelings and opinions about respect forcefully and in the same words (Owen, 1984). If patients perceived that respect was not part of the ongoing patient–physician relational dynamic, then patients left the relationship. Several patients considered issues of respect important enough to constitute a turning point, that is, "any event or occurrence that is associated with change in a relationship" (Baxter & Bullis, 1986, p. 470; see also Rawlins, 1992). Because of the frequency, forcefulness, repetition, recurrence, and reported ramifications of respect, we feel that respect must serve important functions in establishing and maintaining patients' communication satisfaction.

After revisiting the interview transcripts, we found that respect serves two primary functions: enabling information processing and facilitating physician–patient relationship building and maintenance (see Table 10.1). First, respecting the patient as an intelligent and autonomous human being plays an important role in helping the patient to process information and in letting the physician know when and how to share information. The three subthemes of respect aid in information processing by having a calming or comforting effect on the patient, making the situation seem more manageable, allaying patients' fears or concerns, and providing coping strategies (e.g., how to get antinausea drugs or a wig after hair loss) that can help the patient sort through options with her physician. If patients perceive that physicians do not respect them, then they can experience anger or resentment that can interfere with processing.

The second function of respect is to facilitate relational maintenance. The physician–patient relationship is vital to the patient's recovery. If the patient feels she is not respected by the physician, she may be unable to trust or to express her needs to the physician. Sensing physicians' respect helps ease the vulnerability the patients are experiencing by letting them know that their physicians see them as active participants in their own recovery.

Caring. Caring is the second process in patient satisfaction with physician–patient communication (see Table 10.1). Aspects of caring described by participants include (a) touching and other nonverbal behaviors beyond that required for examinations, (b) expressing concern verbally, (c) spending time with patients, (d) treating patients as persons rather than as problems to be solved or diseases to be eradicated, and (e) having a caring staff and hospitable office atmosphere.

Nonverbal cues, such as physical touch, are ways to demonstrate caring. Participant B was 8 months pregnant when her breast tumor was found. When asked what she liked best about her physician, she explained how much it meant to her to have him be close to her: "He gave me the biggest hug. . . . He softly said in my ear, you're going to be fine, we're going to take care of you. And all I could think of was, I love you! [laughs]." Besides touching, patients mentioned more eye contact so they would feel as though their physicians were talking to them instead of to their X-rays and charts (e.g., Participant F) as well as facial expressions (e.g., tears, sad expressions) showing patients that physicians cared about them when physicians told them of the diagnoses (e.g., Participant A).

Participants described verbal assurances as a second type of caring behavior. Participant B's physician offered both a comforting message ("You're going to be fine.") and a promise that "we're going to take care of you." Participant H explained how her physician verbally comforted her by providing a home phone number and messages that invited patients to tell her what was bothering them, indicating that she was willing to listen to and do something about her patients' concerns.

Participants also mentioned physicians' willingness to spend time speaking with patients in person and on the phone as a third form of caring. Several women expressed anger at having to communicate with their physicians via a nurse or receptionist; they wanted to be able to talk directly to their physician within a reasonable period of time. Participant E said that her physician could be reached "24 hours a day everyday." In addition to wanting physicians to return telephone calls, almost all participants mentioned that they wanted someone who took time to be with patients and did not appear rushed. Participant F contrasted her physician, who was "rushed," with the relaxed and friendly nurses at the clinic she went to for treatment as a way to explain caring.

In addition, Participant F brought in another important aspect of caring: being treated as an individual. She noted that the nurses asked her about her kids and husband and other aspects of her life, and she wished her physician would do the same. When the nurses asked her how she was, they treated her as a unique person rather than as a diseased body. The metaphor of friend was used by several of the research participants. Friends have a personal relationship; in a friendship each person is a unique individual who cares about another unique individual. No one could be friends with a disease or with an abstract problem. In contrast, when one doctor referred to her patients as "my ladies," Participant C felt that this phrase was patronizing and possibly dehumanizing.

Finally, several participants remarked about the positive impact of a caring staff, that is, nurses, receptionists, and other providers, who made a big difference in their visits with their physicians. Participant E used the metaphor of an extended family to describe the staff at the clinic where she saw her physician: "it's like a big extended family caring for you." The atmosphere provided by the caring and well-coordinated staff had a very positive effect on her. Participant G added that this same type of treatment made her feel special: "I mean they treated me like I was really really somebody special. And you know, they really did."

In sum, there are five caring behaviors identified by research participants. These caring behaviors work individually and together to communicate to the patient that the physician cares about her. The primary function of the caring theme is to enable relationship building. Wood (1997) explains that women's friendships are based on closeness through talking and sharing personal feelings and experiences. There is a "high level of responsiveness and caring in women's talk, which lends a therapeutic quality" to their friendships (Wood, 1997, pp. 222–223). When the physician acts in a caring manner consistent with a feminine experience of friendship, female patients tend to feel more satisfied with physician–patient communication.

Reassurance of expertise. A third and final theme in conceptualizations of patient satisfaction with physician–patient communication is the desire for reassurance of the doctor's expertise through cutting-edge, thorough, and individualized treatment. In addition to wanting their physicians to have cutting-edge knowledge, most participants stressed that they wanted their physicians to use this knowledge and expertise to "cover all the bases" in their treatment and follow-up care (see Table 10.1). Several participants pointed out that their physicians were affiliated with prestigious research institutions, were "leading breast cancer surgeons," or both. Participants H, B, and E said that they received recommendations from loved ones and friends to go to particular clinics or institutes for treatment. Participant E liked "the fact that he really seems to have done his homework and [that] he talks to you." Participant C mentioned board certification and knowledge that her physician was "in touch" with a research hospital as factors that reassured her that her physician was "on top of things." However, reassurance of expertise is more than patients' desire to have the "best" physician; it is also an ongoing assessment and assurance that the physician is dedicated to checking every possible medical angle for her (e.g., Participants B and C).

Several participants described reassurance of expertise as their belief that their physicians thought through alternatives and derived optimal individualized treatment. As a result, Participant D expressed her gratitude that her physician removed much of her need to worry through this thoroughness. She trusted this physician with her life and felt secure that she was okay as long as her physician said so: "She'll say, I'm paranoid. . . . That's just how I want you [physician] to be. You be paranoid, I'll just live my life." This trust was based on a combination of her physician's cutting-edge knowledge of "all the tests" and her willingness to "use all of them" to detect anything amiss.

Reassurance of expertise serves functions of role differentiation, task allocation, and trust in the physician (see Table 10.1). These women envisioned their roles as equal, but not identical to, their physicians' roles. They relied on the medical practitioner to be on the cutting edge, to know all the options, and to be able to communicate them. The woman's role was to get through the treatment, to make assisted decisions, and to take care of herself and the rest of her life. When the patient wants her physician to cover all bases and to explain all options (but know the best one), she is asking him or her to communicate expertise. Through information sharing, the patient develops expertise herself and can feel comfortable placing trust in her physician.

Root Themes

In response to RQ1, we found that simply identifying the three themes of respecting, caring, and reassuring patients of expertise was insufficient for understanding how the patients conceptualized their satisfaction with physician–patient communication. Although these themes always were present in each woman's stories, the themes operated differently for individual women and became more or less salient at different times in their cancer treatment. To understand these processes, we derived two root themes, or underlying dynamics: (a) dialogic of power and control within the physician–patient relationship and (b) contextualization (see Table 10.2).

Dialogic processes of power and control. The themes of respecting, caring, and reassuring expertise coalesce in a struggle for power or control between physician and patient. Patient satisfaction is the ongoing process of managing this dynamic relationship during changing circumstances, including a great deal of stress. Baxter (1994; see also Baxter & Montgomery, 1996) described *dialogic processes,* a variation of dialectical theories, as relational maintenance in which contradictory tensions emerge throughout the history of a relationship. Each party or voice retains its uniqueness. At any moment, one or the other voice (e.g., patient or physician, ownership of body [ultimate decision making entity] or medical expertise) may emerge as dominant, or neither may be dominant. According to Rawlins (1992), a dialectical view of social processes involves totality, contradiction, motion, and praxis. There is interconnection and mutual influ-

Table 10.2
Root Themes in Conceptualization of Patient Satisfaction With Physician-Patient Communication

Root Theme	*Description*	*Functions*
Dialogic of power and control	Patients engage in a dynamic process of continual renegotiation of power with their physicians as their treatment, health, emotions, and knowledge evolve during the physician–patient relationship.	To make decisions.
Contextualization	Patients see the context of their lives (e.g., children, husband, work, friends) as intimately connected to themselves, their treatment, and their recovery.	To enable them to cope with the disease and to establish and maintain relationships.

ence by which patients (and physicians) actively choose among possibilities (e.g., treatment, relational issues).

In the physician–patient relationship, the tension is between the need to surrender decision-making power to the physician and, at the same time, to retain control over treatment decisions. The process of continually negotiating a balance between retaining and sharing control with the physician is crucial to patient communication satisfaction. When control is shared, participants feel as though they are in partnerships, that they know why actions are taken or decisions made, and that they are treated as unique, intelligent, full human beings. For breast cancer patients, retaining control and utilizing support groups are associated with survival (Keeley, 1996).

This framing of patient satisfaction with physician–patient communication as being a change-driven, tension-balancing process is quite different from traditional definitions of patient satisfaction. Patient satisfaction definitions resemble our findings only insofar as both have similar components (e.g., physician's communication style, personal and professional qualities; DiMatteo & Hays, 1980; Hulka et al., 1971; Ware & Hays, 1988). Although patient satisfaction aspects seem similar to our themes, prior research has not explored patient communication satisfaction as a process of continually negotiating and changing tensions between the parties. Moreover, a dialogic approach is empowering, because it enables women not only to thrive in a medical climate that devalues the feminine but also to maintain their integrity as intelligent, capable, feeling women. Communication is the process whereby the tensions inherent in the physician–patient relationship are managed. At times, some themes are more prominent than others, but all are essential to the patient's satisfaction with physician-patient communication.

Contextualization. A second root theme is the ways in which the patients situated their treatment and recovery within the broader context of their lives (see Table 10.2). Treatment was not divorced from other aspects of these women's lives. Rather, patient satisfaction with physician–patient communication meant that physician interaction and treatment were integrated within and became inseparable from their "ordinary" lives. There are two primary ways in which patients integrated their physicians in their lives: (a) The women wanted their physicians to be able to identify with their life contexts, and (b) they wanted their physicians to respect their inclusion of their support systems (family and close friends) in their interactions with physicians.

Participants expressed the desire that their physicians identify with and understand their patients' lives. Rather than simply being known as individuals, participants wanted to connect with their physicians as whole, situated, fully contextualized persons. Participant B found the point of connection in the fact that she and her physician both had young children. For other patients, the notion that physicians might be able to imagine their own wives in breast cancer treatment enabled them to feel as though their physicians could empathize with and be sensitive to their experiences (e.g., Participant A's physician's wife had breast cancer). Knowing physicians before diagnoses and living in the same communities made patients, like Participant A, feel more comfortable.

A second aspect of context is inclusion of the patients' support systems. Participants commonly brought their husbands, mothers, sisters, and grown daughters with them to checkups and treatments not only to gather and record information but also to enable their physicians to envision their lives. When loved ones were asked to leave a discussion, women, such as Participant B, wanted their physicians to provide concrete reasons why they were asked to leave, to acknowledge patients' need for support, and to recognize the effect that this disease had on the patients' whole family so that physicians would see themselves as involved in "family treatment." Participant E appreciated her physician even more when this physician actually welcomed her husband and considered his presence to be an advantage, particularly in processing treatment information.

Contextualization functioned to enable these patients to continue their lives while coping with the disease, to deal with instrumental components of physician–patient communication, and to maintain relationships with physicians. By contextualizing the disease, treatment, and interaction with the physician into their lives, participants could make sense of their experiences and the implications of their disease and treatment for their relationships and for other aspects of their lives, or both. Feeling that physicians respect patients' support systems helps patients to cope with their recovery while maintaining other aspects of their lives. At the same time, patients can use important people in their lives to deal with instrumental components of physician–patient communication, that is, to help obtain and process information (e.g., Participant E). Finally, identification with and respect for patients' lives can improve the physician-patient relationship. Similarities (e.g., having young children) can make the patient feel closer to the physician, not unlike the ways similarity influences attraction processes (e.g., Berscheid & Walster, 1978).

Gendered Patient Satisfaction With Physician–Patient Communication

Our second RQ asked how patients' satisfaction with physician–patient communication might be gendered. We approached RQ2 by examining transcripts individually and together to see if a gendered pattern emerged. Specific gendered processes were not anticipated ahead of data analyses but emerged consistently in the women's stories. We found that there were two ways in which gender operated as a backdrop for patients' constructions of their interactions with physicians and for their conceptualizations of patient communication satisfaction: (a) gendered ways of knowing and (b) feminine communication styles (see Table 10.3).

First, because these women had different ways of knowing, learning, experiencing, and expressing their realties, there were differences in the ways they conceptualized patient satisfaction with physician–patient communication. Belenky, Clinchy, Goldberger, and Tarule (1986) developed five knowledge orientations that are characteristic of many women (and men): silence, received knowing, subjective knowing, procedural (connected and separate) knowing, and constructed knowing.[5] They explored how and why some women relied on external knowledge bases, such as expert opinion (silence and received knowing; e.g., Participant B), whereas others utilized primarily "gut-level beliefs" or intuition (subjective knowing; e.g., Participant C), and still other women combined knowledge obtained from multiple sources when making decisions. Ways of knowing shift throughout lives and within and across contexts and cultures (Goldberger, 1997).

Although we found evidence for all of the knowledge orientations, most of our breast cancer patients fit within Belenky et al.'s (1986) construct of procedural knowledge, whereby they placed a great deal of faith in medical authority but also saw themselves as capable of processing information and making decisions with their physicians, Most of our respondents, when they found themselves feeling silenced by their physicians, disengaged from the physician–patient relationship and developed relation-

Table 10.3
Gendered Communication and Storytelling Processes

Process	*Description*	*Function*
Ways of knowing	Patients want concrete examples and reasoning: Patients use a combination of subjective, expert, and connected knowing—women's style of talk.	To provide backdrop for interaction.
Feminine communication style	Talk generally involved emphasis on equality, relationships, support for others, and concrete details.	To provide backdrop for interaction.
Unfolding structure	Participants' stories are richly detailed, not plot related, but unfolding, tangential, relational, and emotional.	To make sense of their experiences and to contextualize their experiences.

ships with other physicians. For example, Participant D decided to leave her physician after her biopsy but feared possible retaliation if she told the physician her intentions right away. She felt that if she voiced her displeasure, she risked punishment.

A few women, such as Participant E, processed their physician–patient interactions and communication satisfaction at the constructed level of knowledge in which they acted as authorities, and they drew on physicians and other experts to help them construct treatment that was right for them. They worked with their physicians to decide among various options available for treatment, not doubting their ability to know and understand but placing a lot of faith in their physicians' studies and test results. Participant G expressed her trust in her physician: "When I was sitting in the office, and I could hear him talking about things and that just, I really feel like he really knows what he's doing." She relied not only on rational or objective proof of his expertise but also on her personal evaluation of him, including an overheard telephone call that apparently made him sound credible and knowledgeable.

This openness to different approaches and the acknowledgment that there is no one right way for everyone was vital to Participant E's recovery. She saw herself, her physician, and a large number of other caregivers as creating knowledge. She had faith in her physician but also in herbal treatments, exercise, meditation, reading, and alternative therapies. She chose a physician who was willing to work with her in a holistic approach toward recovery. Here, the physician was not the expert but one authority on whom she could draw to help her construct knowledge.

In sum, what constituted satisfaction for each of these women was determined partly by their view of themselves as knowers and part[l]y by the relative trust they had in themselves as receivers, and possibly creators, of knowledge. Each woman negotiated communication satisfaction in her relationship with her physician according to her needs, identity, and epistemological viewpoint.

Feminine communication style. A second gendered aspect that emerges from the interview data is the use of a feminine communication style (see Table 10.3). The feminine communication style described by Wood (1997; see also Buzzanell, 1995; Tannen 1993, 1997) states that many women, but not all, share several speech patterns. First, talk is the primary way that most women create and maintain relationships. Prioritization of talk was displayed in our interviews when most participants stressed their desire to have physicians spend time talking with them. Participant D described how her physician "sat down with me and talked . . . mother, my husband, and myself, talked to all three of us. Um, for about 90 minutes without interruption." The process of talking as well as what they were talking about (i.e., giving the woman information about breast cancer and treatment options) helped Participant D feel more satisfied with her physician–patient communication. Several women expressed difficulty in forming a relationship with physicians who spent insufficient time talking to them and who instead gave verbal and nonverbal signals that they were not interested in talking with patients (e.g., avoiding eye contact, remaining standing).

Another aspect of talk that tends to be characteristic of women's communication style is the emphasis on showing support for others (Wood, 1997). Offering support involves hopeful and encouraging messages, indicating sympathy verbally and nonverbally (e.g., facial expression, touch), and providing examples of similar situations that the other has experienced to indicate understanding. Third, our respondents used a personal, concrete style including details, personal disclosure, anecdotes, and concrete reasoning. Participants described what prompted feelings of comfort and care from coffee in the waiting room to small talk with nurses and hugs from physicians. Participants disclosed personal aspects of their lives, such as the reactions of their children to their illness, how their body image was affected by the treatment, and how their husbands showed support for them. Anecdotes frequently were nested within answers to questions that provided as much insight into the woman's experience with breast cancer as did the information that related directly to the interview question. If a woman shares stories of her experiences with her physician and that physician attends to these details and, perhaps, reciprocates with some of his or her own anecdotes or stories, she is likely to feel a lot more satisfied with her physician's communication style.

A final aspect of a feminine style of talk is equality.[6] Equality is fostered through matching experiences to indicate that others are not alone in their experiences. The goal of equality lends itself to a "participatory mode of interaction in which communicators respond to and build upon each other's ideas" (Wood, 1997, p. 170). Our participants sought give and take in their conversations with their physicians. They expressed considerable satisfaction when they were encouraged to ask questions, bring up new topics, and relate personal experiences to their physicians rather when the physicians controlled the interaction.

In short, women's talk tends to have several patterns. The degree to which these patterns are associated with aspects of physician–patient communication seems to correspond with the satisfaction patients feel about their physicians' communication with them. These ways of communicating and knowing indicate how our breast cancer patients initiated, developed, and maintained relationships with their physicians. When these women were acting within a relationship with their physician that validated them and their experiences, they felt safe and grew in the ways in which they acquired, used, and created knowledge. The role of women's ways of knowing and talking was sometimes prominent, such as during the establishment of physician–patient relationships or during relational turning points. At other times, women's ways of knowing and talking were subtle aspects of the ongoing relational dynamics between physician and patient. As their relationships continued, many women experienced changes in how they negotiated satisfaction with physician–patient communication.

Structure in Women's Stories About Physician–Patient Communication

When we addressed RQ1, we found that an interplay of content (themes) and processes (root themes or underlying dynamics) described patient's satisfaction with physician–patient communication. For RQ2, we returned to our data and found that the women negotiated their communication satisfaction with physicians within women's ways of knowing and feminine communication styles. These themes, root processes, and gendered epistemologies and communication preferences addressed their conceptualizations of patient communication satisfaction. Yet these findings did not display how the women interwove their concerns, made treatment decisions with physicians (and others), and brought elements of their lives together so that they could integrate cancer treatment into the rest of their lives. As we again returned to our data, we found that how they told their stories was just as important as what they said.

M. M. Gergen (1992) proposed that "womanstories" are distinct from "manstories" in that womanstories reflect many women's propensity toward connected, nonlinear, "tangential" storytelling that reflects ambiguities about what is good and bad. Through womanstories, women converse about critical matters of identity and of relationship (Buzzanell, 1995), such as the ways breast cancer and treatment affect so many aspects of their lives. Hence, it is not just the product of singular or multiple retellings that provides insight into women's experiences with physician–patient communication; it is also the process of women speaking that reveals the meaning of their personal experiences. Our participants used unfolding or nested narratives to display structurally how satisfaction emerged for them throughout interactions with physicians.

Patients' stories were generally nonlinear, weaving many different subplots, themes, and characters together in a form that can be represented as unfolding rather than as conforming to the traditional construction of a linear, event focused narrative (e.g., "the epic quest;" M. M. Gergen, 1992; see also

Wood, 1994, 1997; see Table 10.3). Without being asked, participants included incredible detail, such as who was taking care of their children while they went to physician visits, which friends or family members they brought with them, and how they treated themselves to shopping and a frozen yogurt after each physician visit. This storytelling reflects many women's tendencies to incorporate various aspects of their lives into stories because they see aspects as closely related to each other and to their illness and recovery (see Gabbard-Alley, 1995; Sharf, 1993). For example, participant G responded to a request for a particular interaction with her physician by talking about how she wanted her physician to prescribe a higher dose of sleeping pills, then she veered off into her divorce and remarriage. The disease, unhappy marriage, and subsequent divorce and remarriage were linked for her in thought, speech, and daily life.

Another aspect of the unfolding structure is the use of a story to describe a person. The women, when asked to describe their physicians, told stories instead of listing characteristics. Participant F talked about the first time she met her physician and the physician joked with her about who (her husband or herself) found the lump. This story revealed the characteristics that the participant liked about her physician, such as a sense of humor, calmness, and easygoing or laid-back attitude. The remembered incident, just a brief part of her initial visit with a particular physician, was recalled when the woman was trying to put into words her feelings about her physician. It appears that telling the story better served her goals of describing the physician as a unique person than providing information in list form. Several other women told stories rather than providing lists of physical and psychological characteristics. It appears that they were more interested in concrete actions taken by physicians than in abstract characteristics.

Another way in which these women structured their stories was to jump immediately to the part of the story in which they were interested. Women tended to resist starting their narratives at the point suggested by the interviewer (i.e., preparing to leave home to go to a visit with their physicians), instead preferring to skip to the part that was meaningful for them. Interestingly, many stories not only were nonlinear in plot sequence but also had no discernible beginning or end. Very few of the women were interested in telling complete, step-by-step stories. For example, when Participant G presented an issue that she was upset about, that is, wanting a stronger prescription for sleeping pills, she described a part of a particular phone call and jumped to the resolution of the problem. Apparently, Participant G included only the aspects of the interaction that were relevant to the point she wanted to express.

In sum, participants' stories generally were richly detailed, nested or unfolding rather than following a linear plot, and focused on relationships and emotions. Unfolding structures enabled them not only to make sense of and to contextualize their experiences but also to formulate and present connections among ideas by integrating aspects of their life context into their stories. Because stories are not static, they cannot be evaluated for stability overtime (Sandelowski, 1991). Instead, they can be assessed by the ways stories perform other functions in people's lives. Narratives are ways in which people make sense of their experiences and create knowledge about self and others (Bochner & Ellis, 1995; Stivers, 1993) and are key to conceptualization of self and everyday life (K. J. Gergen & M. M. Gergen, 1988). Stories tell others what is significant in our lives, as well as how we revise our understandings of ourselves, others, and our experiences. The stories that the gendered self tells differ across context and time (Bochner & Ellis, 1995; Brison, 1997; Charon, 1989; North, 1996; Sandelowski, 1991); stories are revised repeatedly to express themes central to one's self, such as patient satisfaction with physician–patient communication.

Discussion

The purpose of our study was to examine the concept of patient satisfaction with physician–patient communication by using women's stories about their breast cancer treatment. We posed two interrelated RQs: (a) How do women conceptualize satisfaction with physician–patient communication?, and (b) How are these conceptualizations gendered? In general, patients experienced communication satisfaction as a dynamic, ongoing negotiation process with their physicians. Three themes emerged within and across interviews: respecting the patient as an intelligent, autonomous human being; caring about patients as unique individuals; and reassuring patients of medical expertise. Two root themes operated as underlying processes by which the three themes became more or less prominent over the course of the physician-patient relationship: (a) dialogic of power and control and (b) contextualization. Furthermore, how patients conceptualized satisfaction was linked to their epistemologies and to feminine communication styles. They displayed these themes, root themes, and gendered ways of knowing and talking in an unfolding structure of their cancer treatment narratives.

Our findings diverge from results of traditional physician–patient communication satisfaction research in several ways. First, our findings focus on women and their experiences, whereas traditional research either has focused on men or has ignored gender. Second, our study is grounded in women's descriptions and stories of their communicative experiences with their physicians, whereas traditional research has used quantitative instruments to measure communication, satisfaction, and effectiveness variables. Third, our goal was to understand women's experiences, whereas the aim of most traditional studies has been behavioral prediction. Overall, we found that women develop patient communication satisfaction as an ongoing relational process with their physicians in a relationship marked by power imbalances and initiated by a life-threatening and potentially disfiguring disease. Their gendered discourse and narrative structure display their ongoing struggles for respect, care, and reassurance in interactions with physicians. In sum, our research used a different and fruitful approach to patient communication satisfaction.

However, our study had two main limitations, namely, sample homogeneity and a relatively small number of research participants. Our findings reflect the perspectives of some White, middle-class, female cancer patients in the United States. Men and women from other racial or ethnic groups, sexual or social orientations, and socioeconomic backgrounds, and with different forms of cancer (or other illnesses) and ways of knowing, may experience and express patient satisfaction with physician–patient communication differently (e.g., Goldberger, Tarule, Clinchy, & Belenky, 1996; Wood, 1996). Our findings do provide descriptive information about a group generally underrepresented in scholarly health communication research (i.e., women) as well as possible directions for further research and practice.

Certainly, our understandings of patient satisfaction with physician–patient communication would benefit from larger and more diverse samples, including consideration of health insurance coverage and of patients' (and family members' or friends') prior long- and short-term interactions with health care providers. Moreover, research designed specifically to examine contextual and interactional relational dialectics (Rawlins, 1992), relational turning points (e.g., Baxter & Bullis, 1986), and strategic responses to relational contradictions (Baxter, 1988, 1990) would enable researchers to diverge from static notions and dimensions of patient satisfaction with physician-patient communication. How these dialectical tensions emerge throughout the course of cancer treatment could provide direction for oncologists, pain management specialists, and others to engage in communication that would be more satisfying for both parties. They also could enable physicians to communicate more effectively with patients (see Mann, 1998). Future research should address the ways female (and male) patients manage these tensions in same-sex and cross-sex physician–patient interactions. Furthermore, sensitivity to these and other tensions (e.g., cultural and economic differences) in physician–patient relationships could assist researchers and practitioners in finding more effective ways of encouraging preventive care and treatment of breast cancer (and other diseases), particularly in women of color who historically have lower treatment and survival rates (Anders, 1997; Kahl & Lawrence-Bauer, 1996; Keeley, 1996; Lagnado, 1997).

Finally, pragmatic implications from our study reside in the main finding that these women wanted to be treated as intelligent and unique persons with lives and relationships of their own that were inherently valuable. Integration of details and context of patients' (and physicians') lives helped these women maintain dignity and satisfying relationships with physicians and others under life-threatening conditions. Just as their stories wove together many aspects of their lives and identities, so should their cancer treatment.

Acknowledgments

This article is based on Laura L. Ellingson's master's thesis, completed under the direction of Patrice M. Buzzanell at Northern Illinois University in Spring 1997. We thank Martha Cooper, Kathleen Propp, Steve Wilson, Glenn Ellingson, Vicki Pasch, and the remarkable women who participated in this study.

Notes

1. Many different scales have been used to obtain quantitative measures of satisfaction. Buller and Buller (1987) used an adapted version of Hecht's (1978) 16-item Interpersonal Communication Satisfaction Scale. Cardello et al. (1995) measured patient satisfaction with the Medical Interview Satisfaction Scale that was developed by Wolf, Putnam, James, and Stiles (1978). Street and Wiemann (1988) measured patient satisfaction using the Personal Qualities subscale of Zysanski, Hulka, and Cassel's (1974) Medical Care Satisfaction Measure. Ware and Hays (1988) designed the Visit-Specific Satisfaction Questionnaire; Linder-Pelz and Struening (1985) developed the Patient Satisfaction Scale. All of these Likert-type scales have been found to be reliable and valid, and most continue to be used in research.
2. There is evidence that women tend to be more verbal than men in interactions with physicians, that women spend more time than men interacting with physicians, and that physicians take women's concerns less seriously than men's (Gabbard-Alley, 1995). A meta-analysis of 41 studies on doctor-patient interaction found that more information was given to female patients (Hall et al., 1988). However, women's own experiences, concerns, and language are largely missing from current research.
3. The racial and relative class homogeneity of our participants was an unintentional result of our sampling techniques. We recruited participants from local support groups made up entirely of White women. Likewise, our snowball technique yielded White middle-class participants.
4. Our processual themes of respect, caring, and reassurance are recurring ideas and ways of describing people and interactions that are derived directly from talk. Themes differ from images, schemas, and frames-reframing processes because of their direct grounding in language choices (see Buzzanell & Burrell, 1997, for distinctions). We use the term *root themes* to represent the underlying communicative dynamics by which participants connect and use themes differently as physician-patient relationships and contexts change. Root themes embody patients' life situations, reasoning, and dialectic structuring as derived from and underlying what they say. For instance, we can not interpret the theme of respect without also looking at the dialogical nature of the physician-patient relationship or the importance of the context of the women's lives.
5. Belenky et al. (1986; see also Goldberger, 1997) described five ways of knowing. In *silence,* women and men feel powerless and voiceless. People who employ *received* knowing expect to learn from perceived omniscient authority and knowledge figures, whereas those who experience *subjective* knowing base knowledge on feelings and intuition, rather than on evidence and thought. In *procedural* knowing, women and men utilize techniques for gaining and evaluating claims; *separate* procedural knowers use a skeptical, "reasoning against" approach and *connected* procedural knowers use an empathic, "reasoning with" approach. Finally, *constructed* knowers understand knowledge as tentative, situated, and socially constructed. Each way of these five main ways of knowing is neither better nor worse than others, just different.

6. One of our reviewers suggested that the term *reciprocity,* as used by Rosenfield, Hayes, and Frentz (1976), better captures the ways in which our respondents matched experiences conversationally. Although *reciprocity* more accurately represents the mutual give-and-take (Rosenfield et al., 1976, p. 74) aspects of our respondents' interactions with physicians, reciprocity often occurs in conversations between people of unequal status. There are degrees of reciprocity from practically none, in which one does almost all the giving and another virtually all the taking, to considerable, in which both give and take equally (Rosenfield et al., 1976). We chose *equality* because our participants expressed their satisfaction with physician–patient communication that enabled them to feel that they were equal contributors to the exchange with a degree of power equal to that held by the physician (Wood, 1997; see also S. K. Foss & Griffin, 1995). Given that traditional medical settings place patients in a passive and powerless role that is further exacerbated when the physician is male and the patient is female (Borges & Waitzkin, 1995; S. Fisher, 1984, 1986; Gabbard-Alley, 1995), the notion of equality best reflects the meaning conveyed by our research participants.

References

Anders, G. (1997, September 4). Doctors learn to bridge cultural gaps. *Wall Street Journal,* pp. B1–B2.

Baxter, L. A. (1988). A dialectical perspective on communication strategies in relationship development. In S. W. Duck (Ed.), *A handbook of personal relationships* (pp. 257–273). New York: Wiley.

Baxter, L. A. (1990). Dialectical contradictions in relationship development. *Journal of Social and Personal Relationships, 7,* 69–88.

Baxter, L. A. (1994). A dialogic approach to relational maintenance. In D. Canary & L. Stafford (Eds.), *Communication and relational maintenance* (pp. 233–254). New York: Academic,

Baxter, L. A., & Bullis, C. (1986). Turning points in developing romantic relationships. *Human Communication Research, 12,* 469–493.

Baxter, L. A., & Montgomery, B. M. (1996). *Relating: Dialogues and dialectics.* New York: Guilford.

Belenky, M. F., Clinchy, B. M., Goldberger, N. R., & Tarule, J. M. (1986). *Women's ways of knowing: The development of self, voice, and mind.* New York: Basic Books.

Bennett, K. C., & Irwin, H. (1997). Shifting the emphasis to "patient as central": Sea change or ripple on the pond? *Health Communication, 9,* 83–93.

Berscheid, E., & Walster, E. H. (1978). *Interpersonal attraction* (2nd ed.). Reading, MA: Addison-Wesley.

Bertgen, Y., & Costermans, J. (1994). Time, space, and action: Exploring the narrative structure and its linguistic marking. *Discourse Processes, 17,* 421–446.

Bochner, A. P., & Ellis, C. (1995). Telling and living: Narrative co-construction and the practices of interpersonal relationships. In W. Leeds-Hurwitz (Ed.), *Social approaches to communication* (pp. 201–216). New York: Guilford.

Borges, S., & Waitzkin, H. (1995). Women's narratives in primary medical care encounters. *Women and Health, 23,* 29–56.

Boston Women's Health Book Collective. (1984). *The new our bodies, ourselves.* New York: Simon & Schuster.

Brison, S. J. (1997). Outliving oneself: Trauma, memory, and personal identity. In D. T. Meyers (Ed.), *Feminists rethink the self* (pp. 12–39). Boulder, CO: Westview.

Buller, M. K., & Buller, D. B. (1987). Physicians' communication style and patient satisfaction. *Journal of Health and Social Behavior, 28,* 375–388.

Burgoon, J. K., Pfau, M., Parrott, R., Birk, T., Coker, R., & Burgoon, M. (1987). Relational communication, satisfaction, compliance-gaining strategies, and compliance in communication between physicians and patients. *Communication Monographs, 54,* 307–324.

Buzzanell, P. M. (1995, May). *The telling of women's life experiences: Conversational functions of women's metaphoric language.* Paper presented at the annual International Communication Association Convention, Albuquerque, NM.

Buzzanell, P. M., & Burrell, N. A. (1997). Family and workplace conflict: Examining metaphorical conflict schemas and expressions across context and sex. *Human Communication Research, 24,* 109–146.

Cardello, L. L., Ray, E. B., & Pettey, G. R. (1995). The relationship of perceived physician communicator style to patient satisfaction. *Communication Reports, 8,* 127–137.

Cecil, D. W, (1998). Relational control patterns in physician-patient clinical encounters: Continuing the conversation. *Health Communication, 10,* 125–149.

Charon, R. (1989). Doctor–patient/reader–writer: Learning to find the text. *Soundings, 72,* 137–151.

Cook, J. A., & Fonow, M. M. (1990). Knowledge and women's interests: Issues of epistemology and methodology in feminist sociological research. In J. M. Nielsen (Ed.), *Feminist research methods: Exemplary readings in the social sciences* (pp. 69–93). Boulder, CO: Westview.

DeVault, M. L. (1990). Talking and listening from women's standpoint: Feminist strategies for interviewing and analysis. *Social Problems, 37,* 96–116.

DiMatteo, M. R., & Hays, R. D. (1980). The significance of patients' perception of physician conduct. *Journal of Community Health, 6,* 18–19.

DiMatteo, M. R., Hays, R. D., & Prince, L. M. (1986). Relationship of physician's nonverbal communication skill to patient satisfaction, appointment compliance, and physician workload. *Health Psychology, 5,* 581–594.

DiMatteo, M. R., Taranta, A., Friedman, H. S., & Prince, L. M. (1980). Predicting satisfaction from physician's nonverbal communication skills. *Medical Care, 18,* 376–387.

Evans, B. J., Stanley, R. O., & Burrows, G. D. (1992). Communication skills training and patients' satisfaction. *Health Communication, 4,* 155–170.

Fisher, S. (1984). Doctor–patient communication: A social and micro-political performance. *Sociology of Health and Illness, 6,* 1–29.

Fisher, S. (1986). *In the patient's best interest: Women and the politics of medical decisions.* New Brunswick, NJ: Rutgers University Press.

Fisher, W. R. (1987). *Human communication as narration: Toward a philosophy of reason, value, and action.* Columbia: University of South Carolina Press.

Fitch, K. L. (1994). Criteria for evidence in qualitative research. *Western Journal of Communication, 58,* 32–38.

Foss, K. A. (1989). Feminist scholarship in speech communication: Contributions and obstacles. *Women's Studies in Communication, 12,* 1–10.

Foss, K. A., & Foss, S. K. (1994). Personal experience as evidence in feminist scholarship. *Western Journal of Communication, 58,* 39–43.

Foss, S. K., & Griffin, C. L. (1995). Beyond persuasion: A proposal for an invitational rhetoric. *Communication Monographs, 62,* 2–18.

Gabbard-Alley, A. S. (1995). Health communication and gender: A review and critique. *Health Communication, 7,* 35–54.

Gergen, K. J., & Gergen, M. M. (1988). Narrative and the self as relationship. *Advances in Experimental Social Psychology, 21,* 17–56.

Gergen, M. M. (1992). Life stories: Pieces of a dream. In G. C. Rosenwald & R. L. Ochberg (Eds.), *Storied lives: The cultural politics of self-understanding* (pp. 127–144). New Haven, CT: Yale University Press.

Goldberger, N. (1997). Ways of knowing: Does gender matter? In M. R. Walsh (Ed.), *Women, men & gender: Ongoing debates* (pp. 252–260). New Haven, CT: Yale University Press.

Goldberger, N., Tarule, J., Clinchy, B., & Belenky, M. (1996). *Knowledge, difference, and power: Essays inspired by Women's Ways of Knowing.* New York: Basic Books.

Hall, J. A., Roter, D. L., & Katz, N. R. (1988). Meta-analysis of correlates of provider behavior in medical encounters. *Medical Care, 26,* 657–672.

Heath, C. (1984). Participation in the medical consultation: The coordination of verbal and nonverbal behavior between the doctor and patient. *Sociology of Health and Illness, 6,* 311–338.

Hecht, M. L. (1978). The conceptualization and measurement of interpersonal communication satisfaction. *Human Communication Research, 4,* 253–264.

Hulka, B. S., Zysanski, S. J., Cassel, J. C., & Thompson, S. J. (1971). Satisfaction with care in a low income population. *Journal of Chronic Disability, 25,* 661–678.

Janesick, V. J. (1994). The dance of qualitative research design: Metaphor, methodolatry, and meaning. In N. K. Denzin & Y. S. Lincoln (Eds.), *Handbook of qualitative research* (pp. 209–219). Thousand Oaks, CA: Sage.

Kahl, M. L. & Lawrence-Bauer, J. (1996). An analysis of discourse promoting mammography: Pain, promise, and prevention. In R. L. Parrott & C. M. Condit (Eds.), *Evaluating women's health messages: A resource book* (pp. 307–321). Thousand Oaks, CA: Sage.

Keeley, M. P. (1996). Social support and breast cancer: Why do we talk and to whom do we talk? In R. L. Parrott & C. M. Condit (Eds.), *Evaluating women's health messages: A resource book* (pp. 293–306). Thousand Oaks, CA: Sage.

Korsch, B. M., & Alley, E. F. (1973). Pediatric interviewing techniques. *Current Problems in Pediatrics, 3,* 3–9.

Korsch, B. M., Gozzi, E. K., & Francis, V. (1968). Gaps in doctor–patient communication. *Pediatrics, 42,* 855–871.

Lagnado, L. (1997, June 25). When racial sensitivities clash with research. *Wall Street Journal,* pp. B1, B6.

Lincoln, Y. S., & Guba, E. (1985). *Naturalistic inquiry.* Beverly Hills, CA: Sage.

Linder-Pelz, S., & Struening, E. L. (1985). The multidimensionality of patient satisfaction with a clinic visit. *Journal of Community Health, 10,* 42–54.

Linn, L. S., & Greenfield, S. (1982). Patient suffering and patient satisfaction among the chronically ill. *Medical Care, 20,* 425–431.

Mann, D. (1998, January 8). Doctors, patients need to talk more. *The Medical Tribune, Family Physician Edition,* pp. 1, 6.

Mishler, E. G. (1984). *The discourse of medicine: Dialectics of medical interviews.* Norwood, NJ: Ablex.

Mishler, E. G. (1986). *Research interviewing: Context and narrative.* Cambridge, MA: Harvard University Press.

Montini, T. (1996). Gender and emotion in the advocacy for breast cancer informed consent legislation. *Gender & Society, 10,* 9–23.

Nechas, E., & Foley, D. (1994). *Unequal treatment; What you don't know about how women are mistreated by the medical community.* New York: Simon & Schuster.

Nielsen, J. M. (1990). Introduction. In J. M. Nielsen (Ed.), *Feminist research methods: Exemplary readings in the social sciences* (pp. 1–37). Boulder, CO: Westview.

North, C. L. (1996, November). *Narratives as health communication research.* Paper presented at the 1996 Annual Speech Communication Association Conference, San Diego, CA.

Owen, W. F. (1984). Interpretive themes in relational communication. *Quarterly Journal of Speech, 70,* 274–287.

Rawlins, W. K. (1992). *Friendship matters: Communication, dialectics, and the life course.* New York: deGruyter.

Reinharz, S. (1992). *Feminist methods in social research.* New York: Oxford University Press.

Riessman, C. K. (1993). Qualitative research methods: Vol. 30. *Narrative analysis.* Newbury Park, CA: Sage.

Roghmann, K. J., Hengst, A., & Zastowny, T. R. (1979). Satisfaction with medical care: Its measurement and relation to utilization. *Medical Care, 17,* 461–479.

Rosenfield, L., Hayes, L., & Frentz, T. (1976). *The communicative experience.* Boston: Allyn & Bacon.

Sandelowski, M. (1991). Telling stories: Narrative approaches in qualitative research. *Image: The Journal of Nursing Scholarship, 23,* 161–166.

Schneider, D. E., & Tucker, R. K. (1992). Measuring satisfaction in doctor-patient relations: The doctor-patient communication inventory. *Health Communication, 4,* 19–28.

Sharf, B. F. (1993). Reading the vital signs: Research in health care communication. *Communication Monographs, 60,* 35–41.

Stewart, C. J., Jr., & Cash, W. B. (1991). *Interviewing: Principles and practices* (6th ed.). Dubuque, IA: Brown.

Stivers, C. (1993). Reflections of the role of personal narrative in social science. *Signs: Journal of Women in Culture and Society, 18,* 408–425.

Street, R. L., Jr., & Wiemann, J. M. (1987). Patient satisfaction with physicians' interpersonal involvement, expressiveness, and dominance. In M. L. McLaughlin (Ed.), *Communication Yearbook 10* (pp. 591–612). Newbury Park, CA: Sage.

Street, R. L., Jr., & Wiemann, J. M. (1988). Differences in how physicians and patients perceive physicians' relational communication. *The Southern Speech Communication Journal, 53,* 420–440.

Tannen, D. (1993). The relativity of linguistic strategies: Rethinking power and solidarity in gender and dominance. In D. Tannen (Ed.), *Gender and conversational interaction* (pp. 87–114). New York: Oxford University Press.

Tannen, D. (1997). Women and men talking: An interactional sociolinguistic approach. In M. R. Walsh (Ed.), *Women, men & gender: Ongoing debates* (pp. 82–90). New Haven, CT: Yale University Press.

Todd, A. D. (1989). *Intimate adversaries: Cultural conflict between doctors and woman patients.* Philadelphia: University of Pennsylvania Press.

Vanderford, M. L., Jenks, E. B., & Sharf, B. F. (1997). Exploring patients' experiences as a primary source of meaning. *Health Communication, 9,* 13–26.

Waitzkin, H. (1990). On studying the discourse of medical encounters: A critique of quantitative and qualitative methods and a proposal for reasonable compromise. *Medical Care, 28,* 473–487.

Ware, J. E., & Hays, R. D. (1988). Methods for measuring patient satisfaction with specific medical encounters. *Medical Care, 26,* 393–402.

Ware, J. E., & Synder, M. K. (1975). Dimensions of patient attitudes regarding doctors and medical care services. *Medical Care, 13,* 669–682.

West, C., & Zimmerman, D. H. (1987). Doing gender. *Gender & Society, 1,* 125–151.

Wolf, M. H., Putnam, S. M., James, S. A., & Stiles, W. B. (1978). The Medical Interview Satisfaction Scale: Development of a scale to measure patient perception of physician behavior. *Journal of Behavioral Medicine, 1,* 391–398.

Wood, J. T. (1994). Engendered identities: Shaping voice and mind through gender. In D. R. Vocate (Ed.), *Intrapersonal communication: Different voices, different minds* (pp. 145–167). Hillsdale, NJ: Lawrence Erlbaum Associates, Inc.

Wood, J. T. (Ed.). (1996). *Gendered relationships.* Mountain View, CA: Mayfield.

Wood, J. T. (1997). *Gendered lives: Communication, gender, and culture* (2nd ed.). Belmont, CA: Wadsworth.

Wyatt, N. (1991). Physician–patient relationships: What do doctors say? *Health Communication, 3,* 157–174.

Zastowny, T. R., Roghmann, K. J., & Hengst, A. (1983). Satisfaction with medical care: Replications and theoretical reevaluation. *Medical Care, 21,* 294–313.

Zysanski, S. J., Hulka, B. S., & Cassel, J. C. (1974). Scale for the measurement of "satisfaction" with medical care: Modifications in content, format, and scoring. *Medical Care, 13,* 611–620.

Discussion Questions

1. What does it mean to take a feminist approach to studying health communication? How does this approach differ from the biomedical approach?
2. How does gender influence health-care interactions and attitudes? What are the influences of gender on patient-provider interactions?
3. Ellingson and Buzzanell argue that dialogue between physicians and patients leads to greater satisfaction. What is meant by dialogue, and how does it differ from traditional interactions? How can dialogue be facilitated? ✦

Part III

THE CHANGING ROLE OF PATIENTS IN HEALTH CARE

Chapter 11
Reconceptualizing the 'Patient'

Health Care Promotion as Increasing Citizens' Decision-Making Competencies

Rajiv N. Rimal, Scott C. Ratzan, Paul Arntson, and Vicki S. Freimuth

Part III consists of three chapters that focus on the ways in which patients today are entering into interactions with health-care providers in more active and participatory roles. If the chapters in this section are read along with Parts II and Parts IV and V, the full scope of communication's role in breaking the barriers that often divide health-care providers from patients will be understood. These barriers place the providers in the expert role and patients in the role of the passive recipients of the experts' knowledge. Part III begins with Chapter 11, which discusses the traditional ways in which patients enacted their roles in health care and how, if at all, that is changing. The authors argue, in fact, that we should shift to a view of patients as "health citizens" and examine the broader physical, social, and mediated environments that influence our health. The authors' intent is to create health campaigns that are more effective and health citizens who are more actively involved in their own health care.

Related Topics: culture, ethical issues, groups, health campaigns, health-care behaviors, media, patient-centered communication, patient-provider communication, patients' perspectives, role of the patient, social support

In this article, we argue that our current understanding of "patient," which is based on unidirectional models of influence from health care providers to recipients, is inadequate for a broader conceptualization of health. We propose instead the use of "health citizen" to capture individual and collective group decision-making processes that are intimately connected with individuals' well-being. Traditional illness-centered models assume health professionals "know" what is in patients' best interests, and research questions center around factors that inhibit or promote rates of compliance. Communication, in this approach, is seen as a one-way flow of influence from the health professional to the patient.

Carey (1989) distinguished between the transmission (or instrumental) and ritual conceptualizations of communication. Although the approach just outlined can be classified as an instrumental model, one in which information "flows" from the source to the receiver (e.g., from the doctor to the patient) and one in which information is used as an instrument to bring about change (e.g., compliance), the ritualistic model defines *communication* as the symbolic exchange of meaning, one in which the emphasis is on interaction and participation more than on influence and persuasion. Communication, in this approach, is said to occur to the extent that interactants build on shared experiences and meaning.

The inadequacies of the instrumental model of communication in health have been pointed out elsewhere (see, e.g., Dervin, 1990). Primary criticisms of this line of work have centered around its neglect of the patient's perspective in health decision making. By holding the health professional's intentions and prescriptions in primacy, it relegates the patient's experience and interpretation to a secondary role and simultaneously ignores the multiple goals present in the physician-patient encounter, thus en-

From "Reconceptualizing the 'Patient': Health Care Promotion as Increasing Citizens' Decision-Making Competencies" Rajiv N. Rimal, Scott C. Ratzan, Paul Arntson, and Vicki S. Freimuth, 1997, *Health Communication*, Vol.9:1, pp. 61–74.

hancing the likelihood of misunderstanding and dissatisfaction (Sanders, 1991).

Recent thinking presents a much more dynamic role for both the provider as well as the consumer of health information (see, e.g., Ratzan, 1996). By replacing the term *patient* with more participatory terms such as the *health citizen* or *health decision maker* (Arntson, 1989), it recasts health as a wellness-centered phenomenon (Tinsley & Parke, 1984). By conceptualizing health as a multifaceted concept that includes biomedical, psychosocial, and environmental determinants (Jessor, 1993), a wellness-centered approach is adaptive to problems faced by the population in the latter half of this century, especially as it relates to chronic diseases (Ratzan, 1996), the leading cause of morbidity and mortality in the United States.

Public health efforts to combat the threat of chronic diseases concentrate on life-style factors that are amenable to change. Although some diseases have a strong genetic component, others are preventable with a behavioral change, which could prevent over two million deaths each year in the United States (*Healthy People 2000,* 1991). Many psychological theories that focus on both intra- and interpersonal processes have been utilized over the last few decades to enhance our understanding of and bring about a change in individuals' behaviors. Cognitively based approaches, such as the health belief model (Becker, 1974), protection motivation theory (Maddux & Rogers, 1983), elaboration likelihood model (Petty & Cacioppo, 1981), extended parallel processing model (Witte, 1994), stages of change model (Prochaska, 1979), and social cognitive theory (Bandura, 1986) have all contributed significantly in this process.

At the heart of these approaches is the assumption that health behaviors can be changed only to the extent that individuals are empowered with effective psychological tools that promote learning, some of which include enhanced perceptions of self-efficacy, greater knowledge and awareness of health issues, realistic appraisals of barriers, and positive attitudes toward healthier life-styles. Because the individual's well-being is at stake and health behaviors center around what individuals do, health promotion efforts, for the most part, have taken an individual-centered approach.

Whereas reliance on psychological processes to modify health behaviors have resulted in positive outcomes in diverse domains, many researchers have raised concerns that these approaches are too individual focused, that they disregard the powerful roles played by institutional forces in shaping individuals' health (Weinstein, 1987). Examples of such institutional forces include those connected directly with medical care facilities, including hospitals and public health departments, as well as others that indirectly impact individuals' health choices and behaviors, such as social service systems, immigration service, educational and legal institutions and so forth (Sharf & Kahler, 1996).

An exclusive focus on individuals places the onus of change on individuals and disregards the wider societal-level factors that may inhibit change (Salmon, 1989). By implication, those who do not practice healthy behaviors are perceived to be irresponsible, unmotivated, or incompetent. However, for a variety of reasons, health behaviors may not be amenable to individual change as long as structural and societal barriers persist. Without taking into account environmental constraints, we run the risk of "blaming the victim" (Minkler, 1978). In many urban settings, for example, indigent individuals may have to travel long distances to access affordable health care facilities, and many impoverished citizens have to forego routine primary care to offset additional expenses incurred in making such trips.

Researchers who have pointed out the need to incorporate societal-level phenomena in health promotion emphasize that a more effective approach would concentrate on community and institutional changes that tackle health problems at the source (National Research Council, 1989). As noted by Weinstein (1987), for example, urging workers to wear expensive and cumbersome protective gear, in the long run, is a less effective strategy than requiring manufacturers to design equipment and workplace environments with workers' safety in mind.

This article is based on a three-part premise: (a) the individual, community, and institutional approaches previously noted are not mutually exclusive, (b) concepts that bridge these approaches will be most effective in understanding and improving citizens' well-being, and (c) the researcher's role is to increase citizens' health decision-making competencies. By building on shared experiences and collective action, this approach promotes participation and blurs the distinction between concepts, such as source and receiver, that signify a one-way flow of information.

A Multilevel Approach

Pointing out the need for a multilevel approach for a better understanding of health has become somewhat of a cliche. Researchers have often noted that effective health promotion efforts, from both a practical and theoretical perspective, have to incorporate individuals; families, peers, and other community groups; work and school environments; institutions; and national policies (National Research Council, 1989; Rimal, Fogg, & Flora, 1995). And yet, we have few theoretical frameworks for incorporating these multiple levels in our health promotion efforts. Our concepts are often operationalized and confined to one level of analysis, despite calls for more holistic strategies.

The first step in synthesizing and applying the disparate research from micro- and macrolevel work to health promotion is the recognition that health is an individual-level outcome whose causes can be traced to individual, community, and institutional levels. At the individual level, antecedents include such variables as self-efficacy (Bandura, 1977), knowledge (Chaffee & Roser, 1986), and socioeconomic status (McGauhey & Starfield, 1993). These individual-level factors, however, cannot in and of themselves make substantial changes in individuals' health if community and institutional barriers persist. Efforts to improve individuals' health have to focus concomitantly on more than one antecedent, such as health policy, community activism, and affordable access to medical care.

Role Definition

Given the changing dynamics of the doctor-patient relationship, it is incumbent on researchers to assume a greater responsibility in helping citizens navigate through the impending complexities of modern day health care. Indeed, the Federal Government's report, *Healthy People 2000* (1991), calls on increased participation in health decisions by all sectors of society. As a starting point, researchers can highlight the citizen role in health care. The traditional patient role can be reframed as citizens making decisions with other people about health and well-being (Arntson, 1989). However, to make these decisions, not only do citizens have to be made aware of their rights and *responsibilities* (Arntson, 1989), they have to assume and perceive control over their lives (Makoul, Arntson, & Schofield, 1995), and feel empowered to bring about change (Wallerstein, 1992).

Citizens make decisions in a variety of health-engendering contexts that can be grouped into three interrelated environments: physical, social, and media. In each context, a different set of decisions is made that can affect citizens' well-being. Not only can failure in any of these contexts lead to adverse health consequences, but an overall healthy life-style is predicated on decision-making competencies in all three environments.

Before elaborating on each of these environments, we point out an important caveat: The distinction we make among them is for heuristic purposes only. In reality, it is difficult to classify, for example, the domestic environment as either a physical or a social one. It is likely both; the domestic environment is shaped by the physical structure as well as by the relationships among its inhabitants. Furthermore, imposing on both these environments is the media environment. It is our contention, however, that all three environments can contribute to individuals' decision-making competencies, and, to varying degrees, individuals can shape each of the three environments for their own well-being.

Physical Environment

Health care decisions are made ubiquitously. For our discussion, three primary locations include the household, where most day-to-day decisions about life-style factors and health are made, and where individuals spend much of their life; the workplace, where many of the positive (e.g., exercise facilities) and negative (e.g., stress) determinants of health reside; and health care institutions, where adverse health outcomes are treated and preventive measures prescribed.[1]

The roles of individuals across these settings involve different decision-making scripts and strategies. However, extant research on decision making falls short on two counts. First, it has ignored the impact of the environment on the nature of decisions made by individuals. Psychological theories about decision making and judgment (Tversky & Kahneman, 1974), for example, strip from the decision-making process any potential impact of the environment within which the individual functions. Second, communication approaches that incorporate the physical environment study one environment (e.g., schools or organizations) in isolation from others. Hence, we know a great deal about communication patterns within one location, but little about how those patterns may work across locations.

The research prescription here is one for including individuals' environments as the unit of analysis, not only individuals. Instead of asking, "Which individuals change health behaviors?" for example, this line of research would ask, "How do various physical environments aid in judgment and decision?" Are factors that individuals incorporate in making health-related decisions in the home different from those they use in making similar decisions in the workplace?

Take, for example, decisions regarding the adoption of exercise routines. The nature and duration of such activities will undoubtedly be different in the two settings; exercise routines taken up in the workplace will likely be more structured—ones that can be undertaken in a fixed amount of time (e.g., during lunch hour) will be preferred over other, open-ended ones. Those taken up at home will likely depend on external factors, such as the weather and personal safety, for execution. As a result, the latter group of activities may be more irregular. The point is not so much that we distinguish health behaviors according to physical settings in which they occur, but rather that we acquire a better understanding of how physical environments affect health-related decisions.

How might criteria individuals use in making health decisions differ according to where those decisions are made? We offer three considerations. First, each environment imposes *its own set* of options and restrictions, some of which may be health friendly, whereas others may not. Promoting healthy practices by allowing flexibility in employees' daily routines, making available nutritious foods in the cafeteria, or providing access to child care are just a few examples of workplace environments that can be expected to influence employees' health decisions. Similarly, proximity to exercise facilities, prevalence of crime in the neighborhood, and threat of domestic violence are realities that will impinge on individuals' health decisions.

Second, physical environments are closely associated with informational normative cues.[2] Individuals are less likely, for example, to litter in a clean, as opposed to an already littered, environment (Cialdini, Reno, & Kallgren, 1990), supposedly because the former informs the individual about the inappropriateness of littering. In other words, cues individuals receive from the environment, which might include observation of others' behavior, are often internalized and used as decision-making tools. Similarly, we might expect overcrowded health facilities to engender feelings of impersonal care.

Third, some environments are associated with habitual and routine behavior, whereas others promote more conscious decision making. We might hypothesize, for example, that certain work environments, relative to the domestic environment, would promote more mindful and less routinized behavior. Knowledge about the nature of behavior (e.g., mindful vs. habitual) as a function of physical environment can provide a deeper understanding of the criteria individuals use in making health-related decisions.

Although we have so far focused primarily on barriers to and facilities for healthy behaviors imposed by the physical environment, we need also to consider individuals' perceptions of their environment. Physical environments do not explain completely individuals' choice of health practices. We know, for example, that how individuals construe their environment and their abilities to overcome extant barriers shape, to a large extent, their choice of activities, likelihood of persevering in the presence of setbacks, choice of social networks, and attributions for success and failure (Bandura, 1986). Our explanations of health behaviors will remain incomplete to the extent that we fail to incorporate both psychological and physical realities in our models. Health communication research adopting a multilevel approach can bridge the gap between subjective perceptions and objective realities by enhancing individuals' decision-making competencies and raising their awareness about their rights and responsibilities.

Social Environment

Individuals' social environments are determined by the nature of their relationships with others (Chaffee, McLeod, & Wackman, 1973; Meadowcroft, 1986). With regard to health decision making, important social environments are those that either promote or inhibit health outcomes. Adolescents' acquisition of health behaviors, for example, can be traced to the makeup of their social circle, including peers (Lau, Quadrel, & Hartman, 1990) and parents (Fischoff, 1990).

Two implications emerge from this understanding. First, health promotion efforts cannot neglect the power of injunctive social cues. Conversely, those that incorporate individuals' social environments as a channel of influence are likely to increase their effectiveness (see, e.g., Aspinwall, Kemeny, Taylor, Schneider, & Dudley, 1991). Second, influences that exist between individuals and their social environments are reciprocal (Bandura, 1977). That is, not only do social environments shape, but they are also shaped by, individuals' behaviors, as is revealed by studies that demonstrate the role of minority influence (Kitayama & Burnstein, 1994), as well as those of opinion leaders (Rogers, 1983) on groups. It is, after all, the collective behavior of individuals in groups that shapes culture.

Each of the physical environments noted previously—the home, the workplace, and the professional health setting—is also associated with social processes that citizens have to negotiate, and each environment acts as a potential socializing agent. The community, the family, and key social institutions are also socializing agencies that can help influence individuals' health scripts. Relevant here are questions pertaining to how these social entities impact decisions reached by citizens.

There is now a large body of literature to suggest that the family plays an important role in shaping individuals' health. Many health behaviors that have long-term consequences, such as smoking, exercise, and dietary practices, can be traced to childhood behaviors that are influenced by the family (Chassin, Presson, Sherman, & Edwards, 1990).

Parents are children's primary socializing agents for political (Dennis, 1986) and health issues (Lau et al., 1990), and children's learning from television is augmented by parental presence (Chaffee & Tims, 1976). Furthermore, there is also evidence that children themselves shape parental attitudes and behaviors (Bell, 1979).

The implication from these studies is clear: Health behaviors have to be studied in the context within which health decisions are made with the realization that the role of the family in shaping those decisions is crucial. Fitzpatrick and Wamboldt (1990) proposed that we treat the family, as opposed to the individual, as the unit of study by investigating the transactional processes that occur within it. According to this perspective, a family is "a group of intimates who generate a sense of home and group identity, complete with strong ties of loyalty and emotion, and an experience of a history and a future" (Fitzpatrick & Wamboldt, 1990, p. 425).

Applied to the health promotion perspective being proposed here, this definition of family includes a collective decision-making process that is rooted in a common purpose for all members: that of maintaining and improving the family's well-being (Ell & Northen, 1990). By implication, efforts to enhance the quality of individuals' health have to discover and improve the decision-making processes within which individuals function.

The school and the workplace comprise two other social environments that affect individuals' health and provide them with health decision-making scripts. School-based efforts to change children's health practices have had some success (see Bartlett, 1981, for a review; Schall, 1994), especially when health issues are presented as an integral part of the school curriculum (Bartfay & Bartfay, 1994). Once individuals are out of school, or beyond the primary and secondary school age, the workplace provides a common context for acting on health issues. The importance of including the role of the workplace environment in shaping individuals' health decisions emerges from a more pragmatic concern employees increasingly face: Employers are the major providers of health insurance in the United States. Accordingly, as health insurance costs continue to rise, individual health decisions are likely to be made at a collective level, with fewer inputs available for the individual citizen. The increasingly prominent roles played by health management organizations will likely propel this move further.

Beyond school and workplace environments, citizens are also community members with rights and responsibilities. Expanding to a community-oriented model of health communication stresses that the shared experiences of individuals can be a motivating factor for a community group to address common health related issues through collective action (see Medoff & Sklar, 1994, for an example of how one community turned itself around through collective citizen action). Discovering and mobilizing community members' gifts and capacities together with enhancing the *level* of trust among neighbors while engaged in collective health action are healthy outcomes regardless of the action's success (see, e.g., Kretzmann & McKnight, 1993, for a guide on how to rebuild communities based on members' assets). Through participatory learning and shared experiences, group members can develop a heightened critical awareness of the social, psychological, political, and economic factors affecting specific health issues and the overall public good (Reed, 1994). Citizens can discover that they have the power and capacity to improve their health rather than to depend on health professionals to fix them (McKnight, 1994; see also United Way of America, 1995, for seven stories of how communities have improved their well-being). Further, citizens often contribute to society collectively, working in social advocacy groups (e.g., breast cancer coalitions) to affect health and policy. The overall goal of these models is to enhance the health status and the community's quality of life through concerted action (Wallerstein, 1992). The picture emerging from this conceptualization of health promotion is one that is driven by the common goal to imbue within the population the virtue of good health and to increase the quality of life: Healthy people living in a society that encourages healthy homes, schools, and neighborhoods; workplaces and communities prospering in a clean environment; a nonviolent society encouraging disease prevention, family support, education, meaningful work, and exercise; and a society with an abiding value in collective decision making as a primary determinant of the quality and duration of life expectancy of its population (Ratzan, 1994).

Media Environment

Much of the research on the role of the media on individuals' decision-making processes has asked questions about the unidirectional flow of influence from media institutions to individuals. This line of work is concerned with what media do to individuals, not what individuals do with the media. Uses and gratifications (Blumler & Katz, 1974) and media advocacy (Wallack, 1990) are exceptions and are discussed subsequently.

The socializing role of the media has been extensively documented (Chaffee, Nass, &

Yang, 1990; Minow, 1991). Mass media are by far the leading source of information for public affairs for most citizens (Chaffee, Ward, & Tipton, 1970). The media are also perceived by parents to be one of the most credible sources of health information, after doctors and other parents (Bruhn & Parcel, 1982). Prominent media-based public health campaigns (e.g., the Stanford Five City Project, Farquhar et al., 1990, and the Minnesota Heart Health Program, Pavlik et al, 1993) have met with moderate success. Their success can in large part be attributed to the mobilization of community groups in their media campaigns (Bracht, 1990).

Although media are excellent vehicles for propagating messages and enhancing people's awareness of various issues, a number of problems still persist. First, the mass media have proven to be largely ineffective in motivating people to change their high-risk behaviors, especially with regard to AIDS. Second, the prevalence of unhealthy behaviors depicted in the media—for example, the preponderance of "junk food" consumption and violence—are closely associated with either corresponding practices in real life (Gerbner, Gross, Morgan, & Signorielli, 1981), or, at a minimum, skewed perceptions of reality. Third, there is growing concern in the research community that media-based efforts to improve individuals' health practices are not reaching the underserved population (National Institutes of Health, 1992) and thus are perpetuating the knowledge gap (Freimuth, 1990) between the haves and the have-nots in society. And fourth, efforts to counter the preponderance of negative media images (such as those promoting tobacco use through sponsorships of various sporting and cultural events) are severely handicapped by a lack of corresponding public funds, which presents further barriers in setting a healthy media agenda.

These realities paint a rather gloomy picture for health promotion efforts that rely on the media to propagate their messages. However, even though most of our current understanding of media influences is one of a unidirectional flow of information in which societal agendas mirror those of the media's (McCombs & Shaw, 1972), efforts to reverse this direction through media advocacy (Blum, 1994; Wallack, 1990) show promise. Media advocacy efforts are concerned with providing individuals and communities with a voice in the media environment in order, ultimately, to change public policy.

Similarly, the uses and gratifications approach (Blumler & Katz, 1974) offers another perspective on how individuals actively seek and utilize the media. It suggests that individuals can and do engage in active decision-making processes with regard to the media (Katz, Gurevitch, & Haas, 1973) and are not mere passive recipients of information. Further, individuals can be mobilized to make their voices heard by media institutions (Freimuth, Greenberg, DeWitt, & Romano, 1984). The long-term implication and efficacy of these approaches are still unclear, but, by attempting to engage the media in a dialogue, this line of work certainly opens the door for bottom-up processes.

Implications

This article has examined some of the problems in our current models of health promotion and has pointed out the need for a fundamental change in our conceptualization of the traditional term patient. We have argued that the term is no longer suitable for people who must decide how to be healthy in their physical, social, and mediated environments. Rather, our view of the patient is an active citizen who is involved in individual and collective health decision making. A number of implications emerge as a result of this reorientation, especially as they pertain to the roles of health care providers and researchers.

Our models of health have to be more comprehensive in terms of how citizens make health care decisions within and across various physical and social environments. Researchers need to identify the functional decision-making scripts that are necessary for citizens to maintain and enhance their well-being in their various physical and social contexts. The processes by which citizens acquire, enact, and evaluate these scripts must also be understood (Arntson, 1989).

Given the perspective we have outlined here, the role of health professionals, particularly primary care providers, will have added health promotional importance (David, 1994). Not only will it be necessary to provide citizens with the information they need to make functional health care decisions (Makoul et al., 1995), it will also be necessary for health professionals to encourage patients to accept responsibility during the encounters; to make decisions about their health; to develop with their patients decision-making scripts so that their patients can, as citizens, make functional health care decisions in their homes and communities; and to provide feedback to patients about the decisions that were made. For many people, we need to help transfer the decision-making authority for their health from professionals to themselves in a way that creates a sense of self-efficacy.

We also need to look at the media's role differendy. Whereas traditional public information campaigns have sought to increase people's knowledge about health issues with the hopes that such changes would subsequently lead to healthier behaviors, the emphasis on education that we propose is one that improves citizens' decision-making skills about their well-being. The media need to provide models of functional decision-making processes for how people can be healthy, not merely disseminate health information.

Another implication of this understanding is the recognition that we can no longer measure client compliance and consumer satisfaction as our two most important health communication outcomes. Citizens' competencies to make individual and collective health care decisions become the outcome of choice. Citizens' assessments of professional services and whether or not they adhere to treatment plans are all aspects of how competently they make decisions about their well-being.

Our research methodologies also need to reflect this change in thinking. If citizens are their own change agents, questions about their state of health and means of improving their quality of life cannot be answered according solely to the researchers' definitions. As others have pointed out (see, e.g., Jensen, 1987; Liebes, 1988), we need an audience-centered perspective that incorporates subjective experiences and meanings (Dervin, 1990). Our unit of analysis must also change. Besides talking to individuals, we must also record the collective health understandings and decisionmaking scripts of family, community, and work groups. Results from such qualitative endeavors can serve as stepping stones for developing more representative measurement instruments to incorporate quantitative methodologies as well.

Acknowledgments. We are grateful to editors Barbara F. Sharf and Richard L. Street, Jr., for their suggestions and comments on earlier drafts of this article.

Notes

1. We do not imply that these are the only physical environments pertinent to the health consumer. These three settings were chosen to highlight the differences that locations have in aiding or hindering health decision making.
2. Cialdini, Reno, and Kallgren (1990) distinguished between descriptive and injunctive normative cues. Descriptive cues provide information on what is normal; it "is what most people do, and it motivates by providing evidence as to what will likely be effective" (p. 1015).

References

Arntson, P. H. (1989). Improving citizens' health competencies. *Health Communication, 1,* 29–32.

Aspinwall, L. G., Kemeny, M. E., Taylor, S. E., Schneider, S. G., & Dudley, J. P. (1991). Psychosocial predictors of gay men's AIDS risk-reduction behavior. *Health Psychology, 10,* 432–444.

Bandura, A. (1977). *Social learning theory,* Englewood Cliffs, NJ: Prentice-Hall.

Bandura, A. (1986). *Social foundations of thought and action.* Englewood Cliffs, NJ: Prentice-Hall.

Bartfay, W. J., & Bartfay, E. (1994). Promoting health in schools through a board game. *Western Journal of Nursing Research, 16,* 438–446.

Bartlett, E. E. (1981). The contribution of school

health education to community health promotion: What can we reasonably expect? *American Journal of Public Health, 71,* 1384–1391.

Becker, M. H. (Ed.). (1974). The health belief model and personal health behavior. *Health Education Monographs, 2,* 324–473.

Bell, R. Q. (1979). Parent, child, and reciprocal influences. *American Psychologist,* 34, 821–826.

Blum, A. (1994). Paid counter-advertising: Proven strategy to combat tobacco use and promotion. *American Journal of Preventive Medicine, 10* (Suppl. 3), 8–10.

Bracht, N. (Ed.) (1990). *Health promotion at the community level.* Newbury Park, CA: Sage.

Bruhn, J. G., & Parcel, G. S. (1982). Preschool Health Education Program (PHEP): An analysis of baseline data. *Health Education Quarterly, 9,* 20–23.

Carey, J. W. (1989). *Communication as culture: Essays on media and society.* Boston: Unwin Hyman.

Chaffee, S. H., McLeod, J. M., & Wackman, D. B. (1973). Family communication patterns and adolescent political participation. In J. Dennis (Ed.), *Socialization to politics: Selected readings* (pp. 349–364). New York: Wiley.

Chaffee, S. H., Nass, C. I., Yang, S. M. (1990). The bridging role of television in immigrant political socialization. *Human Communication Research, 17,* 266–288.

Chaffee, S. H., & Roser, C. (1986). Involvement and the consistency of knowledge, attitudes, and behaviors. *Communication Research, 13,* 373–399.

Chaffee, S. H., & Tims, A. R. (1976). Interpersonal factors in adolescent television use. *Journal of Social Issues, 32*(4), 98–115.

Chaffee, S. H., Ward, S., & Tipton, L. (1970). Mass communication and political socialization. *Journalism Quarterly, 47,* 647–659.

Chassin, L., Presson, C. C., Sherman, S. J., & Edwards, D. A. (1990). The natural history of cigarette smoking: Predicting young-adult smoking outcomes from adolescent smoking patterns. *Health Psychology, 9,* 701–716.

Cialdini, R. B., Reno, R. R., & Kallgren, C. A. (1990). A focus theory of normative conduct: Recycling the concept of norms to reduce littering in public places. *Journal of Personality and Social Psychology, 58,* 1015–1026.

David, A. K. (1994). Challenges in personal and public health promotion: The primary care physician perspective. *American Journal of Preventive Medicine, 10*(Suppl. 3), 36—38.

Dennis, J. (1986). Preadult learning of political independence: Media and family communication effects. *Communication Research, 13,* 401–433.

Dervin, B. (1990). Audience as listener and learner, teacher and confidante: A sense-making approach. In R. E. Rice & C. K. Atkin (Eds.), *Public communication campaigns* (2nd ed., pp. 67–86). Newbury Park, CA: Sage.

Ell, K. & Northen, H. (1990). *Families and health care: Psychosocial practice.* New York: Aldine de Gruyter.

Farquhar, J. W., Fortmann, S. P., Flora, J. A., Taylor, C. B., Haskell, W. L., Williams, P. T., Maccoby, N., & Wood, P. D. (1990). Effects of community-wide education on cardiovascular disease risk factors: The Stanford Five-City Project. *Journal of the American Medical Association, 264,* 350–365.

Fischoff, B. (1990), Risk taking: A developmental perspective. In J. F. Yates (Ed.), *Risk taking.* New York: Wiley.

Fitzpatrick, M. A., & Wamboldt, F. S. (1990). Where all is said and done? Toward an integration of intrapersonal and interpersonal models of marital and family communication. *Communication Research, 17,* 421–430.

Freimuth, V. S. (1990). The chronically uninformed: Closing the knowledge gap in health. In E. B. Ray & L. Donohew (Eds.), *Communication and health: Systems and applications* (pp. 171–186). Hillsdale, NJ: Lawrence Erlbaum Associates, Inc.

Freimuth, V. S., Greenberg, R. H., DeWitt, J., & Romano, R. M. (1984). Covering cancer: Newspapers and the public interest. *Journal of Communication, 34,* 62–73.

Gerbner, G. Gross, L., Morgan, M, & Signorielli, N. (1981). Health and medicine on television. *The New England Journal of Medicine, 305,* 901–904.

Healthy People 2000: National health promotion and disease prevention objectives. (1991). Washington, DC: U.S. Department of Health and Human Services.

Jensen, K. (1987). Qualitative audience research: Toward an integrative approach to reception. *Critical Studies in Mass Communication, 4,* 21–36.

Jessor, R. (1993). Successful adolescent development among youth in high-risk settings. *American Psychologist, 48,* 117–126.

Katz, E., Gurevitch, M., & Haas, H. (1973). On the use of the mass media for important things. *American Sociological Review, 38,* 164–181.

Kitayama, S., & Burnstein, E. (1994). Social influence, persuasion, and group decision making. In S. Shavitt & T. C. Brock (Eds.), *Persuasion: Psychological insights and per-*

spectives (pp. 175–193). Needham Height, MA: Allyn & Bacon.

Kretzmann, J. P., & McKnight, J. L. (1993). *Building communities from the inside out: A path toward finding and mobilizing a community's assets*. Chicago: ACTA.

Lau, R. R., Quadrel, M. J., & Hartman, K. A. (1990). Development and change of young adults' preventive health beliefs and behavior: Influence from parents and peers. *Journal of Health and Social Behavior, 31,* 240–259.

Liebes, T. (1988). On the convergence of theories of mass communication and literature regarding the role of the reader. In B. Dervin & M. Voigt (Eds.), *Progress in communication sciences* (Vol. 9, pp. 123–143). Norwood, NJ: Ablex.

Maddux, J. E., & Rogers, R. W. (1983). Protection motivation and self-efficacy: A revised theory of fear appeals and attitude change. *Journal of Experimental Social Psychology, 19,* 469–479.

Makoul, G., Arntson, P., & Schofield, T. (1995). Health promotion in primary care: Physician-patient communication and decision making about prescription medications. *Social Science and Medicine, 41,* 1241–1254.

McCombs, M. E., & Shaw, D. L. (1972). The agenda-setting function of the mass media. *Public Opinion Quarterly, 36,* 176–187.

McGauhey, P. J., & Starfield, B. (1993). Child health and the social environment of White and Black children. *Social Science and Medicine, 36,* 867–874.

McKnight, J. L., (1994). Two tools for well-being: Health systems and communities. *American Journal of Preventive Medicine, 70*(Suppl. 3), 23–25.

Meadowcroft, J. M. (1986). Family communication patterns and political development: The child's role. *Communication Research, 13,* 603–624.

Medoff, P., & Sklar, H. (1994). *Streets of hope: The fall and rise of an urban neighborhood*. Boston: South End Press.

Minkler, M. (1978). Ethical issues in community organization. *Health Education Monographs, 6,* 198–210.

Minow, N. (1991, May 9). "How vast the wasteland now?" Keynote address delivered at the Gannett Foundation Media Center, Washington, DC.

National Institutes of Health. (1992). *Health Behavior research in minority populations: Access, design, and implementation*. Washington, DC: U.S. Department of Health and Human Services.

National Research Council. (1989). *Improving risk communication*. Washington, DC: National Academy Press.

Pavlik, J. V., Finnegan, J. R., Jr., Strickland, D., Salmon, C. T., Viswanath, K., & Wackman, D. B. (1993), Increasing public understanding of heart disease: An analysis of data from the Minnesota Heart Health Program. *Health Communication, 5,* 1–20.

Petty, R. E., & Cacioppo, J. T. (1981). *Attitudes and persuasion: Classic and contemporary approaches*. Dubuque, IA: Brown.

Prochaska, J. O. (1979). *Systems of psychotherapy: A transtheoretical analysis*. Homewood, IL: Dorsey Press.

Ratzan, S. C. (1994). Health communication as negotiation: The Healthy America Act. *American Behavioral Scientist, 38,* 224–247.

Ratzan, S. C. (1996). Effective decision making: A negotiation perspective for health psychology and health communication. *Journal of Health Psychology, 1,* 323–333.

Reed, J. (1994). Health promotion: A community-based perspective. *American Journal of Preventive Medicine, 10*(Suppl. 3), 26–29.

Rimal, R. N., Fogg, B. J., & Flora, J. A. (1995). Moving toward a framework for the study of risk communication: Theoretical and ethical considerations. In B. R. Burleson (Ed.), *Communication yearbook* (Vol. 18, pp. 320–342). Thousand Oaks, CA: Sage.

Rogers, E. M. (1983). *Diffusion of innovations*. New York: Free Press.

Salmon, C. T. (1989). Campaigns for social "improvement": An overview of values, rationales, and impacts. In C. T. Salmon (Ed.), *Information campaigns: Balancing social values and social change* (pp. 19–53). Newbury Park, CA: Sage.

Sanders, R. E. (1991). The two-way relationship between talk in social interactions and actors' goals and plans. In K. Tracy (Ed.), *Understanding face-to-face interaction: Issues linking goals and discourse* (pp. 167–188). Hillsdale, NJ: Lawrence Erlbaum Associates, Inc.

Schall, E. (1994). School-based health education: What works? *American Journal of Preventive Medicine, 10*(Suppl. 3), 30–32.

Sharf, B. F., & Kahler, J. (1996). Victims of the franchise: A culturally sensitive model of teaching patient-doctor communication in the inner city. In E. B. Ray (Ed.), *Communication and the disenfranchised: Social health issues and implications* (pp. 95–115). Mahwah, NJ: Lawrence Erlbaum Associates, Inc.

Tinsley, B. J., & Parke, R. D. (1984). The historical and contemporary relationship between developmental psychology and pediatrics: A review and empirical survey. In H. E. Fitzgerald, B. M. Lester, & M. W. Yogman (Eds.), *Theory and research in behavioral pediatrics* (pp. 2–30). New York: Plenum.

Tversky, A., & Kahneman, D. (1974). Judgment under uncertainty; Heuristics and biases. *Science, 185,* 1124–1131.

United Way of America. (1995). *United Way's community capacity-building stories. Key issue papers on community building.* Alexandria, VA: Author.

Wallack, L. (1990). Improving health promotion: Media advocacy and social marketing approaches. In C. Atkin & L. Wallack (Eds.), *Mass communication and public health: Complexities and conflicts* (pp. 147–163). Newbury Park, CA: Sage.

Wallerstein, N. (1992). Powerlessness, empowerment, and health: Implications for health promotion programs. *American Journal of Health Promotion, 6,* 197–206.

Weinstein, N. D. (1987). Introduction: Studying self-protective behavior. In N. D. Weinstein (Ed.), *Taking Care: Understanding and encouraging self-protective behavior* (pp. 1–13). New York: Cambridge University Press.

Witte, K. (1994). Fear control and danger control: A test of the extended parallel process model (EPPM). *Communication Monographs, 61,* 113–134.

Discussion Questions

1. The authors propose a shift from the term *patient* to *health citizen.* What are the implications of the term *patient* in the health-care setting? Does shifting to *health citizen* have different implications for the role of health consumers? If so, are these new roles an improvement?
2. What social environments most directly affect your own health behaviors? How does this broader, contextual view of health aid your understanding of what influences the health behaviors of others?
3. Rimal et al. argue that citizens can (and should) have a more active role in their own health care. What implications could a more active role have for different social groups? How would this shift be viewed by health-care providers? ✦

Chapter 12
'E-Health'
The Internet and the Transformation of Patients Into Consumers and Producers of Health Knowledge

Michael Hardey

Michael Hardey's chapter examines the ways in which the changing role of the patient is a product of the Internet and the ways in which it allows for more pluralistic and democratic processing of health knowledge and experiences. The Internet has given rise to many innovations regarding public access to health information. This transformation of "patients" in need of health services to "consumers" who are empowered to make their own decisions is the focus of this chapter. Using data from two different sources, this chapter suggests that the Internet offers a valuable resource in the consumption and production of health information. The Internet allows for more pluralistic and democratic processing of health knowledge and experiences.

Related Topics: e-health, health-care behaviors, Internet, media, patient-centered communication, patients' perspectives, qualitative methods, role of the patient

> A Pandora's box has been opened and there is no closing the lid now. Medical lore has been let loose. It is no longer the secret preserve of physicians. It is out there for anybody and everybody to possess. (Boseley 2000)

Since Parsons (1951) developed the concept of the 'sick role,' the patient has been defined in relation to the more powerful role of the doctor. More broadly Foucault (1990) and others have argued that medicine creates and maintains a 'social monopoly of expertise and knowledge' (Turner 1995: 47). The development of information and communications technologies (ICTs), and in particular the Internet, is collapsing the boundary fences around previously carefully guarded information domains that form the basis for professional monopolies such as medicine. Indeed, Giddens (1999) amongst other commentators has argued that the Internet is the most significant technological advance since the development of the printing press. This new technology arrived at a time when health policy in the UK was emphasizing 'the needs of individual patients, rather than the connivance of the system or institution' (DOH 1996: 29). Within both health and social services, an emphasis on the 'patient' or 'user' as 'consumer' with the implied ability to make decisions based on information and experience has emerged. The ease with which information can be accessed on the Internet has encouraged the UK and other Western governments make use of it to provide information in support of consumer-based policies (Loader 1997). However, the Internet provides far more than a simple conduit for government and medical information that it is considered desirable for consumers to access. Users can seamlessly pass through the divisions between different knowledge, professions and practices. They can also move from being consumers to producers of information by participating in Usenet newsgroups or chat rooms or by constructing their own web pages. What has been described as the 'new medical pluralism' (Cant and Sharma 1999) is, therefore, embodied in the Internet. This pluralism echoes the time before the hegemony of Western medicine when the emergent medical profession was seeking to mark out a territory of expertise by identifying and marginalizing competing therapists though a discourse about 'quackery' (cf. Porter 1998).

From "E-Health: The Internet and the Transformation of Patients into Consumers and Producers of Health Knowledge," Michael Hardy, 2001, *Information, Communication, & Society*, Vol. 4:3, pp. 388–405.

The public response of the medical profession to public access to health information on the Internet has ranged from caution to hostility. However, an increasing number of doctors are involved in the development and maintenance of Internet sites. Indeed, the content of many health-focused sites is primarily authored by health professionals. Much of the debate in medical journals has been framed in terms of the reliability and quality of Internet health material. In this, medicine can be seen to act out the role of guardian of the public interest and safety. As Saks (1995) has shown, this was a significant strategy in defining the boundaries around orthodox and non-orthodox approaches to health. This has given rise to stories in both the popular and medical journals about 'bogus therapies' being promoted on the Internet. Efforts to establish boundaries have produced a plethora of individuals and organizations that claim to provide, or be developing, ways of assessing health information on the Internet. These include private initiatives such as 'Quackwatch,'[1] institutions and organizations such as the Health Information Technology Institute[2] and the British Healthcare Internet Association.[3] A commercial UK site headlines its main page with:

> Welcome to HEALTHINFOCUS—Your comprehensive resource for trustworthy, independent health information.[4]

However, there are links and information about alternative health that would be derided by organizations such as Quackwatch. Despite such concerns the number of consumers using the Internet for health information is growing rapidly. One survey has reported that over half the online adult population in the USA has sought health care material (Cyber Dialogue 2000). The online population in the UK continues to expand and increasing availability of digital technology is making the Internet accessible in many homes through the television.

The Research

This paper draws on data from two related research studies. The first consisted of a case study often households in the south of the UK. The households were recruited through e-mails to subscribers of a locally based ISP and to members of e-mail discussion groups. An invitation to take part in the study was sent to subscribers of three different e-mail lists that contained members largely confined to the south of Britain. This invitation contained information about the study and appeared in users' e-mail utility as a 'health on the Net study.' People who responded to this initial request were sent a letter outlining the project and a short questionnaire so that they could be screened for inclusion in the research. The households included in the research described themselves as 'healthy' although some households contained members who had asthma and eczema. All the households contained at least one school-aged child and none of the participants regarded themselves as an 'expert' in relation to computers. No household had owned a home computer with a modem link for more than sixteen months. Reflecting the relationship between social class and the ownership of home computers the occupations of the main income earners fell into the categories of social class one and two. During the course of a year, two interviews in participants' homes were undertaken with each household. The majority of interviews lasted between one and two hours each and focused on a range of topics related to health and the Internet. The interviews were tape-recorded and transcribed. Analysis followed a grounded theory approach whereby themes are identified through the 'constant comparative method' that validates the categories against the data they are grounded in (Strauss and Corbin 1990). This involves the systematic analysis of data in order to identify phenomena which are defined as categories (Bartlett and Payne 1997). The data are then examined for further cases of the categories and associations made with existing theory. Extracts from this data are indicated by the prefix 'int/.'

The second study involved an examination of home pages constructed by people that contain accounts of their experiences of ill health. The pages were identified through search engines, newsgroup correspondence and chat room exchanges. Yahoo, Alta Vista and the meta search engine Dogpile were used to identify web pages that contained the words 'my' and 'illness.' The subsequent reports identified many thousands of pages of which a few were personal pages. The first 100 pages from each search engine were scanned to identify relevant personal pages. In addition, a search was undertaken using the words 'asthma' and 'multiple sclerosis.' Again this produced a large number of web sites and so the first 100 were scanned to identify personal pages. In addition, where links were made to other personal pages these were followed.

Home page authors can 'inform' search engines about their page but many do not do this and the protocols of the various search engines may not identify individual home pages. Therefore, thirty-eight newsgroups formed around health and illness topics were monitored in order to identify any home pages that were posted by participants. Finally, ten chat rooms about health and identified through 'ICQ chat' and were monitored for six hours over five evenings to provide further personal pages that participants note during the course of exchanges. A final total of 132 personal pages were identified through this combination of strategies. Just over half of these pages originated in the USA. The web pages were printed and saved onto a computer hard drive. The analysis of the content followed the grounded approach adopted in the first study that this paper draws on. It is not claimed that the sample is representative of the entire population of personal web pages but it will not be untypical of those concerned with health illness. The decision to use two common chronic conditions to help identify web sites clearly introduced a bias towards these conditions so that the choice of other key words would have changed the composition of the sample to some degree.

A simple questionnaire was constructed and sent via e-mail to those authors who published their e-mail address on their home page. Ninety-eight people were sent the questionnaire and seventy-four responded to it within four weeks. This response rate is congruent with that reported by other researchers who have used e-mail-based questionnaires and for the purposes of this study, enable data to be collected from participants who were spread across the globe (Selwyn and Robson 1998). In this paper, I have followed the convention of making the responses to the questionnaire anonymous. It would have been easy to link responses to the authors of individual pages that are cited in the paper. However, the questionnaire may often involve participants in contributing information that they had not included on their web pages. It was decided, therefore, to ensure that confidentiality would be maintained and that it would not be possible to identify individuals through associating their questionnaire with their web pages. Material quoted from the e-mail questionnaire is identified by the prefix 'eq/.' Given that the home pages used in this study are in the public domain, these have be cited where relevant by providing the URL from which the page was originally accessed. It should be noted that, owing to the dynamic nature of the Internet these home pages may have been removed or subject to wholesale reconstruction since they were accessed for the purposes of this paper. Spelling and punctuation have been retained unless they make it difficult to understand a particular extract. The home pages used in this study are in the public domain and so the Universal Resource Locations (URLs) of those that have been cited have been given. Given the dynamic nature of the Internet, home pages may have been removed, associated with a different Internet Service Provider or subject to wholesale reconstruction since they were accessed for the purposes of this paper.

Consuming Health Information

From the analysis of data from the study of Internet users it is evident that the most common route into health information is through a search engine. David provides a typical account of the process:

> When I looked up hay fever I just typed the word into Yahoo and away it went. I got back a load of sites about hay fever and allergies. As you know you get a short description so I just picked some sites that looked interesting. From then

> on I could go Web hopping by following links or going back to my original search.

As David went on to explain how such searches tap into the health pluralism of the Internet:

> I found sites from all over, you know, medical stuff and some really loony ideas someone has put on their web page. What I found most useful was the information about homeopathy and allergies which I didn't know much about before. This came off a personal page from a guy in the States who had the problem and had put together a load of useful links. You know how you just use antihistamine without question and put up with feeling tired. I had no idea that there were treatments that could get rid of the sneezing and itching with no side effects.

These extracts show how users identified and used information from the Internet in a way that complements the role of a consumer of health care. Note that David's use of the word 'loony' implies some form of critical appraisal of the content of web sites.

In the UK and other western countries, health care provision has come under increasing pressure to be 'cost effective' and ensure the patients are seen and treated as soon as possible (RVZ 1999). Consultation times within general practice have an average duration of eight minutes although within individual practices this may range from just over a minute to five minutes (Barry et al. 2000). The exchange of information that takes place is largely 'biomedical' with the patient cast in the role of 'a person with disconnected bodily symptoms, wanting a label for what is wrong and a prescription to put it right' (Howie et al. 1999: 1246). It is not surprising therefore that dissatisfaction with the medical encounter and the user centredness of ICTs is a significant factor in encouraging people to use the Internet for health information and advice (Eysenbach and Diepgen 1999). Mary explains the opportunities offered by the Internet:

> My GP is very busy and does not have time to answer questions fully. Actually, it is much easier to think about what you want to ask when you look things up on the Net. I don't get that nagging feeling that I'm needlessly taking up his time.

The Internet also provides an anonymous space within which the 'gamble' (Giddens 1991) involved in sharing intimate feelings and embarrassing problems is minimized.

> I'll tell you something . . . my eczema keeps flaring up and the GP gave me some steroid ointment that didn't do much good. I kept going back and I could see he was thinking I was making a fuss . . . it is embarrassing . . . going on thirty with eczema in places I'm not going to talk about (laughs). So you could say the Net has been more use than my GP. I get advice off some really good pages and I find those which have people explaining how it is for them especially good. You know, they have the experience and some have got ways of dealing with it that I never thought of. . . . Oh yes I looked at those groups (newsgroups) and I even emailed some doctors in America and they came back with some handy suggestions. So yes the Net is the place for me!

This apparent anonymity offered by the Internet was reflected in a recent advertisement displayed on the London Underground for a commercial medical internet site that stated 'Embarrassing itch? Anonymity assured at www. . . .' As in other areas of commerce the Internet provides a new way of advertising and delivering and products and services to consumers. In addition, the growth of the NHS and private 'walk-in' surgeries and the popularity of the NHS Direct suggests that consumers are increasingly obtaining information and advice from sources other than the General Practitioner. However, the structure of the health care system that is founded on the primacy of the medical profession ensures that patients are dependent on health care professionals for the majority of clinical treatments and services. An editorial in a leading dermatology journal has noted that 'it is becoming increasingly common for patients to arrive at the office with printouts of information of varying quality depending on the source' (Huntley 1999: 198). As Hardey (1999) has noted, patients use Internet-derived information to negotiate treatment with doctors when their health problem cannot be addressed by self-care.

The consumption of information is not confined to those who are experiencing symptoms or who have a diagnosed condition. Health-related sites such as that provided by the BBC[5] or the NHS[6] in the UK and,[7] in the USA, On Health and Health Gate[8], contain information based around disease categories as well as broad lifestyle advice. This includes material within the tradition of health education about healthy diets and ending smoking as well as interactive exercises such as 'yoga at your desk' and 'how to be younger.' This proliferation of advertising and advice which offers to enhance the body and allow people to 'improve' their lifestyle or leisure activities reflect the central place of the body within consumer culture (Featherstone 1982). Internet sites that promote diets and other ways of losing weight are common:

> You know I'm bit of a diet freak. So after yet another round of Weight Watchers I had a look at their web page. Before long I had spent an evening wondering around diet sites on the Net. You should take a look (laughs) if you see what I mean! Maybe its because I'm a skeptic but I found some seriously odd ideas. . . . My favourite is God's diet and I won't tell you about sex diets (laughs) very kinky. Anyhow I have got into cyberdiet because I quite like the routines and as it is from America the recipes are unusual.

Debbie's experience highlights the diversity of information on any one topic. This very diversity encourages users to be 'skeptical' about the material that is presented to them. Giddens (1991: 141) in a fictional account of a search for health information has noted how people make 'a reasonably informed choice' from a mass of competing and sometimes contradictory information. The evaluation noted earlier in the usage of the word 'loony' is again reflected in the extract below:

> There were some stories in the papers about autism and the MMR jab which Jane was due for. We belong to a parent group and this was quite a topic at the time. I remember I looked up MMR on Alta Vista and got one of those answer boxes that somehow take you to a direct response to your question. Couldn't tell you how it works but anyway this and the links gave loads of stuff about MMR. . . . In the end we decide to go with the MMR. Most advice showed that there was not a big risk of autism and that the benefits were far more. I looked at papers from medical journals and other reports. It was important to us that we could make a proper discussion about the jab and not be unquestioning parents.

At the time of the interview there had been a lot of media coverage of potential health risks associated with the combined Measles, Mumps and Rubella (MMR) vaccination. Newsgroups arranged around parenting topics also actively discussed the MMR issue (Burrows et al. 2000). Access to medical journals and other medical resources connect users directly to medical knowledge. This is not mediated by the press, public relations expertise or, in this case, health promotion professionals. This has implications for the 'quality' debate within medicine that through the application of various protocols seeks to 'protect' users from some health information. The problem here is that 'protect' can be translated as 'restrict.' By reducing the diversity of the resources available users may become more skeptical about the nature of the information they can easily access. What users define as 'loony' and 'odd' help to define what they regard as credible and the basis for making choices about health.

Producing Health Information

Little attention has been paid to consumer or lay production of health information on the Internet. The simplest form of user-produced health information can be found within newsgroups and chat rooms. Dedicated to topics such as dieting, anorexia and alcoholism these resources are largely controlled by the members. The exchanges provide advice and support for others in a way that has been described as forming a 'virtual community of care' (Burrows and Nettleton 2000). Few technical skills are required to construct a web page and many ISPs provide simple type, cut and paste systems. In the most basic form, a home page consists of information about the author's health problem so that others will understand the changes that have taken place since the onset of a chronic illness. Home pages titles like 'Everything you ever needed to know about poor, diseased, Teresa!'[9] and 'My illness for which there is no cure: but I'm not gonna die so there!' [10] are typical and indicate the nature of the contents. Within the sociology of health there is a long tradition of research into 'health narratives' and how people explain and come to understand chronic illness model (Bury 1991; Kleinman 1998; Frank 1995; Radley 1999). The interweaving of personal experience and knowledge with advice about health has long been recognized within lay referral networks (Hyden 1997). These home pages take the illness narrative into a new genre where individuals publish their stories that are not mediated by health professions or health researchers (Hardey forthcoming). The shift from a narrative about an individual illness to the broader provision of health information is captured in the following extract from the opening of a web page:

> This page has been designed to provide information to people who want to learn more about paraplegics. On this page I will tell you about my life as a paraplegic and provide links to other information sources, as well as links to pages of other paraplegics. It wasn't long ago that my girlfriend was doing searches on the internet for information about paraplegics and disabilities. After much time and effort she found very little information. Hopefully this page can be a starting point of information for those people in situations like hers and mine.[11]

This indicates the way consumers who feel that existing information fails to meet their needs find resources on the Internet and pass their experiences on to others. The advice offered is, therefore, embedded in personal experience.

The process of assessing Internet resources noted earlier is also evident in the care that authors take in providing links and other information on their own web pages:

> Putting up links on the (Web) page is too easy. I only use links that I think are useful and I go back and check these regularly. There is nothing as frustrating as hitting on a good link and finding that it is dead. It takes time but my belief is that you have to take responsibility for the information you give out. I have a good understanding of I.B.S. (Irritable Bowel Syndrome) but it is a very personnel disease. So I offer what I find useful to others and they can email me if they want.

This cautious approach extends to providing assessments of treatments or approaches to health and illness. However, the degree to which the 'if you link to my site, I will link to your site' culture influences health web pages has yet to be assessed. There are echoes here of the 'quality' debate within medical circles in that consumers of health are producing their own assessments of treatments and health products:

> What about Theratec in Mexico?
>
> They claim: 'there will be no more episodes or exacerbations' after their treatment, and they claim their therapy 'terminates the MS virus.' But, Karan was treated at this clinic twice, and her exacerbation never left! Karan was also told that the treatment would eliminate her burning nerve pain, but instead it has increased. This very expensive therapy may have improved some patients, but it obviously doesn't work as well as they claim. Their post-treatment recovery also requires diligent long-term physical therapy in most cases.[12]

The extract above shows that home pages can be just as critical of non-orthodox medicine as medical sites. However, this critique is more evaluative and based on personal experience rather than medical research (Williams and Popay 1994). Home pages may contain not only a critique but also clear warnings about what the author perceives as unfair or inappropriate treatment he or she has received from a medical practitioner.

Experience leads many authors to reinforce the importance of medical care as the text bellow illustrates:

> Over the last two years I have received thousands of e-mails from people all over the world asking advice on how to

> deal with panic attacks and most of the time my advice is the same. Find a qualified psychologist in your area for a complete diagnosis and STAY in therapy. I believe that medication should be used to help deal with the attacks as you learn how to control the attacks through therapy. The medication should be used along with therapy, not alone. Please remember, I am not a doctor and this advice is just my opinion.[13]

The broad advice offered by the home pages considered so far contrasts to the more focused advice offered by those who used their web page to advocate a particular approach to health. Like Internet resources constructed within a biomedical perspective, these web pages provide advice and links to other sites within a specific paradigm. The home page, from which the extract below is taken, provides a large number of annotated links and other information about chiropractice:

> In 1998 I went to a holistic health fair. Well, OK, my wife took me along as I was not keen this alternative stuff! So I had a free examination and the chiropractor told me I had spinal curvature and that she would do a contour analysis (hyperlinked to an explanation) for me if I came to see her. Odd thing was that afterwards my back and breathing did seem easier. Or was it the meal in the pub? At the consolation [sic] I had a Contact Reflex Analysis (hyerplinked to an explanation) and contour analysis . . . changed my life in ways that doctors never had.
>
> It can change yours. Take a look at my links and find out about chiropractic.
>
> Go on I was a skeptic too. You have read my story so now why don't you use a chiropractor?[14]

Amongst the links that follow the extract above are a number of medical web sites that are highly critical of chiropractice and dismiss 'contour analysis' as pseudoscience. The author introduces these sites by informing readers that:

> You must make up your own mind. This page will warn you about the risks as seen by medicine. Remember not all chiropractors are trained. Do not allow anyone to violently manipulate your neck. This can cause serious injuries and should be avoided.[15]

There are interesting similarities here with medical web pages that include links and information about non-orthodox treatments. In this instance, the author is reflecting on his own experiences and passing these on so that others can evaluate and perhaps challenge expert knowledge (cf. Lupton 1997). Variations of the term 'make up your own mind' combined with the provision of resources that provide a critique of the approach advocated by the author, are congruent with this consumerist discourse.

The rise of e-commerce has attracted much attention and so it is not surprising that some home pages advertise and sell health products and treatments. It is difficult to know the degree to which commercial considerations influence the contents of home pages. In the USA a web page offering medical advice constructed by a former US surgeon-general was criticized by the American Medical Association for failing to indicate that he had a financial incentive to sell certain products through his page (Burkeman 2000). One respondent to the e-mail questionnaire explained how he was approached by a pharmaceutical corporation:

> I received an email from a manufacture who offered me a percentage if I recommended or helped to sell their products on my page. I was quite flattered that they had noticed my little page. I was tempted but I didn't do this to make money. The point of my page is that it offers help from a fellow sufferer. I'm not a doctor or a salesman.

Such 'covert' commercialism may be hard to detect. The more overt kind is represented by those who offer products directly from their home page:

> When I was diagnosed with CFIDS (Chronic Fatigue and Immune Dysfunction Syndrome) I just added some stuff to my home page to explain what had happened to people I knew. . . . I know more than most doctors now and I hope that my web site will answer people's questions and get them to buy things I recommend. It is a full time job for me and I make a living out of dispatching orders to people around the world.

Marketing health products is undertaken in a way similar to any commercial web site:

> I have used Bio-MagneticTherapy (hyperlink to detailed explanation) since 1999. It uses the magnetic fields of the human body end stiffness in the limbs and more importantly to improve the peripheral blood flow. Order online or call.[15]

The extract above is taken from a home page that also offers to enter into e-mail correspondence, and contains advertisements from therapists and health food companies. Such marketing mixed with health information and advice can also be found in medically oriented commercial sites. The UK-based 'healthinfocus' site contains advertisements for private health care, popular magazines and an Internet book store. Some home pages have links to commercial 'lifestyle' products that are also found on commercially based health pages. For example, 'Imagine' capsules that claim to provide a 'natural weight loss' were present as links on several home pages and commercial medical sites in the USA. Like commercial concerns, home page authors can generate an income by including such links on their pages. The 'direct-to-consumer' advertising of prescription drugs is a rapidly growing part of e-commerce (Alan and Holmer 1998). The text below is taken from a site originating in the USA that sells prescription drugs.

> SafeWeb Medical is proud to bring you prescription medicine through an easy, secure and confidential environment. Save time with our convenient online pharmacy. Receive your order in 24–48 hours after your prescription is approved by the medical doctors.
>
> Get a prescription and order securely online.
>
> No appointment
>
> No embarrassment
>
> No waiting rooms
>
> Confidential SSL Secure Ordering

What is significant here is that the outcome for the consumer in terms of the provision of prescription drugs matches that which most patients desire from a conventional medical encounter (Britten and Ukoumunne 1997). In the UK this cycle cannot be completed because doctors have to physically sign a prescription form. However, consumers in the UK may try and import drugs from other countries. Indeed a number of Internet sites provide the online translation of drug names available in different countries under various labels.

Conclusion and Discussion

The Internet provides a new rich source of health information, advice and treatment. As a resource for the publication and consumption of health information it is essentially pluralistic, democratic and both global and local. What has been described as 'glocalization' provides users with health information and advice that is not constrained by geographical or national boundaries (Featherstone et al. 1995). The previously closed and exclusive domain of Western medical information is open to consumers. Medical resources such as National Institute for Clinical Excellence (NICE) that provides guidance on 'best practice' and key medical journals are equally available to health professions and consumers of health care. Such material can be difficult for those without medical training to assimilate but the seamless nature of the Internet provides the means to find more accessible information. Health care provision and medical encounters in the UK have been described as endemically paternalistic (Coulter 1999). This reflects a culture in which 'assumptions that doctor (or nurse) knows best, making decisions on behalf of patients without involving them and feeling threatened when patients have access to alternative sources of medical information' is widespread, despite policy initiates to the contrary (Coulter 1999: 319). A recent report that looked at the future of UK general practice noted that:

> The informed health consumer is already a reality in certain socio-economic groupings, and with the growth of Internet and electronic libraries this trend can only accelerate. Is the informed patient a threat or an opportu-

> nity? Presumably GPs will have to become even more guides and translators of a mass of unfiltered information to help patients gain accurate knowledge about their condition. (Mihill 2000: 1405)

This suggests the potential transformation of the doctor/patient relationship in the face of the end of the medical monopoly over medical information. There are, however, certain notes of caution that need to be made concerning the role of the Internet and health. The first note of caution relates to inequalities of access to the Internet experienced by people located in different parts of the globe and in different social class categories. There are well-known social and economic inequalities that arise that form chronic illness and disability that may exclude individuals from using the Internet. The second area of concern is that those who use the Internet may be able to make disproportionate demands on health care resources to the detriment of others. This may allow relatively technologically rich middle classes to maintain advantages in terms of access and use of health resources. The final reservation relates to the organization and delivery of health and social services. Doctors and other health professionals act as gatekeepers to treatments, services and, in some instances, social benefits. Indeed this is a significant aspect of the 'sick role' that maintains the dependence of patients on doctors. What remains uncertain is whether the use of the Internet by consumers will increase pressure to improve the quality of health services and promote patient-centered medical practice, or encourage professional and organizational closure in the face of challenges to the status quo.

This paper has shown that consumers may also be producers of health information and advice to a global audience. This forms a hitherto neglected, but significant, part of the pluralization of health on the Internet. It has been noted that the use of the term 'quality' is seen, in part, as a means of ensuring users are not exposed to the 'risks' of pluralistic health knowledge. Seen from another perspective, the use of such terms as 'quality' (or 'evidence-based') may be regarded as an attempt to maintain boundaries around medical knowledge. As various protocols or quality filters to determine 'quality' become established the term may be confined to evidence-based medicine. The fact that potentially dangerous or inappropriate health information, advice and services are available does not underwrite the unambiguous usefulness of 'quality' to shape what is available to users. Despite difficulties with both the idea of 'quality' and the identification of particular information, it may well be argued that ethical considerations give medical professionals little choice in this matter. Indeed the assumption that 'the physician operates as a general trustee of the interests of the general population' (Crossley 1998: 509) remains a central plank of the professional status of medicine. It also underpins the privilege relationship the profession enjoys with the state (Saks 1995). The potential reproduction of a knowledge hierarchy on the Internet does not necessarily mean that it will be formative in shaping how users identify, use or produce health information on the Internet. Indeed, it is the diversity of information and choices that are available to users that characterize post-traditional society where choices are not constrained by the status accorded to a limited number of 'experts.' Well-publicized medical 'scandals' and a general public disenchantment and cynicism towards science and expertise suggests that Internet users do not desire to be confined to resources that been judge to be suitable for a lay audience (Giddens 1991; Lupton 1997). In what has been described as the 'risk society,' the interpretation of information and advice from a broad range of 'experts' forms part of a wider reflexivity (Beck 1992). As this paper has shown, the reflexive construction and publication of health narratives forms part of the reconfiguration of health expertise that is available to Internet users.

The erection of boundaries around what might be termed 'orthodox' or 'legitimate' knowledge and the 'non-orthodox' does not necessarily exclude both from occupying space within the Internet. As demonstrated in this paper, producers of health resources include both approaches within the same web pages. Users value and use medical information, personal narratives and other resources to make sense of their illness and to shape their health and lifestyle. More complex, however, is the emergent reconfiguration of the doctor—patient/consumer—health professional relationship. It would seem likely that we would wish to preserve some aspects of the traditional relationship where trust is developed through a negotiation of diagnosis and treatment. The question is not one of whether Internet health information is 'legitimate' but rather the more pragmatic one of how health and illness is understood and the forms of social relationships that stem from this. In some cases the answer may be that users gain a great deal, while in other cases the consequences may be less faith in medical care and greater exposure to risk.

References

Alan, F. and Holmer, J.D. (1998) 'Direct-to-consumer prescription drug advertising builds bridges between patients and physicians,' *Journal of the American Medical Association,* 281: 380.

Barry, C. A., Bradley, C. R., Britten, N., Stevenson, F. A. and Barber, N. (2000) 'Patients' unvoiced agendas in general practice consultations: qualitative study,' *British Medical Journal,* 321: 78–82.

Bartlett, D. and Payne, S. (1997) 'Grounded theory: its basis, rational and procedure' in G. McKenzie, J. Powell and P. Usher (eds) *Understanding Social Research: Perspectives on Methodology and Practice,* London: Falmer Presss.

Beck, U. (1992) *Risk Society: Towards a New Modernity,* London: Routledge.

Boseley, S. (2000) 'Virtual healing: Life Online,' *Guardian Unlimited,* 18 January.

Britten, N. and Ukoumunne, O. (1997) 'The influence of patients' hopes of receiving a prescription on doctors' perceptions and the decision to prescribe: a questionnaire survey,' *British Medical Journal,* 315: 1506—10.

Burkeman, O. (2000) 'Outright quackery,' *The Guardian,* 18 January. Online. Available: http://lifeonline.guardianunlimited.co.Uk/week/story/0,6457,123729,00.htm

Burrows, R. and Nettleton, S. (2000) 'Reflexive modernization and the emergence of wired self-help,' in K.A. Renninger and W. Shumar (eds) *Building Virtual Communities: Learning and Change in Cyberspace,* New York: Cambridge University Press.

Burrows, R., Nettleton, S., Pleace, N., Loader, B. and Steven, N. (2000) 'Virtual community care? Social policy and the emergence of computer mediated social support,' *Information, Communication and Society,* 3: 95–121. Online. Available: http://www.infosoc.co.uk/current/feature.htm

Bury, M. (1991) 'The sociology of chronic illness: a review of research and prospects,' *Sociology of Health and Illness,* 13: 451–68.

Cant, S. and Sharma, U. (1999) *A New Medical Pluralism?,* London: UCL Press.

Coulter, A. (1999) 'Paternalism or partnership?', *British Medical Journal,* 319: 719–20

Crossley, M. (1998) 'Sick Role' or 'Empowerment': the ambiguities of life with an HIV-positive diagnosis,' *Sociology of Health and Illness* 20: 507–31.

Cyber Dialogue (2000) Survey of Net Health Sector, Cyber Dialogue. Online. Available: http://www. Cyber Dialogue / surveys

Department of Health (1996) *A Service with Ambitions,* London: Stationary Office.

Eysenbach, G. and Diepgen, T. L. (1999) 'Patients looking for information on the Internet and seeking teleadvice: motivation, expectations, and misconceptions as expressed in e-mails sent to physicians,' *Archives of Dermatology,* 135: 151–6. Online. Available: http://www.ama-assn.org/scipubs/journals/archive/derm/vol_l35/no_2/

Featherstone, M. (1982) 'The body in consumer culture,' *Theory Culture and Society,* 1: 18–33.

Featherstone, M., Lash, S. and Robertson, R. (eds) (1995) *Global Modernities,* London: Sage.

Frank, A. W. (1995) 'The rhetoric of self-change: illness experience as narrative,' *The Sociological Quarterly* 34: 39–52.

Giddens, A. (1991) *Modernity and Self-Identity,* Cambridge: Polity Press.

Giddens, A. (1999) *Runaway World: How Globalisation is Reshaping our Lives,*Cambridge: Polity Press.

Hardey, M. (1999) 'Doctor in the house: the Internet as a source of lay health knowledge and the challenge to expertise,' *Sociology of Health and Illness,* 21: 820–35.

Hardey, M. (forthcoming) ' "The story of my illness": personal accounts of illness on the internet,' *Health: An Interdisciplinary Journal for the Social Study of Health and Illness and Medicine.*

Howie, J. G. R., Heaney, D. J., Maxwell. M., Walker, J. J., Freeman, G. K. and Rai, H. (1999) 'Quality at general practice consultations: cross sectional survey,' *British Medical Journal,* 319: 738–43.

Huntley A. C. (1999) 'The need to know patients, e-mail, and the Internet,' *Archives of Dermatology,* 135: 198.

Hyden, L. C. (1997) 'Illness and narrative,' *Sociology of Health and Illness,* 9: 48–69.

Kleinman, A. (1998) *Illness and Narrative: Suffering Healing and the Human Condition,* New York: Basic Books.

Loader, B. D. (ed.) (1997) *The Governance of Cyberspace,* London: Routledge.

Lupton, D. (1997) 'Doctors on the medical profession,' *Sociology of Health and Illness,* 19:480–97.

Mihill, C. (2000) *Shaping Tomorrow: Issues Facing General Practice in the New Millennium,* London: British Medical Association.

Parsons, T. (1951) *The Social System,* Glenco: Free Press.

Porter, R. (1998) *Health for Sale: Quackery in England 1650–1850,* Manchester: Manchester University Press.

Radley, A. (1999) 'The aesthetics of illness: narrative, horror and the sublime,' *Sociology of Health and Illness* 21: 778–796.

Saks, M. (1995) *Professions and the Public Interest,* London: Routledge.

Selwyn, N. and Robson, K. (1998) 'Using e-mail as a research tool,' *Social Research Update,* 21.

Strauss, A. and Corbin, J. (1990) *Basics of Qualitative Research: Grounded Theory Procedures and Techniques,* London: Sage.

The Dutch Council for Health and Social Service (RVZ) (1999) *Advisory Report on the Patient and the Internet,* Amsterdam: RVZ. Online.

Turner, B. S. (1995) *Medical Power and Social Knowledge,* London: Sage.

Williams, G. and Popay J. (1994) 'Lay knowledge and the privileging of experience,' in J. Gabe, D. Kelleher and G. Williams (eds) *Challenging Medicine,* London: Routledge, pp. 61–84.

Websites

1. http://www.quackwatch.com (Accessed 29 October 1999)
2. http://hitiweb.mitretek.org/ (Accessed 29 October 1999)
3. http://www.bmia.org/ (Accessed 25 November 1999)
4. http://www.healthinfocus.co.uk/cms_anon.pl/home (Accessed 18 January 2000)
5. http://www.bbc.co.uk/health/ (Accessed 28 January 2000)
6. http://www.nhsdirect.nhs.uk/ (Accessed 28 January 2000)
7. http://www.onhealth.com/home/index (Accessed 25 November 1999)
8. http://www.healthgate.com/ (Accessed 28 January 2000)
9. http://www.princeton.edu/~tgmiller/log/initial.html (Accessed 28 January 2000)
10. http://members.tripod.co.uk/~timlang/illness.html (Accessed 28 January 2000)
11. http://www.goes.com/~paraplegics.html (Accessed 15 November 1999)
12. http://heskco.com/karan/home.htm (Accessed 29 October 1999)
13. http://home.pacbell.net/eah/mypage/index.htm (Accessed 25 November 1999)
14. http://hometown.aol.com/chan/page.htm (Accessed 29 October 1999)
15. http://www.SafeWebMedical.com/ (Accessed 28 January 2000)

Discussion Questions

1. Should consumers have increased access to public health information? What are both the benefits and drawbacks of using the Internet to learn about our individual health status?
2. What does it mean to "consume" and "produce" health information? What are some examples of consumption and production via the Internet?
3. What does it mean to take a "paternalistic" approach to health care? How might consumers use the Internet to transform this approach? ✦

Chapter 13 Uncertainty in Illness

Merle H. Mishel

Chapter 13 completes the third part of this anthology and considers uncertainty as a major emotion that shapes so much of how patients see themselves and determines the way they seek information from health-care providers. When dealing with health-related issues, both providers and consumers inevitably encounter a great deal of uncertainty. This chapter frames uncertainty as the absence of meaning and suggests that individuals construct meaning to cope with uncertain situations like illness. Uncertainty is often associated with increased psychological and emotional stress during times of illness; therefore, a greater understanding of uncertainty might help both providers and consumers manage its effects.

Taken together, the chapters in Part III open up the complex set of dynamics that need to be examined when looking at health-care provision and the ways in which patients are no longer seen as passive vessels that medical experts "pour" their knowledge into.

Related Topics: health-care behaviors, media, patient-provider communication, role of the patient, social support

Uncertainty concerning what will happen, what the consequences of an event are, and what the event means, are important to a person with any illness. Managing the uncertainty associated with an illness and its treatment may be an essential task in adaptation.

From "Uncertainty in Illness," Merle H. Mishel, 1988, *Image—the Journal of Nursing Scholarship*, Vol. 20:4, pp. 225–232.

Uncertainty is defined as the inability to determine the meaning of illness-related events. It is the cognitive state created when the person cannot adequately structure or categorize an event because of the lack of sufficient cues. Uncertainty occurs in a situation in which the decision maker is unable to assign definite value to objects or events and/or is unable to predict outcomes accurately (Mishel, 1984). The middle-range nursing theory of uncertainty in illness is discussed in this paper. The theory contains knowledge derived from nursing and other disciplines, addresses clinical phenomena derived from the practice arena (Roy, 1985) and offers an interactionist perspective for explaining the process of determining meaning in the illness experience.

Uncertainty in Illness

The uncertainty theory explains how patients cognitively process illness-related stimuli and construct meaning in these events. Uncertainty, or the inability to structure meaning, can develop if the patient does not form a cognitive schema for illness events. A cognitive schema is the patient's subjective interpretation of illness, treatment and hospitalization. As can be seen in Figure 13.1, stimuli frame, cognitive capacity and structure providers precede uncertainty and offer the information that is processed by the patient.

The primary antecedent variable, stimuli frame, refers to the form, composition and structure of the stimuli that the person perceives; the stimuli frame has three components: symptom pattern, event familiarity and event congruence. These three components provide the stimuli that are structured by the patient into a cognitive schema, which creates less uncertainty. *Symptom pattern* refers to the degree to which symptoms present with sufficient consistency to be perceived as having a pattern or configuration. Based on this pattern, the meaning of the symptoms can be determined. *Event familiarity* refers to the degree to which the situation is habitual, repetitive, or contains recognized cues.

When events are recognized as familiar, they can be associated with events from memory and their meaning can be determined. *Event congruence* refers to the consistency between the expected and the experienced in illness-related events. This consistency implies reliability and stability of events, thus facilitating interpretation and understanding. These components of the stimuli frame are inversely related to uncertainty; they reduce uncertainty.

The three components of the stimuli frame are influenced by two variables: cognitive capacity and structure providers. *Cognitive capacity* refers to the information-processing abilities of the person. Only a limited amount of information can be processed at any one time (Warburton, 1979). Information overload occurs when this capacity is exceeded. Limited cognitive capacity will reduce the ability to perceive symptom pattern, event familiarity and the congruence of events.

The second variable influencing the stimuli frame is *structure providers*—the resources available to assist the person in the interpretation of the stimuli frame. Structure providers are proposed to reduce the state of uncertainty both directly and indirectly. Uncertainty is reduced directly when the patient relies on the structure providers to interpret the events. The reduction in uncertainty occurs indirectly when structure providers aid the patient in determining the pattern of symptoms, the familiarity of events and the congruence of experiences. Structure providers are educational level, social support and credible authority.

Stimuli are processed by patients to construct a cognitive schema for illness events. Uncertainty results when a cognitive schema cannot be formed. In the illness experience, uncertainty has four forms: (a) ambiguity concerning the state of the illness, (b) complexity regarding treatment and system of care, (c) lack of information about the diagnosis and seriousness of the illness, and (d) unpredictability of the course of the disease and prognosis.

Uncertainty is not inherently a dreaded or desired state until the implications of the uncertainty are determined. Under conditions of uncertainty, there is great potential for diverse evaluations and outcomes because the situation lacks form or structure, thus leaving it open to multiple definitions. Because of the amorphous nature of the stimuli, they can be shaped by the person's appraisal and reformed like putty. According to this theory, uncertainty can be appraised as a danger or as an opportunity. Uncertain events evaluated as a danger

Figure 13.1
Model of Perceived Uncertainty in Illness

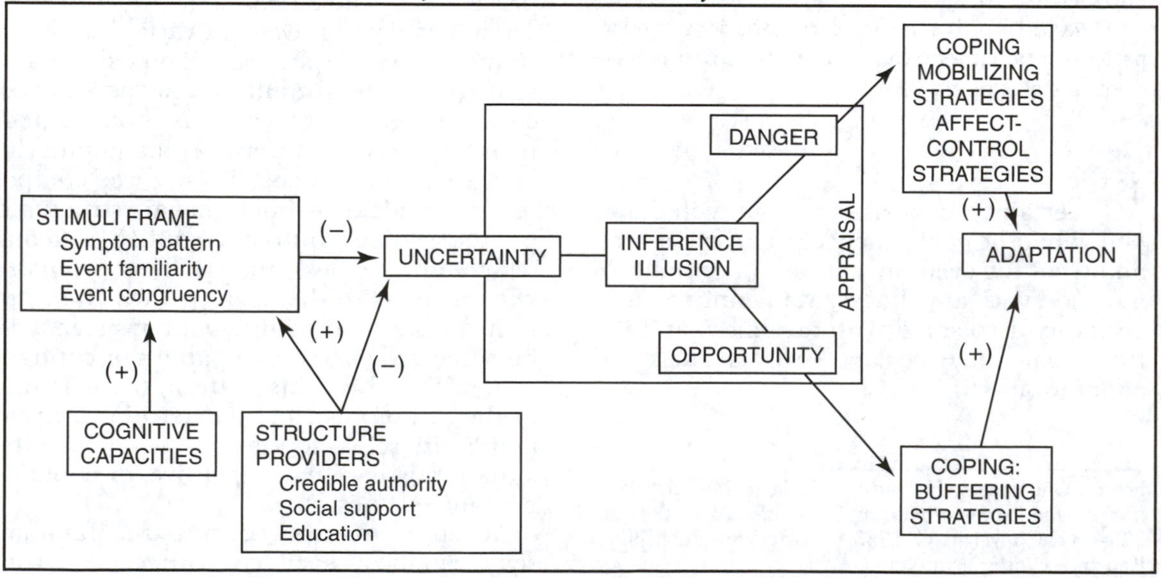

imply harm, and coping strategies to reduce the uncertainty are implemented. Uncertain events evaluated as opportunity imply a positive outcome, and coping strategies to maintain uncertainty are implemented. If the coping strategies are effective, then adaptation will occur. Signs of difficulty in adapting, rather than indicating uncertainty itself, indicate individuals' inability to manipulate the uncertainty in the desired direction. When the theory is applied to patient's experience with specific illness, selected linkages in the theory are singled out for study. Following the model, the theory of uncertainty will be elaborated using current findings from a series of uncertainty studies from nursing and related fields.

Stimuli Frame

Symptom Pattern

Symptom pattern, one component of stimuli frame, refers to the degree to which symptoms present with sufficient consistency to form a pattern or configuration. When symptoms form a pattern, less uncertainty exists, particularly less ambiguity about the state of the illness (Mishel & Braden, 1988). To appraise symptoms, patients evaluate their number, intensity, frequency, duration and location. To generate a hypothesis, this sensory information is used along with generalized information from their own illness experience, culture and social network as well as from health care practitioners. Multiple factors can interfere with the normal process of symptom appraisal such as the characteristics of the stimuli, the accuracy of the appraisal and the saliency or distinguishability of symptoms.

When symptoms are characterized by inconsistency in intensity, frequency, number, location and/or duration, such as occurs in some chronic illnesses, a pattern is not discernable. Inconsistent symptoms cannot be used to gauge reliably the state of the illness; thus they generate uncertainty. Illnesses characterized by remissions and exacerbations, having flares indicating symptom reoccurrence and disruption of previous symptom pattern, are associated with elevated levels of uncertainty (King & Mishel, 1986). Braden and Lynn (1987) found that, in persons with rheumatoid arthritis, lack of a consistent symptom pattern was the greatest predictor of uncertainty. Patients with diseases characterized by symptom variability such as immunological conditions, systemic lupus erythematosus and heart disease have higher levels of uncertainty than do persons with illness characterized by symptom consistency (Mishel, 1981).

Accuracy of symptom perception is frequently limited because of perceptual and cognitive biases such as selective attention and emotional arousal. Levanthal, Nerenz and Steele (1984) note that emotions play a role in the accuracy with which individuals scan their symptoms. If a person is depressed or threatened by an illness, symptoms of actual or presumed illness may be interpreted to be more severe than they actually are. Also, a sense of helplessness surrounding the cause or persistence of symptoms may make it difficult to discern the seriousness of the physical state (Rowat & Knafl, 1985).

Symptom appraisals may also be difficult because symptoms lack saliency. Symptoms must be sufficiently prominent to be included in the symptom pattern. Absence of salient symptoms with no guarantee of cure can generate more uncertainty than does the existence of symptoms (Mishel, Hostetter, King & Graham, 1984). Distinguishability also affects assessment of a symptom pattern. To assess the characteristics of each symptom, patients must be able to differentiate one symptom from another. In treatments such as those given for cancer, when symptoms of illness blend with symptoms generated by treatment, distinguishability of symptoms becomes an issue.

Because of the large number of internal sensations that are vague, diffuse and subjective, monitoring the body to identify symptom pattern is a continual activity. If symptoms are consistent, predictable, salient and distinguishable, then a symptom pattern can be identified, and uncertainty will be less. Mishel and Braden (1988) found that the presence of a symptom pattern was a significant predictor of less uncertainty among women undergoing treatment for gynecological cancer.

Event Familiarity

The second component of stimuli frame, event familiarity, refers to the habitual or repetitive nature of the structure of the environment. Whereas symptom pattern refers to the structure of physical sensations, event familiarity refers to patterns within the health care environment. Familiarity of events is developed over time and through experience in a setting.

Familiarity is generated through a cognitive map built on experience with the environment. New events are related to the cognitive map and, if they fit the general nature of individuals' schematic knowledge, the event is evaluated as being familiar. Cognitive maps are generated from personal experience, cultural input, social sources and health professionals (Levanthal et al., 1984). Information about the environment stored in cognitive maps enables persons to sense the expected performance in various circumstances. With event familiarity, uncertainty is prevented.

In the health care environment, novelty and complexity of events impede development of event familiarity. According to Budner (1962), novelty indicates a substantially new situation in which there are few familiar cues such as first admission to a hospital or initiation of chemotherapy, radiation or other treatments. Complexity is a situation in which there are a great number of cues to be taken into account, for example, in a diagnostic work-up.

Novelty resulting in higher uncertainty levels occurs in family members of patients suddenly admitted to intensive care. When patients and family members are oriented to the unit prior to admission and gain a degree of familiarity, this reduces the novelty of the environment (Mintun, 1984). With a sudden admission, patients and family members are thrust into a novel and complex treatment setting. Mishel (1981) found that complexity and novelty of events resulting in uncertainty can also occur in patients undergoing diagnostic tests that are unfamiliar such as a cardiac catheterization. When treatment is more routine and consistent, for example, a medical treatment or a routine invasive treatment such as hemodialysis, the events are familiar and associated with lower levels of uncertainty (Mishel, 1981). Novelty appears to be the aspect of unfamiliarity that generates uncertainty, and, as novelty abates, uncertainty decreases. The longer patients live with a disease, the less uncertainty they experience (Braden & Lynn, 1987; King & Mishel, 1986). Yet, when novelty does not abate over time and the treatment setting remains strange and alien, higher levels of uncertainty are evidenced (Mishel, 1987).

Event Congruence

Event congruence, the third component of stimuli frame, refers to the consistency between what is expected and what is experienced in illness-related events. Lack of congruence between the expected and the experienced creates questions concerning the predictability and stability of the event. The generation of uncertainty through the lack of congruence can occur when expectations of cure are shattered by an unforeseen reoccurrence of disease. Webster and Christman (in press) noted that patients who had a history of coronary artery disease, experienced more uncertainty in recovering from a myocardial infarction than did patients having their first exposure to coronary artery disease. Likewise, unmet expectations of cure also generate uncertainty when a treatment effect is not achieved by a predetermined time (Mishel, 1985). Another source of incongruence resulting in uncertainty can occur when treatment does not produce a change in how a person feels, therefore they have no indication of any change in their physical status, for example, undergoing radiation. Unexpected rapid changes that are inconsistent with expectations also exemplify a lack of congruence. Levanthal et al. (1984) noted that when cancer patients' nodes shrank in one or two treatment cycles, the recovery was associated with levels of distress twice that reported by patients whose lymph nodes shrank more gradually. The former group had difficulty coping with the inconsistency between the absence of concrete symptoms and the continuation of treatment.

Cognitive Capacity

Since cognitive capacity refers to the information-processing abilities of persons, any physiological malfunction will lessen these abilities and have an impact on cognition. The processing abilities most susceptible to disruption are those requiring attentional resources. Demands on the attentional capacity disrupt the processing of stimuli frame information, thus eliciting uncertainty. Physical illness itself is a potent attention-seizing distraction and can reduce the total amount of attention that individuals can devote to a cognitive task. Attentional resources are also reduced by pain, drugs and poor nutritional state. Internal stimuli such as pain, discomfort, danger, and such internal physiological events as autonomic nervous system activity can monopolize cognitive capacity and impair problem-solving activity (Mandler, 1979).

When the patient perceives the health-related environment as a danger, cognitive efficiency is lessened, and fewer cues are processed. Dangerous situations tend to increase the level of arousal, which in turn focuses patients' attention more narrowly on aspects of the situation considered most important. Restrictions on cognitive capacities under stress also affect memory function. When these patients attempt to recall events, only the most salient will be accessible, thus weakening the ability to associate incoming stimuli with preexisting cognitive schema (Mandler, 1979).

Changes in cognitive processing abilities also occur through manipulation of corticol activity by cholinolytics. Mandler (1979) reported that persons receiving cholinolytics report loss of awareness or alertness, difficulty in concentrating and shortened attention span. Other drugs, particularly sedatives, have a depressing effect on cognition and weaken particularly the ability to search for information in the long-term memory, to maintain attention and to suppress distractions. Impairment in information processing has also been attributed to the neurotoxic effects of chemotherapy, particularly in older age groups (Silberfarb, 1983). Impairment of memory and thinking, whether the result of demands that monopolize cognitive resources or because of factors that alter cognitive abilities, weaken the accuracy of appraisal, causing environmental events to be perceived as being uncertain.

Structure Providers

Education

Education is proposed to have both an indirect and direct relationship to uncertainty. In the indirect relationship, education can assist in supplying a structure to the events in the stimuli frame by enlarging a patient's knowledge base with which to associate these events, thus providing meaning and context. Support for this position is uneven when education is considered along with other components of structure providers (Mishel, 1981; Mishel & Braden, 1988). When education is examined alone, support for its direct impact on uncertainty is evident, with those having less than a high school education demonstrating higher levels of uncertainty in the form of more perceived complexity concerning treatment and more difficulty in understanding the system of care (Galloway, 1984; King & Mishel, 1986; Mishel, 1985). Those with more education are able to modify the uncertainty more rapidly than are those with less education. Individuals with less education seem to require more time to construct meaning for events, and they experience uncertainty for longer periods of time than do individuals with more education (Christman et al., 1988; Mishel, 1985).

Social Support

Social support acts to prevent uncertainty in various life crisis by supplying feedback on the meaning of events (Wortman & Dunkel-Schetter, 1979). The opportunity to clarify a situation through discussion and supportive interactions with others clarifies contingencies and aids the patient in forming a cognitive schema (Wortman, 1984).

Researchers on social support have found that support systems have both a direct and indirect influence on uncertainty. The result of the direct influence is the modification of three types of uncertainty: (a) the ambiguity concerning the state of the illness, (b) the complexity perceived in treatment and (c) the unpredictability of the future (Hilton, 1986; Mishel & Braden, 1987). The indirect influence of social support is on strengthening the clarity of the symptom pattern (Mishel & Braden, 1988). Sharing information with persons in the social network assists patients in the appraisal of symptoms. Patterson, Freese and Goldenberg (1986) reported that women consult their social network about positive indicators of pregnancy. The significant others add to the repertoire of indicators and notice confirming indicators of pregnancy, thus preventing uncertainty.

The importance of social support as a source of information extends beyond the patients to their caregivers. For patients' caregivers, communication with others who have the same diagnosis as do the patients or are having the same treatment conveys support by providing shared meaning for an initially unfamiliar and seemingly hostile treatment environment. Among caregivers, lack of such support is associated with higher levels of uncertainty (King, 1983).

Aside from providing information, social support also functions as a means of avoiding uncertainty by establishing a network where each member depends on another member's expertise to handle various threatening events. After treatment for gynecological cancer ends, having persons one can rely on for life's daily tasks reduces patients' unpredictability about the future (Mishel & Braden, 1987). Social support in the form of material aid may reduce uncertainty by providing assurance of the stability of the environment. Hilton (1986) reported that women with breast cancer found that the emotional, physical and resource support provided by relatives was extremely helpful. Assistance such as caring for the household and rides to radiation therapy were important in patients' handling of the uncertainty surrounding their illness. Awareness of a stable core of others to provide concrete services and tangible aid functions to minimize the unpredictability of the outcome.

Credible Authority

Credible authority refers to the degree of trust and confidence patients have in the health care providers. Indirectly, credible authority influences uncertainty by its positive association with the stimuli frame. Credible authority, in the form of the nurse and physician, strengthens the stimuli frame by providing information on the causes and consequences of symptoms. Patients often doubt their appraisal of symptoms and seek confirmation from physicians and nurses (Levanthal et al., 1984). Patterson et al. (1986) found that women sought professional confirmation that their symptoms were indicators of pregnancy. Women expressed little confidence in their diagnostic capabilities and desired professional validation.

Health care providers also share information about the manifestations of the illness and the performance of the health care system, which enhances event familiarity. Consistent contact with the health care providers makes possible a set of expectations about caregiver behavior and the components of the treatment setting (Oberst, 1984).

Health care providers also promote event congruence. Johnson (1984) showed that provision of sensory information focusing upon the patient's impending experiences may influence the structure of the cognitive schema. Sensory information has been found to reduce the patient's emotional response and length of hospitalization. Johnson explained this as promoting congruence between the expected and experienced event. Nurses, as credible health care providers, enhance event congruence by providing patients with a framework for interpreting their experience as they proceed through it. The enhancement of predictability through promoting event congruence can indirectly avoid uncertainty.

In the direct relationship between credible authority and uncertainty, health care providers may work through assumption of power. Often patients do not attempt to understand the technical mechanisms underlying their illness but prefer to rely on health care providers to provide a logical structure to the events. Patients often expect the physician or nurse to take responsibility to provide judgment and recommendations of value. When the authority is evaluated as being highly credible, uncertainty will be lessened. The relationship with the health care provider has been reported as the major means for the prevention of uncertainty (Mishel & Braden, 1988). Trust and confidence in the health care provider leads to a lower level of overall uncertainty, less ambiguity about the state of the illness and less perceived complexity concerning treatment (Mishel & Braden, 1987).

Credible authority and social support assist in the prevention of uncertainty by structuring meaning relative to different sources of cues (Mishel & Braden, 1988). Cues residing in the health care environment are best addressed by the credible authority. Such cues refer to the physical aspects of treatment, the efficacy of treatment, relationships with health care providers, expectations about care outcomes and performance of the health-care system. Cues residing within the individuals are best addressed by interaction with significant others. These cues refer to personal concerns such as interpreting body signs and symptoms and planning for one's life and personal responsibilities.

Uncertainty and Appraisal

When uncertainty exists, the perceptual tasks of recognition and classification are not completed, and formation of a cognitive schema is hampered (Bower, 1978). For recognition and classification of illness-related events to occur, the stimuli must be specific, familiar, consistent, complete, limited in number and clear in boundaries. The stimuli must also correspond with an existing frame of reference and be congruent with a person's expectations of physical and temporal context. When stimuli lack these characteristics, cognitive processing errors occur, and uncertainty results as the predominant cognitive state. The state of uncertainty may be the result of the nature of the stimulus, for example, its random pattern of occurrence, or the result of a deficiency in the perceiver such as the lack of a frame of reference for an event or because of limitations in current medical knowledge. When an event is perceived as being uncertain, one of three situations is operative: (a) the event is not recognized; (b) the event is recognized but not classified; (c) the event is recognized but classified incorrectly.

The experience of uncertainty is neutral; it is neither a desired nor avoided experience until it is appraised. Appraisal in an uncertain situation involves two major processes: inference and illusion. Inference refers to the evaluation of uncertainty using related examples that one can recall and is built on personality dispositions, general experience, knowledge and contextual cues. Illusion refers to the construction of beliefs formed from the uncertainty—beliefs that have a generally positive outlook.

Inference

Inferences built on personality dispositions refer to general beliefs about oneself and one's relationship with the environment. Such dispositions include learned resourcefulness (Rosenbaum, 1983), a sense of mastery (Pearlin & Schooler, 1978) and locus of control (Rotter, 1966). These dispositions refer to persons' beliefs that they have the skills and behavior to deal effectively with major life events. These beliefs are put into effect to appraise uncertainty. However, for learned resourcefulness and mastery to be operative the events must be represented objectively and must correspond to a past experience (Rosenbaum, 1983). In illness, uncertain events lack the clarity and predictability necessary for objective representation, and they may not correspond to past learning. Thus uncertain events, appraised by these personality dispositions, are likely to be viewed as difficult to manage indeed dangerous. Uncertainty significantly reduced the sense of mastery in women treated for gynecological cancer and weakened the learned resourcefulness of chronically ill persons living in the community (Braden, 1986). Likewise, the reduction in a sense of mastery was a cause of uncertainty appraised as a danger.

When stimulus cues are highly ambiguous, the personality disposition of locus of control becomes important in determining the appraisal process. There is a common misconception about the stability of a person's locus of control. Actually, locus of control, either internal or external, becomes active *only* in ambiguous situations (Folkman, Schaefer, & Lazarus, 1979). For those persons who have a disposition toward internal control, uncertainty would likely be appraised as controllable and thus an opportunity. A disposition toward external control would cause uncertain events to be appraised as dangerous in situations where the credible authority is absent or unavailable.

Inference can also be based on general experience and knowledge. General knowledge is used to identify examples of similar situations that, when viewed as having a beneficial outcome, would facilitate uncertainty's being evaluated as beneficial. Recalling related situations can be done by the patients, by significant others, or by the health care providers. The greater the similarity between the recalled situation and the patients' current situation, the greater is the influence of the recall on the appraisal of uncertainty.

Similarly, specific knowledge related to the situation will also influence appraisal. This knowledge can be stimulated by significant others or by health care providers. The influence on a danger appraisal or on an opportunity appraisal will depend on the content of the specific information, be it positive or negative.

Inference can also occur by generalizing from immediate communications, or contextual cues. If prior communications are perceived as being threatening, then the ambiguous events will be interpreted as being ominous by the process of generalization. According to Janis (1962), generalization occurs only in high-threat situations.

Illusion

Uncertainty can also be appraised through the process of illusion. Illusions are defined as beliefs constructed out of uncertainty—beliefs that are viewed in a particular light with emphasis on their favorable aspects (Taylor, 1983). Self-enhancing illusions cannot be constructed out of certainty. Once a situation is clear or certain, it is difficult or impossible to redefine it. Perception of uncertainty provides the foundation on which illusionary meaning can be constructed (Holmes & Houston, 1974). When illusions are generated from the uncertainty, the uncertainty is appraised as an opportunity.

In the past, construction of illusion was likened to denial and was judged as being maladaptive. The recent literature reflects support for illusions, avoidance and denial (Breznitz, 1983; Lazarus, 1983). Support for such palliative responses is seen as being particularly appropriate in situations in which individuals are helpless to influence the outcome or in which the outcome has a negative, downward trajectory. In such situations, it may well be that maintenance of hope depends on the existence of uncertainty. Lazarus suggested that the maintenance of illusion is valuable in protecting persons both in the initial stages of threat and when persons must come to terms with information that is difficult to accept.

The generation of illusion can be fostered by significant others in an attempt to support patients in maintaining hope or by health care providers who respect patients' need to emphasize the ambiguity in a situation in order to perceive a potential positive outcome. Sensitive health care providers can aid patients in constructing supportive illusions; often, however, ambiguous information is considered stressful, and attempts are made to reduce uncertainty by presenting specific treatment-related details that may not be desired by the patients. As patients receive detailed information beyond that requested, situations become more structured, and illusions may be destroyed. Much is still unknown about the conditions under which uncertainty promotes illusion. Yet it is important to consider the positive view of uncertainty and to pursue identification of when it occurs and how it operates.

Uncertainty, Danger, Coping

Based on the appraisal, uncertainty is viewed as being either a danger or an opportunity. When uncertainty is considered a danger, the possibility of a harmful outcome is the result of an inference appraisal. A danger appraisal occurs when the predictive accuracy of the inferences is unknown. Extensive evidence supports the appraisal of uncertainty as a danger. Uncertainty has been associated with a pessimistic outlook and negative evaluation of the future in both newly diagnosed cancer patients and in cancer patients measured at treatment and stabilization (Campbell, 1986; Mishel et al., 1984). Uncertainty is associated with elevated anxiety levels in parents of children in pediatric intensive care units (Mintun, 1984), in spouses of patients admitted to a coronary care unit (Herbst, 1986), in patients with myocardial infarction measured one week after discharge (Webster & Christman, in press), arid in caretakers of persons with lupus (King, 1983). Uncertainty has also been associated with depression in patients following myocardial infarction (Christman et al., 1988) and in cancer patients at diagnosis and at three and six months postdiagnosis (Richardson et al., 1987). Others have not specified the negative affect associated with uncertainty but have noted the relationship between uncertainty and distress (Jessop & Stein, 1985). The specific antecedents found to influence uncertainties being appraised as a danger include loss or absence of a credible authority at diagnosis and during treatment (Mishel & Braden, 1988), event unfamiliarity (recency of diagnosis) and a lack of a symptom pattern, (King & Mishel, 1986).

Uncertainty perceived as a danger is associated with electrocortical arousal, the amount of which is related to the amount of uncertainty in the environment. Electrocortical arousal and corticosteroid release are predicted to be related. Since electrocortical arousal is a response to high uncertainty appraised as a danger, the stress steroid release will be elevated. Evidence from studies on corticosteroid excretion of soldiers under constant threat of attack shows that uncertainty associated with danger seems to be a common factor in multiple situations in which stress steroid is released (Warburton, 1979). Not only are corticosteroids released, but there is also a noticeable release of catecholamines in situations that are unpredictable and possibly require action.

Coping

With a danger appraisal, coping methods are directed toward reducing the uncertainty if possible and managing the emotion generated by a danger appraisal. There are two coping tracks: mobilizing contains the strategies of direct action, vigilance and information seeking, while *affect-management* contains the methods of faith, disengagement and cognitive support.

Within the mobilizing track, there is evidence that, among patients with catastrophic illnesses such as cancer or heart disease, direct action was the least used method for the reduction of uncertainty (Christman et al., 1988; Molleman, Krobendam, Annyas, Koops, & Sleufer, 1984). Vigilance as a coping method for uncertainty reduction has been addressed primarily in social psychology laboratory studies (Miller, 1980; Monat, 1976). In the only work relating vigilance to uncertainty in illness, Jessop and Stein (1985) found that parents of chronically ill children used vigilance to manage the uncertainty stemming from their children's symptoms. Yet, the constant need to be watching their children created emotional disturbance in the mothers and increased the negative impact of the children's illness on family functioning.

The third mobilizing strategy, information seeking, has been proposed as the primary means for reducing uncertainty (Berlyne, 1977; Lanzetta, 1971). Clinical studies on the use of information seeking to modify uncertainty support its effectiveness. Information is used to formulate time tables and probabilities and to form a framework to order the illness-related experiences (Comaroff & Maquire, 1981).

Information is sought from significant others, physicians and nurses. These health care providers function as antecedents to uncertainty by structuring information to prevent uncertainty and also serve as information sources to reduce uncertainty once it has been generated. Molleman et al. (1984) noted that the use of experts is effective in reducing uncertainty.

Significant others also aid in the reduction of uncertainty by providing expert information or interpreting events. The sense of disorganization resulting from uncertainty can be reduced by contact with others who have faced the same experience. Molleman et al. (1984) found that patients used fellow patients for social comparison to reduce uncertainty, with preference being given to fellow patients who were undergoing problems similar to those of the patient or even better off since they were more informative. Mishel and Murdaugh (1987) found that family members of heart transplant patients sought information from each other about how to reduce their spouses' unpredictable susceptibility to infection. In a quasiexperimental study, Bradley and Mikolajczak (1986) reported that the use of two nursing exit interviews providing postdischarge information to medical patients reduced uncertainty, ambiguity and complexity, as compared with the control group subjects.

If the mobilizing techniques are not effective in reducing uncertainty then affect-control strategies are called into action. The major purpose of these coping methods is to manage the emotional responses, particularly the anxiety that occurs when the person believes that nothing can be done to modify the uncertainty.

Studies on affect-control strategies have not addressed each strategy individually but have considered affect management as a whole. There is evidence that strategies to control affect are used to manage uncertainty. Although Christman et al. (1988) did not find a relationship between affective coping and the reduction of uncertainty, Webster and Christman (in press), in earlier pilot work, reported that affective coping was used to manage uncertainty. Support for the use of affective coping was also reported by Viney and Westbrook (1984), who noted that chronically ill persons with higher levels of uncertainty preferred strategies to control negative emotions. Likewise, cancer patients have been noted to try to blunt their negative emotional response to uncertainty by giving themselves pep talks, playing with ideas, attempting to redefine the situation and using wishful thinking (Molleman et al., 1984; Mishel, 1988).

Uncertainty, Opportunity, Coping

When uncertainty is considered as an opportunity, the possibility of a positive outcome is the result of the appraisal. This possibility can result from inference or illusion but more likely emanates from the process of the generation of illusion. The vague and amorphous nature of an uncertain situation allows it to be reformed by persons into a positive situation. Under the umbrella of uncertainty, a new illusionary structure can be developed that portends a more positive outcome. Viewing uncertainty as an opportunity requires preoccupation with the positive rather than the negative.

Folkman et al. (1979) noted that most information-processing models are concerned only with the reduction of uncertainty; the issue of tolerating uncertainty is ignored. A theoretical model is needed that describes the processes by which persons reduce uncertainty and the processes that also permit uncertainty to persist. Attention should be given to the adaptive value of uncertainty in situations where it allows individuals to interpret transactions in a positive light.

Although uncertainty is generally considered a threat that implies danger, while certainty is seen as being beneficial, evidence from the research is inconsistent (Berlyne, 1977; Janis, 1962; Lanzetta, 1971). It has been suggested that patients may desire to maintain uncertainty since it facilitates hope (Folkman et al., 1979; Holmes & Houston, 1974).

An opportunity appraisal occurs when the alternative is a high probability of negative certainty. Negative certainty signifies an illness situation with a known downward trajectory. When the alternative is negative certainty, uncertainty may be a preferable state. An evaluation of uncertainty as an opportunity allows the person to forestall perception of an absolute negative outcome or reoccurrence. Although few studies have explored the possibility that uncertainty can be viewed as a positive state, there is some support for an opportunity evaluation. Evidence suggests that in illnesses with a downward trajectory such as chronic hemodialysis, uncertainty about the outcome influences patients to be more adherent to their treatment regimen since they believe in the potential of recovery (Capritto, 1980). Similarly, among adolescents with cystic fibrosis, those with higher levels of uncertainty had a longer future time perspective (Yarcheski, in press). Among parents of hospitalized children, lack of information (a type of uncertainty) was found to be associated with a more positive interpretation of the seriousness of their child's illness (Mishel, 1983).

Further support for an opportunity evaluation was noted by King and Mishel (1986) who reported that the longer individuals live with the diagnosis of lupus, the more likely they are to evaluate the uncertainty in the disease as an opportunity. Evidence of a physiological basis for opportunity appraisal was reported by Pergrin, Mishel and Murdaugh (1987), who found that caretakers of victims of Alzheimer's disease with higher levels of uncertainty had significantly lower levels of urinary cortisol and catecholomines. The reduced arousal may reflect the caregivers' view that more is yet to be learned about Alzheimer's disease and progress is still to be made.

With an opportunity evaluation of uncertainty, hope is possible and can be an active state. Support for the tie between opportunity and hope was found in family members of heart transplant patients who evaluated the uncertainty of their future as a second chance at life when contrasted with the certain death that had awaited their spouses. They actively utilized hope maintenance methods in order to deflect threats to their perception of reality (Mishel & Murdaugh, 1987).

Based on these findings, it appears that uncertainty can be seen as an opportunity when the alternative is negative certainty. Further study is necessary to identify the persons and situation contingencies that influence opportunity appraisals.

Coping

With an opportunity appraisal, buffering methods are used to support the uncertainty. For the opportunity appraisal to be maintained, it is necessary that uncertainty continue. If uncertainty disappears, the person must recognize the negative certainty, and the belief in a positive outcome is destroyed. The opportunity appraisal is constructed on illusions generated to explain uncertain events. These illusions exist only under the protective veil of uncertainty. If uncertainty is removed, the illusionary structure vanishes.

Buffering serves the purpose of blocking the input of new stimuli that could alter the view of uncertainty as an opportunity. The strategies include avoidance, selective ignoring, reordering priorities and neutralizing. Such forms of coping have found increasing support as the adaptive functions of palliative coping have been rehabilitated (Breznitz, 1983).

The use of these methods involves gathering carefully collated bodies of evidence. Individuals have to manage communication so as to maintain fragile optimism. One such method is to ignore selectively the differences between the patient and others doing better and stress only the similarities (Comaroff & Maquire 1981; Mishel & Murdaugh, 1987). A second method is to minimize new information in order to neutralize threatening content (Hilton, 1986). Comaroff and Maquire suggested that minimization can range from absolute denial to selective misinterpretation. Downward social comparisons, according to Mishel and Murdaugh, is yet another method used to neutralize threatening material by identifying characteristics present in failing patients that are absent in oneself. Other methods include reordering priorities by making changes in life-style and selective ignoring by focusing on only the positive aspects of unpredictability (King & Mishel, 1986).

Uncertainty and Adaptation

If the coping strategies are effective for an uncertain event appraised as either a danger or an opportunity, adaptation will occur. Adaptation is defined as biopsychosocial behavior occurring within persons' individually defined range of usual behavior. It is essentially a neutral zone that contains adequate but not extreme activation and also allows goal-directed behavior to continue. Adaptation difficulty implies behavior outside of the usual range with a level of activation that is higher or lower than the individuals' norm.

In most of the studies on uncertainty and adaptation, appraisal and coping have not been considered. Adaptation has been operationalized as psychosocial adjustment, recovery, stress, life quality, or health. Support exists for the relationship between uncertainty and poor adaptation in cancer patients, who express dissatisfaction with the health care system, problems in family relations and emotional distress plus sexual and work problems (Campbell, 1986; Mishel et al., 1984; Mishel & Braden, 1987), and in discharged myocardial infarction patients, who demonstrate lower levels of physical activity and self-ratings of poor recovery, which were not supported by physicians' evaluations (Christman et al., 1988; Painter, 1981).

The impact of uncertainty on health was investigated in two studies: one with a healthy college-age population (Suls & Mullen, 1981); the other with caregivers of terminally ill persons (Stetz, 1986). In both populations, uncertainty concerning the outcome of aversive events was associated with poorer health. Other evidence indicates that uncertainty is associated with stress in medical patients (Mishel, 1984), lower quality of life in rheumatoid arthritis patients (Braden & Lynn, 1987), and poorer psychosocial adaptation in persons with chronic low back pain (Bidnick, 1986).

In none of the investigations on uncertainty cited has appraisal of uncertainty been considered, and only one study addressed the joint effect of uncertainty and coping on adaptation. In the only study on the appraisal of uncertainty, uncertainty appraised as a danger resulted in the affect-control strategy of wishful thinking and was associated with elevated levels of emotional distress (Mishel, 1988). Further study of the uncertainty appraisal coping-adaptation piece of the model is necessary to explain how adaptation is influenced by uncertainty appraised as a danger or as an opportunity.

Conclusion

The study of uncertainty represents an area of inquiry in which many investigators have studied the same phenomena. Repeated investigations of conceptual relationships specified in the theory plus theoretical support from nursing and related disciplines provide initial confidence in the linkages. However, continued study is necessary to test the theory and confirm its generalizability in nursing practice.

To generalize from the theory, studies are needed with different patient populations in varied settings. Portions of the theory requiring additional empirical validation include (a) the antecedents that influence the appraisal of uncertainty as a danger or opportunity; (b) the influence of cognitive capacity on stimuli frame variables; (c) the conditions under which inference or illusion influence uncertainty appraisal; (d) the coping strategies used in an opportunity or danger appraisal; and (e) the link between effective coping (either reducing uncertainty appraised as a danger or maintaining uncertainty appraised as an opportunity) and adaptation. Following further study, intervention methods can be developed to reduce uncertainty when it is a danger and to support uncertainty when it is an opportunity.

References

Berlyne, D. E. (1977). The affective significance of uncertainty. In G. Serban (Ed.), *Psychopathology of human adaptation* (pp. 319–341). New York: Plenum Press.

Bidnick, M. (1986). *The relationship between perceived uncertainty and adaptation to chronic low back pain.* Unpublished master's thesis, University of Kansas.

Bower, G. H. (1978). *The psychology of learning and motivation: Advances in research and theory.* New York: Academic Press.

Braden, C. J. (1986). *Self-help as a learned response to chronic illness experience: A test of four alternative theories.* Unpublished doctoral dissertation, University of Arizona.

Braden, C. J., & Lynn, M. (1987, October). *Antecedents to and outcomes of uncertainty experienced in chronic illness.* Paper presented at Nursing Advances in Health: Models, Methods and Applications, ANA Council of

Nurse Researchers 1987 International Nursing Research Conference, Washington, D.C.

Bradley, J. C., & Mikolajczak, M. (1986). *The effect of a nursing exit interview on the client's perception of uncertainty in illness.* Unpublished manuscript, University of Illinois, Peoria.

Breznitz, S. (1983). Denial versus hope: Concluding remarks. In S. Breznitz (Ed.), *The denial of stress* (pp. 297–303). New York: International Universities Press.

Budner, S. (1962). Intolerance of ambiguity as a personality variable. *Journal of Personality, 30,* 29–50.

Campbell, L. (1986). *Hopelessness and uncertainty as predictors of psychosocial adjustment for newly diagnosed cancer patients and their significant others.* Unpublished doctoral dissertation, University of Texas at Austin.

Capritto, K. (1980). *The effect of perceived ambiguity on adherence to the dietary regimen in chronic hemodialysis.* Unpublished master's thesis, California State University at Los Angeles.

Christman, N. J., McConnell, E. A., Pfieffer, C., Webster, K. K., Schmitt, M., & Ries, J. (1988). Uncertainty, coping, and distress following infarction: Transition from hospital to home. *Research in Nursing and Health, 11,* 71–82.

Comaroff, J., & Maquire, P. (1981). Ambiguity and the search for meaning: Childhood leukemia in the modern clinical context. *Social Science and Medicine, 15B,* 115–123.

Folkman, S., Schaefer, C., & Lazarus, R. (1979). Cognitive processes as mediators of stress and coping. In V. Hamilton & D. M. Warburton (Eds.), *Human stress and cognition: An information processing approach* (pp. 265–298). New York: John Wiley and Sons.

Galloway, S. G. (1984). *A comparison of the responses of patients with and without a diagnosis of cancer to a bowel resection in the immediate postoperative period.* Unpublished master's thesis, University of Toronto, Department of Nursing.

Herbst, M. C. (1986). *Uncertainty experienced by spouses of patients admitted to the coronary care unit for a definite or suspected myocardial infarction.* Unpublished master's thesis, University of North Carolina at Chapel Hill.

Hilton, B. A. (1986). *Coping with the uncertainties of breast cancer: Appraisal and coping strategies.* Unpublished doctoral dissertation, University of Texas at Austin.

Holmes, D. S., & Houston, B. K. (1974). Effectiveness of situation redefinition and affective isolation in coping with stress. *Journal of Personality and Social Psychology, 29,* 212–218.

Janis, I. J. (1962). Psychological effects of warnings. In G. W. Baker & D. W. Chapman (Eds.), *Man and society in disaster* (pp. 69–79). New York: Basic Books.

Jessop, D. J., & Stein, R. E. K. (1985). Uncertainty and its relation to the psychological and social correlates of chronic illness in children. *Social Science and Medicine, 20,* 993–999.

Johnson, J. E. (1984). Psychological interventions and coping with surgery. In A. Baum, S. E. Taylor, & J. E. Singer (Eds.), *Handbook of psychology and health* (pp. 167–187). Hillsdale, NJ: Laurence Erlbaum Associates.

King, B. (1983). *The psychological impact of systemic lupus erythematosus on the primary caregiver.* Unpublished master's thesis, University of Arizona.

King, B., & Mishel, M. (1986, April). *Uncertainty appraisal and management in chronic illness.* Paper presented at the Nineteenth Communicating Nursing Research Conference, Western Society for Research in Nursing, Portland, Oregon.

Lanzetta, J. T. (1971). The motivational properties of uncertainty. In D. E. Berlyne & D. E. Hunt (Eds.), *Intrinsic motivation: A new direction in education* (pp. 134–147). New York: Holt, Rinehart and Winston.

Lazarus, R. S. (1983). The costs and benefits of denial. In S. Breznitz (Ed.), *The denial of stress* (pp. 1–30). New York: International Universities Press.

Levanthal, H., Nerenz, D. R., & Steele, D. J. (1984). Illness representations and coping with health threats. In A. Baum, S. E. Taylor, & J. E. Singer (Eds.), *Handbook of psychology and health* (pp. 219–252). Hillsdale, NJ: Laurence Erlbaum Associates.

Mandler, G. (1979). Thought processes, consciousness and stress. In V. Hamilton & D. M. Warburton (Eds.), *Human stress and cognition: An information processing approach* (pp. 179–201). New York: John Wiley and Sons.

Miller, S. M. (1980). When is a little information a dangerous thing: Coping with stressful events by monitoring versus blunting. In S. Levine & H. Ursin (Eds.), *Coping and health* (pp. 145–169). New York: Plenum Press.

Mintun, M. K. (1984). *Measurement of parental uncertainty in a pediatric intensive care unit.* Unpublished master's thesis, University of Kansas.

Mishel, M. H. (1981). The measurement of uncertainty in illness. *Nursing Research, 30,* 258–263.

Mishel, M. H. (1983). Parents perception of uncertainty concerning their hospitalized child. *Nursing Research, 32,* 324–330.

Mishel, M. H. (1984). Perceived uncertainty and stress in illness. *Research in Nursing and Health, 7,* 163–171.

Mishel, M. H. (1985, November). *The nature of uncertainty in women with gynecological cancer.* Paper presented at the National Symposium of Nursing Research, San Francisco, CA.

Mishel, M. H. (1987, October). *The existence of uncertainty after treatment ends.* Paper presented at Nursing Advances in Health: Models, Methods and Applications, ANA Council of Nurse Researchers 1987 International Nursing Research Conference, Washington, D.C.

Mishel, M. H. (1988, April). Coping with uncertainty in illness situations. *Proceedings of Conference: Stress, Coping Processes, and Health Outcomes: New Directions in Theory Development and Research* (pp. 51–84). Rochester: Sigma Theta Tau International Epsilon Xi chapter, University of Rochester.

Mishel, M. H., & Braden, C.J. (1987). Uncertainty: A mediator between support and adjustment. *Western Journal of Nursing Research, 9,* 43–57.

Mishel, M. H., & Braden, C.J. (1988). Finding meaning: Antecedents of uncertainty. *Nursing Research, 37,* 98–103.

Mishel, M. H., Hostetter, T., King, B., & Graham, V. (1984). Predictors of psychosocial adjustment in patient newly diagnosed with gynecological cancer. *Cancer Nursing, 7,* 291–299.

Mishel, M. H., & Murdaugh, C. (1987). Family experiences with heart transplantation: Redesigning the dream. *Nursing Research, 36,* 332–338.

Molleman, E., Krobendam, P. J., Annyas, A. A., Koops, H. S., & Sleufer, D. T. (1984). The significance of the doctor-patient relationship in coping with cancer. *Social Science and Medicine, 18,* 475–480.

Monat, A. (1976). Temporal uncertainty, anticipation time and cognitive coping under threat. *Journal of Human Stress, 2,* 32–43.

Oberst, M. T. (1984). Patient's perception of care: Measurement of quality and satisfaction. *Cancer, 53,* 2366–2375.

Painter, P. (1981). *Perceived uncertainty and its relationship to perceived recovery and activity in the post myocardial infarction patient.* Unpublished master's thesis, California State University at Los Angeles.

Patterson, E. T., Freese, M. P., & Goldenberg, R. L. (1986). Reducing uncertainty: Self diagnosis of pregnancy. *Image, 18,* 105–109.

Pearlin, L. I., & Schooler, C. (1978). The structure of coping. *Journal of Health and Social Behavior, 19,* 2–21.

Pergrin, J., Mishel, M., & Murdaugh, C. (1987, April). *Impact of uncertainty and social support on stress in caregivers.* Paper presented at the Twentieth Communicating Nursing Research Conference, Western Society for Research in Nursing, Phoenix, Arizona.

Richardson, J. L., Marks, G. S., Johnson, C. A., Graham, J. W., Chan, K. K., Selser, J. N., Kishbaugh, C., Barronday, Y., & Levine, A. M. (1987). Path model of multidimensional compliance with cancer therapy. *Health Psychology, 6*(3), 183–207.

Rosenbaum, M. (1983). Learned resourcefulness as a behavioral repertoire for the self-regulation of internal events: Issues and speculations. In M. Rosenbaum, C. M. Franks, & Y. Jaffe (Eds.), *Perspective on behavior therapy in the eighties* (pp. 51–73). New York: Springer, 51–73.

Rotter, J. B. (1966). Generalized expectancies for internal versus external control of reinforcement. *Psychological Monographs, 80,* (1, whole No. 609).

Rowat, K. M., & Knafl, K. A. (1985). Living with chronic pain: The spouse's perspective. *Pain, 23,* 259–271.

Roy, C., Sr. (1985). The future of nursing science: Response of the academy. In G. Sorensen (Ed.), *Setting the agenda for the year 2000: Knowledge development in nursing,* American Academy of Nursing.

Silberfarb, P. M. (1983). Chemotherapy and cognitive defects in cancer patients. *Annual Review of Medicine, 34,* 35–46.

Stetz, K. M. (1986). *The experience of spouse caregiving for persons with advanced cancer.* Unpublished doctoral dissertation, University of Washington.

Suls, J., & Mullen, B. (1981, June). Life events, perceived control and illness: The role of uncertainty. *Journal of Human Stress,* 30–34.

Taylor, S. E. (1983). Adjustment to threatening events: A theory of cognitive adaptation. *American Psychologist, 38,* 1161–1173.

Viney, L. L., & Westbrook, M. T. (1984). Coping with chronic illness: Strategy preferences, chances in preferences and associated emotional reactions. *Journal of Chronic Disease, 37,* 489–502.

Warburton, D. M. (1979). Physiological aspects of information processing and stress. In V. Hamilton & D. M. Warburton (Eds.), *Human stress and cognition: An information processing approach* (pp. 33–65). New York: John Wiley and Sons.

Webster, K. K., & Christman, N. J. (in press). Perceived uncertainty and coping post myocardial infarction: A pilot study. *Western Journal of Nursing Research.*

Wortman, C. B. (1984). Social support and the cancer patient: Conceptual and methodological issues. *Cancer, 53* (Suppl.), 2339–2360.

Wortman, C. B., & Dunkel-Schetter, C. (1979). Interpersonal relationships and cancer: A theoretical analysis. *Journal of Social Issues, 35,* 120–155.

Yarcheski, A. (in press). Uncertainty in illness and the future: An empirical test of a theoretical synthesis. *Western Journal of Nursing Research.*

Discussion Questions

1. How is uncertainty reduction or uncertainty management a communication phenomenon?
2. The author seems to suggest that uncertainty is associated with poorer health. Are there any situations in which you would rather be uncertain about your health status?
3. This chapter was written by a professor from a nursing department. Discuss the relationship between communication and other disciplines. ✦

Part IV

HEALTH COMMUNICATION IN ORGANIZATIONS, GROUPS, AND TEAMS

Chapter 14 Interdisciplinary Health Care

Teamwork in the Clinic Backstage

Laura L. Ellingson

Part IV of this volume is a short section consisting of only two chapters. However, it is an important line of inquiry to consider when examining the ways in which communication is part of health and health care. The focus of Part IV is the context in which health care is provided. The primary purpose of this section is to help the reader begin to comprehend the totality of the institution within which health care is provided. This institution contains complex dynamics and structures that shape any communication that can take place among doctors, their patients, and others in health-care services. Each chapter in this section examines how the health organization itself, as well as the groups and teams of health-care specialists within that organization, shapes the communication that takes place in health care. This section reminds us that even though we focus on health communication involving patients and providers, the interactions take place within structures and groups of people that have their own roles within those structures.

Laura L. Ellingson looks at teams who work together to treat cancer patients. Ellingson's focus is on the ways the doctors share a patient's medical information with one another and how that information is communicated differently to the patients. The importance of how communication theory informs research about teams working in health care is illustrated. Interdisciplinary teamwork has become increasingly prevalent across many sites of health care, including hospitals, sub-specialty units, and Health Maintenance Organizations (HMOs).

By focusing on the "frontstage" and "backstage" dynamics of an oncology team, the author argues that health teams find creative ways to organize their daily activities. In doing so, she places an emphasis on context and the "embedded" processes that help interdisciplinary health teams work.

Related Topics: cancer, groups, health-care behaviors, media, organizations, patient-provider communication, qualitative methods

Contemporary health care organizations increasingly rely on interdisciplinary teams for comprehensive diagnosis and treatment of patients (Cott, 1998), particularly in the field of geriatrics (Wieland, Kramer, Waite, & Rubenstein, 1996). By far, the majority of studies of health care teams have sought to establish a correlation between team intervention and measurable patient outcomes. Interdisciplinary teams improve overall care for patients (Cooke, 1997; McHugh et al., 1996) and correlate with specific outcomes such as: decreased length of hospital stay (Wieland et al., 1996); better coordination of patient care (McHugh et al., 1996); fewer nursing home admissions following hospitalization (Zimmer, Groth-Junker, & McClusker, 1985); and decreased mortality one year after discharge (Langhorne, Williams, Gilchrist, & Howie, 1993). Teams improve training of students in medicine and allied health disciplines, as well as enable veteran staff to learn from each other (Abramson & Mizrahi, 1996; Edwards & Smith, 1998) and promote job satisfaction for team members (Gage, 1998; Resnick, 1997). Despite evidence of positive effects of teams on patient outcomes and employee satisfaction, we know relatively little about how health care teams communicate in daily practice (Opie, 2000). Critics of team research argue that despite correlations between use of teams and favorable outcomes, the effectiveness of team communication is often in doubt:

> most literature on health care teams sub-

From "Interdisciplinary Health Care: Teamwork in the Clinic Backstage," Laura L. Ellingson, 2003, *Journal of Applied Communication Research*, Vol. 31:3, pp. 93–117.

> scribes to three basic assumptions: (1) that team members have a shared understanding of roles, norms and values within the team; (2) that the team functions in an egalitarian, cooperative, interdependent manner; and (3) that the combined efforts of shared, cooperative decision-making are of greater benefit to the patient than the individual effects of the disciplines on their own. (Cott, 1998, p. 851)

Research often fails to support the first two assumptions, and the third is unlikely to come true without the others in place. Much team research is "anecdotal, exhortatory and prescriptive . . . there is an absence of research describing and analyzing teams in action" (Opie, 1997, p. 260).

This study uses ethnographic methods to examine a bona fide team in order to understand more fully how teamwork is enacted through communication. Bona fide groups occur naturally in organizations and are "characterized by stable yet permeable boundaries and interdependence with context" (Putnam & Stohl, 1990, p. 248). I focus on dynamic teamwork in the clinic *backstage,* those regions off-limits to patients (Goffman, 1959).

Health Care Teams

Health care teams have fostered and formalized collaboration among members of different disciplines, particularly in the field of geriatrics (Lichtenstein, Alexander, Jinnett, & Ullman, 1997). Increased specialization contributes to the need for collaboration among experts from different specialties (Cooley, 1994; Satin, 1994). Geriatric teams are designed to meet the needs of elderly patients through comprehensive assessment and intervention (McCormick, Inui, & Roter, 1996). Assessment and coordination of services are especially important for older patients because this population is more likely than others to experience complex interactions of medical, psychosocial, and material circumstances (Siegel, 1994; Stahelski & Tsukuda, 1990).

Composition, organization, and functioning of teams vary widely among institutions, specialties, and services provided. Scholars of teamwork use differing terminology but generally represent teamwork as existing along a continuum of collaboration. Representing one end of the continuum, Jones (1997) defines multidisciplinary collaboration as "a multi method, channel type process of communication that can be verbal, written, two-way, or multi way involving health care providers, patients, and families in planning, problem solving, and coordinating for common patient goals" (p. 11). Members of multidisciplinary teams work toward common goals but function largely independently, relying on formal channels (e.g., memoranda, meetings) to keep others informed of assessments and actions (Satin, 1994). Moving along the continuum toward interdependency, Wieland et al. (1996) define interdisciplinary teams as working interdependently in the same setting, interacting both formally and informally to achieve a significant degree of coordination and integration of services and assessments. Some role shifting and evolution may occur over time (Schmitt, Farrell, & Heinemann, 1988). In some cases, interdisciplinary teams evolve into transdisciplinary teams, in which "members have developed sufficient trust and mutual confidence to engage in teaching and learning across disciplinary boundaries and comfortably sharing their "turf" as they work toward common goals (Wieland et al., 1996, p. 656). At their best, teams are synergistic, enabling high quality patient care and a high level of job satisfaction (Pike, 1991).

Effective communication is crucial to teamwork but often lacking (Abramson & Mizrahi, 1994; Gage, 1998). Negotiation of overlapping roles and tasks may be difficult because of territorial behavior; each team member must sacrifice some autonomy for the group to function (Sands, 1993). Role confusion, overlapping responsibilities, and other disciplinary factors can inhibit teamwork (Berteotti & Seibold, 1994; Sands, Stafford, & McClelland, 1990); successful negotiation of boundaries is a hallmark of well functioning teams (Sands, 1993). Additionally, the ideology of teamwork often is not accompanied by egalitarianism. Despite recent changes in medical organizations, physicians remain firmly ensconced as team leaders and administrators, with the majority of the high ranking physicians being (white) men and the vast majority of the lower status professions (e.g., nurses and social workers) being women (including women of color) (Cowen, 1992; Wear, 1997). The power disparity can cause a great deal of resentment and impede successful collaboration (Lichtenstein et al., 1997). Perceptions of teamwork effectiveness vary significantly between prestigious highly paid positions of physician and administrator and relatively low ranking positions, such as nurses (Cott, 1998; Griffiths, 1998).

Backstage of Health Care

Much teamwork among health care professionals takes place in the backstage of the health care system. Goffman (1959, p. 112) defines the backstage region as

> a place, relative to a given performance, where the impression fostered by the performance is knowingly contradicted. . . . It is here that the capacity of a performance to express something beyond itself may be painstakingly fabricated . . . illusion and impressions are openly constructed. Here stage props and items of personal front can be stored in a kind of compact collapsing of whole repertoires.

Atkinson (1995) points out health care researchers have focused the vast majority of research and theorizing of the medical practice on the frontstage of medical care—physician-patient interaction. The predominance of this focus has led to certain limiting tendencies in research. One is the relative lack of problematizing of discourse among health care practitioners that occurs away from patients. Second is a largely unreflected upon preference for bounded communication episodes. Physician-patient interactions are generally very brief, take place in a single, private location, and are easily recorded and transcribed (Atkinson, 1995). Such manageable episodes influence scholars to think of medical interactions as spatially and temporally bound.

Empirical work on health care teams clearly reflects this preference for bounded, convenient chunks of communication in its focus on formal meetings. For example, Opie's (2000) otherwise excellent study of health care teams in New Zealand centered on team meetings and excluded joint work between team members that occurred outside of meetings, positing that such work was only relevant to teamwork to the degree to which it was discussed within team meetings. Researchers' focus on meetings as the site of teamwork also reflects a privileging of formal, public (masculine) discourse over informal, more private (feminine) forms of discourse (Meyers & Brashers, 1994). Meetings have agendas, leaders, systems of turn-taking, and other norms associated with public communication, fitting naturally within researchers' existing schemas for teamwork. Such beliefs and preconceptions reflect a white, middle-class, male bias in communication research (Wyatt, 2002). Moreover, studies of meetings have traditionally focused on decision-making as the crucial task of groups (Barge & Keyton, 1994). Topics such as cooperation, socialization, and connection have been marginalized, socially constructing current conceptualizations of how communication operates in small groups (and teams) that are inherently gender-laden (Meyers & Brashers, 1994).

My extensive interaction with one geriatric team suggests that backstage communication in the clinic is crucial to accomplishing teams' patient care goals. Using a bona fide group perspective, I sought to uncover ways in which team members engaged in teamwork outside of meetings, addressing the following research question: What are the communication processes among team members in the clinic backstage?

Method

Setting and Participants

This study of communication in the clinic backstage is part of a larger ethnographic study of communication within an interdisciplinary geriatric oncology team at a regional cancer center in the southeastern US (Ellingson, 1998). The clinic team included two oncologists (one of whom was the team's director; only one oncologist was in the clinic at a time), a nurse practitioner, a clinical pharmacist, a registered dietitian, two registered nurses (each assigned to one of the oncologists), and a licensed clinical social worker. During the study, the disciplines represented on the team remained constant, but personnel changed: the nurse practitioner, dietitian, and social worker each resigned and was replaced by a candidate already working within the cancer center in another capacity. The introduction of a known member made the transition into the team relatively smooth; only brief explanations at team meetings functioned as overt attempts to socialize new members. Team members worked in clinic space that they shared with health care providers in separate diagnostic areas unrelated to the geriatric program. Clinic nursing assistants escorted patients to rooms and recorded their vital signs for all programs, including the geriatric team.

All new patients over the age of seventy were seen by the geriatric team on their first visit to the cancer center for a comprehensive geriatric assessment. Virtually all patients were accompanied to their visit by one or more companions (e.g., spouses, adult children) who also participated in the interactions (Ellingson, 2002). The visit structure was as follows. After recording of vital signs by a clinic nursing assistant (not considered to be part of the team), a registered nurse conducted an orientation to the comprehensive geriatric assessment. Then, in order of team member availability, the nurse practitioner took a medical history and conducted a physical exam; the dietitian screened for malnutrition, dehydration, eating difficulties, and use of nutritional supplements; the social worker screened for depression and cognitive deficits and discussed psychosocial well-being of patients; and the pharmacist screened for polypharmacy and potential drug interactions. At a given time, three patients occupied examination rooms, and team members cycled through the rooms, communicating with each other in the hallways and desk area. The dietitian, social worker, and pharmacist then reported their findings and interventions to the nurse practitioner, who in turn reported the results of her history taking and exam, along with selected aspects of others' findings, to an oncologist. An oncologist, accompanied by the nurse practitioner, saw each patient and made treatment recommendations. Finally, a registered nurse discharged patients, providing prescriptions and instructions. The process typically took two to three hours. I documented this process through ethnographic field notes, transcripts, and interviews.

Data Collection

Ethnographic field notes. I assumed the participant-as-observer position in my fieldwork (Lindlof, 1995), spending three to five hours, one day per week in the new patient clinic and one hour per week in team meetings of the interdisciplinary geriatric oncology team. Clinic observation was conducted weekly from September 1997 through December 1999. With permission, I observed interactions among patients, companions, and team members; helped with minor tasks (e.g., getting patient a glass of water); relayed messages from one team member to another; offered information if requested by a team member (e.g., explained which team member was with a patient); participated in team members' discussions about patients (e.g. listening to their opinions and offering my own opinions of patients' or companions' affect); engaged team members in discussions about their personal lives and careers; and talked with patients and their companions, particularly when there was a long wait before they saw the oncologist. In the clinic, I kept a notebook or a palm top computer at the desk area, in which I wrote brief notes. Immediately after observing, I typed extensive field notes, producing more than 300 pages of text.

Transcripts. To supplement the field notes, I completed and transcribed nine sets of audio-recordings of initial patient visits from May through July 1999. I selected initial patient visits because initial visits were the only time that patients interacted with the entire team, and hence the primary time in which team members communicated in the backstage as they completed the comprehensive geriatric assessment of patients. The recordings enabled me to discern how backstage communication among team members both resulted from and contributed to communication between team members and patients. Following an Institutional Review Board approved protocol, I approached patients in the waiting room and invited them to participate. I was present during the interactions in order to monitor equipment. Except for a few times when directly addressed by patients or companions, I did not participate in the audio-taped interactions.[1] Each set of recordings included interactions between a patient, his or her companion(s), and each of the team members in turn, for a total of seven interactions per patient (patients saw the registered nurse both upon arrival and upon discharge, and had one interaction each with the oncologist, dietitian, nurse practitioner, pharmacist, and social worker). The interactions were transcribed using transcription guidelines developed specifically for medical discourse (Waitzkin, 1990).

Interviews. As a feminist researcher conscious of the power disparity between researcher and researched (e.g., Reinharz, 1992), I wanted the team to have an opportunity to provide feedback on my preliminary findings. I asked team members to participate in interviews; six of the current team members consented (all the clinic staff except the pharmacist with whom I was unable to schedule a meeting). I also interviewed the nurse practitioner who is no longer with the team but who was my primary informant for the first year of observation, a founding member of the team who continued to substitute occasionally for the current nurse practitioner. Semi-structured interviews (average length = 60 minutes) elicited team members' perceptions of backstage communication and feedback on my findings.

Data Analysis

Charmaz (2000) revised Glaser and Strauss' (1967) classic method of grounded theory, moving it from a positivist to a social constructivist framework. Charmaz explains that researchers can "form a revised, more open-ended practice of grounded theory that stresses its emergent, constructivist elements" and eschews positivist claims of objectivity (p. 510). I followed the steps of traditional grounded theory research outlined by Strauss and Corbin (1990) and Charmaz (2000): coding data, developing inductive categories, revising the categories, writing memos to explore preliminary ideas, continually comparing parts of the data to other parts and to literature, collecting more data, fitting it into categories, and noting where it did not fit and revising the categories (theoretical sampling). To develop categories of communicative processes, I compared interactions in the field notes and transcripts, noting similarities and differences in content and structure of interactions among team members as they communicated in the clinic backstage. I developed preliminary categories based on similarities I observed across interactions and continually refined the typology as I reread notes and transcripts, using constant comparative analysis (Charmaz, 2000). I further explored categories and subcategories of communication processes by explicating relationships among the processes and their context, conditions, and consequences in the communication I observed (paradigm model).

At the same time, I was aware of the constructed nature of knowledge and the influence of my own positionality on my findings, as Charmaz recommends. Reflexive consideration of my own role in data gathering and analysis enhances "theoretical sensitivity," or "an awareness of the subtleties of meaning of data" (Strauss & Corbin, 1990, p. 41). Specifically, my sensitivity to the complex meanings of field notes and transcripts was influenced by my familiarity with literature on team communication and communication theories, lengthy interaction with my data,[2] and my own experiences as a cancer patient. After determining a preliminary typology, I obtained team members' feedback in interviews, which informed the final results (Reinharz, 1992). Through careful data gathering and documentation, systematic analysis, reflexive consideration of my own positionality, and inclusion of participants in generating results, I met Fitch's (1994) criteria for rigor and validity in qualitative research.

Table 14.1
Backstage Communication Processes

Process Category	Subtypes
1. Informal Impression and Information Sharing	Request for information/clarification
	Request for opinion
	Request for reinforcement of message
	Offering of information
	Offering of impression
2. Checking Clinic Progress	Finding out which patients are in rooms
	Finding out who has seen whom
3. Relationship Building	Life talk
	Cancer center troubles talk
4. Space Management	Sharing resources (e.g., phones, computers)
	Physical movement in crowded space
5. Training Students	Reporting
	Offering assistance, answering questions
6. Handling Interruptions	Patient care related (e.g., answering patients' calls)
	Personal or family issues
7. Formal Reporting	Reading charts
	Reporting to nurse practitioner
	Reporting to physician
	Writing clinic notes
	Dictating
	Communicating treatment plan and discharge instructions

Results

In the following section, I explore backstage categories of communication individually for ease of discussion. However, the communication categories are interdependent and often overlap or occur simultaneously, rather than discretely. The following seven inductively derived categories describe the communication involved in daily backstage communication among team members: informal impression and information sharing, checking clinic progress, relationship building, space management, training students, handling interruptions, and formal reporting (see Table 14.1). Due to space constraints, I have selected an excerpt of the data to serve as an extended example. I will refer to line numbers periodically in the results. All names are pseudonyms.

Data Excerpt

1. "Hey," said Susan [pharmacist], catching Ashley's [dietitian] eye. "Great dress."

2. "Hi! Thanks—I went on a shopping spree last weekend." She opened her white

3. lab coat further and tossed her long brown hair over her shoulder so Susan

4. could get a good look, "I bought two of these dresses in different flowered prints, both long but with

5. short sleeves, very comfortable," said Ashley.

6. Susan nodded but then shook her head, her brow furrowed with concern, "Have

7. you seen Mr. Walker yet?" she asked abruptly.

8. Gesturing to Mr. Walker' paperwork on the counter before her, Ashley said,

9. "I'm just getting ready to go in now. Why?"

10. "He's got a real problem with his Coumadin [blood thinner] levels; they're all

11. over the place."

12. "Excuse me," said a technician trying to work his way down the crowded hall.

13. "Sure," replied Susan and Ashley in unison, flattening themselves against the

14. slate blue counter to make more room as he passed.

15. "Let me guess" said Ashley. "He' s taking the Coumadin with food?"

16. "Yes," continued Susan. "And he is

eating greens, you know, some days, and then

17. none on other days. I tried to tell him he has to keep a consistent intake of food rich in

18. [vitamin] K, but he didn't seem to go for it. He's stubborn. Could you say something?"

19. Ashley picked up her pen and made a note on her nutrition screening form. "I'll

20. be sure to stress that he needs to take the Coumadin by itself, not with food. That should

21. help make absorption more consistent, even if we can't get the K intake completely

22. under control. When did he say he was taking it?"

23. "With lunch," answered Susan, "I suggested midmorning or midafternoon as an

24. alternative. . . ."

25. "All right, well, I'll make sure I repeat what you've said and push him to find a

26. time at least a couple of hours after he has eaten to take the Coumadin," said Ashley.

Informal Impression and Information Sharing

Informal impression and information sharing involved discussion of patients, patients' companions, and related topics. This process includes five subprocesses: request for information/clarification, request for opinion, offering of information, offering of impressions, and request for reinforcement of a message. The line between fact and impression is somewhat slippery. Impressions used more emotion and description to accompany information and judgments, whereas information involved more precise, observable facts.

Request for information/clarification. Team members requested a specific piece of information that was missing, in doubt, or a source of confusion. Thus, in the excerpt above, line 22, the dietitian requested a piece of information—the timing of the medication—that she needed before speaking with the patient. An unfortunate prompt for this process was when team members discovered that patients or their companions had provided contradictory or inconsistent information; they then questioned each other to resolve disparities. For example, the pharmacist said to the dietitian about a diabetic patient, "I recommended that this man see his primary care physician in regard to testing and controlling his blood sugar. He said he didn't test it regularly." The dietitian replied, "He told me that his blood sugar was well controlled, and he tested it twice a day." Then the pharmacist asked, "Did he say he was taking insulin?" Through questioning each other about the information the patient supplied, the team members determined how best to address the problem.

Request for opinion. Team members solicited opinions on issues such as affect, depression, and patients' relationships with companions both to obtain confirmation of their own uncertain impressions and to initiate discussions about patients whose perceived problems could be addressed by one or more team members' expertise. For example, the social worker collaborated when a patient did not screen at a clinical level of depression, but she sensed distress intuitively. By asking others, "Do you think she is depressed?" she effectively conducted her psychosocial assessment. Another way to request an opinion was to offer an opinion (discussed below) in a clearly questioning tone, inviting discussion. For example, after seeing a patient, the pharmacist said to the nurse, "This patient seemed frightened of her husband?"

Offering of information. Specific pieces of information about a patient or a companion were offered to other team members when team members perceived that such information would provide practical assistance to facilitate another team member's communication with a patient. In the excerpt above (lines 10–11, 16–17), the pharmacist tells the dietitian that a patient's blood thinner medication levels were unstable and that this was due in part to his diet, an issue the dietitian would be discussing with him. Mentioning that a patient was hard of hearing enabled the team member to be prepared to speak loudly and enunciate carefully. Also, explaining patients' and companions' relationships avoided possible embarrassment. For example, a team member once explained that a male patient was accompanied by his sister, since others assumed that she was his wife. In one unusual case, two friends accompanied a woman patient. One was a much younger man, for whom she used to work and with whom she now shared a house. He helped to care for her, but was not related to her, nor were they romantically involved. The man's cousin accompanied them—a woman who spent considerable time with both the patient and her friend and caregiver. Clarifying the relationships among the patient and her companion(s) enabled team members to better understand the patient's social support network. Similarly, researchers of a team of medical and educational specialists who provide early interventions to children with disabilities found that passing along pieces of day-to-day information informally helped team members to effectively accomplish their work (Hinojosa et al., 2001).

Offering of impressions. Team members offered each other positive or negative impressions, with or without facts to support their judgments. For example, opinions were offered of how patients were sweet, pleasant, sad, angry, uncooperative, or dominated by a companion. In the excerpt, the pharmacist described the patient as "stubborn" (line 18). Offering negative impressions could perform a steam-venting function as much as a collaborative one. Two team members reported in interviews that they expressed frustration over an encounter as much for catharsis as for a desire to facilitate a team member's subsequent interaction. Venting is an important strategy for coping with stress in health care settings (Laine-Timmerman, 1999). On one occasion, an overbearing husband insisted on answering questions directed to the patient, his wife. The dietitian, social worker, and I expressed to each other how angry we felt at the husband's behavior. We did this to warn others of what they would encounter, but it was just as important to have our feelings validated by others and relieve some stress through articulating our anger. Expressing emotions in the backstage (away from patients) assisted team members in controlling their emotional display while in the clinic frontstage, thus preventing team members from disrupting the team's performance of calm professionalism (Goffman, 1959).

Request for reinforcement of message. This process involved asking a team member to repeat information already mentioned to a patient. Each team member was empowered to do interventions: the pharmacist made recommendations on the timing of drugs, and the social worker advised counseling, for example. In order to encourage patients to act on recommendations, team members asked each other to provide reinforcement, as in the interaction in the above excerpt (line 18) where the pharmacist asked the social worker to repeat her recommendation on the timing of the blood thinner medication. Another example was when patients had difficulty sleeping—due to chronic insomnia, anxiety, pain, or medications—the nurse practitioner or social worker recommended a sleeping aid. If they encountered resistance from patients who perceived sleeping aids as addictive and stigmatizing, the nurse practitioner asked the oncologist to reinforce to patients that sleeping pills are safe and effective when used properly. Team members reported that they believed, that repetition increased likelihood that the patients would follow recommendations: "Sometimes it helps when they hear it twice," the pharmacist stated.

In summary, informal information and impression sharing helped to break down barriers by fostering connections and overlap among disciplinary roles and tasks, moving closer to Opie's (1997) ideal of transdisciplinary teamwork. At the same time, this process helped facilitate the frontstage performance (comprehensive geriatric assessment) given by team members to patients and their companions by assisting team members in anticipating and resolving problems through backstage discussion away from the audience's hearing (Goffman, 1959).

Checking Clinic Progress

Checking progress involved asking team members which patients had been seen, and by whom. With so many team and nonteam staff moving through the clinic, it was difficult to keep track of team members' locations. Team members accomplished such tracking through brief questioning (e.g., "Have you seen Mr. Walker yet?"; excerpt lines 6–7). Checking progress was not one team member's job; everyone took part. Angry patients or patient companions also prompted checking, as in the case of a patient and her husband who, after waiting over two and a half hours, threatened to leave if the physician did not appear soon. The nurse practitioner checked to make sure that all of the other team members had seen the patient before placating the couple. The long process of assessment exhausted very ill patients, particularly those who had been undergoing chemotherapy or who were in advanced stages of disease. In such cases, team members requested that the nurse practitioner report on and have the oncologist see a particular patient before the others in order to hasten the fatigued patient's departure. A final motivation for checking progress was that nonphysician team members had competing time commitments and needed to attend to other responsibilities related to other departments or teams.

Checking clinic progress assisted team members in estimating and minimizing the amount of time before they could move on to other tasks. Although not complex, it was vital to keeping the clinic flowing smoothly. Team members valued efficiency not only for making their work easier but also as a kindness to patients.

Relationship Building

Professional and collegial relationships rather than close friendships characterized the team, although team members' relationships varied significantly, including their relationships with me. Team members had time between patients to communicate about issues unrelated to patients. The nurse practitioner and oncologists typically had less free time than others because the oncologists saw established patients in between the new patients being seen by the entire team, and the nurse practitioner had a lengthier set of tasks and more formal reporting than the other team members. Relationship building also occurred outside of the clinic backstage, as team members encountered each other in other cancer center locations during the course of their work and also in some social situations outside of work. Team members' non-task-related communication reflected two primary categories: life talk and cancer center troubles talk.

Life talk included discussing such outside interests as families, vacations, house buying, and clothing. While topics of discussion varied over time and changes in team membership, some topics recurred. Team members who had children discussed their progress in school, sports, and other activities, and shared pictures too. The pharmacist led a children's choir and related humorous stories about choir rehearsal. When the social worker returned from a family emergency leave, team members offered sympathy and support. The pharmacist's and dietitian's discussion of clothes is another example (excerpt lines 1–5). Such talk reflects Goffman's (1959) concept of familiarity, where team members in a frontstage performance assume a level of informality with each other in the backstage that arises from their successful cooperation and may be inconsistent with the frontstage performance, in this case the role of health care professional.

The other primary category of relationship building was cancer center "troubles talk" (Tannen, 1990), which included mild to vehement complaining about scheduling, limited resources, overbooking of patients, overcrowding in the backstage area, and the behavior of clinic staff. One source of annoyance that prompted troubles talk was the scheduling of new patients when one of the oncologists was assigned to conduct rounds for inpatients in the main hospital-building. All cancer center physicians were required to take turns fulfilling this function, even though it interfered with their clinics. The stress level on oncologists' rounding days was noticeably higher, as indicated by more rushing, less relationship building talk, and impatient tones when handling interruptions. Mild griping, rolling one's eyes, and expressing fatigue and frustration were typical at these times. Team members repeatedly offered and received affirmation of the difficulty of their circumstances from each other, performing a verbal ritual of griping (Katriel, 1990). For example, "We're really hectic in here today," the nurse practitioner said to one of the oncologists as she hurried to gather materials to report a patient's case. "I know, it's crazy, don't worry," replied the oncologist. Both the team oncologists made an effort to thank the rest of the team for their hard work and patience on days with rushed schedules, which other team members reported appreciating. Both life talk and troubles talk fostered a sense of connection among team members (Tannen, 1990). Such talk enhanced collegial relations, judging by the initiation of talk among team members.

Space Management

Team members shared limited space and resources with each other and with other health care providers whose practice was assigned to the clinic. A significant number of people (one approximately every five minutes) also passed through the clinic on the way to the break room, restroom, or photocopiers, and technicians were frequently paged to the clinic to attend to patients (e.g., conduct an EKG). The number of people in the small space made it virtually impossible to move around without bumping into others or moving into others' intimate space. Carts of patient charts and equipment also took up room. The noise level became problematic at times as phones rang, the photocopier and printer hummed, and multiple conversations occurred.

Space management involved extensive verbal and nonverbal negotiation. Nonverbal communication included claiming of desk or counter space with charts or other objects, use of facial expressions (e.g., welcoming smile or exasperated frown), pushing past someone, moving (or refusing to move) one's body to allow another to pass, and vacating when a person of higher status approached a space (e.g., chair) or resource (e.g., phone) (nonphysicians made way for oncologists; administrative assistants vacated space for all other staff). The position of the door between the backstage area and the hallway of examination rooms (frontstage) was a hotly contested issue when certain people were in the clinic. Rather than openly discussing the issue, the door would be repeatedly opened and closed by the staff members according to their preference. It was not unusual for the door to be opened and closed four times in an hour, demonstrating how borders are disputed and negotiated (Goffman, 1959). This is particularly prevalent in service professions, where some team members prefer that the audience not be able to view the backstage, and others prefer ease of movement between the two regions. Verbal negotiation of space included asking how long someone would be using a computer; requesting a seat or space; (oncologists) ordering others to be quiet, move to another area, or reposition the door; and asking to be allowed to pass, as in the excerpt (lines 12–14) where team members verbally consented and moved their bodies to accommodate the technician.

Training Students

Another of the team's communication processes involved training students in medicine, social work, nurse practitioner, and pharmacy. Students shadowed team members initially, and some then conducted interviews with patients. The team member who was functioning as a mentor for a given period of time (ranging from a day to a month) introduced her student to the other team members to initiate relationships. Training students took time and effort, although competent students in pharmacy, social work, dietary, and nurse practitioner also took on part of their mentor's workload, interviewing one out of every three patients in place of the mentor. Team members met with their assigned students before and after interactions with patients and helped with needed interventions. For example, when a social work student found that a patient needed a referral for community services, the student informed the social worker, who questioned the patient and her companion further and then made the arrangements herself. Social work, dietary, and pharmacy students reported relevant information directly to the nurse practitioner (e.g., drug interaction risk), with their disciplinary mentor observing the report and offering assistance only if necessary. The nurse practitioner students reported on their patients first to the nurse practitioner and then, with her approval, reported to the oncologist. Medical students shadowed oncologists but did not perform any tasks or communicate with patients.

Team members trained students in their disciplines as they carried out tasks, and socialized students into teamwork as they interacted in the backstage. In addition to reporting to the nurse practitioner (or in the case of nurse practitioner students, to the oncologist) students engaged in informal information and impression sharing and relationship building with team members (and me) as we worked and waited in the clinic backstage. In Goffman's (1959) terms, students experienced both the frontstage performance of providing comprehensive geriatric assessments and the backstage where that performance was dropped in favor of familiarity; they were treated as people in the know and functioned as part of the team.

At the same time, students marked their outsider status by deferring to team members' higher status, as evidenced by students' respectful tones, waiting to be acknowledged rather than interrupting an interaction between team members, and actively listening to and carefully following instructions given by their mentors. For example, "I'm ready whenever you are," a nurse practitioner student said to the nurse practitioner, indicating she had prepared her report and that she would wait for a time that was convenient for her mentor. However, students were treated as trustworthy sources of information and opinions; team members requested information and opinions of students and took seriously information and impressions offered by students, often acting upon them. For example, a student nurse practitioner offered to the dietitian information regarding a patient's hearing loss; the dietitian responded to the information by speaking loudly and slowly to the patient. Likewise, when a nurse practitioner student reported a patient's medical history to an oncologist, her report was accepted as the basis for treatment recommendations. Communicating in the backstage with members of other disciplines is valuable because students learn about differences in disciplinary socialization and terminology. Teamwork is increasingly important in health care as managed care decreases reliance on physicians and promotes the roles of other health disciplines to cut costs (Cooley, 1994). Teams are particularly effective at training health care students (Edwards & Smith, 1998). Having engaged in interdisciplinary collaboration during training, students were better prepared to begin (or advance) their careers.

Handling Interruptions

As in any other workplace, outside concerns intruded. Tangentially related and unrelated tasks were fairly minor interruptions of team members' work. I distinguish between interruptions, and talk about outside concerns within the team, which I consider part of relationship building. Interruptions were either patient-care related, or personal and family concerns. Such interruptions were unavoidable, and while they could delay patient care or interrupt teamwork, they were handled efficiently. Patient-care related activities included calls or pages from team members' departments concerning patients who were not part of the geriatric program but who were under their care in other capacities. Team members, except for the director and nurse practitioner, had only part of their time designated for the team. The rest of the time, they worked with their home department or other teams. Thus, for example, while seeing geriatric patients, the social worker received calls that related to discharge planning for patients she served as a member of the psychosocial oncology department. Handling interruptions from other departments and teams overlapped with checking clinic progress; team members checked with others to see when they could finish their current tasks and attend to the other work. Another patient-care related task that interrupted the oncologists and registered nurses was answering telephone calls from community physicians consulting about established patients' care plans. Established patients also called the registered nurses frequently, who discussed symptoms and requested recommendations from the physicians to address patients' concerns (e.g., nausea).

Personal and family concerns also interrupted team members. Calls from child care providers about team members' sick children and pages by spouses exemplify family concerns. Nonurgent personal messages were left on team members' voicemail to be picked up at their convenience. Team members did not voice resentment of interruptions caused by other team members' personal issues, and I did not observe signs of tension between team members when one was handling an interruption. Both oncologists (the highest status team members) reported being sympathetic to the need for parents to balance work with their children's needs and expressed their understanding to team members. For example, once when the nurse practitioner received a page and had to leave the clinic to collect her sick baby at a day care center, an oncologist smiled and said kindly to her, "Go! Go! It can't be helped. We'll be fine."

Formal Reporting

The final process I identified is the formal reporting of patient information. Team members accomplished such reporting both in writing and through oral communication, and it was both the first and the last aspect of patient care. Written reporting involved reading patient charts and team-specific paperwork completed by patients and either writing or dictating a clinic note after the patient was seen. Oral reporting of information existed in conjunction with the informal system of information sharing.

Formal written reporting. As in all health care settings, record keeping was an essential component of patient care. Preparation for a patient interview involved looking through the chart and, if available, the information provided by the patient on the paperwork sent to patients before their visit. Information from the chart was added to assessment forms (e.g., the patient's weight was recorded on the malnutrition screening instrument). Team members attended to different types of information in the chart, with the nurse practitioner conducting the most thorough review to obtain medical history and to determine patients' current stage of diagnosis and treatment. In the data excerpt, the dietitian was reviewing a patient's chart to learn about his dietary habits, weight, and nutritional level when she was approached by the pharmacist (lines 8–9). She added the information supplied by the pharmacist about blood thinner medication and vitamin K intake to her paperwork (line 19).

Initial gathering of information had a profound effect on how team members constructed images of patients. According to Berg (1996), "the medical record plays an active, constitutive role in current medical work" (p. 501). Charts contain a complex but abbreviated accounting of a patient's history. Medical records reflect a biomedical assessment of the patient that relies on claims of objective data and systematic objective evaluation; records note very little about how patients feel about their diagnosis, how they are coping, or what the illness means to them (Donnelly, 1988). The record not only represented past events (diseases and medical interventions), but actively shaped the current event by shaping the information team members had, their expectations, and even what blanks needed to be filled in (Berg, 1996). Thus interacting with written accounts affected team members' views of patients before they met.

After seeing new patients, team members (except the oncologists and RNs) wrote or dictated a note, the second form of written formal reporting. The dietitian, social worker, and pharmacist wrote brief notes on the computer database, while the nurse practitioner dictated the note for her and the oncologist's visit. This difference in recording medium was due in part to the large volume of information contained within the medical history which the nurse practitioner dictated, as well as her responsibility for dictating some information gathered by other team members, such as the Body Mass Index from the dietitian and the treatment plan developed by the oncologist. The selection and ordering of information determined the official accounts of "what happened," (Berg, 1996) as in this excerpt of a note written by a social worker.

> PT is a 78 YO WWF S/P liver biopsy. She is at [hospital] for evaluation by [team]. Not interested in support groups or counseling. She joined a support group after her husband died but did not find it

> useful. "I can do better by myself." She missed 3 of 30 on the mini mental status: She was unable to count backwards from 100. She scored perfectly on the Geriatric Depression Scale. Pt denied any stressors at this time, seemed relatively unconcerned about possible treatment. Writer briefly discussed psychosocial services available at [hospital] and gave business card to PT . . . Pt is well-groomed with carefully applied makeup. She emphatically answered GDS questions related to happiness.

The sense-making process of choosing details and arranging them directly affected team members' understanding of their just-concluded interactions with patients. Because team members composed separate accounts, the record generated from the initial visit could contain consistent, somewhat variable, or contrasting views of a patient, depending upon the amount and type of communication among team members regarding the patient. Such disparities were discovered when team members shared their summaries of patients in their weekly meeting, two to three days after the interaction with the patients. If disagreements warranted follow-up with a patient, a team member was assigned to contact the patient. Otherwise, the divergent opinions were simply noted before discussion moved on to the next patient on the agenda; team members did not express a need to make the accounts consistent.

Another aspect of formal written reporting was the preparation of the treatment plan and discharge paperwork by the nurse practitioner or oncologist in conjunction with the registered nurse. Team members wrote out instructions, prescriptions, orders for tests, and other forms, which were compiled by the nurse practitioner for delivery to the patient by the registered nurse. The treatment plan was also recorded on the nurse practitioner's dictation.

Formal oral reporting. Set reporting procedures determined in advance were completed routinely for each patient via structured verbal communication. The dietitian, social worker, and pharmacist reported specific pieces of information (e.g., Geriatric Depression Scale score) to the nurse practitioner after interacting with the patient, before the nurse practitioner reported to the oncologist. The nurse practitioner then reported her own findings and aspects of the others' findings (at her discretion) to the oncologist, who then went with the nurse practitioner to see the patient.

At the conclusion of the visit, the nurse practitioner or the oncologist reported both the treatment plan and any orders for prescriptions and diagnostic tests to the registered nurse, who discussed information with patients and saw that they were discharged. This process of reporting was carried out for each patient; however, it occurred within the midst of other types of backstage communication, such as information and impression sharing. Thus, the social worker reported screening scores for a specific patient to the nurse practitioner, but also shared her impression that "[patient] doesn't want to continue treatment, but I think his family was uncomfortable with discussing hospice [palliative care] arrangements." For a high functioning patient whose assessment was more a formality than an in-depth exploration, the dietitian reported to the nurse practitioner the Body Mass Index score along with her impression, "He's fine," accompanied by a casual tone and a dismissive wave of her hand. Thus at times the ritual of formal reporting became a forum for informal impression and information sharing.

Discussion and Implications

Theorizing and Researching Teams

Putnam and Stohl (1990, p. 260) called for research to "improve the ecological validity of our findings" by paying attention to the meaning of bona fide group processes within their specific contexts, a task for which ethnographic methods are well suited (Dollar & Merrigan, 2002). Privileging formal communication (i.e., meetings) in past studies of teamwork has led to a lack of recognition of the crucial roles that informal communication play in teamwork. The ethnographic study reported here demonstrates that the clinic backstage, not just team meetings, must be recognized as a site of teamwork (Goffman, 1959).

The bona fide group model does not adequately account for the capacity for teams to interact informally through a system that they devise or adapt to suit their constraints, communication styles, and goals. The examples of interactions offered in this article represent the creativity of a particular team that developed ways to do its work and meet its goals more effectively. Collectively, these interactions demonstrate clearly that team members conducted significant teamwork in hallways, desk areas, break rooms, and other clinic spaces not designated as meetings. The orderly presentation of these communicative processes in the results section somewhat obscures the contextualization of the processes within the busy clinic, perhaps leading readers to perceive them as much more orderly and organized than they were. Indeed, in our interview, the team's first nurse practitioner called the backstage "controlled chaos," emphasizing that the chaos usually worked quite well in its organic development and constant readjustment. The interactions occurred opportunistically rather than on a schedule; emerged in response to team members' desires to improve patient care and assessment as they went about providing it, not by a preset agenda; were dyadic and triadic rather than including the entire team; and developed within the process of accomplishing comprehensive geriatric assessments in an outpatient clinic, with all the noise, crowding, and simultaneously activities of that space. The opportunities and constraints differed every clinic day, and team members responded to each day's contingencies. A more holistic model would reflect this dynamism and multiple sites of communication in the everyday enactment of teamwork. Therefore, I propose the concept of embedded teamwork. Embedded teamwork acknowledges the discourse between dyads and triads of team members in which disciplinary (or professional) lines are blurred and redrawn; significant variation in teamwork practices occurs; team members' beliefs and attitudes are expressed and change over time; and contextual constraints are reproduced, resisted, and negotiated through communication.

Certainly, some of this negotiation of meaning happens in meetings in which ritualistic reporting of patients' cases occurs. However, the discourse of clinic practice as team members carry out comprehensive geriatric assessments should not be dismissed as joint work (Opie, 2000). Both stage models of teamwork developed by allied health and social services disciplines (e.g., Opie, 1997) and the bona fide group model which focuses on communication (Putnam & Stohl, 1990; see also Lammers & Krikorian, 1997) would be enhanced through incorporation of the embedded teamwork concept; I will discuss each in turn.

Stages of cross-disciplinary collaboration developed by theorists such as Opie (1997) (i.e., multidisciplinary, interdisciplinary, transdisciplinary) function as a useful heuristic for health care researchers and are widely cited by researchers in social work, medicine, nursing, pharmacy, dietary, rehabilitation, and mental health. However, such theories do not account fully for the dynamic nature of teamwork. Teams do not attain the level of interdisciplinary, for example, and consequently work in that mode. While models of interdisciplinary teamwork mention that informal communication occurs in interdisciplinary teams, there is no explication of what that would involve or how it influences the dynamism of teamwork. Realistically, there will be good and bad days for teamwork, and there will be some patients for whom teamwork will be more effective than for others. Moreover, some members of a given team will be more willing than others to blur boundaries, openly negotiate roles, and learn from each other (the team pharmacist blurred disciplinary boundaries with the dietitian much more often than with the nurse practitioner, for example). Such fluctuations can be accounted for and their influence considered more fully with attention to embedded practices. Moving beyond the formal meeting expands what counts as teamwork, and hence enables teams both to work in dyads and triads when they deem such collaboration to be beneficial for patient care and to frame such communication as teamwork.

Moreover, embedded practices are more flexible than meetings for navigating the hierarchical medical system. Authors call for boundary blurring, role flexibility, and dynamic teamwork structures to improve health care teamwork by bridging the gaps that persist when team members socialized in different disciplines dismiss, devalue, or misunderstand each other's discipline-specific knowledge claims (Opie, 2000; Siegel, 1994). If the rigid divisions of health care disciplines, and the hierarchy which privileges physician knowledge and power over other disciplines (e.g., Cott, 1998; Griffiths, 1998), are ever to be renegotiated, embedded teamwork through backstage communication may be a good place to start.[3] The fluidity of backstage settings forms contexts in which disciplinary boundaries can more easily waffle, and micro-negotiations can take place without a large audience (as in a meeting). Despite considerable constraints related to the crowded and hectic environment of the backstage, backstage communication moved the team from a multidisciplinary mode (acting in parallel, keeping each other informed) toward an interdisciplinary or transdisciplinary mode where (some) professional boundaries were blurred and roles negotiated (Opie, 1997). By attending to communication within embedded teamwork practices, researchers using stage models of teamwork will be better able to determine the degree of interdependency and boundary blurring that occurs among team members.

Furthermore, acknowledging and exploring embedded teamwork extends bona fide group theory in a useful direction for communication scholars bringing our unique perspective to bear on the study of groups and teams in a myriad of settings, including health care. Lammers and Krikorian (1997) expanded upon Putnam and Stohl's (1990) original model of bona fide groups by articulating implicit aspects of the model via their study of surgical teams. Lammers and Krikorian argued that studies of bona fide groups must involve attention to the group in its specific institutional context because a given team task or decision "is a manifestation of much individual, small group, organizational, and institutional work that goes on prior to and after [it]" (p. 36). To continue along that path, embedded teamwork practices, those that dyads and triads of team members carry out in the backstages of medical (or other) work, involve communication among team members that is just as much a part of the team's discourse and history as that which occurs in meetings; such embedded practices are part of the ongoingness of the team (Berger & Luckmann, 1966; Lammers & Krikorian, 1997). Attention to ongoing communication among team members outside of meetings enables recognition of the embedded nature of teamwork within a context in which team members spend the vast majority of their time not in team meetings, but in accomplishing the work which is planned, reviewed, and evaluated in team meetings. I do not doubt the centrality of meetings to the discursive accomplishment of teamwork; however, an exclusive focus on meetings suggests an artificial demarcation between team communication in meetings and communication among team members in other backstage spaces. My study of an interdisciplinary geriatric team indicates that team members do not experience these forms of communication as separate, but as co-existing in a dynamic system. Thus the permeable boundaries of bona fide teams should be considered to include communication between dyads and triads of team members whether or not that communication is ever brought into a meeting as a specific point of discussion.

Further studies of bona fide teams would be enriched by qualitative documentation of embedded teamwork communication outside of meetings. In addition to the potential of these findings for theories of teamwork, this typology of backstage teamwork also offers crucial insights into frontstage health care delivery.

Researching and Theorizing Linkages Between Frontstage and Backstage

By expanding the definition of what counts as teamwork, we can envision opportunities for enhancing theory and improving practice of health care provider-patient communication. Goffman (1959) points out that all backstages are, in some sense, frontstages for other performances. An embedded teamwork approach blurs the boundary between the frontstage and backstage of health care delivery, and hence reveals both as performative. As team members repeatedly crossed over the literal doorway between frontstage and backstage, the boundary between the performance for the patient and companion audience and the performance of teamwork was continually blurred. The performances became enmeshed and the exact threshold elusive. Theorizing frontstage and backstage as separate spheres obscures the vital connections between them; Goffman's (1959) dramaturgical theory emphasizes that the frontstage and backstage are adjacent, and both are integral to team performances. Even teams that conduct assessments and interventions asynchronously (not in the clinic backstage at the same time) are likely to carry out joint work in dyads and triads of team members outside of meetings (Opie, 2000; Saltz, 1992). These discourses should be considered as existing in a reflexive, integrated, dynamic relationship that is not only the context for frontstage and backstage forms of communication, but produces the communication. Theories and conceptualizations of health care teamwork must inhabit a crossroads of organizational, team, health care provider-patient, and health care provider-patient-companion communication in order to offer a sufficiently complex view of the daily world of clinics. The daily negotiation of teamwork creates a world in which frontstage and backstage communication are inseparable and mutually productive. Backstage practices such as reading and writing notes, discussing patients' affect, and sharing information and impressions influence subsequent interactions with patients. As this cycle is continually repeated, each interaction contributes to the development the climate and culture of teamwork and health care delivery.

Pragmatic Implications for Health Care Practitioners and Administrators

Because of the interrelation of backstage and frontstage communication, the backstage can be conceptualized as a site for improving patient care. Backstage communication impacted communication with patients and companions in five specific ways that may be useful to teams reflecting on backstage teamwork or considering fostering such communication. For each, I offer pragmatic suggestions to enhance patient care. Like the typology of backstage communication, these processes overlap; they are separated for ease of discussion.

First, team members developed beliefs and attitudes about patients before they met them, and backstage communication contributed to this process. Information and opinions from other team members and from documentation in charts led to preconceived ideas about patients (Donnelly, 1988). Forming at least some ideas about patients is inevitable, and in many ways it had beneficial effects. For example, it was often helpful to know in advance that the patient about to be seen was angry or fatigued; the team member could then enter the room ready to deal with the patient's affect instead of having to react unprepared. On the other hand, advance warnings also may have caused snap judgments or discouraged team members from making up their own minds about a patient. For example, the social worker received negative information from the pharmacist about a couple before she saw them; being warned of the patient's husband's communication style may have helped her to negotiate her tasks more effectively, but it also provided her with an unflattering impression that shaped her views. Team members did not always accept the impressions that were shared with them, however. In interviews, two team members explained that they sometimes used warnings from others as an inspiration to try to be empathic with a patient. Health care providers should be conscious of how the information contained in charts and the information and impressions shared with them by team members has lead them to anticipate certain behaviors. Ideally, health care providers should both be prepared to manage such behaviors, and be open to the possibility of forming a different impression than the one fostered in the backstage.

Second, backstage communication often resulted in a modification of the agenda for a team member's subsequent encounter with a patient. The most significant and consistent example of shaping an agenda was the nurse practitioner's report to the oncologist. For every patient, the nurse practitioner had to make strategic decisions on which details to present, wanting to be comprehensive, but also balancing time constraints and not wanting to give the impression that she was unable to make sound judgments concerning what data was relevant to the oncologist's decisions. Since the oncologist had no prior contact with the patient, the oncologist's view of the patient, and hence the oncologist's agenda, was influenced strongly by the nurse practitioner. Informal collaboration among team members also altered agendas. Recommendations that patients eliminate, reduce, or change dosages of vitamin and herbal supplements were messages that were reinforced frequently by multiple team members following backstage communication. Being prepared to address issues ahead of time, and being able to reinforce pieces of information or an impression, appeared to increase team member effectiveness and patients' receptiveness to messages. Health care providers should consider both formal and informal talk in the backstage as opportunities to adapt their own and each other's agendas for communicating with patients in ways that enhance case delivery.

Team members' backstage communication also provided practical facilitation of encounters. For example, being told that a patient was very hard-of-hearing encouraged team members to speak loudly and more slowly from the outset of their encounter and thus improved communication. Reading of patient records, one aspect of backstage formal reporting, also may have facilitated subsequent communication with patients. For example, the pharmacist always checked the list of over-the-counter and prescription medications before entering a patient's examination room. If the list was lengthy or included drugs that were likely to have harmful interactions, the pharmacist was prepared upon entering the room to spend more time conducting a detailed review with the patient. Diabetics are a good example of patients who often required longer visits from the pharmacist; seeing insulin on a chart facilitated her preparation. Such practical and useful information should be freely shared among health care practitioners in the backstage in order to facilitate others' communication with patients.

A final, and problematic, effect of backstage teamwork on frontstage communication concerns power. Despite its potential for improving patient care, backstage communication increases health care providers' power over patients, undermining patient autonomy. Team members strategize (often extensively) out of patients' presence about how to persuade patients to adopt or discontinue specific behaviors. The paternalism-autonomy dialectic in the health care provider-patient relationship is certainly not unique to team interventions (e.g., Waitzkin, 1984), and is always a significant problem for older patients, toward whom physicians often exhibit ageist attitudes and behavior (Beisecker, 1996; Hummert & Nussbaum, 2001). Additionally, since the team studied works in an outpatient setting, recommendations are made to patients who have time to consider options and make decisions, enhancing their autonomy. Nonetheless, the power (even if benevolent) wielded by team members is problematic because it gives team members further rhetorical advantage over patients who already face status and knowledge differences that privilege medical professionals in their interactions (Adelman, Greene, Charon, & Friedmann, 1992). The exclusion of patients and family members from many teams' meetings has been highly criticized by some scholars of teamwork who object to the marginalization of patients' and families' perspectives (Opie, 1998). A similar criticism could be made of backstage teamwork that fosters repetition and modification of messages designed to move patients toward a particular decision. This ethical issue warrants attention in further research.

In addition to specific implications of backstage communication for frontstage practice, the findings presented here have an important implication for the formation, training, and management of teams in health care settings. Teams should recognize the communication among team members outside of team meetings as part of the fluid process of teamwork, rather than ignoring or discounting such communication as apart from or preliminary to the real teamwork that occurs in meetings. Recognition could include documenting dyadic or triadic interactions by briefly logging date, time, topic, and participants in a team member's daily planner or notebook; compiled periodically, this data would support team members' requests to administrators for (re)allocation of time for teamwork. Periodically bringing such data into meetings for discussion also would enable identification of trends in topics that necessitate frequent out-of-meeting interactions—such knowledge could lead to anticipating and preventing some problems by implementing changes to meeting agendas or procedures to address recurring issues. By recognizing such fleeting, dyadic or triadic communication among team members as impacting on team relationships and process, both team members and administrators can value and reward this professional work, and strategize on how to maximize its effectiveness.

Limitations

Because the typology was developed on the basis of one team's work, the findings can not be generalized to all teamwork contexts. The elite context of a regional cancer center also limits generalizability; all but one of the team members and the vast majority of their patients were white and from middle or upper socioeconomic classes. More culturally diverse medical contexts would present constraints and opportunities largely absent in the team studied. In terms of providing a model or inspiration for future research, this study is limited by its cumbersome methodology. While ethnography of embedded teamwork yielded valuable insights, it is very time consuming, involving long term commitment to an organization. Researchers may find access to informal aspects of teamwork and backstage communication difficult to obtain (Atkinson, 1995; Opie, 2000). Moreover, informal interactions are not bounded geographically or temporally, and do not lend themselves to tape-recording, making them difficult to follow and systematically document, and requiring flexible data gathering strategies (Atkinson, 1995).

Conclusion

The exploration of backstage communication among members of a geriatric oncology team revealed the critical nature of teamwork outside of formal team meetings for both internal team functioning and communication with patients and companions in the frontstage of health care delivery. An embedded teamwork perspective offers important pragmatic and theoretical applications by complexifying the current conceptualizations of teamwork. The backstage of health care delivery will move into the frontstage of health communication research as it becomes increasingly apparent that much of the work of health care teams takes place both in the absence of their consumers and outside of formally designated team meetings.

Endnotes

1. It is, of course, quite possible that my presence impacted the interactions. However, given the research emphasis of the cancer center, my presence was not unusual or disruptive. Staff routinely approached patients about participating in studies, and patients interacted with professionals, students, and interns from many disciplines. It bears mentioning that I walk with a pronounced limp due to reconstructive surgeries for bone cancer in my right leg, and patients and companions often asked about it. I answered all questions about my personal health history and status as a researcher but avoided discussing what I was studying, except to say that I "wanted to understand how patients and team members communicated with each other." While I did not announce my identity as a cancer survivor to every patient, I did reveal it when asked about my limp and leg brace because I believe it would have been unethical to deceive patients and their companions about my survivor status. Patients and companions often said that they were glad that I had some idea of what they were experiencing, and that it was com-

forting to talk with a survivor. See Ellingson (1998) for a discussion of a cancer-survivor-as-researcher positionality.

2. My process of interpreting and analyzing data also included writing ethnographic narratives and an autoethnography of my participant observation; these narrative sense-making processes influenced my understanding of what I had witnessed, and hence affected the meanings I generated in the grounded theory analysis.
3. Systems of social power and privilege in the medical establishment exist in reflexive relationship with backstage clinical communication. Space constraints prohibited full explication of this complex relationship, which I will explore in future publications.

References

Abramson, J. S., & Mizrahi, T. (1994). Collaboration between social workers and physicians: An emerging typology. In E. Sherman & W. J. Reid (Eds.), *Qualitative research in social work* (pp. 135–151). New York: Columbia University Press.

Abramson, J. S., & Mizrahi, T. (1996). When social workers and physicians collaborate: Positive and negative interdisciplinary experiences. *Social Work, 41,* 270–281.

Adelman, R. D., Greene, M. G., Charon, R., & Friedmann, E. (1992). The content of physician and elderly patient interaction in the primary care encounter. *Communication Research, 19,* 370–380.

Atkinson, P. (1995). *Medical talk and medical work.* Thousand Oaks, CA: Sage.

Barge, J. K., & Keyton, J. (1994). Contextualizing power and social influence in groups. In L. R. Frey (Ed.), *Group communication in context: Studies of natural groups* (pp. 85–106). Hillsdale, NJ: Lawrence Erlbaum.

Beisecker, A. E. (1996). Older persons' medical encounters and their outcomes. *Research on Aging, 18,* 9–31.

Berg, M. (1996). Practices of reading and writing: The constitutive role of the patient record in medical work. *Sociology of Health and Illness, 18,* 499–524.

Berger, P. L., & Luckmann, T. (1966). *The social construction of reality: A treatise in the sociology of knowledge.* New York: Anchor Books.

Berteotti, C. R., & Seibold, D. R. (1994). Coordination and role-definition problems in health-care teams: A hospice case study. In L. R. Frey (Ed.), *Group communication in context: Studies of natural groups* (pp. 107–131). Hillsdale, NJ: Lawrence Erlbaum.

Charmaz, K. (2000). Grounded theory: Objectivist and constructivist methods. In N. K. Denzin & Y. S. Lincoln (Eds.), *Handbook of qualitative research* (2nd ed., pp. 509–535). Thousand Oaks, CA: Sage.

Cooke, C. (1997). Reflections on the health care team: My experiences in an interdisciplinary program. *The Journal of the American Medical Association, 277,* 1091–1092.

Cooley, E. (1994). Training an interdisciplinary team in communication and decision-making skills. *Small Group Research, 25,* 5–25.

Cott, C. (1998). Structure and meaning in multidisciplinary teamwork. *Sociology of Health and Illness, 20,* 848–873.

Cowen, D. L. (1992). Changing relationships between pharmacists and physicians. *American Journal of Hospital Pharmacy, 49,* 2715–2721.

Dollar, N. J., & Merrigan, G. M. (2002). Ethnographic practices in group communication research. In L. R. Frey (Ed.), *New directions in group communication* (pp. 59–78). Thousand Oaks, CA: Sage.

Donnelly, W. J. (1988). Righting the medical record: Transforming chronicle into story. *Journal of the American Medical Association, 260,* 823–825.

Edwards, J., & Smith, P. (1998). Impact of interdisciplinary education in underserved areas: Health professions collaboration in Tennessee. *Journal of Professional Nursing, 14,* 144–149.

Ellingson, L. L. (1998). "Then you know how I feel": Empathy, identification, and reflexivity in fieldwork. *Qualitative Inquiry, 4,* 492–514.

Ellingson, L. L. (2002). The role of companions in the geriatric oncology patient-multidisciplinary health care provider interaction. *Journal of Aging Studies, 16,* 361–382.

Fitch, K. L. (1994). Criteria for evidence in qualitative research. *Western Journal of Communication, 58,* 32–38.

Gage, M. (1998). From independence to interdependence: Creating synergistic healthcare teams. *Journal of Nursing Administration, 28*(4), 17–26.

Glaser, B., & Strauss, B. (1967). *The discovery of grounded theory: Strategies for qualitative research.* Chicago: Aldine.

Goffman, E. (1959). *The presentation of self in everyday life.* Garden City, NY: Doubleday.

Griffiths, L. (1998). Humour as resistance to professional dominance in community mental health teams. *Sociology of Health and Illness, 20,* 874–895.

Hinojosa, J., Bedell, G. Buchholz, E. S., Charles, J., Shigaki, I. S., & Bicchieri, S. M. (2001). Team collaboration: A case study of an early intervention. *Qualitative Health Research, 11,* 206–221.

Hummert, M. L., & Nussbaum, J. F. (2001). Successful aging, communication, and health. In M. L. Hummert & J. F. Nussbaum (Eds.), *Aging, communication, and health: Linking research and practice for successful aging* (pp. xi–xix). Mahwah, NJ: Lawrence Erlbaum.

Jones, R. A. P. (1997). Multidisciplinary collaboration: Conceptual development as a foundation for patient-focused care. *Holistic Nursing Practice, 11*(3), 8–16.

Katriel, T. (1990). 'Griping' as a verbal ritual in some Israeli discourse. In D. Carbaugh (Ed.), *Cultural communication and intercultural contact* (pp. 99–117). Hillsdale, NJ: Lawrence Erlbaum.

Laine-Timmerman, L. E. (1999). *Living the mystery: The emotional experience of floor nursing.* Unpublished doctoral dissertation, University of South Florida, Tampa, FL.

Lammers, J. C., & Krikorian, D. H. (1997). Theoretical extension and operalization of the bona fide group construct with an application to surgical teams. *Journal of Applied Communication Research, 25,* 17–38.

Langhorne, P., Williams, B., Gilchrist, W., & Howie, K. (1993). Do stroke units save lives? *Lancet, 342,* 395–398.

Lichtenstein, R., Alexander, J. A., Jinnett, K., & Ullman, E. (1997). Embedded intergroup relations in interdisciplinary teams: Effects on perceptions of level of team integration. *Journal of Applied Behavioral Science, 33,* 413–434.

Lindlof, T. R. (1995). *Qualitative communication research methods.* Thousand Oaks, CA: Sage.

McCormick, W. C., Inui, T. S., & Roter, D. L. (1996). Interventions in physician-elderly patient interactions. *Research on Aging, 18,* 103–136.

McHugh, M., West, P., Assatly, C., Duprat, L., Niloff, J., Waldo, K., et al. (1996). Establishing an interdisciplinary patient care team: Collaboration at the bedside and beyond. *Journal of Nursing Administration, 26*(4), 21–27.

Meyers, R. A., & Brashers, D. E. (1994). Expanding the boundaries of small group communication research: Exploring a feminist perspective. *Communication Studies, 45,* 68–85.

Opie, A. (1997). Thinking teams thinking clients: Issues of discourse and representation in the work of health care teams. *Sociology of Health and Illness, 19,* 259–280.

Opie, A. (1998). "Nobody's asked me for my view": Users' empowerment by multidisciplinary health teams. *Qualitative Health Research, 8,* 188–206.

Opie, A. (2000). *Thinking teams/thinking clients: Knowledge-based teamwork.* NY: Columbia University Press.

Pike, A. W. (1991). Moral outrage and moral discourse in nurse-physician collaboration. *Journal of Professional Nursing, 7,* 351–363.

Putnam, L. L., & Stohl, C. (1990). Bona fide groups: A reconceptualization of groups in context. *Communication Studies, 41,* 248–265.

Reinharz, S. (1992). *Feminist methods in social research.* New York: Oxford University Press.

Resnick, C. (1997). The role of multidisciplinary community clinics in managed care systems. *Social Work, 42,* 91–98.

Saltz, C. (1992). The interdisciplinary team in geriatric rehabilitation. *Geriatric Social Work Education, 18,* 133–143.

Sands, R. (1993). 'Can you overlap here?': A question for an interdisciplinary team. *Discourse Processes, 16,* 545–564.

Sands, R., Stafford, J., & McClelland, M. (1990). 'I beg to differ': Conflict in the interdisciplinary team. *Social Work in Health Care, 14*(3), 55–72.

Satin, D. G. (1994). The interdisciplinary, integrated approach to professional practice with the aged. In D. G. Satin (Ed.), *The clinical care of the aged person: An interdisciplinary perspective* (pp. 391–403). New York: Oxford University Press.

Schmitt, M. H., Farrell, M. P., & Heinemann, G. D. (1988). Conceptual and methodological problems in studying the effects of interdisciplinary geriatric teams. *The Gerontologist, 28,* 753–764.

Siegel, B. S. (1994). Developing interdisciplinary teams. In D. G. Satin (Ed.), *The clinical care of the aged person: An interdisciplinary perspective* (pp. 404–425). New York: Oxford University Press.

Stahelski, A. J., & Tsukuda, R. A. (1990). Predictors of cooperation in health care teams. *Small Group Research, 21,* 220–233.

Strauss, A., & Corbin, J. (1990). *Basics of qualitative research: Grounded theory procedures and techniques.* Thousand Oaks, CA: Sage.

Tannen, D. (1990). *You just don't understand: Women and men in conversation.* New York: Ballantine Books.

Waitzkin, H. (1984). Doctor-patient communication. *Journal of the American Medical Association, 252,* 2441–2446.

Waitzkin, H. (1990). On studying the discourse of medical encounters: A critique of quantitative and qualitative methods and a proposal for reasonable compromise. *Medical Care, 28,* 473–487.

Wear, D. (1997). *Privilege in the medical academy:*

A feminist examines gender, race, and power. New York: Teachers College Press.

Wieland, D., Kramer, B. J., Waite, M. S., & Rubenstein, L. Z. (1996). The interdisciplinary team in geriatric care. *American Behavioral Scientist, 39,* 655–664.

Wyatt, N. (2002). Foregrounding feminist theory in group communication research. In L. R. Frey (Ed.), *New directions in group communication* (pp. 43–56). Thousand Oaks, CA: Sage.

Zimmer, J. G., Groth-Junker, A., & McClusker, J. (1985). A randomized controlled study of a home health care team. *American Journal of Public Health, 75,* 134–141.

Discussion Questions

1. Why would health-care professionals distinguish between the "frontstage" and "backstage" dynamics of communication? What types of communication practices occur on each stage?
2. What does Ellingson mean when she proposes an "embedded" understanding of teamwork?
3. Ellingson argues that she takes a social constructionist approach to her research. How does she communicate that approach in her description of both method and data? What are some specific examples of how the oncology health-care team socially constructs their reality? ✦

Chapter 15
When Social Workers and Physicians Collaborate

Positive and Negative Interdisciplinary Experiences

Julie S. Abramson and Terry Mizrahi

Julie Abramson and Terry Mizrahi examine the impact of communication among health-care teams on health-care provision. They look specifically at interactions across medical and health specializations and the results of effective or ineffective ways of understanding in interdisciplinary teams. Collaboration across disciplines in health care is becoming increasingly important, as seen in interactions between physicians and social workers. This chapter explores the interaction between the disciplines in a hospital setting and the components that lead to positive and negative collaboration. Communication seems to be the key to successful collaboration, which is illustrated as both social workers and physicians comment on past communication experiences in both their best and worst collaborations.

Related Topics: culture, groups, managed care, organizations, qualitative methods, quantitative methods

From "When Social Workers and Physicians Collaborate: Positive and Negative Interdisciplinary Experiences," Julie S. Abramson and Terry Mizrahi, 1996, *Social Work*, Vol. 41:3, pp. 270–281.

Interdisciplinary teamwork and collaboration in health care are assuming greater importance as changes in social and economic conditions, demographics, and diseases converge to focus attention on models of health care delivery. Many major health care reform initiatives in government and in the private sector have emphasized elimination of duplication and fragmentation through referrals, networking, and coordination. In today's climate of cutbacks, managed care, and deprofessionalization, the efficiency of the health care system will increasingly depend on the ability of social workers, physicians, and other health care providers to collaborate effectively in the provision of services to patients.

This article presents a subset of data from a larger study that explores the nature of social worker-physician collaboration in hospital settings. The article will focus on positive and negative collaborative experiences between social workers and physicians to identify factors that facilitate successful collaboration and factors that impede it. We asked members of both professions to share their best and worst experiences with the other profession, expecting that extreme examples would help us address two research questions: First, do the two professions identify similar or different factors in describing their experiences? In other words, are there universal collaborative factors, or does each profession have distinct and separate priorities in evaluating collaborative experiences? Based on our knowledge of differential socialization processes, we hypothesized that social workers and physicians would value different aspects of their experiences. Second, do positive and negative experiences evoke similar or different reactions with respect to the contribution of various factors? We hypothesized that respondents would emphasize different factors in evaluating their positive and negative experiences. Answers to these two questions can increase understanding of collaboration; help professionals improve collaborative skills; and contribute to the development of a well-coordinated, collaborative model of patient care.

Literature Review

Impediments to Collaboration

Much of the literature on collaboration has a negative emphasis, focusing on the obstacles to effective interdisciplinary functioning, particularly in team situations. Conflict among collaborators as a result of varying professional or personal perspectives can undermine collaborative efforts (Lowe & Herranen, 1981; Sands, Stafford, & McClelland, 1990; Schindler, Berren, Hannah, & Belgel, 1981). Role competition, role confusion, and turf issues also cause interdisciplinary tensions because each discipline must sacrifice some degree of autonomy for collaborative problem solving to take place (Abramson & Rosenthal, 1995; Campbell-Heider & Pollack, 1987; Kulys & Davis, 1987; Lowe & Herranen, 1981; Watt, 1985). Role definition poses problems as well. A number of studies have identified discrepancies between the perceptions of social workers and those of physicians regarding functions assigned to social workers. In particular, counseling activities are more often seen as a prime social work responsibility by social workers than by physicians (Carrigan, 1978; Huntington, 1981; Koeske, Koeske, & Mallinger, 1993; Lister, 1980).

Conflict also can arise from variations in professional socialization processes (Mizrahi & Abramson, 1985; Sands, 1989). Members of each profession define their role and the goals of services to clients differently and impart distinct values and culture in training their recruits (Cowles & Lefcowitz, 1992; Huntington, 1981; Mizrahi, 1986; Roberts, 1989). Communication difficulties then arise and often are ascribed to interpersonal dynamics rather than recognized and addressed as interprofessional in nature (Abramson & Mizrahi, 1986).

Physician dominance of team and interprofessional decision making has remained a critical issue for other health professions (Abramson, 1989; Campbell-Heider & Pollack, 1987; Dingwall, 1982; Freidson, 1984; Sheppard, 1992; Watt, 1985). Nurses, pharmacists, and social workers face comparable issues in collaborating with physicians, including a lack of acceptance by physicians of the full breadth of other professionals' roles, continuing status and gender differences, contradictory expectations regarding the autonomy of nonphysicians, and a commonly expressed need for physicians' recognition of their competence (Baggs & Schmitt, 1988; Cowen, 1992; Fagin, 1992; Koeske et al., 1993; Lamb, 1991; Mullaly, 1988; Pike, 1991).

The perception that physicians do not emphasize collaboration with other groups is reinforced by the absence of articles that focus on interprofessional relationships in mainstream medical journals. Articles on teamwork and collaboration in such journals usually refer to the "medical team" (medical student, resident, attending physician) (Rutala, Fulginiti, McGeagh, Koff, & Witzke, 1992), whereas the term "interdisciplinary" generally refers to different specialties within medicine (Murray, Wartman, & Swanson, 1992; Skochelak & Jackson, 1992). Indeed, some physicians actively oppose the role expansion and increasing autonomy of other professionals (Williams, 1992).

Strengths of Collaborative Approaches

Despite broad acceptance of interdisciplinary collaboration and teamwork as the modality of choice in health care settings, the literature usually assumes rather than specifically addresses the strengths of this model of patient care. It is clear that pooling interdisciplinary expertise yields a better understanding of client needs and resources while enhancing the range of options considered and skills applied in problem solving (Abramson & Rosenthal, 1995; Bruner, 1991). Interdisciplinary collaboration also directly benefits collaborators. Individuals expand knowledge and expertise through exposure to other professionals. They can share the burden of dealing with particularly onerous problems or difficult patients; division of responsibility in such circumstances cushions the effect of failure (should it occur), provides necessary support from colleagues, and can even reduce burnout (Abramson & Rosenthal, 1995; Andrews, 1990; Vachon, 1987).

Although obstacles remain, this period of uncertainty and rapid change in the health care field provides opportunities for improved collaborative relationships. Some recent discussions of interprofessional relationships suggest cautious optimism. An expanded role for social work is documented; social work competence is more often recognized; and some reduction in turf battles among social workers, nurses, and physicians is noted as well (Cowles & Lefcowitz, 1992; Trella, 1993; Walton, Jakobowski, & Barnsteiner, 1993). Moreover, a limited number of sources identify teamwork skills that can enhance collaboration (Abramson, 1989; Abramson & Mizrahi, 1986; Lonergan, 1985; Toseland & Rivas, 1984).

However, a more data-based understanding of the issues involved in successful and unsuccessful collaboration is necessary (Schmitt, 1994). For the most part, relationships between social workers and physicians have been presented anecdotally in the social work literature. Furthermore, these articles have rarely emphasized mainstream medical specialties such as internal medicine and surgery. Yet the latter two are the largest and most prestigious medical specializations and are highly influential in shaping the policies, education, and practice of medicine. Therefore, the study presented here examined actual positive and negative collaborative experiences of social workers and physicians in internal medicine, surgery, and related subspecialties.

Method

Two subsets of data were collected as part of this exploratory study of social worker-physician collaboration. Part 1 investigated the perspectives of pairs of social workers and physicians about their actual collaboration on a shared case. Part 2, presented in this article, examined additional cases identified by the same physicians and social workers that reflected their most positive and negative collaborative experiences with the other profession. Both qualitative and quantitative methods were used.

Sample

The nonrandom sample consisted of 51 physicians and 54 social workers working in internal medicine, surgery, or related subspecialties in 12 hospitals (four in the New York City area; five in the Albany, NY, area; and three in western Massachusetts). The hospitals were selected with the purpose of achieving diversity of size, auspice, and location. All but one hospital social work director who was approached cooperated. All social workers asked to participate did so. The hospitals were in urban, suburban, and small-town settings and were divided among medical school-affiliated teaching hospitals, community-based teaching hospitals, and community hospitals. (Medical school-affiliated teaching hospitals had teaching programs for medical students, interns, and residents or house staff. Community-based teaching hospitals were not affiliated directly with a medical school but trained house staff, whereas community hospitals did not have any teaching programs.)

The sample was obtained by first securing participation from social workers with medical or surgical assignments in the various hospital departments. We asked each social worker to identify a complex case in which extensive collaboration with a physician took place. We then recruited the physician on that case to participate in the study; all but three did so.

In the part of the study presented here, we asked each social worker and physician respondent to provide additional case descriptions representing their most positive and negative collaborative experience with the other profession. First, they described the cases and discussed why they viewed these experiences positively or negatively. They were then given a precoded list of items related to collaborative attitudes and behavior; the negative items were in general the inverse of the positive items. The respondents were asked to check those items they felt contributed to their assessment of the positive or negative collaborative experience. They were free to pick as many items as seemed relevant.

The items on the precoded list (Tables 15.1 and 15.2) were based on our prior conceptualization of social worker-physician collaboration (Abramson & Mizrahi, 1986; Mizrahi & Abramson, 1994), on the literature, and on our clinical and participant observations. Some of the items described characteristics or skills of the collaborator such as style, personality, and competence; others emphasized communication between the collaborators, including amount of communication and being kept informed of or involved in decision making. Still a third group of items focused more on characteristics of the patient and family, including type of illness, social status of the patient and family, and the challenge of the case.

We deliberately skewed the social work respondents' selection toward atypical cases—namely, those arousing strong feelings—to obtain richer data regarding collaboration. We were interested in examining extreme examples because we assumed they are highly influential in shaping interprofessional perspectives and would facilitate identification of the most salient features and dynamics of collaboration.

Data Analysis

Data from the precoded lists were analyzed by comparing the frequency of selection of items by each profession; these frequencies were ranked and compared by profession to examine which items were more and less important to each group and whether they varied according to the posi-

Table 15.1

Ranked Percentages of Subjects Selecting Positive Collaboration Items, by Profession

		Social Worker (N = 54)			Physician (N = 47)		
Positive Variables	*Construct*	*n*	*%*	*Rank*	*n*	*%*	*Rank*
Respect for collaborator	a	52	96.3	1	33	70.2	3
Similar perspectives	a	47	87.0	2	32	68.1	4
Positive quality of communication	b	46	85.2	3	35	74.5	2
Your role well understood by collaborator	b	46	85.2	3	23	48.9	10
Amount of communication was positive	a	44	81.5	5	26	55.3	7
Capability acknowledged by collaborator	b	41	75.9	6	16	34.0	23
Collaborator treated you respectfully	a	39	72.2	7	20	42.6	14
Challenging case	c	38	70.4	8	28	59.6	6
Collaborator's positive style with you	a	37	68.5	9	18	38.3	20
Collaborator included you in decisions	a	37	68.5	9	20	42.6	14
Collaborator kept you informed	b	37	68.5	9	32	68.1	4
Collaborator gave you needed information	b	35	64.8	12	25	53.2	9
Positive personality traits of collaborator	a	33	61.1	13	17	36.2	22
Positive personality traits of patient and family	c	32	59.3	14	21	44.7	11
Collaborator's positive style with patient and family	c	27	50.0	15	20	42.6	14
Degree of emotion evoked	c	27	50.0	15	13	27.7	26
Type of patient illness	c	27	50.0	15	20	42.6	14
Your impact on case was positive	c	27	50.0	15	16	34.0	23
Collaborator did not interfere with your autonomy	a	27	50.0	15	8	17.0	30
Collaborator was capable	a	27	50.0	15	37	78.7	1
Collaborator gave timely feedback	b	26	48.1	21	26	55.3	7
Patient was happy	c	23	42.6	22	21	44.7	11
Family was happy	c	23	42.6	22	19	40.4	18
Collaborator did needed paperwork	b	23	42.6	22	18	38.3	20
Success against odds	c	22	40.7	25	21	44.7	11
Your identification with patient and family was positive	c	17	31.5	26	10	21.3	28
Collaborator wrote good notes	b	17	31.5	26	13	27.7	26
Collaborator understood impact of case on you	a	15	27.8	28	15	31.9	25
Social status of patient and family	c	11	20.4	29	9	19.1	29
Collaborator did job independently of you	b	9	16.7	30	19	40.4	18

Note: Items that are tied are given the same rank; items ranked next after tied items are given the rank they would have had if no items were tied. Mann-Whitney rank-order correlation: $Z = -3.6380$, $p = .0003$. a = items included in the interactional construct; b = items included in the competence construct; c = items included in the case construct.

Table 15.2
Ranked Percentages of Subjects Selecting Negative Collaboration Items, by Profession

Negative Variables	*Construct*	Social Worker (N = 53)			Physician (N = 46)		
		n	%	*Rank*	n	%	*Rank*
Dissimilar perspectives	a	40	75.5	1	21	45.7	1
Poor quality of communication	b	36	68.0	2	17	37.0	5
Collaborator's negative style with you	a	33	62.3	3	12	26.1	10
Lack of respect for collaborator	a	29	54.7	4	12	26.1	10
Negative personal traits of collaborator	a	29	54.7	4	11	23.9	12
Your role poorly understood by collaborator	b	27	50.9	6	10	21.7	15
Amount of communication was inadequate	a	24	45.3	7	21	45.7	1
Negative personal traits of patient and family	c	22	41.5	8	15	32.6	7
Your capability not acknowledged	a	22	41.5	8	5	10.9	28
Collaborator left you out of decisions	a	22	41.5	8	14	30.4	9
Disrespectful treatment by collaborator	a	20	37.7	11	6	13.0	24
Challenging case	c	18	34.0	12	7	15.2	22
Needed information not provided	b	18	34.0	12	17	37.0	5
Collaborator did not keep you informed	b	18	34.0	12	18	39.1	4
Collaborator was not capable	b	18	34.0	12	15	32.6	7
Collaborator's negative style with patient and family	c	17	32.1	16	11	23.9	12
Patient was unhappy	c	16	30.2	17	9	19.6	17
Type of patient illness	c	14	26.4	18	5	10.9	28
Collaborator's feedback not timely	b	14	26.4	18	21	45.7	1
Success against odds	c	13	24.5	20	9	19.6	17
Impact of case on you not understood	a	13	24.5	20	8	17.4	21
Family was unhappy	c	12	22.6	22	10	21.7	15
Collaborator interfered with your autonomy	a	12	22.6	22	6	13.0	24
Social status of patient and family	c	11	20.8	24	5	10.9	28
Degree of emotion evoked	c	11	20.8	24	9	19.6	17
Your impact on case was negative	c	11	20.8	24	6	13.0	24
Collaborator didn't do his or her job	b	9	17.0	27	9	19.6	17
Collaborator didn't do paperwork	b	8	15.1	28	11	23.9	12
Your identification with patient and family was negative	c	6	11.3	29	6	13.0	24
Collaborator wrote poor notes	b	4	7.5	30	7	15.2	22

Note: Items that are tied are given the same rank; items ranked next after tied items are given the rank they would have had if no items were tied. Mann-Whitney rank-order correlation: $Z = -3.3695$, $p = .0008$. a = items included in the interactional construct; b = items included in the competence construct; c = items included in the case construct.

tive or negative nature of the experience. Where appropriate, comparisons were examined using rank-order correlations and t tests to locate statistically significant differences.

The positive and negative case descriptions provided open-ended data for qualitative analysis, and the data generated by respondents' selection of items from the precoded list of factors affecting collaboration were analyzed quantitatively. We applied grounded theory methodology to data from the case descriptions to develop categories inductively; we then applied these codes to additional cases to further test their usefulness and relevance. The details of developing these analytic constructs are presented elsewhere (Abramson & Mizrahi, 1993; Mizrahi & Abramson, 1994). All qualitative coding was done separately by two coders (interrater reliability = .81) who reconciled differences where necessary. We also compared related qualitative and quantitative findings to see if similar patterns existed between a category derived from respondents' descriptions in their own words and their responses to categories in the precoded list.

Results

Sample Characteristics

The social work respondents (N= 54 for positive case and N = 53 for negative case) were primarily female (87.0 percent), whereas the physician respondents (N = 47 for positive case and N = 46 for negative case) were primarily male (88.2 percent). Both groups were predominantly white (83.3 percent for social workers and 94.1 percent for physicians). Approximately 48 percent worked in large hospitals (more than 600 beds), 38.8 percent in medium-sized hospitals (350 to 600 beds), and 13.1 percent in small hospitals (fewer than 350 beds), Most social workers had MSW degrees; a few had BSW or other bachelor's degrees. In the physician sample, there were 31 internists, 10 surgeons, two in rehabilitation medicine, two family practitioners, and six house staff (five internists and one surgeon). Social workers varied in years of experience from one to 39 with a mean of seven years; the physicians' experience ranged from one to 46 years with a mean of 16 years since the completion of formal training. We did not find significant differences on any of the dimensions examined between male and female social workers or physicians, nor were there any significant differences by medical specialty among physicians. However, the low number of physicians in each specialty and of female doctors and male social workers in our sample leads us to be tentative about these findings and suggests a need for further research on the effect of gender and medical specialty on collaboration.

Patient Characteristics

The respondents provided some demographic information about the patients involved in their positive and negative experiences; however, such data were not collected systematically. Certain patterns did emerge with respect to patient age and type of illness. Respondents selected higher numbers of patients under 65 years of age than would be expected in light of typical inpatient hospital demographics. Physicians chose such patients (positive cases, 71.5 percent; negative cases, 70.5 percent) even more frequently than social workers (positive cases, 54.6 percent; negative cases, 53.7 percent). Patients were described as having a wide range of primary illnesses, although those with terminal illnesses were selected approximately 33 percent of the time by doctors and social workers in the positive cases and 33 percent of the time by social workers and 20 percent of the time by doctors in the negative cases.

Quantitative Analysis of Positive and Negative Collaborative Factors

The major findings are drawn primarily from quantitative analysis of the social worker and physician responses to the precoded list of the factors contributing to positive or negative collaboration (Tables 15.1 and 15.2). We have included a few illustrative examples from the qualitative data as well. For each profession, we ranked the items from the precoded list by the percentage of each group who selected them to compare the degree to which they did or did not emphasize the same issues. Before discussing these findings, however, we want to note contrasts in the two professions' responses to the precoded items. First, there was greater consensus among the social workers regarding the importance of particular items. In addition, social workers chose many more items on average to explain their collaborative experiences than did physicians; the list of items clearly had greater salience to them. The difference, as measured by *t* tests, reached statistical significance for the combined positive and negative experiences when the professions were compared. The average response for social workers was 45.8 percent of all items, whereas the doctors checked an average of 33.1 percent ($p < .05$). This artifact of the sample encouraged the investigators to choose data analysis strategies such as rank-order correlations in which the higher response rate of the social workers would not distort the meaning of the findings.

For the positive cases, both groups stressed the importance of their respect for their colleague (ranked first for social workers and third for doctors), their similar perceptions (ranked second for social workers and fourth for doctors), and the quality of communication between them (ranked second for doctors and third for social workers). However, social workers focused more than physicians on the other professional's understanding of his or her role (also ranked third in a tie for social workers and 10th for doctors), acknowledgment of the other's capability (ranked sixth for social workers and 23rd for doctors), and respectful treatment by the collaborator (ranked seventh for social workers and 14th for doctors). The physicians focused primarily on the collaborator's capability (ranked first for doctors and 15th for social workers) and also stressed being kept informed more than social workers (ranked fourth for doctors and ninth for social workers). When we compared the overall rankings of items from the precoded list by profession using a Mann-Whitney rank-order correlation, there were significant differences between the two groups ($Z = -2.8360$, $p = .0046$).

In reacting to the negative cases, both groups focused on interaction and relationships with the other profession to a greater extent than when assessing the positive cases. Dissimilar perceptions about the case ranked highly for both professions (first for social workers and tied for first for doctors). Poor quality of communication was second for social workers and fifth for doctors, whereas the amount of communication was tied for first for doctors and seventh for social workers. The doctors' negative style was of great concern to social workers (ranked third), whereas social workers' negative style was ranked by physicians much lower (10th). The same pattern existed regarding lack of respect for the other professional, which was more important to the social workers (ranked fourth) than to the physicians (ranked 10th). Similarly, social workers stressed lack of understanding of their role more than physicians (ranked sixth for social workers and 15th for doctors). In contrast, aspects of competence were highlighted much more frequently by physicians than by social workers; lack of timely feedback was ranked first in importance by doctors and 18th by social workers, and not being kept informed was ranked fourth by doctors and 12th by social workers. Again, when the overall rankings of items were compared by profession, the Mann-Whitney rank-order correlation demonstrated significant differences between the two groups ($Z = -3.3695$, $p = .0008$).

Secondary Analysis of Positive and Negative Collaborative Factors

Patterns in the rankings discussed above indicate that social workers focused more on the relationship with physicians and on what their collaborator thought of them than did the physicians, who concentrated more on what social workers did. In looking at these patterns, certain items seemed to cluster conceptually into constructs that reflected particular aspects of the collaborative experience: those related to the case, to the interaction between collaborators, and to the competence of the collaborator.

We therefore did a secondary analysis to further examine these patterns. The two primary investigators independently assigned all 30 precoded items to one of three conceptually derived constructs (agreement was 97.0 percent) to compare the two professions on these dimensions (see Tables 15.1 and 15.2 for identification of items assigned to each construct). We then redid the rank-order correlation, grouped by construct, for both the positive and negative cases. There were significant differences between the two professions on the interactional construct in both the positive ($Z = -3.6380$, $p = .0003$) and negative ($Z = -2.9997$, $p < .0001$) cases, whereas comparisons on the competence construct were not significant for either. Comparisons on the case-related construct were significant only for the negative case ($Z = -2.4636$, $p = .0138$). The analysis by construct of the rankings of the two groups indicates that the differences between the two professions can be primarily accounted for by greater social worker emphasis on interaction with the physicians.

Examples From Social Workers Focused on Interactional Issues

Social Worker, Positive Case. "One particular staff member came to see me and said, 'This elderly patient would be appropriate for a geriatric consultation team.' . . . I was very impressed . . . I had never heard of a physician making a consult; it was usually the social worker. . . . Several times, we'd sit down and [the doctor] would say, 'What are we going to do with this lady?' and we discussed options."

Social Worker, Negative Case. "Just recently, there was a person who was supposed to return to the nursing home. We needed information from the doctor about the time he was going to be discharged. It was his poor attitude; he kept asking, 'Why are you asking me when this person is going to be leaving? . . . Do you own the case?' He saw me as pressuring him. He said, 'I can't be bothered with you. I'll make my decision when I make it.' "

Social Worker, Positive Case. "I was in a family meeting with a physician. I think my role was to facilitate communication between the doctor and the family in regard to the person's health status and prognosis. There was a question of home care versus nursing home placement, and I felt that he was really utilizing my skills in terms of being able to explain hospital systems. . . . We were working together trying to help the family come to terms with the decisions that were to be made."

Examples From Physicians Focused on Competence Issues

Physician Positive Case. "I had a recent situation with a patient who was in the community with Alzheimer's disease awaiting placement, draining extremely heavily on his wife. He came in the hospital, and [the social worker] intervened very rapidly and helped with his placement in a very expeditious way. It was very positive for me, for the family, for his wife to see that we could do this the way we did. . . . The process worked the way I would like it to work."

Physician, Negative Case. "I did a total knee replacement on a lady. It was a very difficult family. Every night they would get into an altercation with the nurse that she didn't check their mother properly. There was a standoff. . . . Finally the social worker came in. . . . She supported the nurse. It was the hospital on one side and the daughters on the other. . . . I was hoping the social worker would have been more effectual in terms of getting the situation palliated. . . . There was a real standoff between me and the nurses. I didn't get any kind of help from the social worker."

Physician, Positive Case. "I had a guy whose foot I operated on. He told me he couldn't walk around very well. I thought I explained every thing to him. . . . I told him it would take six to eight weeks to get better. . . . He became absolutely outrageous. I made a couple of house calls trying to defuse his anger. . . . I asked [the social worker] if he could help me out with this guy. He started to talk with the guy and explain things to him. I don't know what he did, but within a few weeks, the patient comes in and says he understands. . . . I realized there must be some psychological problem, and eventually [the social worker) turned it around."

Comparing Qualitative and Quantitative Findings on Collaboration Factors

When the precoded ranked findings are compared with the qualitative analysis of the respondents' descriptions of their experiences, similar patterns emerge quite clearly from both sets of data. For the most part, responses were similar whether respondents chose from preset categories or provided information in their own words. Two additional categories emerged from the respondents' qualitative descriptions of their collaborative experiences and were coded using grounded theory methodology. The first was the concept of "shared responsibility," which we used to capture an expressed sense of mutuality, egalitarianism, and interdependence. We found it mentioned more often in the positive case descriptions by both professions, although it was mentioned much more often by social workers than by physicians. The second category, "shared ethics and values," or its opposite, "ethical dilemmas or conflict," was alluded to by both groups, often as a factor contributing to negative collaboration. Although social workers identified it more often than doctors in the negative cases, neither group framed their issues in collaborating with the other profession in ethical terms to any great extent.

Qualitative Analysis of the Focus of Collaboration

To provide a context for understanding their collaborative experiences, we used the brief case descriptions to classify the focus of the physicians' and social workers' collaborative activities. Not surprisingly, both professions stressed planning for posthospital care and obtaining community resources as the focus of collaboration in both the positive and negative cases. At times, the focus of the collaboration addressed the relationship with the collaborator rather than specific professional activities. Activities related to counseling were seen as the focus of collaboration more often in the positive cases than in the negative cases by both professions. When all positive cases were compared to all negative ones without regard to profession, the mean number of counseling activities was significantly higher in the positive cases (1.19 versus 0.58). Although social workers noted the importance of counseling more frequently than physicians, there were no significant differences between the two groups regarding mean number of counseling activities noted for either the positive or negative cases.

Discussion

Contrasts existed in the two professions' response rates to the precoded items. Did the physicians care less about collaboration or about completing the interview in a substantive way? Did our social work background affect the questions we asked as well as the responses given? Our experiences in conducting the interviews belied the first assumption because the physicians, as a group, were generous with their time and gave serious consideration to the questions asked. However, they were likely less familiar with the issues and language of the study than the social workers. Physicians generally give lower priority to collaboration than social workers, whose interaction with physicians is central to carrying out their functions (Mizrahi & Abramson, 1985). Finally, both professions selected fewer items to explain their negative experiences than their positive ones. Perhaps the presence of conflict masks and prevents a more comprehensive analysis of interaction

More of the patients selected were younger and terminally ill than anticipated. Such cases may evoke stronger emotional identification from both groups and thus greater investment, particularly for the positive cases. The intimacy with terminally ill patients and their families also may create an intimacy in the collaborative process that arises from the need for mutual support and shared responsibility.

The sample had at least one characteristic that may have influenced the findings: The pairs of collaborators almost exclusively involved male physicians and female social workers. This sample does not reflect the increasing number of women in medicine. Given the traditional dominance of physicians in interactions with other professionals, the gender pattern in this study would be expected to underscore that dominance. Therefore, evidence of egalitarian collaborative perspectives, particularly on the part of physicians, may indicate some shift in degree of medical dominance and in gender relationships. However, differences in status between the two professions and medical dominance in the collaborative relationship continue to be major factors in the collaborative dynamics between them.

As noted in our secondary analysis, clear patterns emerged from the data that distinguished social workers from physicians in the aspects of collaboration they saw as most critical. Whereas social workers emphasized their interaction with physicians, physicians saw the competence of the social workers as more important than interactional factors. Put another way, social workers seemed to seek validation from physicians, whereas physicians seemed generally unconcerned about receiving validation from social workers. This pattern held for both qualitative and quantitative data and was consistent across both positive and negative cases.

One aspect of the social workers' concern with interaction—their emphasis on shared responsibility as a highly desirable feature of positive collaborations—was quite telling. They clearly valued this presumed rarer form of collaboration with its implication of equality, mutuality, and interdependence. This dimension of collaboration was prized when it was present but was not commented on when absent. No doubt because of continued medical dominance, it is not yet a norm of collaborative behavior to be missed when it does not occur. It was surprising that about one-third of the physicians also stressed the importance of shared responsibility in the positive cases. In an era of increasing accountability and dissatisfaction with practice circumstances, physicians may be willing to give up authority in exchange for sharing some burdens of patient care with social workers, at least those whom they respect and deem competent. The minority of physicians and social workers who practice in this way reflect a transformative, interdependent model of collaboration (Mizrahi & Abramson, 1994).

The extent of physician concern about communication was somewhat surprising. From our previous work and experience, we were aware that social workers perceive many physicians as inaccessible or as valuing brevity in their communication with social workers. Therefore, we did not anticipate the extent to which physicians expressed appreciation of good communication in the positive cases or dissatisfaction with the amount of communication in the negative cases. According to some doctors, it was the social worker who was unavailable or withheld information. This finding might be partially attributed to traditional physician attitudes regarding control over patient care; perhaps the social workers in the negative cases were perceived as undermining physician authority by avoiding communication or obstructing the physicians' efforts to quickly discharge patients. Alternatively, the social workers may have lacked clarity regarding what to communicate or the confidence to express their views effectively.

Given the extent of emphasis by both social workers and physicians on communication in both types of cases, communication appears to be the only intrinsic or universal aspect of collaboration that is equally important to both professions and in positive or negative circumstances. The emphasis on communication by both doctors and social workers reinforces how critical and complex this dimension of collaboration truly is. This finding and others related to the importance of interactional factors suggest that professional training needs to focus more on interactional skills. Although these competencies have always been stressed in social work education and are increasingly a part of medical education, they are most often directed toward improving relationships with patients in the clinical encounter rather than addressing collegial relationships.

We have some concern about the extent to which both groups stressed the importance of respect for their collaborator or, in the negative case, the emphasis by social workers on the negative style and personality traits of the physicians. Patients depend on professionals to work together effectively on their behalf, regardless of professional relationships. Similarly, the importance of similar and dissimilar perceptions in evaluating collaboration deserves attention because it was important to both groups. Whereas similar perspectives can facilitate working relationships, optimum collaboration occurs when interprofessional interaction adds previously unrecognized perspectives or additional options to resolving the situation at hand. Learning from others as well as contributing to their learning is a key objective; merely convincing another professional of one's own views on a specific case is not necessarily the hallmark of success. Indeed, the management of the process and dynamics of collaboration must include the ability to negotiate and compromise as well as to persuade and defend.

We also did not anticipate that close to two-thirds of the physicians (almost as many as social workers) would emphasize at least one aspect of counseling as the focus of collaboration in the positive case. Perhaps physicians valued counseling in those cases based on direct experience with positive outcomes as a result of successful social work interventions with patients and families. However, the literature is consistent in identifying social workers as much more likely than physicians to stress a social work counseling role (Cowles & Lefcowitz, 1992; Lister, 1980). The extent to which social workers in this study sample valued good physician understanding of their role in the positive cases seems to indicate that they did not often encounter physicians who fully understood the breadth of their contribution to patient care.

Implications for Social Work

We suggest caution in generalizing from our findings to the larger population of social worker physician collaborators, even those in medical and surgical specialties, because our sample was not randomly selected. Our sampling method may have been biased toward selection of physicians more open to collaboration with social workers. Additionally, in providing examples of their best and worst collaborative experiences, both social workers and physicians may have selected experiences that portray themselves positively. Yet the patterns that emerged from the data were robust across various hospital settings.

Our results point to the likelihood of significant changes. Whereas most social workers valued collaborative relationships and interaction, so did a substantial group of their physician colleagues, as indicated by the high percentages of physicians who chose interactional items as well (Tables 15.1 and 15.2). If our sample is in any way normative, social workers may increasingly encounter physicians who are invested in having a positive relationship with them based more on collegiality and reciprocity than previously has been the norm. Awareness of this factor, as well as clarity about the increased centrality of the social work counseling, discharge planning, and case management roles, can provide the underpinnings for a more assertive and confident social work approach to collaboration with physicians.

The range of relationships uncovered between social workers and physicians reinforces the need to use a strategic or sociopolitical perspective in interprofessional relationships (Specht, 1985). Social workers must have a repertoire of collaborative strategies that address the remaining inequities in their relationships with many physicians. Yet they also need to remain open to sharing responsibility and relinquishing a quest for autonomy when collaborating with physicians whose interprofessional interactions seem based on assumptions of equality and interdependence rather than hierarchy and control.

The differences we identified in perspectives between the two professions support the importance of understanding the distinct socialization experiences of each profession. Social workers who grasp the action and outcome orientation of many physicians (Huntington, 1981) as well as the emphasis they place on communication will stress these aspects when collaborating. Strategic social workers will attempt to understand the professional experiences and perspectives of physicians if they wish to build interprofessional cohesion. For the present, social workers still need to look to their own profession as well as to other nonphysician reference groups for support and validation. Given traditional physician socialization, the majority of physicians are unlikely at present to offer the degree of shared responsibility and mutuality that many social workers seek. Yet for a significant subset of physicians, collaborative relationships seem to be moving more toward greater reciprocity. This phenomenon is likely to expand in response to the changing health care environment, in which all health care professionals are coming under increasing scrutiny and control by corporate-like structures.

The time is ripe for alliance and coalition building across disciplines. As the health care system moves toward greater emphasis on care provided in ambulatory settings, ongoing rather than episodic collaboration may become the norm. Success in developing collaborative practice requires that all team members understand common barriers and the strategies needed to minimize them. Identifying impediments to effective interprofessional collaboration does not always mean that they are desirable to overcome. Rather, the goal of successful teamwork is to consistently recognize and manage these tensions. Our data indicate that boundaries are permeable and that opportunities to improve collaborative interactions clearly exist. Social workers can assume leadership in shaping, rather than merely responding to, changing conditions and in the process contribute to the development of new and more effective models of interdisciplinary patient care.

References

Abramson, J. S. (1989). Making teams work. *Social Work with Groups, 12*(4), 45–63.

Abramson, J. S., & Mizrahi, T. (1986). Strategies for enhancing collaboration between social workers and physicians. *Social Work in Health Care, 12*(1), 1–21.

Abramson, J. S., & Mizrahi, T. (1993). Examining social work/physician collaboration: An application of grounded theory methodology. In C. Riessman (Ed.), *Qualitative studies in social work research* (pp. 28–48). Newbury Park, CA: Sage Publications.

Abramson, J. S., & Rosenthal, B. B. (1995). Interdisciplinary and interorganizational collaboration. In R. L. Edwards (Ed.-in-Chief), *Encyclopedia of social work* (19th ed., Vol. 2, pp. 1479–1489). Washington, DC: NASW Press.

Andrews, A. (1990). Interdisciplinary and interorganizational collaboration. In L. Ginsberg et al. (Eds.), *Encyclopedia of social work* (18th ed., 1990 suppl, pp. 175–188). Silver Spring, MD: NASW Press.

Baggs, J. G., & Schmitt, M. H. (1988). Collaboration between nurses and physicians. *Images, 20,* 145–149.

Bruner, C. (1991). *Thinking collaboratively: Ten questions and answers to help policy-makers improve children's services.* Washington, DC: Education and Human Services Co-Forum.

Campbell-Heider, N., & Pollack, D. (1987). Barriers to physician/nurse collegiality: An anthropological perspective. *Social Science & Medicine, 25,* 421–425.

Carrigan, Z. (1978). Social workers in medical settings: Who defines us? *Social Work in Health Care, 4,* 149–164.

Cowen, D. L. (1992). Changing relationships between pharmacists and physicians. *American Journal of Hospital Pharmacy, 49,* 2715–2721.

Cowles, L. & Lefcowitz, M. (1992). Interdisciplinary expectations of the medical social worker in the hospital setting. *Health & Social Work, 17,* 57–65.

Dingwall, R. (1982). Problems of teamwork in primary care. In A. Clare & R. Carney (Eds.), *Social work and primary care* (pp. 81–103). New York: Academic Press.

Fagin, C. (1992). Collaboration between nurses and physicians: No longer a choice. *Academic Medicine, 67,* 295–303.

Freidson, E. (1984). The changing nature of professional control. *Annual Review of Sociology, 10,* 1–20.

Huntington, J. (1981). *Social work and general medical practice: Collaboration or conflict.* London: George Allen & Unwin.

Koeske, G., Koeske, R., & Mallinger, J. (1993). Perceptions of professional competence: Cross-disciplinary ratings of psychologists, social workers, and psychiatrists. *American Journal of Orthopsychiatry, 63,* 45–54.

Kulys, R., & Davis, M. Sr. (1987). Nurses and social workers: Rivals in the provision of social services? *Health & Social Work, 12,* 101–112.

Lamb, G. (1991). Nurses practice interaction and decision making with physicians. *Research in Nursing Health, 14,* 379–386.

Lister, L. (1980). Role expectations for social workers and other health care professionals. *Health & Social Work, 5*(2), 41–49.

Lonergan, E. (1985). *Group intervention: How to begin and maintain groups in medical and psychiatric settings.* New York: Jason Aronson.

Lowe, J., & Herranen, M. (1981). Understanding teamwork: Another look at the concepts. *Social Work in Health Care, 7*(2), 1–11.

Mizrahi, T. (1986). *Getting rid of patients: Contradictions in the socialization of physicians.* New Brunswick, NJ: Rutgers University Press.

Mizrahi, T., & Abramson, J. (1985). Sources of strain between physicians and social workers: Implications for social workers in health care settings. *Social Work in Health Care, 10*(3), 33–51.

Mizrahi, T., & Abramson, J. (1994). Collaboration between social workers and physicians: An emerging typology. In E. Sherman & W. J. Reid (Eds.), *Qualitative methods in social work practice* (pp. 135–151). New York: Columbia University Press.

Mullaly, Z. (1988). The application of a social health perspective: A shared social worker-doctor responsibility. *Australian Social Work, 41*(1), 5–9.

Murray, J. L., Wartman, S. A., & Swanson, A. G. (1992). A national interdisciplinary consortium of primary care organizations to promote the education of generalist specialists. *Academic Medicine, 67,* 8–11.

Pike, A. W. (1991). Moral outrage and moral discourse in nurse-physician collaboration. *Journal of Professional Nursing, 7,* 351–363.

Roberts, C. (1989). Conflicting professional values in social work and medicine. *Health & Social Work, 14,* 211–218.

Rutala, P., Fulginiti, A., McGeagh, E., Koff, N., & Witzke, D. (1992). Validity studies using standardized patient examinations: Standardized patient potpourri. *Academic Medicine, 67*(10, Suppl.), S60–S62.

Sands, R. (1989). The social worker joins the team: A look at the socialization process. *Social Work in HealthCare, 14*(2), 1–14.

Sands, R., Stafford, J., & McClelland, M. (1990). 'I beg to differ': Conflict in the interdisciplinary team. *Social Work in Health Care, 14*(3), 55–72.

Schindler, F., Berren, M., Hannah, M., & Belgel, A. (1981). A study of the causes of conflict between psychiatrists and psychologists. *Hospital & Community Psychiatry, 32,* 263–266.

Schmitt, M. H. (1994). Focus on interprofessional practice, education, and research. *Journal of Interprofessional Care, 8,* 9–18.

Sheppard, M. (1992). Contact and collaboration with general practitioners: A comparison of social workers and community psychiatric nurses. *British Journal of Social Work, 22,* 419–436.

Skochelak, S., & Jackson, T. (1992). An interdisciplinary clerkship model for teaching primary care. *Academic Medicine, 67,* 639–641.

Specht, H. (1985). Managing professional interpersonal interactions. *Social Work, 30,* 225–230.

Toseland, R., & Rivas, R. (1984). *An introduction to group work practice.* New York: Macmillan.

Trella, R. (1993). A multidisciplinary approach to case management of frail, hospitalized older adults. *Journal of Nursing Administration, 23*(2), 20–26.

Vachon, M. (1987). *Occupational stress in the care of the critically ill, the dying and the bereaved.* New York: Hemisphere.

Walton, M., Jakobowski, D., & Barnsteiner, J. (1993). A collaborative practice model for the clinical nurse specialist. *Journal of Nursing Administration, 23*(2), 55–59.

Watt, J. W. (1985). Protective services teams: The social worker as liaison. *Health & Social Work, 10,* 191–198.

Williams, C. (1992). Everybody wants to play doctor. *Medical Economics, 69,* 42–45.

Discussion Questions

1. Why is interdisciplinary work in health care important?
2. When different professionals work collaboratively in the health-care system, such as physicians and social workers, does one profession have more credibility than other? Does one have more responsibility than the other?
3. How does collaboration work effectively? How does the stress of dealing with someone's health affect the situation? ✦

Part V

BEYOND HEALTH-CARE PROVIDERS: SOCIAL SUPPORT

Chapter 16
Bonding and Cracking
The Role of Informal, Interpersonal Networks in Health Care Decision Making

Rebecca W. Tardy and Claudia L. Hale

Part V of this anthology goes outside the boundaries of the health-care provider-patient relationship to look at the social networks that surround patients, their families, and friends. These other people to whom patients turn for information, advice, and support provide an additional area to examine in learning about health communication. More than ever, patient-provider communication in health care is impacted by patients' social networks. These networks extend the support that patients have as they address their health issues. There are three chapters in this section, and each in its own way reminds us that the role of communication in health care is not limited to the interactions that take place within the walls of health-care institutions.

Part V begins with Rebecca W. Tardy and Claudia L. Hale looking at informal communication networks and the ways these groups function to help members better understand health and illness. This is the first chapter in this part of the reader that takes health communication outside the specific patient-provider relationship to look at the various other factors, both face-to-face and mediated, that are part of contemporary health communication. Through their study of an informal playgroup, Tardy and Hale discuss the ways in which health understandings are constructed and social support is enacted in a less conventional setting. Through this discussion, we see how interpersonal interactions outside of medical institutions can have significant impacts on health behaviors and attitudes.

Related Topics: culture, groups, health-care behaviors, organizations, patient-centered communication, patients' perspectives, qualitative methods, social support

Throughout health communication research we see the continuing assumption that at the center of the health experience is the institution. Although acknowledging that the concept of health has been dominated by medicine (making the terms almost synonymous), Pettegrew and Logan (1987) explicitly situated health communication within the institutional world of hospitals, physicians' offices, and mass media campaigns. Nussbaum (1989) also supported this position, urging communication scholars to leave the comfort of their classrooms and focus on communication as it takes place within the organizations of health services. Although conversations among interpersonal networks are an appealing site of research, he situated health communication within the institutions of medicine and encouraged researchers to venture out into that strange, new territory.

Communication scholars have ventured out, in profuse numbers, into that strange land, especially investigating what Smith (1989) referred to as the conditions that enhance patient participation with institutional directives. Considerable health communication research has focused on the primary, institutional relationship between physicians and their patients (e.g., Ballard-Reisch, 1990; Beisecker, 1990; Burgoon et al., 1990; Conlee & Vagim, 1992; Geist & Hardesty, 1990; Klingle, 1990; O'Hair, 1989; Street, 1989, 1991; Thompson, 1981). Throughout current health communication research there has continued the perspective outlined by Smith (1989) that the physician (or other institutional speaker or source) occupies a position of power and

From "Bonding and Cracking: The Role of Informal, Interpersonal Networks in Health Care Decision Making," Rebecca W. Tardy and Claudia L. Hale, 1998, *Health Communication*, 10:2, pp. 151–173.

control when interacting with passive patients. Based on this body of research, the prevailing suggestion has been for physicians to increase their interpersonal communication skills to be more in accordance with other interpersonal encounters, such as between friends or coworkers (Korsch, 1989). This recommendation has been accompanied by promises of lowered malpractice suits and increased patient satisfaction and compliance (e.g., O'Hair, 1989; Rouse, 1989). In essence, then, more effective interpersonal skills (i.e., such as the expression of empathy and establishing trust) serve as a second insurance policy (Zook & Spielvogel, 1992).

Although effective communication should increase the likelihood of more effective medical treatment, there is no established, direct link between communication and health status at the individual level (Zook & Spielvogel, 1992). Achieving competency in communication would be a wonderful deterrent to disease, if only that connection existed. However, better communication does not necessarily hinder the onset or progression of disease, and communication scholars who sell such a tale to practitioners and consumers are tantamount to "snake oil" salesmen peddling panaceas.

Finally, we have a voice (Burgoon, 1992) within our own discipline telling communication scholars to check their participative, prescriptively prosocial ideologies at the door when they enter the institutionalized domain of medical science. Burgoon declared that we must "abandon the assumption of the communicationally incompetent physician" (p. 105), focus on variables deemed more scientifically serviceable (such as physician aggressiveness), and establish a more direct connection between health status and communication.

This directive supports the unwavering acceptance of the dominant voice of medical institutions in decreeing what behaviors people should practice with regard to their health. In spite of all of our allegiance and efforts to enhance physician control, patients, although satisfied with their physicians, still do not completely comply with the established order. McKnight (1988) offered some unique insights into the dilemma of patient noncompliance. As Smith (1989) brought up the issue of power, McKnight suggested that we turn our attention away from the institutionalized voices toward more mundane interactions that potentially have a greater impact on health status. McKnight illustrated how it is that someone who has certainly heard the messages of what to eat, how to live, and what to do regarding her health, chooses not to listen or obey the institutionalized "loudspeakers" of physicians, health departments, schools, and mass media campaigns in an effort to establish some personal control in her powerless situation. As he states, "Perhaps the only affirmation of her selfhood that remains is to defy the alien voices that would tell her how to live" (p. 43). What is labeled *noncompliance* in the institution could be labeled *strength* or *surviva*l outside the institution; not survival of the body, perhaps, but survival of identity and spirit.

What results from the traditional, dominant line of research is the continuing construction of health communication as discussions of physiological "data," medically established options, physician adoption of a more collaborative model of decision making, and patient adaptation to the medical environment. Although this construction is not without merit, what appears not to be recognized is that health decisions occur outside the establishment and that consumers have their own language and practices of health. If patient empowerment is the desired goal, then understanding the language of "health consumerism" should begin not with the primacy of the medical establishment, but with investigating what is essentially the daily lived experiences and perceptions of health for consumers.

Even the health belief model (Becker, 1974; Janz & Becker, 1984; King, 1983; Meischke & Johnson, 1993; Rosenstock, 1974; Smith, 1989), which outlines the effects of forces existent in everyday life on health care choices, has been utilized to gain greater patient cooperation. The question has been not how reality (regarding health, illness, and medicine) is understood and shared by consumers, but how health services practitioners can develop practices oriented around these beliefs in order to increase rates of patient compliance. The point is that we have allowed medical practitioners, the institution, to shape our discipline's research agenda. As such, our research does have sociopolitical consequences (Arntson & Droge, 1983; Pettegrew & Logan, 1987) as we continue to privilege institutional voices of health over the mundane practices of consumers.

This study, therefore, investigated the conversations of members of a social network regarding the health and illnesses of themselves, their family members, and their friends. In this article, the content and impact of these women's conversations are presented in light of practical and narrative qualities. Before presenting an analysis of these conversations, however, the phenomenon specifically under investigation (i.e., health information-seeking) must be defined.

Health Information-Seeking Among Informal Interpersonal Networks

Termed *health information-seeking,* the basic construct under investigation is defined as verbal and nonverbal messages ascertained via everyday interaction, either purposeful or serendipitous, by members in a self-defined network that serve not only to reduce uncertainty regarding their health status, but also to construct a social and personal (cognitive) sense of health. This definition is based on several bodies of research including mass media channel selection and social support (i.e., Albrecht & Adelman, 1987; Dervin, 1978; Edgar, Fitzpatrick, & Freimuth, 1992; Freimuth, 1987; Freimuth, Stein, & Kean, 1989; Johnson, Meischke, Grau, & Johnson, 1990; Levanthal, Safer, & Panagis, 1983). Information-seeking among informal, interpersonal channels is thought to be utilized as frequently as other channels, including physicians and organizations (37 to 38%; Connell & Crawford, 1988; Johnson et al., 1990); therefore, these connections are at least as potentially influential as more formal sources.

Among informal, interpersonal networks, information-seeking and sharing is considered one category of the multidimensional construct termed *social support.* Other categories include esteem, tangible assistance, emotional, and network (Cutrona, Suhr, & MacFarlane, 1990). House (1981) and House and Kahn (1985) presented four categories of social support including informational, emotional, appraisal, and instrumental. Although it identifies the existence of information-seeking and sharing within informal, interpersonal networks, research does not appear to have fully investigated the content of this type of support. The bulk of research has focused on how interpersonal interactions serve to enhance relational growth or facilitate coping with emotions and stress. Other investigations have focused on negative outcomes of informal support systems in an effort to balance out the overwhelmingly positive approach to social support (particularly when the network members are overly controlling, abusive, or depressing; La Gaipa, 1990).

This approach to investigating the social construction of illness is based largely on suggestions by Zook and Spielvogel (1992; cf. Brody, 1987; Engel, 1977,1979; Frank, 1993; Friedson, 1970; Kleinman, 1988; and Smith, 1989) in which they recommend hinging the contribution of communication researchers on the "making and managing" of illness through social interaction. Based on the biopsychosocial model of medicine (Engel, 1977,1979), language and social interaction are seen to reify experiences and subsequently create perceptions of health states. We name symptoms and signs as diseases, making the unidentified less unknown and therefore more manageable (Smith, 1989). *Disease* is defined as the evidence gleaned from the interaction of the physician with the patient's body (Friedson, 1970; Kleinman, 1988); illness is the individual's or patient's perception of and response to the physical symptom (Brody, 1987); and, finally, sickness is designated to represent others' perceptions (Friedson, 1970; Kleinman, 1988). These three terms assist us in understanding the various ways in which our illness and wellness status is determined biologically, psychologically, and socially.

Leatham and Duck (1990) reviewed how social support talk (or conversation) is best conceptualized as situated, symbolic, social, and strategic. Talk, as they explained, involves processes of shared meaning that not only serve to construct reality, but also to develop relationships. Leatham and Duck (1990) suggested investigating social support via four specific areas, including the network structure, the nature of the relationships, the content of interaction, and the impact of support. The first of these areas, the network structure, is explored in another report by the current authors (Tardy & Hale, in press); this article will focus on the latter three areas.

Method

The fundamental goal of this study was to observe, collect, and analyze mundane conversations regarding health issues by members of a social system. Therefore, this study used ethnographic methods typical of anthropological explorations (i.e., Basso, 1990; Carbaugh & Hastings, 1992; Fetterman, 1989; Geertz, 1973; Philipsen, 1975/1990) including participant observation, personal interviews, and an open-ended survey.

Participants

The participants in this study were members (mothers) of a local playgroup for infants and toddlers. The playgroup was one benefit offered through a community outreach program to integrate newcomers. Membership in this playgroup was contingent upon having recently moved to the city or having recently become a mother. The members paid a nominal fee for membership. In addition, some members of the playgroup also attended meetings of a local breastfeeding support group which met once a month in the basement of the local hospital.

There were approximately 30 women involved in this playgroup at any given time; however, only 24 women were identified as regular participants for the interviews and surveys. Characteristically, the women in this study were predominantly "stay-at-home" moms who had given up work or a career (some temporarily) to rear their children. Former occupations ranged from cosmetology, social services management, computer operations, x-ray technology, obstetrical nursing, elementary education, and advanced biological research. The women were all European American, with 2 women from other countries (Peru and Russia) and ranged in age from 23 to 43. All of the women had at least one child, with a maximum of three children. Socioeconomic status was estimated to range from lower class (graduate students' wives) to upper middle class (their specific incomes were not solicited). Finally, half of the women were native to the location, whereas the rest had been relocated because of their husbands' occupations.

Procedures

As Fetterman (1989) defined ethnography, the primary purpose is to provide a cultural interpretation that describes local practices. However, in this study, the researcher did not make these observations in isolation—that is, she related her observations to the participants and sought verification. Therefore, the data were not collected via a single observation, but through repeated observations and conversations with the participants. As such, the researcher served as the instrument, refining her observations and using the participants' perspectives to develop a contextualized theory. Inherent to this process is the identification of key informants who assist the researcher in refining observations. Fetterman (1989) explained this process as using the subjective experiences of the observed participants inductively to discover cultural patterns. Based on Glaser and Strauss's (1967) grounded theory, this approach sought not to use objective typologies or theories as a template for investigation but, rather, sought to develop a materialistic theory (Fetterman, 1989) based on observed behavioral patterns (i.e., Carbaugh & Hastings, 1992).

Participant Observation

The members met every week for approximately 2 to 2.5 hr, first in a church basement and then, with the change in seasons, alternating between a park and a restaurant chain with a playground. The members also met once a month for a "mom's night out," varying between members' homes on two occasions and a restaurant on two occasions. In all, 14 playgroup meetings and four mom's night out meetings were attended. The nature of the research and participants' rights to deny access was announced at three consecutive meetings with newcomers introduced and informed of the research as needed.

At the weekly playgroup meetings the women typically gathered in small groups, sitting or standing, talking with each other and playing with their children. The noise level at all of the sites precluded any possibility of audiotaping the interactions. As such, the attending researcher sat as unobtrusively as possible near conversations and, essentially, "eavesdropped." Notes were made regarding how they gathered, who gathered with whom most often, the tone of conversations, and the content of their interactions. Further, the field notes were openly displayed so that anyone could read the notes, thereby lessening the sense that the notes were secret and the women were being spied upon.

It is important to explain how efforts were made to ensure cooperation and reduce the participants' anxiety about being observed. First, the nature of this research was thoroughly explained and other relevant personal information was provided (e.g., the researcher shared personal stories and frequently joined in conversations about taking care of children). In addition, care was taken to engage in the group activities (by bringing refreshments, dressing casually, sitting on the floor, and playing with the children). In light of Fetterman's (1989) observations of ethnography, the women were informed of some "hunches" and were asked what they thought. Subsequently, the women would clarify what was going on in their interactions. Further, they began to engage in their own observations and report with such comments as "Oh, I heard a lot of interesting health talk going on tonight!" (this comment was made at a mom's night out). Although all these actions sound rather manipulative, based on responses from the members ("Thank you for not just being there—but enjoying yourself and not making us uncomfortable!", a survey response) the observation proved to be a pleasant experience.

Interviews

In addition to the observation, the participants were asked to engage in personal interviews to solicit their narratives with respect to health concerns and examples of information-seeking behaviors. The participants were offered a sign-up sheet if they were interested in assisting in the research by agreeing to a personal interview. The women provided their telephone numbers and were subsequently contacted and appointments made for the interviews. Efforts were made to include a variety of women in terms of age, socioeconomic status, and background.

Located in the participants' homes at their convenience, the personal interviews lasted a minimum of 1 hr to a maximum of 3 hr. All of the interviews were audiotaped with the participants' consent. In all, 13 women and 1 man participated in interviews. The man was included as the husband of one of the participants who happened to be present during the interview. Questions included ones associated with reflections of their own conversations with others about health issues: "What health-related issues do you talk about with only a few people?" "Where do these conversations take place?" "Can you tell me about a time when what someone said made you seek medical care?" "What purpose do these conversations serve for you?" Subsequently all relevant dialogue was transcribed by the researcher and subjected to inductive analysis.

Survey

The third step of this study included a survey to solicit more information regarding their impressions of health information-seeking:

> Think about people with whom you frequently discuss health issues and explain why you talk with this person.
>
> What are the characteristics of this person?
>
> In light of your health-oriented discussions, what is it that you want most?

What are "taboo," inappropriate, or difficult health topics to discuss?

The surveys were distributed to the members at a playgroup meeting and included a self-addressed, stamped envelope for them to return at their convenience. Four weeks after the distribution of the survey, those women who had not yet returned their surveys were contacted by telephone to request that they fill out and return the survey, resulting in a response rate of 62.5% (15 out of 24 surveys). These responses were also transcribed according to each question and coded for analysis. Finally, the field notes, interview transcripts, and survey responses were all analyzed and coded for emergent themes; that is, recurrent topics were identified and examined. The resulting categories include pregnancy and delivery, physicians and hospitals, breastfeeding, illnesses and accidents, diet and nutrition, and exercise. The various transcripts, notes, and surveys were also examined for the sense of impact friends and family members had upon the participants' health care decisions. Subsequently, the role of these conversations in the lives of these women was further determined. The conversations were found to serve distinctive functions. On one level, the conversations served a function of "bonding" the women together. The conversations are not only exchanges of information but are also narratives through which shared experiences are created and maintained. On this latter level, the women's conversations serve a rather practical function of informing the women of their options and others' experiences; their conversations help the women "crack the code" of institutional bureaucracy.

Results

The women's health-oriented conversations are reported here according to the aforementioned functions. Throughout this report, the names of the participants have been changed, with other names used to facilitate comprehension. In addition, the initials "ER" are used to indicate the interviewer.

Health Information-Seeking as Bonding Narratives

The primary topics especially noted for their narrative quality included pregnancy and delivery and breastfeeding. Conversing about pregnancy and delivery took two essential forms: first, in light of very serious exchanges of information and, second, as the sharing of experiences rather publicly with much humor and drama. The shifting back and forth between these two styles of delivery are noteworthy as they exemplify the different modes of conveying information.

First, the very serious exchanges of information focused on medical "facts" based on one's own reading, conversations with a doctor, midwife, or nurse, and one's own experience or the experience of another shared secondhand. Typically, these conversations were conducted dyadically in quiet tones and very little laughter. Difficult to overhear, the exchange could shift very suddenly to a much louder conversation marked by jokes and laughter. For example, Sharon and Angela, during a mom's night out event, found that they had the same obstetrician, whom Sharon recently visited due to her new pregnancy. Sharon had discussed rather openly—that is, to all present—that she had just visited her doctor. Angela asked who it was, and they discovered their commonality. Then, the conversation turned from including all present to a dialogue just between the two of them. The conversation lasted for about 10 min before they moved along to less serious and personal issues, such as the physician's own, unplanned pregnancy.

More seriously, discussions of pregnancy also focused on decisions regarding more intrusive tests than an ultrasound, such as amniocentesis. Repeatedly, two women engaged in discussions about the safety of these tests. Apparently, the test can result, in some instances, in fetal death. In addition, the issue of whether they would terminate the pregnancy if the baby was "defective" was discarded. Both women stated that they were not comfortable making such a decision and would carry their babies as long as possible, despite any complications. The distinction between louder and more inclusive conversations to quiet conversations indicates the need for privacy regarding some health issues. Essentially, the serious, dyadic conversations were before the fact, before the decisions had been made, and before a "story" had been constructed.

These stories or narratives were told repeatedly with much detail and embellishment. Pauses were strategically placed with expectations for sympathetic head nods, raised eyebrows, and verbal inducements to continue. Occasionally questions were posed for clarification. For example, Jackie had been trying to get pregnant for several months and announced at one playgroup meeting that her period was late. Another woman commented that she did not know that Jackie and her husband were trying. The response was a humorous retort that she thought she had been trying harder than her husband who was in the process of finishing his dissertation. "Poor man, he has to work so hard!" The other group members were curious about how she was feeling and what symptoms she had had so far. Head nods and "yep, that sounds like you're pregnant" provided confirmation of her suspicions with questions then turning to what doctor and hospital she would use.

On another occasion, Sylvia had arrived with her ultrasound pictures very clearly indicating that her unborn baby was a boy. With two girls already, she was very happy to be having a boy. The ultrasound pictures became a source of humor in that the word boy had been printed in the picture near an enlarged view of his genitalia. Sharon, also pregnant, expressed her admiration in an observation that he would make some woman very happy one day. Accompanied by laughter, Sylvia responded that he must have gotten it from her side of the family, but that her husband was very proud.

Further exemplifying the narrative nature of these conversations, at one mom's night out Sylvia reported the arrival of Marsha's baby. With all the mothers present and attentive, Sylvia stood centrally to the group, raised her arms and said loudly that she had an announcement. She paused for everyone to quiet and then said: "Marsha has had her baby." Pausing again for the questions and expressions of excitement, she announced that Marsha had had an 8 lb, 14 oz boy—again pausing for expressions of concern because he was a big baby—and was 21 inches long. "He was born this morning and his Apgar score was at first an 8 but then was up to 10 within a few minutes. Marsha is doing well; she only had Grade 4 tears." Sylvia had not been able to speak with Marsha and had just heard the news on her answering machine—so no more details.

Based on this revelation, we note that not only did Sylvia present the information very dramatically, but also she provided details using medical jargon. The observation regarding the grade of tears was in reference to tissue damage of the vagina during delivery. This type of comment was not made with embarrassment or enthusiasm, but concern. To an outsider, the term has rather gruesome connotations; however, for the women, terms such as these constitute the language of pregnancy. Another unfamiliar term was that of being four fingers along which is more commonly a reference for how many centimeters dilated. These two terms provide some sense that there is a language for the experience of pregnancy. Although perhaps familiar to outsiders, the language of pregnancy is laden with such expressions and shortcut codes such as asking someone how far along she was (usually expressed in weeks), if she has been sick (referring to morning sickness rather than any other sickness), and whether she was planning on nursing (breastfeeding).

Breastfeeding conversations observed in the playgroup, the breastfeeding support group, and in the personal interviews revolved around breastfeeding on demand, when to wean the baby, how to respond to mastitis, what medications a mother can safely take while pregnant and breastfeeding, when to introduce solid foods, how to breastfeed a toddler, how to handle colic, what to do about birth control and getting pregnant while breastfeeding, and how one's own diet can affect the breastfeeding infant or toddler. Although the bulk of conversations revolved around the sharing of information and advice about breastfeeding, conversations also focused on rather humorous, emotional, and sentimental aspects. One example of humor in breastfeeding was explaining to young children what is breastfeeding. Very often little children will imitate their mothers or other women and "breastfeed" their dolls or stuffed animals. One young woman tried to explain breastfeeding to her 6-year-old brother by comparing herself to a cow. This comparison is fairly common as women express feeling like a cow when breastfeeding on demand and nursing around the clock. The child found the comparison humorous and, in a sibling manner, began teasing his sister and calling her "Bessie." The sharing of this event provides some reduction of the seriousness and stress of breastfeeding and making light of others' impressions.

On the more emotional and sentimental side, women breastfeeding toddlers commented on having their children request to breastfeed, for example, by asking to "nur-nur." The toddler further complimented her mother and said, "umm, good nur-nur." Another woman, who got pregnant while still breastfeeding her toddler and experienced pain and tenderness, explained how she had to deny her daughter's request to nurse. Later, when she did breastfeed her, the toddler thanked her mother and gave her a kiss on her breast. To those not familiar with the experience of breastfeeding, the whole notion of conversing with the child seems odd and uncomfortable. To the women breastfeeding, the story was an example of the very close bonds between a mother and her nursing child. In addition, the sharing of these stories further created closer bonds between the women.

Finally, as with pregnancy, the women created special terms and, essentially, a language centering around the breastfeeding experience. Becoming indoctrinated into breastfeeding required learning this language and using the terms. For instance, when a baby is first born, a mother has *colostrum,* which is not milk, but is a fluid the mother's body produces full of antibodies and special nutrients for the newborn baby. Within about three or four days, the colostrum is replaced with milk and this event is referred to as the *milk coming in.* Often the mother's breasts will become *engorged,* which is extremely painful and potentially serious in the case of mastitis. In response to this event, mothers must continue to nurse, use a breast pump, or hand express their milk to relieve the pressure.

When the baby first begins nursing, he or she has to learn how to suck sufficiently so that the milk will "let down" or begin to flow. The women laughed about how, once adept at breastfeeding, just the sound of a baby crying would cause the milk to release from the ducts and, of course, they would have a wet shirt. Another term references the difference between the milk the baby receives initially upon breastfeeding, which is rather watery, and the *hindmilk* which is creamier. Mothers were taught to keep the baby nursing until the hindmilk was produced at each sitting. *Nipple confusion* is when infants are allowed to use a bottle (usually introduced by a well-intentioned nurse at the hospital wanting to give the mother a break) and have difficulty adapting to the work required by them to breastfeed (i.e., getting the milk to let down). Referred to as *mother's milk,* there are several myths surrounding the benefits of breastmilk. The women at the support group commented on breastmilk being a "miracle fluid," as it is sometimes used to reduce ear and eye infections. Whether supported scientifically or not, these terms and ideas help support the women in their convictions that all the symptoms and experiences of breastfeeding are natural and that they should continue nursing.

Women sharing stories about pregnancy, childbirth, and breastfeeding is hardly a remarkable finding. However, although women have been having children (and talking about their experiences) for millennia, now, more than ever before, women are highly dependent upon medical technology and guidance. In their efforts to understand the changes in their lives, such as for those who have left a career to become stay-at-home moms, women have found more than just good advice in their conversations. These mundane conversations are the stories or narratives of their lives. They portray them in dramatic tones, embellishing them with greater significance. Further, their conversations and narratives are important to the establishment of new connections. The notion that women value connectedness is well supported by research (i.e., O'Connor, 1992), and the women of this study were no exception. Based on the need to relieve their isolation, the playgroup was established in order for women to develop connections and friendships. Removed from their family and friendship networks, these women recognized their vulnerability and the importance of developing new friendships. Having left careers, these new stay-at-home moms had a greater need for social support. In a time when women are still striving for equal rights and equal pay, they must defend their positions and clarify that the "job" of motherhood is not simple or stress free. As Betty observed regarding having children, "It's a topic that just bonds us women together."

Cracking the Code and the Practical Impact of Health Information-Seeking

The focus of this section is on the extent to which the conversations had an impact. What happened subsequent to discussions of health? Did the women go to the referred physician? Did they try out a new product or try a new technique? Observations and interviews overwhelmingly indicated that the women not only followed their friends' "prescriptions" and advice, they purposefully solicited that assistance. The impact was also rather accidental when guidance was modified to best meet the mothers' unique situation. Finally, the impact could emerge after years of exposure to information and practices that the woman found detrimental or not in keeping with her own convictions.

Direct impact was evident as the women asked each other about feeding their families healthier foods. Patty provided an example when her daughter appeared rather pale, listless, irritable, and lethargic. She mentioned her concerns to her neighbor, a nutritionist, who thought the problem might be low iron because her own son had exhibited similar behavior with the resulting diagnosis. The neighbor suggested getting a blood count, but because Patty disliked taking her daughter to the pediatrician, she opted for feeding her daughter a breakfast cereal high in iron. Whether the problem was actually low iron is unknown; however, Patty changed her daughter's diet in direct connection with her neighbor's observation with positive results.

Although some of the women changed their practices to meet recommendations, both Betty and Jackie told stories of their childhood when their families' diets were not consistent with their own preferences for vegetarianism and low-fat consumption. Although both of their families continued in their long-standing practices, these women conferred regularly not only on how to handle their families' disparaging comments, but also on new recipes for a healthier diet.

Annie's, Jackie's, and Betty's encounters are all examples of how previous experiences have affected health care choices and philosophies. Annie also explained how her former network of friends, prior to moving, had not breastfed their children, so that her decisions to bottle feed was shaped by that exposure. She had given birth to two children previously with this former circle of friends. Even though she moved and developed affiliations through the playgroup, in which the women predominantly breastfed, she still chose not to breastfeed. The practice was not in keeping with her own level of comfort and former role models. So, although she felt somewhat isolated, she continued with her previous practice. (A = Annie, ER = interviewer).

> ER: Did you breastfeed her at all?
>
> A: No, I never did . . . I thought about her—it's just something that—my family never did it—and none of my friends ever did—I really didn't understand anything about it and I would have felt like an outcast—and here—I feel like an outcast because I feed her with a bottle. It's just how different just from here to there.
>
> ER: But you were here when she was born.
>
> A: Yea, and I thought about it . . . but I never did with them two and I was like . . . so I just didn't. When they were little, no one I was around ever nursed. I never knew anybody that ever . . . You know . . . so that was just the thing to do. And here—everybody does! And you feel like such an outcast because she drinks from a bottle!

Based on these accounts, there is the sense that the social network can potentially affect the women's choices, but their decisions are ultimately based on what is the most comfortable choice.

The women in this study also conferred with their friends and family members about childhood illnesses, colds, broken limbs, spider and tick bites, gynecological problems, and more serious illnesses, such as cancer and heart disease. Childhood illnesses included such problems as chicken pox, ear infections, allergies, and childhood development (colic, teething, walking, etc.). Gynecological problems included having a mammogram, mastitis (breast infections), fibroid cysts, lumpectomies, hysterectomies, tubal ligations (sterilization), and routine pap smears. Discussions with friends and family assist the women in knowing when a problem is serious enough for an appointment or the emergency room. Sylvia told the story about when, at the physician's office, one of her daughters tripped and severely bit her tongue. The bite was deep, but the physician explained that the child should be given acetaminophen for the pain and popsicles or other cool liquids. Although some bites are severe enough to require stitches, her daughter's wounds were not that severe. During the past year, she recalled that the same thing had happened to Amy's son during a visit. Amy was all ready to take her son to the emergency room, and had Sylvia not been there, she probably would have taken him. However, Sylvia was able to assist in this instance by providing her own experience, enhanced no doubt by having had medical advice at the time of the earlier incident.

In addition to soliciting advice regarding an illness or accident, the women also asked for physician referrals. However, asking friends or network members for a referral is not always positive. For example, Doris received a recommendation for a pediatrician from her best friend. The pediatrician recommended was a popular one among the network of women ("You have probably heard of Dr. Smith. Everyone takes her child to him"), but Doris was dissatisfied with him, feeling that he tended to treat her child as "eardrums," rather than as a child.

That a physician's reputation (and subsequent business) can be determined by members of a social network was evident in the story of a new physician who had moved into town during the course of this research. Because she was unknown, little was known about her abilities, and until the participants knew someone who had experienced treatment from her, she was a dubious candidate. Finally, someone went to see her and reported some inadequacies. The inquiry continued with another member talking with her cousin, a physician in another town, who had trained the new physician and claimed that she was "good," thereby increasing the new physician's credibility. It is doubtful that the physicians realize the extent or power of the women's network in ensuring the success of their practice.

Another observation of discussions regarding physician treatment included comments on the appearance and attire of a physician. Maria expressed her views of her gynecologist who did not wear the traditional garb of white coat over a business suit when he examined her:

He looked like a rock star! He was wearing jeans and a shirt—with no lab coat. And he had a pony tail! I liked him but it felt strange to have him examine me.

Although informal appearances are important in making a positive impression, the women were more comfortable with the way that the nurses and receptionists express their familiarity than with the physicians. Positive impressions of physicians were based more on the doctor's ability to explain a problem, understand and respect individual philosophies, and accommodate individual expectations. The women expressed an interest in having their physicians recognize them and know their individual cases and ease the explanation of personal information.

Obtaining a referral from a network member was just half the battle; getting in to see the physician became another issue. Maria (M) and Amy (Am) shared their amusement at "cracking the code" and getting immediate access to a physician.

> M: My biggest frustration is needing someone immediately.
>
> Am: I need to get in . . . I was sick with a sinus infection. I was taking boxes of

over-the-counter medication—it was getting so bad that

M: I had to do what she did . . . I was sick twice this past winter and I never went to the doctors—and someone told her to go to. . . .

Am: Someone told me that they are always looking for GOOD patients . . . is how they phrase it and what that means is payment.

M: Insurance.

Am: Right, that pay their bills

ER: Who told you that?

Am: The receptionist said, oh, you want to go to the M.D.—like that was the way to go. Tell them that you are a patient of Dr. Smith's and I referred you . . . and it was almost like you needed the code word to get in. . . .

M: Cause I called and they said—you're sick today?—we can get you in in 3 weeks on such and such a date. And my husband said, I'm sick now—I'll be better by then! And that has happened to me twice where I have called and I made the appointment for a month later and I'll be better by then. So I did what Amy did and I never talked to Smith's office but called the other office and I said . . .

Am: Did they ask you what kind of insurance you had?

M: I said that I go to Dr. Smith's and they recommended that I see you—now I'm sick from my kids. I mean—they didn't ask about the physical but they did say that normally new patients—uh, we have no new appointments—and she kept putting me on hold . . . and I know darn well she was checking my insurance! I know she did—I know she did! So she came back on and got me in the next morning or that afternoon. I don't remember but they got me in.

ER: So, you figured out the trick . . . was . . .

M: Well, I did what she did and I hoped that they didn' t call Smith's office and check—well, they know me but they didn't really refer me . . . I just did what she did. And I am telling you that is probably the only way I got in there.

ER: You sound like you all cracked the code in the system.

M: SHE cracked the code!! I mean we wouldn't have gotten in anywhere . . . because they say that you are a new patient. We don't take new patients.

Am: And I had to get in to someone . . .

M: You need an antibiotic and you can't wait for 3 weeks—or go into the emergency room! You're not a new patient anymore (very excited)!

Am: I'm not a new patient anymore!

M: I m so proud that I can call now when I am sick and stuff and they are going to say are you a new patient? And I can say—NO!!

The use of informal network members for physician referrals is well known; what is not known are the strategies behind gaining information and the outcomes of such searches. The women revealed a number of strategies for referrals including asking strangers, their husbands' coworkers, and members of the playgroup and breastfeeding support group. Betty, when asked how she found referrals, admitted that she asked everyone—everyone with a small child of similar age to her own. Maria also expressed this same dogmatic inquiring:

ER: How did you find out about what to do when you lived in XXX?

M: Umm . . . I started off with the realtor . . . I always start off with the realtor

ER: That is the first person you ask?

M: Yep, and as soon as we move into the neighborhood I start asking right away—EVERYBODY—and then plus—some of this is driven by our insurance plan—and they give you a book of names and then you just start asking everybody.

ER: Through your husband's work?

M: I ask when visiting his work—who does your wife use for a pediatrician—who is your wife's OB/GYN—who is . . . you start getting names and uh . . . you hear oh, this guy is great, this lady is nice and that type of thing. It is pretty much a process of elimination, too. And then, I moved here and I needed to go for my OB checkup, after I had Christina and I asked around and I knew I didn't want to go to anybody around here because I hadn't heard one positive thing and whoever went to the doctors here—went out of sheer desperation or they didn't want to drive anywhere else. So, Amy told me that she loved her OB and just raved about him—so I went up to see him in XXX—and loved him. It was great.

The search for physicians was moderated by the women's personal degree of expertise regarding health services. Sylvia and Marsha both had previously worked in hospitals, whereas Linda and Doris, new not only to the town, but also to the country, were reliant upon women from their native countries who had information. Both women, with fairly distinct accents, were approached by women who recognized their accents and inquired into their needs. Unfortunately, both of these women had difficulties within the playgroup due to their accents.

Using the informal network was not without its hazards and strains. When asked what type of system they would develop to ease the "finding" process, no one suggested a system similar to their support group. The primary reason was that the process was quite time consuming, and the women did not express any recognition of the potential power they had through their interactions. Instead of a more formal or organized interpersonal network, the women suggested telephone referral systems as experienced in larger cities or a publication of physicians complete with biographical information including philosophical approaches to medicine and child development. The complaint is that using the informal network is not only time consuming, but also requires substantial energy on their parts. Lastly, if we consider isolated women or career women who are not part of a network, then relying upon an informal network is not a very efficient means.

Conclusion

There were two, intertwined goals guiding this research project: First, there was the practical goal of investigating the significance of informal, interpersonal networks in health care decision making; and, second, there was an ideological, political goal of seeking to expand the scope of health communication research beyond the boundaries of institutionalized settings. The women's conversations were determined to serve both practical and interpersonal needs; that is, while sharing health information, they not only found out more about their options, but also developed connections with other women.

Although the interaction taking place within institutions is undoubtedly of major importance, decisions are mulled over, reevaluated, and determined outside the institutional context. It could be that these mundane conversations occurring in homes, in church basements, at the playground, or even in baseball bleachers (i.e., Nussbaum, 1989) are not merely appealing to health communication scholars, but are important in the sense of revealing how consumers sift through various alternatives, determine their paths of action, and make choices. It is in these conversations that we hear rationales shaping the choices and behaviors in light of compliance and noncompliance.

Furthermore, as the health services industry seeks to provide better ways of managing care, there is much that can be gleaned by empirical studies of health information-sharing in informal, interpersonal networks for improving the provision of service and facilitating appropriate access to medical services. First, it is evident that these informal networks do serve to shape perceptions not only of themselves as patients, but also of how and when to access practitioners and services. As previously explained, new residents of communities solicit information from a variety of sources. Furthermore, in conversation the reputation of practitioners and facilities are established. The participants of this study, although not cognizant of their own power, could bring a tremendous number of customers to any agency. The well-known adage regarding the power of word-of-mouth advertising was integral to the utility of this playgroup. What was not recognized by the medical community was how to access and fully utilize existing interpersonal networks.

How, then, can any agency best access the power of these networks, not to co-op the women per se, but to provide information, guidance, and legitimate support for the groups? As Vickery and Lynch (1995) pointed out in their application of "demand management" to patient care, although morbidity is perhaps the most objective aspect with which to measure effective utilization of health services, "perceived need is the primary basis upon which individuals make decisions to seek medical care" (p.

553). Variables considered to reflect perceived need include knowledge of the procedures, as well as knowledge of the potential risks and benefits of the prescribed treatment. Furthermore, the sense that someone has of her own ability to assess the problem and handle the consequences and cure of the medical condition is a key issue. These impressions stem from one's education, sex, social support systems, cultural norms, as well as the knowledge and attitudes of medical practitioners within the community.

Within this particular community, the women were not very trustful of the local physicians. Only the uninformed and desperate could rationalize not leaving the town and traveling at least 30 min to a physician and hospital for her prenatal, delivery, and postnatal care. New physicians were scrutinized and their practices and values surmised in light of the women's own value systems and preferences. However, the notion of how to assess the credentials of a particular physician tend to be mysterious at best and presumptuous at worst. Although consumers can be encouraged to have a consultation with a physician prior to actually engaging him or her for treatment, such practice is very expensive, time-consuming, and often not even procurable. Most people engage a practitioner's services when they are ill and must have treatment. The treatment itself serves as the assessment; thus, the service becomes tantamount to a "crap shoot." If I win, great; but, if I lose, then I must suffer the consequences, pay the bill, and seek another physician.

There is not much available, beyond telephone physician referral services, that provides information to prospective consumers. In essence, however, these services operate more like a match-making service, incumbent upon the referral provider's knowledge and expertise in making suggestions. Furthermore, often referral providers are not permitted to disclose negative information (due to nature of the business arrangement these services have with their clients, i.e., the physicians), but attempt to steer consumers to a more viable service provider. A consumer must contact her state's medical licensing bureau and investigate a physician's reputation. When checking a practitioner's credentials, most patients do seem to notice rather aesthetic qualities of attractiveness, orderliness, and interpersonal communication skills (e.g., Schneider & Tucker, 1992), with little comprehension of how to question medical knowledge. When credentials and knowledge are questioned, the practitioner might respond with defensiveness, resulting in a negative experience noted by hostility and power struggles (e.g., Beisecker, 1990).

As such, Vickery and Lynch (1995) reviewed the impact of patient preference on selection of care. This notion is both reflective of and constrained by legal expectations. As Vickery and Lynch (1995) stated, "patient preference is incorporated into the legal standard for informed consent with the resultant applications for medical malpractice" (p. 553). A discussion of patients' preferences for medical treatment has less, initially, to do with their comprehension of the technical language and procedures than with their notion of how to engage in negotiated decision making. Research (e.g., Emanuel, Barry, Stoeckle, Ettelson, & Emanuel, 1991) indicates that patients who are more informed not only choose less costly treatments, including surgery, but also desire to provide advance directives.

Pragmatically, there are several ideas one can glean from this study in light of demand management, managed care, and more effective utilization of health services.

1. Health service organizations (HSOs) could seek out these informal networks and provide informed representatives to visit and present talks or guide discussions on particular health concerns (i.e., diagnoses and treatments) and provide references to a variety of relevant services.

2. HSOs could tap into the opinion leaders within these networks, offering training, education, and information that they can take back to their networks.

3. HSOs could provide more comfortable, physical support for networks in terms of meeting rooms and facilities.

4. HSOs could consider that after the provider's socialization into the discipline

during medical school, there is another socialization into the community of practice. The goal of this activity would not be for providers to teach the community so much as for the community to teach the practitioner about common assumptions, practices, and so forth (e.g., Arntson, 1996).

5. HSOs should not try to eradicate the networks or offset the "contamination" of the information shared. As demonstrated in this study, the bonding and cracking functions are cultural practices that serve to distinguish and probably empower the participants.
6. The providers could solicit information regularly from these networks on how the services can be improved.
7. HSOs could provide information (such as in a pamphlet) about the staff and the philosophy or mission of any agency or institution to realtors and the local chamber of commerce, not to mention physician referral services.

These are only a few ideas on how the identification of informal, interpersonal networks can be useful to the dissemination of medical knowledge. Further, facilities can consider their role not just to be one of dispensing medical care and information but also one that receives information via these networks. As noted previously, Artnson (1996) outlined a program to "deinstitutionalize" medical students,—practiced at Northwestern University—in which students are oriented toward recognizing the assets of their community. As Artnson outlined in these four steps, the students ultimately determine

1. How the institutional and community views of health compare and contrast.
2. How attempts to "fix" individuals, vis-a-vis institutional expectations, can be "dangerous."
3. How to delineate an "asset-based" approach to community health.
4. How to work within the community, focusing on wellness projects in which the institution is one part of the system.

The playgroup used in this study is only one type of network available. Tapping into and "capturing" mundane conversations regarding health issues, at the outset of this study, was like trying to bottle fog. The desired group was one that ostensibly did not gather just to discuss health issues, but health concerns needed to be a salient issue. Essentially, for the mothers in this group, their whole world and identities, once pregnant, began to revolve around their family members and respective health conditions. Given how important prenatal and postnatal care are to health, not to mention a lifelong commitment to maintaining health, the mother role inherently involves decisions regarding medical treatment.

The health communication phenomenon is often reduced to a simplistic panacea of mutual decision making and shared power (use negotiation and call me in the morning), when the reasons for noncompliance are complex (e.g., McKnight, 1988). As Pettegrew and Logan (1987) indicate, there is a vast array of areas to include under the rubric of health communication; limiting ourselves in some aspects is necessary to maintain our uniqueness as a discipline. Health communication, however, does not have to be confined to the physical institutional terrain; instead, researchers can examine health and illness as it occurs and crosses over three distinctive areas, including the medical, the personal, and the public or societal. The combination does not just make for interesting research, but enables us to gain a greater vision of how people symbolically make and manage their experiences of health.

References

Albrecht, T. L., & Adelman, M. B. (1987). Communication networks as structures of social support. In T. L. Albrecht & M. B. Adelman (Eds.), *Communication social support* (pp. 40–63), Newbury Park, CA: Sage.

Arntson, P. (1996, July). *The role of community in "deinstitutionalizing" medical students.* Paper presented at the international conference on Teaching About Communication in Medicine, Oxford, England.

Arntson, P., & Droge, D. (1983, May). *The sociopolitical consequences of health communication research.* Paper presented at the meeting of the International Communication Association, Dallas, TX.

Ballard-Reisch, D. (1990). A model of participative decision making for physician-patient interaction. *Health Communication, 2,* 91–104.

Basso, K. (1990). "To give up on words": Silence in western Apache culture. In D. Carbaugh (Ed.), *Cultural communication and intercultural contact* (pp. 303–320). Hillsdale, NJ: Lawrence Erlbaum Associates, Inc.

Becker, M. H. (1974). The health belief model and personal health behaviour. *Health Education Monologue, 2,* 328–335.

Beisecker, A. E. (1990). Patient power in doctor-patient communication: What do we know? *Health Communication, 2,* 105–122.

Brody, H. (1987). *Stories of sickness.* New Haven, CT: Yale University Press.

Burgoon, M. (1992). Strangers in a strange land: The ph.d. in the land of the medical doctor. *Journal of Language and Social Psychology, 11,* 101–106.

Burgoon, M., Parrott, R., Burgoon, J. K., Coker, R., Pfau, M., & Birk, T. (1990). Patients' severity of illness, noncompliance, and locus of control and physicians' compliance-gaining messages. *Health Communication, 2,* 29–46.

Carbaugh, D., & Hastings, S. O. (1992). A role for communication theory in ethnography and cultural analysis. *Communication Theory, 2,* 156–164.

Conlee, C. J., & Vagim, N. N. (1992, October). *Dimensions of physician interpersonal communication competence as predictors of patient satisfaction with physician care.* Paper presented to Speech Communication Association Convention, Chicago, IL.

Connell, C. M., & Crawford, C. O. (1988). How people obtain their health information—A survey in two Pennsylvania counties. *Public Health Reports, 103,* 189–195.

Cutrona, C. E., Suhr, J. A., & MacFarlane, R. (1990). Interpersonal transactions and the psychological sense of support. In S. Duck & R. C. Silver (Eds.), *Personal relationships and social support* (pp. 30–45). Newbury Park: Sage.

Dervin, B. (1978). Strategies for dealing with human information needs: Information or communication? *Journal of Broadcasting, 20,* 324–333.

Edgar, T., Fitzpatrick, M. A., & Freimuth, V. S. (1992). *AIDS: A communication perspective.* Hillsdale, NJ: Lawrence Erlbaum Associates, Inc.

Emanuel, L. L., Barry, M. J., Stoeckle, J. D., Ettelson, L. ML, & Emanuel, E. J. (1991). Advance directives for medical care—a case for greater use. *New England Journal of Medicine, 324,* 889–895.

Engel, G. L. (1977). The need for a new medical model: A challenge for biomedicine. *Science, 196,* 129–136.

Engel, G. L. (1979). The biopsychosocial model and the education of health professionals. *Annals of the New York Academy of Sciences, 310,*169–181.

Fetterman, D. M. (1989). *Ethnography: Step by step.* Newbury Park, CA: Sage.

Frank, A. W. (1993). The rhetoric of self-change: Illness experience as narrative. *The Sociological Quarterly, 34,* 39–42.

Freimuth, V. S. (1987). Diffusion of supportive information. In T. L. Albrecht & M. B. Adelman (Eds.), *Communicating social support* (pp. 212–237). Newbury Park, CA: Sage.

Freimuth, V. S., Stein, J. A., & Kean, T. J. (1989). *Searching for health information: The cancer information service model.* Philadelphia: University of Pennsylvania Press.

Friedson, E. (1970). *Profession of medicine: A study of the sociology of applied knowledge.* New York: Harper & Row.

Geertz, C. (1973). *The interpretation of cultures: Selected essays.* New York: Basic Books.

Geist, P., & Hardesty, M. (1990). Reliable, silent, hysterical, or assured: Physicians assess patient cues in their medical decision making. *Health Communication, 2,* 69–90.

Glaser, B. G., & Strauss, A. L. (1967). *The discovery of grounded theory: Strategies for qualitative research.* New York: de Gruyter.

House, J. S. (1981). *Work stress and social support.* Reading, MA: Addison-Wesley.

House, J. S., & Kahn, R. L. (1985). Measures and concepts of social support. In S. Cohen & S. L. Syme (Eds.), *Social support and health* (pp. 83–108). Orlando, FL: Academic.

Janz, N. K., & Becker, M. H. (1984). The health belief model: A decade later. *Health Education Quarterly, 11,* 1–47.

Johnson, J. D., Meischke, H., Grau, J., & Johnson, S. (1990, October). *Cancer-related channel selection.* Paper presented at the Speech Communication Association Convention, Chicago, IL.

King, J. (1983). Health beliefs in the consultation. In D. Pendleton & J. Hasler (Eds.), *Doctor-patient communication* (pp. 109–125). New York: Academic.

Kleinman, A. (1988). *The illness narratives: Suffering, healing, and the human condition.* New York: Basic Books.

Klingle, R. S. (1990, November). *Physician compliance-gaining strategies: The impact of identity management objectives on strategy usage.*

Paper presented at the meeting of the Speech Communication Association, Chicago, IL.

Korsch, B. M. (1989). Current issues in communication research. *Health Communication, 1,* 5–9.

Kretzmann, J. P., & McKnight, J. L. (1993). *Building communities from the inside out: A path toward finding and mobilizing a community's assets.* Chicago: Acta Press/Center for Urban Affairs and Policy Research.

La Gaipa, J. J. (1990). The negative effects of informal support systems. In S. Duck & R. C. Silver (Eds.), *Personal relationships and social support* (pp. 122–139). Newbury Park, CA: Sage.

Leatham, G., & Duck, S. (1990). Conversations with friends and the dynamics of social support. In S. Duck & R. C. Silver (Eds.), *Personal relationships and social support* (pp. 1–29). Newbury Park, CA: Sage.

Levanthal, H., Safer, M. A., & Panagis, D. M. (1983). The impact of communications on the self-regulation of health beliefs, decisions, and behavior. *Health Education Quarterly, 10,* 3–29.

McKnight, J. (1988). Where can health communication be found? *Journal of Applied Communication Research, 16,* 39–43.

Meischke, H., & Johnson, J. D. (1993, May). *Using the health belief model to predict breast cancer-related information seeking from physicians and other health professionals.* Paper presented at the meeting of the International Communication Association, Washington, DC.

Nussbaum, J. F. (1989). Directions for research within health communication. *Health Communication, 1,* 35–40.

O'Connor, P. (1992). Friendships between women: A critical review. New York: Guilford.

O'Hair, D. (1989). Dimensions of relational communication and control during physician-patient interactions. *Health Communication, 1,* 97–115.

Pettegrew, L. S., & Logan, R. (1987). The health care context. In C. R. Berger & S. H. Chaffee (Eds.), *Communication yearbook 10* (pp. 675–710). Beverly Hills, CA: Sage.

Philipsen, G. (1990). Speaking "like a man" in Teamsterville: Culture patterns of role enactment in an urban neighborhood. In D. Carbaugh (Ed.), *Cultural communication and intercultural contact* (pp. 11–20). Hillsdale, NJ: Lawrence Erlbaum Associates, Inc. (Original work published 1975).

Rosenstock, I. M. (1974). The health belief model and preventive health behavior. *Health Education Monographs, 2,* 354–386.

Rouse, R. (1989). A paradigm of intervention: Emotional communication in dentistry. *Health Communication, 1,* 239–252.

Schneider, D. E., & Tucker, R. K. (1992). Measuring communicative satisfaction in doctor-patient relations: The doctor-patient communication inventory. *Health Communication, 4,* 19–28.

Smith, D. H. (1989). Studying health communication: An agenda for the future. *Health Communication, 1,* 17–27.

Street, R. L. (1989). Patients' satisfaction with dentists' communicative style. *Health Communication, 1,* 137–154.

Street, R. L. (1991). Physicians' communication and parents' evaluations of pediatric consultations. *Medical Care, 29,* 1146–1152.

Tardy, R. W., & Hale, C. L. (in press). Getting "plugged in": A network analysis of health-information seeking among "stay at home moms." *Communication Monographs.*

Thompson, S. C. (1981). Will it hurt less if I can control it? A complex answer to a simple question. *Psychological Bulletin, 90,* 89–101.

Vickery, D. M., & Lynch, W. D. (1995). Demand management: Enabling patients to use medical care appropriately. *Journal of Occupational Environmental Medicine, 37,* 551–557.

Zook, E. G., & Spielvogel, C. (1992, May). *The management & making of illness: Toward a broader legitimation of health communication.* Paper presented at the convention of the International Communication Association, Miami, FL.

Discussion Questions

1. What is meant by "cracking the code"? When women in the group understand these codes, how does this understanding affect how the women relate to health professionals?
2. This study focused on mothers who primarily discussed health issues related to motherhood (e.g., pregnancy and breastfeeding) and their children's health. What other areas of health do people have significant informal and interpersonal conversations about? What are the impacts of these conversations?
3. What could health providers gain from a better understanding of how people communicate informally about health? ✦

Chapter 17
Sisters and Friends

Dialogue and Multivocality in a Relational Model of Sibling Disability

Christine S. Davis and Kathleen A. Salkin

Chapter 17 addresses one specific area where more than professional health-care support is needed: families who have members with disabilities. Families who have members with disabilities face a unique set of challenges. The chapter addresses the unique set of challenges, which are often centered on the health-care issues of the disabled person, by looking at two sisters and their own experiences. Christine Davis and Kathleen Salkin, who are themselves sisters, co-construct a narrative of their experiences growing up together with Kathleen's disabilities. They argue that disability is experienced as a family and that this view can lead to a better understanding of family relationships in which disability is involved.

Related Topics: body image, culture, disability, family communication, groups, health-care behaviors, patients' perspectives, qualitative methods, social support

> "What seems clear to me is that any disability Kathy had was a 'family disability,' experienced in relationships with our family members."

Prologue

In February 1952, when my mother was 5½ months pregnant with my older sister Kathy, she met a fortune teller. The woman put her hand on mom's abdomen. "I see dancing legs," she predicted. "Your child will be a dancer."

Two weeks later, my sister was born. She was baptized immediately. She was weighed for the first time when she was five days old; she weighed 2 pounds, 4 ounces. When she was eighteen months old, her inability to walk, muscle spasticity, and lack of response to sounds was given a name: cerebral palsy. The cerebral palsy was thought to be caused by a lack of oxygen at birth. Her cognitive functioning was fine, but she was partially deaf and moved around only by vigorous crawling. It took two leg surgeries, huge leg braces and crutches, and years of physical therapy before she was able to walk.

As the younger sister, I was born to exhausted, preoccupied parents with stored-up expectations for their children. I learned independence as I used the physical therapy workroom as a playhouse, running up and down the stairs, along the parallel bars, and over the treadmills, as Mom and the physical therapist worked with Kathy. I developed a fear of doctors as I sat alone in waiting rooms of doctor's offices, listening to Kathy's terrified screams down the hall as the doctor used an electric saw to remove yet one more cast. I acquired patience when I had to wait because it took Kathy longer to do things. I gained responsibility because it was my job to pick up both of our toys; after all, Kathy is "handicapped."[1]

Research Question

In this article, I want to examine my relationship with Kathy. In my research on this subject, I looked for evidence that others have shared my experiences. I found research that says that siblings of people with disabilities are less well adjusted and are more likely to experience severe behavioral problems than children without a sibling with a disability; that siblings of children with severe emotional disturbances tend to feel overlooked or ignored, suffer from a disproportionately lower share of parental attention, and a disproportionately higher share of parental expectations; and experi-

From "Sisters and Friends: Dialogue and Multivocality in a Relational Model of Sibling Disability," Christine S. Davis and Kathleen A. Salkin, 2005, *Journal of Contemporary Ethnography*, Vol. 34:2, pp. 206–234.

ence "survivor's" guilt for their better health (Cuskelly 1999; Fisman, Wolf, and Ellison 1996; LeClere and Kowaleski 1994; Lobato and Kao 2002; Pitten Cate and Loots 2000; Nixon and Cummings 1999; Schulman 1999; Seligman and Darling 1997; Wolf, Fisman, and Ellison 1998). Other researchers have found, however, that siblings of children with disabilities are more well adjusted than other siblings—many show more maturity, responsibility, altruism, tolerance, self confidence, and independence (Pitten Cate and Loots 2000). I relate to all of those findings.

Researchers have looked at sibling caregiving—something I have never had to do for Kathy—and found that sisters are more likely than brothers to provide care for siblings with mental retardation (Krauss, Seltzer, and Gordon 1996; Orsmond and Seltzer 2000). Some siblings of children with disabilities report increased homecare and caregiving responsibilities over other children, while others do not (Damiani 1999; Seligman and Darling 1997). Kathy's disability is physical and not cognitive, and she lives independently, so this is not an experience I share. What I do share, however, is a concern about Kathy's future and an awareness as I was growing up that I might be assisting her when we got older.

Nonetheless, there is little research that looks at the relationship between the sibling with the disability and the nondisabled sibling as it is experienced by the two of them. How did Kathy's disability and impairment affect how we related to each other, I wondered? How much of our relationship was based on being sisters, and how much was based on her physical condition? And can these issues even be separated? Also, I wanted to get clues to whether her disability had in some way affected my relationship with my parents. I wanted to hear an excuse—exhaustion, stress, overload—for my experience of emotional neglect as I was growing up. I decided to use Kathy's and my relationship to write this; to together produce a co-constructed narrative, with the two of us writing and talking together, discovering together as we write, what our relationship is about. I was hopeful that as we wrote about our relationship, we could in fact enhance it.

Disability and Stigma

Of course, disability and impairment are not the same thing. Kathy's body has impairments—cerebral palsy and hearing impairment. Impairment turns into disability through a process of exclusion from social activities in a society that stigmatizes individuals who are physically different (Goffman 1963; Marks 1999, Oliver 1990; Oliver 1996; Shapiro 1993). Stigma has been defined as an "undesirable different-ness" (Goffman 1963), and the stigmatization results not from the differentness itself but from a society that constructs disability and normalcy, one that says that people who are different are somehow "invalid" (Barnes 1996; Marks 1999; Oliver 1990, 1996; Zola 1982). The disability itself often overshadows the person's self-identity (Susman 1993). It seems to me, though, that the differentness of our family overshadowed not just Kathy's identity, but everyone's. It is the hegemonic influence of "able-bodied" society that separates people into categories of "normal" and "deviant" and therefore pushes people with impairments to attempt to behave more like "normal" people—submitting to medical procedures designed to help them "overcome" their physical impairments (Oliver 1990). This traditional "medical model" of care involves professional hegemony in which people with physical disabilities, and sometimes their families, are viewed as deficient objects, responsible for their problems. This perspective emphasizes loss and inability and contributes to a picture of the child and family as being dependent and results in a disempowerment and marginalization of people with physical impairments (Barton 1996; Foucault 1995; Marks 1999; Oliver 1990, 1996; Seligman and Darling 1997). I suggest that to study Kathy's disability within the context of our family and our relationship—studying our collective experience of disability—yields a richness to the understanding of the social aspects of impairment and disability that has yet to be examined. I further suggest that families of people with disabilities and physical impairments also undergo a process of normalization in which they try to live up to society's image of a "normal" family. I also want to make it clear that I am not attempting to classify Kathy or myself into categories of normal versus disabled. I believe that as we age, we are all simply disabilities waiting to happen (Zola 1982). I also believe that each of us has conditions that are at times disabling and are at other times enabling. What seems clear to me is that any disability Kathy had was a "family disability," experienced in relationships between our family members. This is what I wanted to find out with this research—how was Kathy's disability experienced in our relationship, and how was it experienced in my relationship with our parents?

Methodology

I am aware of the moral ethics of speaking for Kathy, and I am sensitive to letting the voice of people with disabilities be heard (Barton 1996). This is why, in writing this article, it was important to me that I not attempt to give my accounts of Kathy's experiences (Oliver 1996). Instead, this article attempts to let each of us give our own accounts of our own experiences. I have made a conscious effort to give both of us voice. My goal in this research was to be a "dialogic researcher" who engages dialogically with Kathy through acknowledging both of our humanities and our vulnerabilities (Czubaroff and Friedman 2000; Mizco 2003; Patton 2002; Reed-Danahay 2001). In essence, this is a case study methodology in which I study one case—my family— within the context of being a family with one member that has a physical impairment. I am attracted to a case study approach to research because it takes a postmodern ethnographic orientation in its basic epistemology. It sees knowledge as experiential, it pays attention to socio-political contexts that influence the meaning within the case, it seeks to understand multiple realities, it takes a radical constructionist position that is interested in the ways that everyone involved is touched by the situation, and it focuses on interpretive knowledge from the human being who is the research instrument. Rather than generalizing to a population, case studies provide naturalistic generalizations so that readers are able to experience the case vicariously along with us. A case study looks at a situation in its contextual complexity and typically focuses on understanding actions, processes, patterns, and problems through interpretation and narratives (Lincoln and Guba 1985; Stake 1995).

Our parents are both deceased, and my other sister Kelli is much younger than us and therefore did not participate in much of our joint childhood experiences. In addition, Kathy has completed graduate work in a social science discipline and has expressed interest in my research. Thus, I decided to invite her to write this article with me. Since we live in two different cities 800 miles apart, and because Kathy is hearing impaired, we discussed these issues via e-mail and America Online Instant Messenger. We also had one in-person conversation during a trip I took to visit her. I sent her this article as I wrote it and invited her to write about her own memories, as well as comment on mine. We performed this article exchange two times. I had hoped that she would feel comfortable putting her voice forward as strongly as mine. I am aware, however, that the hegemonic influence of the academic publishing guidelines gives my academic and narrative voice more "weight" than Kathy's conversational voice and that the editorial necessities of writing such an article give more room for my voice than hers. However, I do believe that the writing is also multivocal and moving toward the dialogic. To preserve the multivocal quality of this article, I have included the exact words from each of us as much as possible. Editing only consisted of removing conversation that did not pertain to the research topic. Methodologically, this article is a combination of in-depth interviewing, interactive interviewing, co-constructed narrative, and a conversation between sisters. Practically, the reader is being taken on a journey inside our relationship.

This article presents recollections, feedback, and conversations. Thoughts constructed after the conversation are in parenthesis.

The Conversation Begins

Kathy: I am the eldest of three sisters and have considered us all to be relatively close—that is, until they moved down to Florida this past year. I do miss them but my life is so full that I keep myself busy, so I don't have time to mope.

I am both excited and apprehensive at this project. Excited because it's always good to learn new things about yourself and those you interact with. Apprehensive because I'm afraid negative things will come up and I don't take criticism very well sometimes. However, this is a good learning opportunity for us and I'm pleased Cris asked me to be a part of it.

Cris: I had the exact same concerns that you did; I was concerned that we might talk about something that might be hurtful, or painful, or we'd bring something up that might insult the other person. If I said something that hurt your feelings, that might cause a problem in our relationship, and one of my goals in doing this is for us to talk about stuff and get closer. I'm hopeful, and I hope you agree, that we can agree to work through anything that gets difficult and make sure that it does make us closer.

Kathy: I don't have a rose colored vision of us as a perfect family. I tend to shy away from confrontations because I don't like them. I don't like being hurt and I don't like hurting people. I'm a little apprehensive.

Cris: One of my goals in studying this for myself is to determine how much of our "weirdness" growing up had to do with the fact that somebody in the family was disabled, nothing personal against you.

Kathy: Yeah, that's the dynamics, there's no getting around it.

The Early Years

I look through the family photo album until, finally, I find the picture I am looking for. This picture is the epitome of our childhood. We are dressed up, posing for pictures, pretending to be perfect. Easter Sunday. I am probably five and Kathy is probably ten. We are in the backyard of our house in California. The sun is casting shadows in front of us. The grass is green. A palm leaf peeks in the corner of the picture. We are dressed in pastels; me with baby blue ruffles running along the bodice of the dress and white chiffon skirt beneath and Kathy in a turquoise blue lace dress with a pink sash. We both have on white socks with lace tops and white Mary Janes. We are both squinting into the sun. Kathy, at least a foot and a half taller than me, is leaning on me ever so slightly. Her feet are turned just a little bit funny, away from the rest of her body.

I wonder how many of my feelings of parental indifference and adjustment problems stem from Kathy's disability, how many stem from my place as a younger sibling, and how many stem from the combination of the two factors? It is interesting to note that research on birth order has found that older siblings have more access to parental time, energy, and engagement in their lives (Steelman et al. 2002), reinforcing my birth order hypothesis. On the other hand, other research has identified difficulties younger siblings have in adjusting to having an older sibling with a disability (Cuskelly 1999).

Cris: I remember playing dress up and I got to be the princess and you had to be the prince, you were the older sister and you had to be the prince.

Kathy: I remember that; that was a lot of fun. I remember I hated the way Mom used to always make me wear pink and you always got the blue dress.

Cris: I always hated dressing up like that anyway. Regardless of what it looked like.

Kathy: It was kind of cute.

Cris: It was so uncomfortable.

Kathy: She made those dresses; she worked hard on those dresses. She put all of her love into those dresses. She wanted the best for us. She just loved to dress us up. She loved us. That I never doubted.

(Cris: [To myself]. I did doubt that. I guess that's why I'm on this journey; to find out that her perceived indifference wasn't about her not loving me. Throughout the years, Kathy and I have had this same conversation, and it always ends the same way, with me saying I didn't feel love from Mom, and Kathy bringing out all sorts of evidence to prove she loved us. Kathy saw her dressing us up as being about love; I saw it as being about her trying to mold us into something we weren't; proof that I wasn't good enough for her the way I was.)

More pictures of us together: Kathy posing with me at my kindergarten graduation; I'm wearing a white graduation gown, holding a white rolled up parchment. Kathy and I held safely in Dad's arms, one on each side of him, sitting on the living room couch. Posing in front of our Christmas stockings, in our matching red and blue dresses. At the beach, sitting side by side. Playing in our playhouse. Playing with our cat. Posed in matching dresses, standing side by side. Playing with dolls. Playing in the backyard. Kathy on her tricycle, me in my "HotRod" toy car. On family vacations. Always side by side. Usually in matching clothes.

Kathy was my first friend, I guess. Long before I went to nursery school, long before I made friends in the neighborhood, Kathy played with me. I was her real-life baby doll and she was my big sister.

Looking back over the pictures, stories, and memories, I can see my conflicted feelings about Kathy. I loved her, and when we were young, I did not see any impact of her disability on her or on our relationship. She was my big sister, and that was just the way she was. As I got older, though, I resented having to take on additional responsibilities to make up for things she could not do. And I was jealous of the time that Mom and Dad seemed to spend with her and not me. Other siblings also seem to have these conflicts. Siblings in Pitten Cate and Loots' (2000) study reported both positive and negative aspects of their relationship with their sibling with a disability. They reported love and affection toward their sibling, perks awarded to the family as a result of the disability (special holidays, going to the head of a line, etc.), and enjoyment in playing together. But they also reported difficulties in playing physical games and in communicating with each other. Part of the communication difficulty was because of the impairment itself, but part was due to the fact that the siblings, because of the impairment, had less in common, and because they were not comfortable discussing the disability itself. Inability to discuss the disability in the family may result in increased loneliness and isolation for the nondisabled sibling (Seligman and Darling 1997). I wonder if this may result in loneliness and isolation for both siblings. I wonder if Kathy ever felt isolated because we could not discuss her disability. I wonder if she still does.

Kathy: It's interesting what you said about the family photos, for there is a family photo of us taken just before I broke my leg back in 1997. You and Kelli are in the back while Jerry, Mom, and I are in the front. I usually am in front in most group photos, as it is an "advantage" of being the shortie—ha. I realize the photographer posed us, but I think it it's interesting that you and Kelli are together because I've felt sometimes that the two of you are closer together than either of you are with me. I've felt the outsider sometimes as we got older, especially after Dad died. However, that might be because Mom got more sharp tongued and divisive after Dad's death, I don't know. *Shrug* However, I don't really obsess about it because it's not really important. We're all that's left of the family, and we need to stick together.

Kathy: I've often wondered; somehow some of the expectations that come with being the number one child got passed on to you because of my disability.

Cris: That's interesting you say that, because I felt often that I was born the oldest child. I've often felt that from the time I was old enough to remember, I was expected to know things that I wasn't old enough to know, know how to do things that I wasn't old enough to do.

Kathy: I don't know about that. Sometimes they say the expectations of the oldest child is that you do well, they have higher expectations of the first born. That's not to say that they didn't have high expectations for me.

Cris: I always felt that their expectations for both of us were put on me to some extent.

Kathy: I think that once that Dad realized that I could do pretty much what I wanted to with my brain, he increased his expectations of me.

Cris: What I'm referring to, for instance, is usually the older sister is expected to kind of watch out for the younger sister, and I think I always felt, whether it was right or not, that it was my responsibility.

Kathy: Oh, yeah, Mom expected you to look after me. I remember I kind of fought that. That's probably one reason I'm so independent. Because I hated feeling like you guys had to watch out for me. I didn't ask to be disabled. You didn't ask to be the middle child. You didn't ask to have expectations higher of you than were normal.

As I look through the photo album, I see a picture of Kathy in her leg braces. I remember them. They were huge metal things, constructed with two flat metal slats fastened into a top thick, tan leather band that fit around her leg above her knee. At the bottom of each metal side slat was a flange that fit into a notch in the side of her specially made, huge, heavy, brown leather lace-up shoes. With the braces on, she walked stiff legged and awkwardly, lunging forward with each step. Spasticity in her legs caused her to walk mostly on her toes. She kept her balance with the aid of arm braces, a combination of canes and crutches that fit to a leather strap fitted around each arm. I don't know how she felt about walking with these braces, but as her little sister, I loved playing with them. To me, they were toys, big-sister props that she had, and I did not, reason enough for me to want to play dress up with them.

Cris: What influence do you think your disability had on all of our family relationships?

Kathy: That's kind of hard to say, because I was the center of it. Kids tend to be centrist; when you're a kid, you don't tend to think of other people's feelings. I do know that it put a lot of money pressures on Mom and Dad. They had to worry about therapies for me, and braces. But they did have help with a lot of that stuff. From Easter Seals. But just the tension of dealing with a disabled child; finding out what schools to send her to and everything. How to get me to school, therapy, and all. I guess we were extremely lucky we lived where we did. LA [Los Angeles] County had an extremely good program for disabled kids. Lowman School was the best academically speaking that I could have gotten, as good a program as any. At least they never ever talked about sending me away. A lot of parents were encouraged to send disabled kids away to boarding school. I remember Mom telling me several times that her doctor told her that I would never be able to be educated, I would have to be institutionalized. This was when I was a baby, before they knew the extent of my disability. She said she refused to believe that. Knowing Mom, I could believe that. She said she was determined to make me be the best I could. And she did. She was the best mother she could have been. A problem with that was, I think it took so much of her energy. And dealing with a disabled child.

Kathy and I certainly had different experiences of mom and dad. I wanted to know if their seeming inattention was caused by a lack of love toward me or their preoccupation with raising Kathy. I wanted to hear evidence that they meant well and that their indifference toward me was out of their control. I wonder what evidence would change my feelings. I look through my research. Parents of a child with a disability have to contend with the loss of their anticipated familial narrative. Their narrative must be transformed to accommodate the disability, which in a systemic sense affects the entire family. Family life is normalized around the disability, as barriers are faced and overcome (Green 2002). Families with a child with a disability tend to have more stress, conflict, financial burden, maternal depression, and marital distress than do families without a child with a disability (LeClere and Kowaleski 1994; Nixon and Cummings 1999). Mothers of children with a disability are more vulnerable to stress and have a diminished sense of mastery (Seligman and Darling 1997). I could say that we experienced all of that.

(Cris: The following interview [done using America Online Instant Messenger] illustrates, I think, how much sometimes Kathy and I are simply big sister and younger sister roles.)

Cris: So, do you want to finish that interview we were in the middle of, at your birthday? We could do it now if you want.

Kathy: Right now?

Cris: Uh huh. For awhile at least. As long as you have time.

Kathy: I was planning to go to bed early.

Cris: For a few minutes? Whine whine. (Sometimes it helps to play "little sister.")

Kathy: OK if it's not too long.

Cris: OK; thanks!

Kathy: Shoot.

Cris: I think I was asking you to describe your relationship with Mom and Dad, and you were in the middle of answering that when we left for dinner, so do you have anything to add about that? So, the question was, how would you describe your relationship with Mom, especially when you were younger, elementary school age?

Kathy: It was pretty good when I was a kid. Not bad at all.

Cris: What made it pretty good?

Kathy: Happy times, and so forth.

Cris: Tell me about a happy time.

Kathy: When she gave me a surprise birthday party and invited my Girl Scout troop and school mates, when I was eleven, I think. There were about ten or so girls, and we had a blast. Mom made one of her cool cakes and it was all very nice.

Cris: Do you remember if I was there?

Kathy: I think you were. You were at all my birthday parties.

Cris: Do you remember the birthday where the magician pulled the rabbit out of the hat? That was a birthday party for you.

Kathy: Oh yeah. I was about seven or eight that year; you were just two or three.

Cris: That was really traumatic for me because I got left out and didn't get to pet the rabbit; for some reason I remember that. (I was the baby; preschool age. Everyone was so busy with Kathy and all her friends with disabilities that I got pushed to the back. I stood in the corner and cried and nobody noticed me.)

Kathy: Awww. . . . I don't remember that part.

Cris: I remember going with you and Mom to your physical therapy. What age did you start going to physical therapy?

Kathy: That was a special thing when I went to St Paul's.

Cris: What age were you diagnosed with cerebral palsy?

Kathy: Diagnosed at two; started physical therapy at three.

Cris: What was physical therapy like for you?

Kathy: I hated it!

Cris: Why?

Kathy: Because I had a mean physical therapist when I was six or so and never got over it.

Cris: Huh! I always thought it was fun to tag along; kind of like playtime.

Cris: What did he/she do to make him/her mean?

Kathy: She would shake me roughly when she thought I wasn't moving fast enough and it scared me.

Cris: Yuck.

Cris: How much extra time as parents do you suppose Mom and Dad spent doing stuff related to your cerebral palsy as opposed to regular parent stuff they would do with any child?

Kathy: Hard to say. I know they put a special effort into the PTA [parent-teacher association] because it was one area where they had a voice.

Cris: Were there issues that you took longer to get dressed in the mornings and stuff?

Kathy: They just got me up earlier, etc.

Cris: My memories are that they were burdened and didn't have time for me, and I'm wondering how much of that was the cerebral palsy and how much of that was them and how much of that was just being a younger child.

Kathy: I remember sometimes they'd have to hurry me up to catch the bus. Dad was a very busy man. . . . He was in PR [public relations] for Technicolor, and he traveled sometimes.

Cris: Yeah, and my memories are that Mom was really busy too.

Kathy: I remember Mom being there all the time.

(Cris: For who? You?)

Cris: Do you remember my relationship with Mom?

Kathy: All I remember early on is that you were a cranky kid at times. You were, you know.

(Cris: Ouch! So much for sympathy! What a big sister thing to say! I feel my old competitiveness rising up!)

Cris: What age, in what way?

Kathy: Well, when you were like two or three you had horrible temper tantrums. You would sit there and cry and cry because you were so mad.

Cris: All two-year-olds have horrible temper tantrums! That's what the phrase "terrible twos" means! (I'm feeling very defensive here! I can see that after forty-five years, you're still able to push my "anger" buttons! I wonder why?)

Kathy: I'm sure you drove Mom crazy.

(Cris: Phew! Sometimes Kathy can be really "know it all," and even at our ages now, she can make me so mad! Why does she have to say something mean like that? As I read through this, I story myself as the little sister to her, who looked up to her, and at the same time as a sort of big sister to her, who watched out for her. Why does she have to have such negative memories of me?)

Kathy: You were stubborn, that I remember too.

Cris: In what way?

Kathy: Always wanted to get your way. You and I used to have these fights in our room all the time, over silly things like who would turn out the lights, who would get which bed, whose stuff went where—usual stuff like that. And Mom would get fed up because she would have to come in and settle things.

(Cris: Yeah, well, it takes two to fight!)

Cris: I remember she used to say that she always wanted us to be close because she had been an only child and had missed that.

Kathy: You were a good kid, basically, but sometimes you could get stubborn and refuse to do something.

Cris: Like what?

Kathy: Oh, jeez I don't know. I can't remember a specific time; it's just a general memory, you know?

Cris: Uh huh. (It's probably time to end this interview before we get into a fight about whether or not I was a brat at age three!) OK. Let's go to bed. Goodnight. Thanks for your time.

Kathy: You're welcome. Good night. Love ya. Bye.

Cris: OK, love you! (I sure hope our relationship survives this project!)

Both: Signed off.

I feel like I am ten years old again! I feel vindicated to read that first-born siblings have been found to be less agreeable than later born siblings. Later born siblings tend to be more agreeable, partly as a strategy to minimize confrontation with their older siblings (Michalski and Shackelford 2002). Nixon and Cummings (1999) found that siblings of children with disabilities experience greater emotional distress in reaction to family conflicts and develop extra sensitivity to family conflict and concerns, perhaps even becoming negatively biased toward social cues in interactions. I wonder if that is true of me. Siblings of children with disabilities tend to use more coping (rather than avoidance) when dealing with family conflict; that is, they try to take the responsibility to "fix" the problem. I wonder if some of our conflicts are a power-resistance dialectic, in which, having both been put in an "older sibling" role, we are both resisting the other. If power in a sibling relationship is an entitlement, then which of us is entitled to it? The one first in the birth order or the one who had the primary sibling responsibility?

Cris: Part of what was up with me was that they didn't have time to teach me things, so I . . .

Kathy: I don't understand what you mean.

Cris: Like tie my shoes.

Kathy: Mom didn't teach me those things; Nana did.

Cris: No one taught me. An older girl in elementary school taught me because she thought it was ridiculous that someone my age didn't know how. No one had time to teach me. I think that I just learned to be good and keep out of the way because Mom had her hands full and didn't have time to mess with me, so I just learned to be the "good daughter."

Kathy: I always thought that before I was the age of age, Nana was the one who was the main . . . of course, Mom was there.

Cris: Why was Nana the one who did that? Was Mom not a nurturing mother?

Kathy: I don't remember. I think Nana sort of spoiled me rotten. I remember Mom used to tell me that anytime she wanted to punish me for something, Nana would say, "Don't do it! She can't help it!"

The Middle Years

When Kathy was ten and I was five, she had the second of three surgeries on her legs to cut the tendons in her calves and allow her to walk more easily. I tagged along when she got the leg casts removed.

Mom helped Kathy out of the car as I waited patiently next to our black 1960 Buick Roadmaster. With the toe of my shoe, I played with a crack in the sidewalk as Mom helped Kathy pull her huge leg casts out of the car and moved her to a waiting wheelchair. I followed behind the wheelchair as Mom wheeled Kathy into the doctor's waiting room.

"Sit over there," Mom said, pointing to a seat, a middle seat in a row of black, olive green, harvest gold, and burnt orange plastic cushioned seats. I complied. Immediately behind me, in the next row of seats, were two nuns. Their eyes, nose, lips, cheeks, and chins stood out from their black starched habits and headpieces. I tried not to stare, but it was hard. I loved nuns. They seemed to be similar to angels, and I figured that they prayed all the time, so they must have more direct access to God than the average person. Direct access to God was a good thing. God could answer prayers. If He wanted to, He could heal impairments like my grandmother's blindness or Kathy's cerebral palsy. I wondered what these nuns were thinking. I tried not to stare as I stole glances at their faces.

"Kathleen Salkin." The nurse at the door called Kathy's name. "Stay here and read your book," Mom whispered as she handed me *Tip and Mitten,* my favorite reading book about a cat and a dog. "We'll be back as soon as we can."

I looked at the book. Suddenly, I heard a commotion coming from the other side of the waiting room door, echoing from far away. First, the loud whirring, whining, screaming sound of a saw. Then, almost instantaneously, the high-pitched sound of a human scream. The scream of the saw and the scream of the human merged in a disharmony of sharps and flats as my hair stood on end. I recognized that scream. It was Kathy, screaming as they were sawing off her cast. I wanted all the screaming to stop; I wished they would stop. Couldn't someone make them stop?

Mercifully, the screaming did finally stop, the nuns were called in to see the doctor, and I got a lollipop from the nurse even though I had not had to scream to earn it.

Kathy: I only had three surgeries as a child—a tonsillectomy at the age of five and the two on my right foot at the ages of eleven and twelve, not four.

Cris: Whatever (she always has to be right!)

Cris: Talk about your relationship with Granddad.

Kathy: He kind of spoiled me too. He was an inventor. He did things that helped me increase my mobility. He built things. When I was a little kid, I couldn't walk very well, so he built a little walker for me. You know those bar stools, he cut the seat and cut a hole in the seat and put wheels on the end of the legs. I'd pull myself up by the shoulders and then just wheel myself all over the place.

Cris: Tell me about your relationship with Mom.

Kathy: She's my mother, and I don't remember having any problems with her when I was a little girl; she was the quintessential housewife. We lived in this really nice house in California, beautiful house; Mom was a very house-proud woman. She loved decorating, and she was very good at keeping things neat and tidy, unlike me. Appearances were very important to her. She'd always fuss at you if you didn't look your best. She always had this picture of what things should look like.

Cris: Let me ask you this. I agree with you, and I'm thinking as I'm doing this writing. Outward appearances were so important to her, how do you think she was affected by your disability? That's an appearance thing.

Kathy: The thing about me is, unless you see me walking or see me in a wheelchair, I don't look disabled. A lot of disabled kids have funny looking teeth or funny looking features. My disability is in my legs; it's not in my face. I've been told I'm pretty.

Cris: I think so.

Kathy: It's not like she had a horrendous child to contend with. She coped with my not being able to walk very realistically. She knew I couldn't do certain things and she made certain allowances. But I will say this for her: when I was a kid, I would have to do the dishes, I would have to help with the housework.

And I hated it, They didn't let me get away with murder. Now you and Kelli may have different opinions.

Cris: I do, but that's alright. (My memory is she did get away with murder!)

Kathy: I got away with as much as I could. That's kids. That's normal for a kid. I don't think, I don't remember Mom or Dad letting me slack off in school just because I was disabled. At least in schoolwork.

Cris: You were always very good in school.

Kathy: Now physically, I remember they made some allowances for me, but I remember Mom would make me help with the dishes, and she would let me help with the cooking. I cleaned rooms, but I admit I'm awful at cleaning rooms. But that's just laziness on my part; it wasn't from lack of effort on Mom's part to teach me. If I had been an only child, she might have made more of an effort with me, but when you were born and Kelli was born, she concentrated on teaching you guys how to clean the house. Maybe she thought it was less of an effort to teach you than to teach me.

The Later Years

Kathy's series of surgeries helped, and she was able, for many years, to walk unaided. She still had a strong limp, still favored walking on her toes, and had balance problems that caused her to fall frequently, which finally convinced her to begin using crutches to help her walk.

When I was twenty-two and Kathy was twenty-seven, we went on a river tubing trip with some of my friends from the single's group at church. I didn't want her to go.

"Mom, they're MY friends! Why do I have to invite Kathy along?" I whined. They were my friends, from my church, in my life, separate from my parents and my sisters. Having her come would ruin everything! I couldn't enjoy myself if Kathy were there. I felt like a teenager whose younger sister wanted to tag along on a date.

"She's your sister! She's met your friends before and they get along great! This is a great opportunity for her to do something she's never done before! This is a church group outing. Why wouldn't you want to take her?" Mom's logic and my guilt fused together and I reluctantly agreed to bring her along. I wasn't quite sure why I was so irritated at including her, but I was. I fought off the ominous feeling creeping into my consciousness.

The day dawned beautifully. It was a sunny July day, not unbearably hot, but hot enough to enjoy floating in the river. The outfitter guys dropped us and our big black rubber inner tubes off at the riverbank. They helped lower Kathy into the river, so all I had to do was watch fretfully as they tried to balance her in the mud and she landed in the inner tube with a plop. I watched as they drove off with her crutches.

"We'll meet you at the end in a few hours!" They waved as we set off.

The water was calm and we settled into a rhythm of lazy floating, letting the current carry us slowly along. I closed my eyes and let my hands drag in the water as I relaxed. I could hear the rest of the group chattering and laughing in the distance as the sun warmed my face and the breeze gently blew through my hair.

"Hey, look!" A shout woke me up. I looked up. Dark, black clouds filled the sky. "We're fixing to get rained on!" someone yelled. Almost immediately, big plops of raindrops fell on the water, created shiny black dots on the inner tubes, and hit our heads. "What should we do?" someone asked, just as a bright flash of lightening hit the water in front of us. "Get out! Now!"

I paddled through the crowd of churning water and flailing arms and reached Kathy. She had a look of alarm on her face. "Here," I said. "Hang on to my tube." We paddled together as I pulled her to shore. The other people were already heading for a path along the side of the river as I struggled to pull her tube and her out of the water.

"Thank you," she whispered. I brushed off the comment and, with great effort, balanced her in one arm and the two inner tubes in the other.

"Here, hold onto me," I said, as we tried to find the path the other people were following. We inched along, one step at a time, as she fought to keep her balance in the rough terrain. "Use me as the crutch," I said. I could see the heads of the rest of the group in the distance. Why couldn't they wait for us? Why didn't they slow down? Why didn't they help?

Step. The thunder cracked in the distance as the rain pelted down. Step. Our bare feet stumbled on brambles and pebbles as I fought to catch my breath while dragging the two tubes and holding up Kathy. Step. Mercifully, the storm finally stopped, and we were able to get back in the water after a while. "Thank you," Kathy said with a hug, after the outfitters helped her back into the van.

I still get a visceral reaction in my gut when I remember that day. I was so scared—scared for Kathy and scared for me. I was scared that I would get struck by lightening helping her and scared she would get struck by lightening while I was helping her. I was angry at my friends for abandoning us and angry at Kathy for holding me back. And I felt guilty for being angry at Kathy for something she couldn't help. Still looking for research that helps explain my experiences and feelings, I continue reading. "The mere expectation of having to carry the role the parents had established with the disabled sibling throws a shadow on the relationship between the well sibling and the handicapped [sic] sibling. This can also be expressed in an antagonistic attitude against the caretaking parent, who is often criticized by the adult well child for overprotective handling and sometimes for further crippling the sibling" (Schulman 1999, 5). I wonder if my feelings toward having to be overresponsible for Kathy have caused antagonistic feelings toward Kathy and toward Mom and Dad. I wonder if it is time to let go of them.

Today

I sent Kathy a draft of this article. I wanted her to respond to it. Days went by and I had not heard from her. I began to get nervous. I sent her an e-mail:

> Hi,
>
> I haven't heard from you since I sent you the article, so I'm wondering if you've been busy or if I said something to upset you in what I wrote. Hope you're doing well and I'm looking forward to hearing/reading your feedback. Love, Cris

Her response came a few hours later:

> Kathy: Well, a couple of things did need pondering over and I'm still trying to figure out how to word my response. But to reassure you I'm not upset, just taken aback. I'll try to get it to you tonight. Is that OK?
>
> (Cris: Taken aback? Oh, no!)

In the past several years, Kathy's legs and joints have become weaker and her falls had become more frequent and more serious. Finally, she had a fall that broke her leg. She has used a wheelchair to get around ever since.

Two years ago, Kathy and I went to see a movie. She drove herself in her hand-control equipped car and met me there. I was running late as usual; she was waiting patiently for me in her car. I watched as she operated the wheelchair carrier on top of her Honda Civic. The carrier looked like a white camper top. It was almost as large as the car itself and added a double-decker look to the roof of her car. The carrier was operated by a mechanical device that lowered the wheelchair to the side of the driver's door where Kathy could reach it.

She proficiently got herself in the chair and wheeled off toward the theatre. I followed behind. People in wheelchairs get in free to the movies, and so do their companions. That has always embarrassed me, and every time I go to a movie with her, I expect someone to stop me for doing something wrong. Kathy walked in the door as if she was right at home, and I just followed along behind. I pushed her chair through the door, to make it look like she needed a companion and there was a reason for my being there, especially for getting in free.

We walked through the nearly empty lobby, wheeling over the red carpet and past the whiffs of popcorn, butter, and salt. "This one," Kathy pointed to a closed door. "Here's the movie."

I opened the door quietly as she maneuvered her wheelchair inside. Since we were a few minutes late, the previews had already begun, and the theatre was dark. About halfway down the aisle, there was one row with a cutout for a wheelchair, and Kathy knew exactly where it was. She headed straight for it, rolling rapidly. I tried to keep up with her, in case she needed help stopping. She didn't. A couple sat in the two seats next to the cutout.

"Excuse me," said Kathy, touching the man's arm to get his attention. "Would you mind moving over one seat, so my friend can sit with me?"

The couple looked up. "What?" the woman said, loudly. "She wants us to move," said the man.

"It's so my friend can sit with me," Kathy said, pointing to me.

"I suppose we can move if we have to," said the woman, as they picked up their coat and made an unnecessary show, I thought, of moving to another row in the theatre.

"I'm sorry if they're upset," Kathy said to me.

"Don't worry," I said in a loud whisper so the people sitting around us could hear. "They must not know that this is the only seat for a wheelchair. They had plenty of seats to choose from. They'll get over it."

We enjoyed the movie, a romantic comedy. When the movie was over, Kathy let me push her up the aisle. "It's hard to push uphill," she admitted. I was glad to have something to do.

"I have to go to the bathroom," I said as the light in the lobby hit our eyes.

"Me too," she said and pointed me to the right direction.

Still pushing her wheelchair, I struggled with opening the bathroom door and pushing her in. A woman leaving pushed the door out and held it so we could enter. The room was long and narrow, with a line of stalls on the left and a line of sinks on the right. Kathy rolled herself down to the handicapped stall. "Oh, shoot!" she said. "The door won't close!" Despite being labeled as a handicapped stall, the door opened in, and the space was too small to allow the door to close with a wheelchair in there.

"I'll stand here and keep anyone from coming by," I offered. I stood with my back to the stall and guarded the space so no other women would walk down to that area.

"Thanks!" Kathy said, as she wheeled out.

"Not a problem!" I responded, speaking loudly so the other women in the room could hear. "It's not your fault that they don't build bathrooms to accommodate wheelchairs!"

We chatted outside our cars for a few minutes, catching up on our lives and promising to get together again soon. I hesitated in my car as she expertly put her wheelchair into the carrier, and waited for her to pull out of the parking lot. I followed her out, just in case she needed my help. She didn't. I thought about how well she has constructed a world that enables her, rather than disables her.

Kathy: The bathroom scene happened in JC Penney's bathroom, not at the theatre.

Cris: I distinctly remember it happening in the theatre!

Reactions

I think back over our family relationships and the issue of normalcy versus difference. In our family, normal was the different. What was normal in our family? To me, when I was a small child, it was about falling down. Kathy fell a lot, and she was my older sister, and I fell a lot too, maybe just to be like her. It was getting angry at her friend Marilyn for cutting the hair off of my Barbie doll, and I don't care if Marilyn was blind. It was chasing Kathy around the house, who could somehow outrun me even with leg braces on. It was being yelled at by my grandmother for chasing Kathy. It was hating Jerry Lewis and the Three Stooges for making fun of people who were different and disabled. It was being embarrassed by having a sister who was different but fiercely protective of anyone who dared say anything against her. To my mom, it was driving Kathy to her special school, to the doctor, to the hospital, to physical therapy. It was finding sources of funding for crutches, braces, and medical care. It was finding help and support from family, friends, professionals, and other parents of children with disabilities. It was making physical therapy for Kathy as normal as ballet lessons for me, hospital trips as normal as Girl Scout camping trips. It was about accepting what life had given us and about taking that life one step at a time—just doing what had to be done, together, as a family.

Kathy: The thing that took me most by surprise (and I confess hurt a bit) was that you were embarrassed by me. I've never been embarrassed by my disability. Yes, I hated being different, but it was so much a part of me I was never embarrassed, and I've never thought anyone in the family was embarrassed because of it.

And I can't believe you still remember Patti and I cutting off your Barbie doll's hair! But Patti wasn't blind, she had a heart defect that was corrected by surgery not long afterwards, and she transferred to a "normal" school. Never saw her again.

Cris: I confess that my first reaction to your comment about your feelings being hurt was to take back saying I had been embarrassed. I'm ashamed to admit that I was embarrassed by your disability, and now I feel bad that I hurt your feelings. But then I think again. Why should I deny my feelings? If this article is about being honest with each other, why shouldn't I admit what it was like from my point of view?

Disability carries a stigma (Goffman 1963). It does. I know you experienced stigma; we've talked about how other people treated you in strange ways. Why should it surprise you that I shared your stigma? We shared everything else! I was "family-wise," and as such had a "courtesy stigma." That is, I "shared some of the discredit of the stigmatized person" (Goffman 1963, 30). As your younger sister, I looked up to you, and identified deeply with you. "Every relationship implies a definition of self by other and other by self (Laing 1961). I am who I am, at least partly based on my relationship with you. We receive our personal identity from our referent group (Goffman 1963). If there was something "discrediting" about you, then I had to have it too! After all, we were sisters! The essence of our self is always in reference to others (Cooley 1964; Mead 1934). I understand my self by seeing myself reflected from the other. Our sense of our selves occurs in community. If the self I see reflected back is different, or, in the eyes of others, "less than," this certainly could affect my self-concept and self-esteem.

You, at least, had others you could identify with. You had all your friends at Lowman School, who were disabled also. You had people who shared your experience and people who spent a lot of time and energy helping you get over being stigmatized. I didn't. I was out there all alone. Talk about being different! I didn't know anyone else who had a sister who was disabled. I didn't have anyone I could relate to, swap stories with, commiserate with. This is probably the first time I've ever admitted this to anyone! I've never had anyone with whom I could talk about this before.

Kathy: As you've probably heard by now, John Ritter died Thursday, It was a shock to me, as he was only fifty-four and was way too young to die. But also, it was more of a personal thing for me as his older brother, Tom, has CP and our parents knew their parents while Tom was a student at Lowman School. Since reading this article, I've wondered upon occasion if John had the same sort of issues with Tom as you did (and other siblings) with CP sibs like me. Tom is a success in his own right, as a lawyer in Nashville, so I'd say he's been successful in dealing with his disability.

Kathy: Hmm . . . what do I remember? I remember being worried about you at St. Paul's because of Nancy Spiker and her bullying you.

Cris: I can't believe you remember that! Nancy used to terrorize me, and I didn't know that anyone in the family even knew about it! It kind of feels nice to think that my "big sister" was in the background, keeping an eye on me. Wish I'd known it then.

Kathy: I remember going to ballet classes with you at Miss Ness's (I was a student there, too) and going to ceramic class with you at Ollie's. We used to go to the library together and we'd sit there and browse while waiting for Mom to come back from running her errands to pick us up.

Cris: I don't remember the library at all, but I do remember ballet class, and now that you mention it, I vaguely remember hanging around during your class which was either right before or right after mine. I do remember ceramics; I loved that!

Kathy: I think we had a lot of fun together—we'd play dress up and play school—I was the teacher and you were the student. I also remember almost killing Mom by shooting an arrow through the house one time— boy was she pissed!

Cris: Yeah, I used to love playing dress up. I remember that because I was younger, you would let me be the princess and you would be the prince. I also remember playing school, but my memory is that I was the teacher! The time you shot the arrow past Mom, I confess, it was great to see you get in trouble for a change!

Kathy: I'm not famous and don't make a lot of money, but I think I've done pretty well—got two degrees and have a job I really like working with good people. It's not a bad life at all! Being disabled is just a part of me and I deal with it.

Cris: As Schulman (1999, 1) points out, "Sibling relationships are the only relationships that last a lifetime." You know, your disability will always be a part of me also, and, like you, I just deal with it.

Kathy: When one has CP, one doesn't overcome it for it never goes away, one simply deals with it and does the best he/she can.

Reflections

In the end, I think this article illustrates the difficulty both Kathy and I have in talking about our feelings. We both admitted at the outset that we were afraid we would hurt our relationship by bringing up painful memories, and one can see throughout the article many missed opportunities for candidness and conversation. We simply were not comfortable saying some things to each other directly, although I think that it is interesting that some of our disagreements were communicated with each other via the exchange of this article. I think we were both afraid that saying more, especially disagreeing with each other directly, would worsen our relationship. I wonder why, and I wonder how we can come to a place where we can disagree with love, empathy, and understanding. I think too that the ethnographic conversation creates an artificiality that makes it safer, in some ways, to say some things, and more difficult, in other ways, to be completely open.

This article ended up being much more of my story than the co-constructed narrative that I had hoped it would be. I know that my voice is more prominent in this article and her voice is more muted, possibly subordinated to the forms of writing dominant in the academy (Ardener 1978; Orbe 1998; Wall and Gannon-Leary 1999). Even with my inviting Kathy numerous times to critique my writing, and to contribute more narratives herself, in retrospect, many of her contributions were more of an interviewee than a coauthor. Perhaps in the context of my searching for love, reassurance, and positive regard, she was afraid that any criticisms or negative stories on her part would be seen as thwarting that. Perhaps in a published ethnography, the academic voice will always be dominant. Perhaps this was resistance on her part against the hegemonic dominance of that academic voice. Perhaps this simply reflects the fact that this was my article, my field of study, my agenda, my project, and my timeline, and not hers. Perhaps she was simply and powerfully giving me my voice, something that I have felt was lacking throughout much of my childhood.

What I wanted for this article was a dialogue, a common understanding (Pearce and Pearce 2000), including creating new ways of understanding ourselves, the other, and our common world (Wood 2003). In dialogic communication, self-disclosure is not a tool but instead is a process of "coauthoring" (Wood 2003) a conversation with the other. We may not have been comfortable verbalizing all of our different points to each other, but we wrote them, read them, heard them. We may not have reached consensus, but we did reach multivocality. Dialogue requires an openness to different voices as well as different ways of enacting voice (Hawes 1999; Wood 2003). In dialogue, the emphasis is on "mutuality, community, transformation . . . and inclusiveness of contexts, perspectives, and individuals" (Stewart, Zediker, and Black 2003, 8). Dialogue does not require overcoming tension, rather it requires "engaging the tension in dialogic encounters" (Stewart, Zediker, and Black 2003, 12). This point of view acknowledges differences, accepts them, and suspends judgment on them as they understand how they create perspectives and interactions. Dialogue goes beyond understanding to transforming the issue and the relationship into something new. Dialogue explores how we think what we think (Cayer 1997). Kathy and I are not all the way there yet, but we are talking. We are listening. We are engaging in dialogue.

As I look over what we've written and discussed, I see the striking difference between the dependent person I was afraid Kathy would be when I was a teenager and the independent person she actually is. I think that much of our relationship dynamics during our lifetimes can be attributed to a sibling rivalry tension, a big-sister/little-sister sort of thing. Maybe her disability got in the way a little bit. Maybe my jealousy got in the way. Maybe her needs got in the way. But you know, we are all mutually interdependent (Marks 1999; Oliver 1990)—that is what makes us human. And maybe it's my needs that got in the way also. And I know that Kathy would help me any way she can, such as helping me with this article. I think there will always be power dynamics at work in our relationship, as in any relationship. As the younger sister, I suppose I hold a certain power over her (remember how I "whined" my way into an interview!). I think Kathy's disability also in some ways gives her power over me—in our mixed-up who-is-really-the-older-sister dynamics, I tend to look out for and worry about her. Yet she told me in a conversation that she has always looked out for me too. When we were both very young, I really didn't see her as disabled. Her cerebral palsy and hearing impairment were simply part of the way she was. When I didn't see her as different, I think our relationship was built more on our being siblings. When I became a teenager, and saw her through the eyes of peers who saw her differentness, I think power dynamics did come into play. Now that I see her for her strengths, for what she can do and for what she has accomplished, I think we're closer, and I think that our relational dynamics are again based on our being siblings rather than on a consciousness of disability.

Conclusion

Research on impairment as a family systems and relational disability is scarce but crucial. Seeing disability in a relational mode takes us one step beyond the social model of disability identified by Oliver (1996), and conducting research that is multivocal and participatory is essential to understanding the relational and systemic nature of family disability.

Identity is formed through relationships, and every identity as a person who is disabled or enabled, disempowered or empowered, is built in relation to others. In our family, Kathy's physical condition and disability was interrelated with our interactional patterns—both the result and the cause of the types of interactions we had. These interactional patterns shaped our individual and group identities. It made us better, perhaps, in some ways, and worse, perhaps, in others. In the end, I think we probably have a pretty normal sibling relationship. We fight, like all siblings do. We make up. We watch out for each other. And, we care.

Note

1. I use the term "handicapped" here purposely. Although this term is not used today to refer to people with physical impairments, when we grew up in the 1950s, it was the language used.

References

Ardener, Shirley. 1978. Introduction: The nature of women in society. In *Defining females,* edited by S. Ardener, 9–48. New York: John Wiley.

Barnes, Colin. 1996. Theories of disability and the origins of the oppression of disabled people in western society. In *Disability and society: Emerging issues and insights,* edited by Len Barton, 43–60. New York: Longman.

Barton, Len. 1996. Sociology and disability: Some emerging issues. In *Disability and society: Emerging issues and insights,* edited by Len Barton, 3–17. New York: Longman.

Cayer, Mario. 1997. Bohm's dialogue and action

science: Two different approaches. *Journal of Humanistic Psychology* 37:41–66.

Cooley, Charles Horton. 1964. *Human nature and the social order.* New York: Schocken.

Cuskelly, M. 1999. Adjustment of siblings of children with a disability: Methodological issues. *International Journal for the Advancement of Counseling* 21:111–24.

Czubaroff, Jeanine, and Maurice Friedman. 2000. A conversation with Maurice Friedman. *Southern Communication Journal* 65:243–55.

Damiani, Victoria. 1999. Responsibility and adjustment in siblings of children with disabilities: Update and review. *Families in Society* 80:34–40.

Fisman, Sandra, Lucille Wolf, and Deborah Ellison. 1996. Risk and protective factors affecting the adjustment of siblings of children with chronic disabilities. *Journal of American Academy of Child and Adolescent Psychiatry* 35:1532–41.

Foucault, Michel. 1995. *Discipline and punish: The birth of the prison.* Trans. A. Sheridan. New York: Random House.

Goffman, Erving. 1963. *Stigma: Notes on the management of spoiled identity.* New York: Simon & Schuster.

Green, Sara. 2002. Mothering Amanda: Musing on the experience of raising a child with cerebral palsy. *Journal of Loss and Trauma* 7:21–34.

Hawes, Leonard. 1999. The dialogics of conversation: Power, control, vulnerability. *Communication Theory* 3:229–64.

Krauss, Marty Wyngaarden, Marsha Mailick Seltzer, and Rachel M. Gordon. 1996. Binding ties: The roles of adults siblings of persons with mental retardation. *Mental Retardation* 34:83–93.

Laing, R. D. 1961. *Self and others.* New York: Routledge.

LeClere, Felicia B., and Brenda Marstellar Kowaleski. 1994. Disability in the family: The effects on children's well-being. *Journal of Marriage and the Family 56* :457–68.

Lincoln, Yvonna, and Egon Guba. 1985. *Naturalistic inquiry.* Newbury Park, CA: Sage.

Lobato, Debra J., and Barbara T. Kao. 2002. Integrated sibling-parent group intervention to improve sibling knowledge and adjustment to chronic illness and disability. *Journal of Pediatric Psychology* 27:711–16.

Marks, Deborah. 1999. *Disability: Controversial debates and psychosocial perspectives.* London: Routledge.

Mead, George Herbert. 1934. *Mind, self, and society: From the standpoint of a social behaviorist.* Chicago: University of Chicago Press.

Michalski, Richard L., and Todd K. Shackelford. 2002. An attempted replication of the relationships between birth order and personality. *Journal of Research in Personality* 36:182–88.

Mizco, Nathan. 2003. Beyond the "fetishism of words": Considerations on the use of the interview to gather chronic illness narratives. *Qualitative Health Research* 13:469–90.

Nixon, Charisse L., and E. Mark Cummings. 1999. Sibling disability and children's reactivity to conflicts involving family members. *Journal of Family Psychology* 13:274–85.

Oliver, Michael. 1990. *The politics of disablement: A sociological approach.* New York: St. Martin's.

——. 1996. *Understanding disability: From theory to practice.* New York: St.Martin's.

Orbe, Mark P. 1998. *Constructing co-cultural theory: An explication of culture, power, and communication.* Thousand Oaks, CA: Sage.

Orsmond, Gael I., and Marsha Mailick Seltzer. 2000. Brothers and sisters of adults with mental retardation: Gendered nature of the sibling relationship. *American Journal on Mental Retardation* 105 (6):486–508.

Patton, Michael Quinn. 2002. *Qualitative research and evaluation methods.* Thousand Oaks, CA: Sage.

Pearce, W. Barnett, and Kimberly Pearce. 2000. Combining passions and abilities: Toward dialogic virtuosity. *Southern Communication Journal* 65:161–75.

Pitten Cate, Ineke M., and G. M. P. Ineke Loots. 2000. Experiences of siblings of children with physical disabilities: An empirical investigation. *Disability and Rehabilitation* 22:399–08.

Reed-Danahay, Deborah. 2001. Autobiography, intimacy and ethnography. In *Handbook of ethnography,* edited by Paul Atkinson, 407–25. Thousand Oaks, CA: Sage.

Schulman, Gerda L. 1999. Siblings revisited: Old conflicts and new opportunities in later life. *Journal of Marital and Family Therapy* 25 (4): 517–24.

Seligman, Milton, and Rosalyn Benjamin Darling. 1997. *Ordinary families, special children: A systems approach to childhood disability.* New York: Guilford.

Shapiro, Joseph. 1993. *No pity: People with disabilities forging a new civil rights movement.* New York: Random House.

Stake, Robert. 1995. *The art of case study research.* Thousand Oaks, CA: Sage.

Steelman, Lala Carr, Brian Powell, Regina Werum, and Scott Carter. 2002. Reconsidering the effects of sibling configuration: Recent advances and challenges. *Annual Review of Sociology* 28:243–311.

Stewart, John, Karen E. Zediker, and Laura Black. 2003. Relationships among philosophies of dialogue. In *Dialogue: Theorizing difference in communication studies,* edited by Rob Anderson, Kenneth N. Cissna, and Leslie A. Baxter, 21–38. Thousand Oaks, CA: Sage.

Susman, Joan. 1993. Disability, stigma, and deviance. *Social Science Medicine* 38:15–22.

Wall, Celia J., and Pat Gannon-Leary. 1999. A sentence made by men: Muted group theory revisited. *The European Journal of Women's Studies* 6 (1):21–29.

Wolf, Lucille, Sandra Fisman, and Deborah Ellison. 1998. Effect of sibling perception of differential parental treatment in sibling dyads with one disabled child. *Journal of the American Academy of Child and Adolescent Psychiatry* 37:1317–41.

Wood, Julia. 2003. Forward: Entering into dialogue. In *Dialogue: Theorizing difference in communication studies,* edited by Rob Anderson, Kenneth N. Cissna, and Leslie A. Baxter. Thousand Oaks, CA: Sage.

Zola, Irving Kenneth. 1982. *Missing pieces: A chronicle of living with a disability.* Philadelphia: Temple University Press.

Discussion Questions

1. In what ways is disability a family issue? Do you think this differs with the age and status of the disabled person (child or parent)? What other health problems are experienced as a family?
2. Davis explains that she tries to create a "multivocal" story, or co-constructed narrative, in this article. Does she succeed in doing so? What are the benefits and drawbacks of this approach?
3. What is the difference between disability and impairment? How is stigma related, and in what ways does society enact stigma? ✦

Chapter 18 Social Support as Relationship Maintenance in Gay Male Couples Coping With HIV or AIDS

Stephen M. Haas

Part V is completed by considering another contemporary social unit: homosexual couples. Stephen M. Haas discusses how these couples deal with the diagnosis of a life-threatening disease. Social support can function as a vital component of success when dealing with illness. This chapter investigates the effects that social support has on relationship maintenance in gay male couples living with HIV or AIDS. Partners, friends, and family can all be sources of social support with unique levels of effect.

Related Topics: chronic care, culture, family communication, HIV/AIDS, patients' perspectives, qualitative methods, social support

HIV and AIDS continue to affect the lives of an estimated 41.8 million persons infected with the disease worldwide (with an estimated 850,000 residing in the US) (UNAIDS, 2000), as well as the millions of individuals whose lives are interconnected with those who have the disease. For couples in which one (HIV-discordant) or both members (HIV-concordant) are HIV infected, managing life with the disease brings new challenges to maintaining an intimate relationship. Advances in combination drug therapies have given hope for longer survival to those infected with HIV, but the possibility of extended life brings with it a whole new set of uncertainties surrounding living with HIV as a chronic illness (Brashers et al., 1999; Nokes, 1991). Increased relationship strain can occur in these couples surrounding such issues as: (i) life expectancy, (ii) the threat of infecting an HIV-negative partner, (iii) dealing with recurring health problems and medication side-effects, (iv) autonomy and dependence, (v) financial strain if an HIV-positive partner cannot work, (vi) emotional intimacy and sexual activity, and (vii) dealing with the social stigma associated with HIV or AIDS (McLean & Roberts, 1995; Moore et al, 1998; Powell-Cope, 1995; van der Straten, Vernon, Knight, Gomez, & Padian, 1998). Levels of uncertainty related to HIV or AIDS also vary across stage of illness and symptom severity (Brashers, Neidig, Reynolds, & Haas, 1998); individuals fluctuate through periods of relatively good health, followed by opportunistic infections and increased stress. Thus, learning to manage chronic uncertainty is a continuing challenge for those living with HIV (Brashers et al, 2000).

The purpose of this study was to explore the importance of particular sources of social support (partners, friends, and family) and how these sources affect relationship maintenance in gay male couples as they live with HIV or AIDS. The following review of literature explores social support for persons living with HIV or AIDS, the existing research on maintaining couple relationships and same-sex relationships, and, finally, relationship maintenance issues facing gay male couples coping with HIV or AIDS. Results from a study exploring the role of social support in the relationship maintenance of male couples coping with HIV is then presented.

HIV and Social Support

Studies have consistently found evidence

From "Social Support as Relationship Maintenance in Gay Male Couples Coping with HIV or Aids," Stephen M. Haas, 2002, *Journal of Social and Personal Relationships*, Vol. 19:1, pp. 87–111.

that social support serves to buffer the negative effects of physical and psychological HIV-related stress (Kessler et al., 1991; Leserman et al., 2000). In particular, Kessler et al. (1991) found that social support was positively associated with a higher quality of life for persons living with HIV. Social support also has been positively correlated with the ability of persons living with HIV to maintain hope (Rabkin, Williams, Neugbauer, Remien, & Goetz, 1990) and reduce anxiety and depression (Hays, Turner, & Coates, 1992). For example, one study found that persons living with HIV who did not have someone to talk to about serious health problems were significantly more distressed than those who did (Ostrow et al., 1989). Severe stress has been found to predict early HIV progression (Evans et al., 1997), and social support has been shown to buffer stress to help reduce impairment of the body's immune function (Kennedy, Kiecolt-Glaser, & Glaser, 1990; Kessler et al., 1991). These findings underscore the importance of social support in the lives of those dealing with stress and illness, in general, and immune-dysfunction diseases, such as HIV, in particular.

Several types of social support have been proposed by scholars. In general, five primary types have been widely agreed upon:

> *Informational support* (providing information about the stress itself or how to deal with it); *tangible aid* (providing or offering to provide goods or services needed in the stressful situation); *emotional support* (communicating love, concern, or empathy); *social network support* (communicating belonging to a group of persons with similar interests or concerns); and *esteem support* (communicating respect and confidence in abilities). (Cutrona & Suhr, 1994: 120)

One important aspect that may influence the effectiveness of any type of social support is the receiver's *perception* of what type of support is considered helpful and desirable from whom. Some researchers have suggested that the same type of social supportive behavior may not be equally helpful from all individuals (Dakof & Taylor, 1990; Gottlieb, 1981; Shinn, Lehmann, & Wong, 1980). Wethington and Kessler (1986) also suggested that *perceived support* may be more important than actual *received support* in adjusting to stressful life events. These researchers found that received support may, in fact, be mediated by one's interpretation of the perceived helpfulness and potential availability of various sources of support. In other words, if certain communicative behaviors are intended to be supportive by a source but are not perceived as helpful by the receiver, then social support has not successfully occurred. In addition, Jacobson (1986) found that the timing of different types of social support influenced whether they were perceived as supportive or not; for example, the same type of expressed support (e.g., emotional concern) may not be perceived as helpful at a time when a person is seeking informational support.

The HIV and AIDS social support literature (focusing primarily on gay males) indicates that close intimates, such as a spouse, partner/lover, friends, and family, have been perceived as having an important impact in providing support by persons living with HIV (Greif & Porembski, 1988). Specifically, research has shown that persons living with HIV most frequently turn to relational partners and close friends when seeking support (Powell-Cope, 1995, 1996; Turner, Catania, & Gagnon, 1994; Wrubel & Folkman, 1997). Family members, in contrast, have been found to provide a combination of helpful and harmful social support attempts to people living with HIV (Barbee, Derlega, Sherburne, & Grimshaw, 1998; Hays, McGee, & Chauncey, 1994). In studies of HIV-positive individuals, however, the *perceived* value of each of these sources of support remains unclear. For example, Barbee et al. (1998) found that friends were described by persons living with HIV as most supportive, with 62% of friends' supportive acts being considered helpful, whereas only 50% of intimate partners' supportive acts were described as helpful, and the majority (62%) of acts by family members were considered unhelpful. Kimberly and Serovich (1996), in contrast, found no significant difference between the perceived support provided by friends and family members to persons living with HIV. Still other evidence has suggested that, because of the unique element of *relational intimacy* (a combination of emotional, intellectual, and physical closeness), a spouse or relational partner provides social support that cannot be substituted by others (Coyne & Delongis, 1986; Lowenthal & Haven, 1968).

The research reviewed here has focused primarily on sources of support for individuals who are HIV-positive, and the inconsistent findings indicate that further investigation is needed to understand the perceived importance of particular sources of support in the lives of persons living with HIV. In addition, few studies have examined the sources of support utilized by *couples* dealing with HIV, and, in particular, the sources of support for HIV-negative partners in a mixed-HIV status relationship have not been investigated. To explore the sources of support for couples dealing with HIV, the following research question is proposed:

> *RQ1:* Who are perceived to be the predominant sources (e.g., partners, friends, family) of social support by gay male *couples* dealing with HIV or AIDS?

Relationship Maintenance

In addition to exploring the relative importance of sources of support, a second goal of this study was to investigate the effects of social support on the relationship maintenance of gay male couples coping with HIV or AIDS. *Relationship maintenance* refers to employing communicative strategies and behaviors to prevent relationship dissolution through 'parties' efforts to sustain a dynamic equilibrium in their relationship definition and satisfaction levels as they cope with the ebb and flow of everyday relating' (Baxter & Dindia, 1990, p. 188). Over the past 15 years, interpersonal communication researchers have begun to explore how romantic partners communicatively define and maintain their intimate relationships (Duck, 1994), and social exchange theory has formed the basis of much of this research. In its most basic form, social exchange theory posits that a relationship consists of resources that are exchanged between two persons (Thibaut & Kelly, 1959). Preferred resources are considered rewards, and lost resources are costs. The theory proposes that as long as there are excess rewards, or profit, for both partners after incurring relational costs, they will seek to maintain the relationship.

Applying social exchange theory, Stafford and Canary (1991; Canary & Stafford, 1992, 1994) developed a typology of five strategic behaviors (defined as purposive communicative behaviors) that both married and dating individuals perceive exchanging in maintaining their intimate relationships. These five categories have been expanded by Stafford, Dainton, and Haas (2000) to encompass seven maintenance behaviors reflecting both strategic and routine aspects of maintenance: (i) positivity (e.g., cheerfulness and being optimistic); (ii) openness (e.g., self-disclosure and meta-relational communication); (iii) assurances (e.g., expressions of love and comfort); (iv) shared tasks (e.g., household duties and relationship responsibilities); (v) advice (offering opinions and problem-solving assistance), (vi) conflict management (engaging in constructive conflict strategies), and (vii) social networks (e.g., seeking mutual friendships and kinship ties).

The research on relationship maintenance has focused almost exclusively on U.S., White, middle-class, heterosexual couples. Though this research has revealed important insights into the ways these couples maintain their relationships, additional research is needed to explore the generalizability of these findings to other types of couples (e.g., couples that differ on the basis of race, ethnicity, or sexual orientation). In particular, to date, research exploring the maintenance of gay and lesbian relationships has been sparse (Clark & Serovich, 1997). One recent study by Haas and Stafford (1998), however, attempted to expand the populations studied by exploring relationship maintenance in gay and lesbian couples. Using an open-ended survey approach, Haas and Stafford found that gay and lesbian partners utilized many of the same basic maintenance behaviors as the heterosexual couples in Canary and Stafford's (1992) study. Examples of these common maintenance behaviors were positivity, openness, assurances, affection, shared tasks, and social network support. Several unique maintenance behaviors also emerged such as (i) being 'out' as a couple to one's social networks, and (ii) seeking out gay/lesbian supportive environments. These unique maintenance behaviors were seen by partners as a means of strengthening their relationship in the face of a general lack of acceptance in U.S. society.

Although the study of communicative behaviors utilized in maintaining gay and lesbian couples has not been studied extensively, limited research does exist outlining general characteristics of gay and lesbian relationships. These characteristics, as well as those of gay male couples dealing with HIV or AIDS, are addressed in the following sections.

Research on Gay and Lesbian Relationships

Gay men and lesbian women face several relationship challenges that may affect their ability to successfully sustain long-term, romantic relationships. First, gay and lesbian relationships are not recognized by legal or social sanctions that recognize heterosexual married couples (although the state of Vermont has recently sanctioned 'civil unions' between same-sex couples, the national ramifications of which remain unclear). Second, gay and lesbian relationships generally lack shared social norms regarding role models for same-sex relationship structures. Research has found that traditional, heterosexual 'masculine' and 'feminine' roles do not provide the relational structure for gay and lesbian couples; instead, same-sex relationships have been found to be characterized by role flexibility and turn-taking (Kurdek, 1987, 1993; Kurdek & Schmitt, 1986a; Lynch & Reilly, 1985/86; Marecek, Finn, & Cardell, 1983; Peplau, 1991). McWhirter and Mattison (1984), for example, found that gay male couples tended to distribute household duties based on skill, interest, and work schedules. Similarly, Kurdek (1993) found that gay and lesbian couples worked to balance household tasks, although this did not mean that each partner performed every task equally. In heterosexual relationships, sex-based roles often make task assignments easier to coordinate and reduce the amount of negotiation required. Although no differences have been found in relationship quality and satisfaction between same-sex and heterosexual relationships (Blumstein & Schwartz, 1983; Kurdek & Schmitt, 1986b; Peplau & Cochran, 1981, 1990), the added role flexibility in same-sex relationships does require additional communicative coordination and may, therefore, increase the potential for relational conflict. Third, when major conflicts do arise, gay and lesbian relationships do not face many of the same barriers that help prevent relationship dissolution in married couples (Attridge, 1994) (e.g., the expensive costs of divorce, child custody and child support disputes, separating combined finances and debt, and the prospect of paying alimony to an ex-spouse). Despite lacking these 'ties that bind,' many gay men and women have been able to establish and maintain long-term, intimate relationships (Berger, 1990; Blumstein & Schwartz, 1983; Mendola, 1980; Ossana, 2000; Peplau, 1991).

Gay Male Couples Coping With HIV

Although they deal with the same challenges facing other gay and lesbian couples, ongoing gay male relationships where one (HIV discordant) or both (HIV concordant) are HIV infected typically have additional health-related stress within the relationship. Couples coping with HIV must deal with a series of complex issues, such as: (i) the possible death of a partner to AIDS, (ii) the threat of infecting an HIV-negative partner, (iii) recurring health and independence issues, (iv) financial strain if an HIV-positive partner cannot work, (v) relational intimacy and privacy issues, and (vi) dealing with the social stigma associated with HIV or AIDS (McLean & Roberts, 1995; Moore et al., 1998; Powell-Cope, 1995; van der Straten et al., 1998).

During periods when physical symptoms increase, persons living with HIV often need others to provide increased care for them, which frequently raises independence issues (Wrubel & Folkman, 1997). Caregiving is rooted in providing tangible support to persons who are not completely capable of self-care (and also likely encompasses other types of social support as well). The amount of caregiving required varies based on symptom severity and individuals' ability to sustain self-care. Research has demonstrated that caregiving of persons living with HIV most often is taken on by relational partners, friends, and family members (Folkman, Chesney, Cooke, Boccellari, & Collette, 1994; Powell-Cope, 1996; Wrubel & Folkman, 1997). When an intimate partner assumes the caregiving role in a gay relationship, he often takes on health care responsibilities that he is unprepared, ill equipped, and/or unaccustomed to perform (Ferrari, McCown, & Pantano, 1993; Greif & Porembski, 1988; Grieco & Kowalski, 1987). Moreover, when one member of a couple becomes ill, relationship roles and responsibilities may shift dramatically; this type of role restructuring (Pearlin, 1989) and relationship renegotiation (Powell-Cope, 1995) often may change and strain the very nature of the relationship (Rolland, 1994).

Over an extended period, as in the case of chronic illness, the added responsibilities involved with caregiving can result in role overload (Corbin & Strauss, 1988). In addition to stress from caregiving itself, HIV-discordant partners may experience uncertainty about their own future health status because they often have been exposed to the risk of HIV infection (Moore et al., 1998; Pearlin, Semple, & Turner, 1988). If partners are also HIV-positive, they may experience psychological stress over who will care for them if their relational partner is too ill or has died (Kalichman, 2000).

A primary factor that affects HIV caregiving, and how couples deal with the disease overall, is coping with the social stigma that accompanies HIV and AIDS (Alonzo & Reynolds, 1995; van der Straten et al., 1998). Almost 40 years ago, Goffman (1963) argued that stigma is rooted in issues of a 'spoiled identity' (p. 6). He suggested that the stigmatized individual is seen as tainted, discredited, or abnormal with respect to three types of 'abnormality': (i) physical irregularities, such as illness or disease; (ii) psychological abnormalities viewed as unnatural (e.g., mental disorders, addiction, or homosexuality); and (iii) group stigma rooted in differences of race, ethnicity, nationality, or religion. Leary and Schreindorfer (1998) pointed out that stigmatized persons, such as those with HIV or AIDS, are avoided, excluded, and ostracized, resulting in personal disassociation and isolation from others.

Persons living with HIV have described feeling subjected to a double or even triple stigma related to the AIDS disease and its association with homosexuality and intravenous drug use. Powell-Cope and Brown (1992) also found that relational partners and family members often take on the social stigma of AIDS through 'guilt by association' because of their close interpersonal ties to the person living with HIV stigma has a strong influence on the willingness of persons living with HIV to openly disclose their HIV status to others (Greene & Serovich, 1996). Family members often are also hesitant to reveal an affected family member's AIDS illness to others for fear of rejection, isolation, and harassment by co-workers, acquaintances, friends, and even other family members (Powell-Cope & Brown, 1992). The fear of social isolation can be highly stress provoking and can produce emotional suffering in the already difficult situation of caring for a terminally ill loved one (Biordi, 1995).

The effects of intense social stigma on persons living with HIV and their intimate partners may lead to a failure to seek out social support and, thereby, isolate them from needed support and increase relationship strain. The loss of desired social relationships and activities outside of the relationship also may result from care responsibilities. Partners holding outside jobs may feel stress from being torn between the duties of both employment and caring for their loved one (Pearlin, 1989). Thus, relational partners are in particular need of social support themselves and need assistance in caring for their HIV-positive partners (Powell-Cope, 1994; Powell-Cope & Brown, 1992; Wight, LeBlanc, & Aneshensel, 1995).

Couples dealing with chronic illness face increased stressors in their relationships due to the presence of the disease and its impact on their lives. HIV and AIDS has increasingly taken on long-term chronic illness characteristics, but unique issues are also present because of the large gay male population affected and the stigma attached to both HIV and AIDS and homosexuality.

Who provides support, as well as the type of support provided, can affect the reduction of strain in those coping with HIV, but few studies have explored the impact of social support in maintaining the relationships of gay male couples coping with HIV, specifically. Thus, a second research question was posed:

> *RQ2:* How does social support affect relationship maintenance in gay male couples coping with HIV or AIDS?

Method

This study employed a qualitative grounded theory approach (Glaser & Strauss, 1967; Strauss, 1987) to explore the two proposed research questions. According to Glaser and Strauss (1967), grounded theory is the generation of theory through inductive analysis of qualitative data. Rather than imposing theory a priori to an area of study, hypotheses and theory emerge from the data and are 'systematically worked out in relation to the data during the course of the research' (Glaser & Strauss, 1967, p. 6). The method of *constant comparative analysis* (Glaser & Strauss, 1967) is used to compare and examine qualitative data for dominant themes and categories. According to Stern (1980), 'Considerable similarity exists between treatment of data in the continuous comparative method and in the computer method of factor analysis . . . data are coded, compared with other data and assigned to clusters or categories according to obvious fit' (p. 21). Categories are, thus, inductively derived in the sense that they are grounded in the data. Glaser and Strauss, however, stressed that this process is not divorced from deduction. In fact, Strauss (1987) has argued that the 'misconception' that grounded theory is purely inductive is inaccurate (p. 55). Throughout the analysis, themes, categories, and subcategories constantly are compared with other data, as well as the researcher's knowledge of pertinent existing research. Thus, constant comparative analysis combines elements of both inductive and deductive methods of theory generation.

Procedure

A semi-structured interview schedule generated from literature on couples dealing with chronic illness (including HIV), and preliminary data from pilot studies, was approved by the author's institutional Human Subjects Internal Review Board. Audiotaped, in-depth interviews (range 50–80 minutes) were conducted in the winter of 1998. The general questions asked included, 'What do you feel has kept your relationship together as you and your partner deal with HIV?,' 'Who do you turn to for support in dealing with HIV?,' 'Are some sources of support more important to you than others?,' and 'What role do you and your partner's families play in dealing with HIV?' Additional follow-up questions were generated during the interviews to further explore these concerns.

In anticipation that some relational partners may not wish to discuss their support provision and relational maintenance openly in front of their partner, participants were interviewed separately. Both partners, however, were interviewed. While each partner was being interviewed, the other waited in a private room and was asked to complete a short questionnaire to provide demographic data. Couples' interviews were matched for comparative analysis, so that both the individual and the dyad were units of analysis. A total of 41 hours of audio-taped interviews was completed, resulting in 459 pages of transcription.

Participant Recruitment

Participants were recruited primarily through an AIDS Clinical Trials Unit (ACTU) at a large Midwestern university hospital, with subsequent recruitment through a second ACTU, also part of another large Midwestern university hospital. Couples were recruited such that both partners agreed to participate in the study. Fliers were placed in ACTU waiting room areas, and clinic nurses personally informed patients of the study. Fliers also were placed at community AIDS service organizations, and an advertisement for the study was run for six months in a monthly newsletter of one AIDS service organization in the primary data-collection metropolitan area. An incentive of $30 per person was paid to participants for engaging in a 60-minute in-depth interview.

Participants

Study participants were 20 couples (*N* = 40) in an ongoing intimate romantic relationship in which one (HIV discordant) or both (HIV concordant) partners were HIV-positive or had AIDS. All names and identifying information have been changed to protect anonymity and confidentiality. In this sample, 15 couples were discordant and 5 were concordant. Fourteen couples were aware of their partner's HIV status upon initiating the relationship. Thus, 70% of the couples in this sample did not face dealing with feelings of betrayal that are frequently experienced when a relational partner tests HIV-positive (the implications of prior knowledge of a partner's HIV status on relationship maintenance are discussed in more detail in Haas, 1999).

All couples reported living together in the same residence. In addition, when asked if they considered their relationship to be (i) dating, (ii) seriously dating, or (iii) committed, all participants responded 'committed.' The mean length of relationship was 7 years, 6 months (*SD* = 7 years, 8 months, range = 4 months–35 years, 2 months). Eighty percent (*n* = 32) of the sample reported the relationship to be sexually monogamous. The mean age of the sample was 38 years (*SD* = 8 years, 3 months, range = 23–58 years). Thirty-seven participants were Caucasian and three were African American. Twenty-seven percent (*n* = 11) of the sample had only completed a high school education; the majority of the sample (73%) had completed some college education, with 15 having a two-year college degree, 10 a four-year college degree, and 3 persons holding a master's degree. Ten of the persons living with HIV were currently working at the time of the study while experiencing problematic HIV-medication side-effects on the job (e.g., fatigue, hot flashes, and nausea), and 15 were unemployed and receiving some form of state-funded disability or Social Security Income. Only one of the 15 HIV-negative partners was not employed at the time of the study because of a work-related injury.

Regarding the health status of the HIV-positive participants, the mean time since diagnosis was 6.5 years (*SD* = 4 years, range = 7 months–12 years). The mean CD4 count (the level of T-helper white blood cells in the bloodstream) was 306 (*SD* = 189, range = 0–750). A normal CD4 count is in the range of 800–1500, with a mean CD4 count roughly around 1000. In this sample, 11 individuals were classified as having AIDS (a CD4 count < 200) at the time of the study. However, several participants' CD4 counts recently had rebounded above 200 due to the inclusion of protease inhibitors in their medical regimen.

Another indicator of the progression of the disease is an individual's viral load (the amount of virus in the blood stream). For this sample, the mean viral load was 30,200 (*SD* = 102,424, range = under 400–500,000). The viral load of 12 individuals was below 400 at the time of this study, which is below the detectable levels of current HIV blood tests; all of these individuals were taking a protease inhibitor in combination with other HIV medications (commonly referred to as a 'drug cocktail'). Three participants were not taking any HIV medications at the time of this study because they could not withstand persistent physical side-effects (e.g., consistent vomiting, fatigue, fever, and chills). Correspondingly, these individuals' viral loads were considerably higher.

Analysis

Transcripts were analyzed and coded using constant comparative analysis. Burnard (1991) proposed a process of several steps for conducting this analysis. This process is used in qualitative analysis to 'produce a systematic detailed report of themes and issues contained in the interviews' (Katz, 1996, p. 23). Following Burnard's steps, theoretic notes were compiled, sorted, insights compared, and conceptual linkages made throughout the data collection. Next, audiotapes were transcribed, and the transcripts were examined for themes and strategies until repetition, or saturation (Strauss, 1987), occurred. Dominant themes and strategies then were grouped into higher order categories.

Content face validity, subsequently, was sought for the categories. In qualitative analysis, participants' responses are retained and presented as evidence for categories. Validity of the categories largely is determined by the reader through confirmation of the data as evidence. In addition, Guba and Lincoln (1989; Lincoln & Guba, 1985) have suggested several means of seeking content validity of dominant themes and categories in constant comparative analysis: audibility, fittingness, credibility, and confirmability. Audibility (audio clarity) was established by the author matching audiotapes to the transcripts. Fittingness is achieved through a separate researcher in the content area reviewing the themes for accuracy. An HIV and AIDS research colleague reviewed and agreed with the fittingness of the data to the emergent themes. Credibility is achieved by having research participants review the dominant themes and categories to verify the applicability to their lives. Toward the end of the study, after completing their interview, 15% of the sample (n = 6) was asked to review the themes and categories. In post-interviews, these participants confirmed the applicability of the categories to their life experience. Finally, confirmability can be claimed if credibility, fittingness, and audibility are achieved (Katz, 1996). A written analysis tying the emergent themes to relevant research literature and a discussion of findings from the study then was undertaken.

Results and Discussion

To maintain their relationships, couples coping with HIV infection must manage the effect of HIV, stigma, and social isolation in their lives. This study sought to explore the sources of social support couples perceived to be most important in coping with HIV, and also explored the impact of illness-related social support on efforts at relationship maintenance for these couples. Findings related to these two areas are discussed in the following sections.

Sources of Social Support in Gay Male Couples Coping With HIV or AIDS

To gain an understanding of the current sources of social support utilized by gay male couples dealing with HIV, RQ1 asked, 'Who are perceived to be the predominant sources of social support by gay male couples dealing with HIV or AIDS?' Consistent with previous research on individuals with HIV (Catania, Turner, Choi, & Coates, 1992; Powell-Cope, 1995, 1996; Turner, Hays, & Coates, 1993; Wrubel & Folkman, 1997), relational partners and very close friends were reported to be the predominant sources of social support by *both* HIV-positive and HIV-negative partners in this sample. In addition, evidence of support from family members (especially mothers) was found. Each source (partners, friends, and family) and types of support provided will be described in the following sections.

Partner support. Past research has implied that partners and friends are fairly equivalent as sources of social support for persons living with HIV (Turner et al., 1994). In this study, however, when asked to rank supportive sources, there was clearly an indication by both members of the couples that relational partners were perceived as the primary source of support in dealing with HIV In general, couples indicated extreme emotional closeness and a great deal of shared time together in joint activities. Though few of these couples completely lacked support from outside of the relationship, there was a clear sense that the relational partner was the person who helped most in coping with HIV or AIDS. This finding is consistent with Coyne and Delongis's (1986) finding that intimate partner relationships were the most crucial sources of support for couples dealing with a spouse recovering from a heart attack and that other sources of support could not compensate for deficiencies in the relationships. Relationships with partners also appear to be a particularly important source of social support because of their overall level of ongoing involvement, quality, and caring for the relationship (Sarason, Shearin, Pierce, & Sarason, 1987).

Relational partners were a source for all forms of social support proposed by Cutrona and Suhr (1994): emotional, informational, tangible, esteem, and network support. For most of the couples in this study, relational partners served the crucial role of confidant and companion that aided them in coping with the stress of HIV, and life in general. One HIV-positive partner, Adam, described his HIV-negative partner Ken's emotional support this way, 'He definitely provides me with support. Just by being there and not running from me. He's very concerned about my health and that I stay healthy. If he weren't, he wouldn't be there, he would be gone.' Ted, who is in a concordant relationship, explained, 'Chris is my primary support. If something was stressing me out, he's the first person I'd talk to.' Chris, Ted's partner, echoed this sentiment, stating that Ted is his primary confidant, and his mother is second: 'If I was worried about my health, I would talk to Ted first, but I would then call my mom. There's two other people I'd call, too, but first I would talk to Ted.' William, who is HIV-positive, described how important his HIV-negative partner Peter's emotional support and companionship is in his life:

> With Peter, things are so easy. I've had other relationships. I've been HIV-positive for 10 years, and I've had two other relationships in that time. With him, nothing ever seems to bother him. He's always there, he's always attentive, he's always compassionate and loving. I mean, I would be hard pressed to say that things could be much better or worse than they are now. He's just always there, which sometimes amazes me even now being together for over a year and a half, and I'm just amazed sometimes that he deals with things as well as he does.

Jake, an HIV-positive individual, explained how his HIV-negative partner, Bill, showed him emotional and tangible support by coming to visit him in the hospital, despite the fact that Bill was at home in a wheelchair with a broken leg at the time:

> I was amazed with him. You know, I knew how much he cared, but I was hospitalized and he was still in his wheelchair at the time. He wheeled himself down to the hospital, which is about a mile. That said so much, and showed his concern.

When asked who he turns to for support, Gary, an HIV-negative partner, stated simply, 'Usually Daryl [his partner] first, and then my mother. He's always first.'

In general, relational partners were reported to provide the most consistent day-to-day social support for each other in dealing with HIV or AIDS. This finding underscores the benefit of entering and maintaining a happy long-term relationship for persons living with HIV, as well as demonstrating that partners turn to one another as the primary source of support, regardless of HIV status. Interestingly, in a sample of primarily gay men, Barbee et al. (1998) found that friends were described as 'most supportive' in stories of supportive interactions, whereas relational partners were described as engaging in a combination of positive and negative interactions. On the surface, this might make sense because relational partners are more likely to openly criticize one another than are friends. Higher conflict likely occurs in couple's interactions because relational partners' needs, desires, and goals have become intertwined, and, therefore, there is a greater need to openly negotiate mutually satisfying outcomes in those interactions. Thus, although the support of friends is important, there is increasing evidence that the support of a relational partner is unique and cannot be compensated for by other sources. In addition, being in a relationship seems to add important esteem support. For instance, Kurdek and Schmitt (1986a) found that, for same-sex couples, being in a relationship strengthened a positive, gay identity and increased those individuals' self-concept over those not in a relationship; maintaining a relationship also led to a greater belief in one's ability to have control over life events and lowered levels of anxiety and depression. The couples in this study described these types of relational benefits as well.

Friend support. Close friends served as the second most important source of support for the couples in this study. For instance, Jerry, who is HIV-positive, explained the importance of his close friend in providing him tangible and emotional support. Specifically, Jerry detailed how his friend prevented him from committing suicide when he was diagnosed HIV-positive:

> I wanted to commit suicide that night when I found out, but I had a friend that

> I went over to and we got drunk 'til we passed out. She helped me through that. It's so funny, I mean, looking back at it now after all this time. Now I'm fighting for my life, now that I have AIDS and stuff, and there I wanted to end it.

Jerry went on to explain that when he was hospitalized with an opportunistic infection and feared he was near death, he turned to his friends for emotional support. He described how his closest friend provided emotional and tangible support by coming to see him from another state:

> Well, I've got friends. That's why my one friend flew here from Louisiana. She didn't really have the money to come but I just told her on the phone that I'd probably never see her again, you know, so she came. And I was pretty depressed when I was in the hospital, so I called people and talked to them.

Dennis, a partner in an HIV-concordant relationship, addressed the fact that in addition to supporting each other, his partner Todd relies on his best friend who lives out-of-town for emotional support. Thus, proximity was not a requirement for this person to be considered part of Todd's perceived support network. As Dennis explained:

> He has a friend, I think she's in Indiana or something like that. Well, that's where he's from, Indiana, so she lives in Indiana. He goes to visit her sometimes. I think he's going to be able to visit her next weekend when he visits his dad. But other than that, it's basically just the two of us.

Similarly, Steve, who is HIV-positive, felt that he has access to a network of several close friends who are sources of support:

> Scott [his partner], or my two friends Tom and Jim, and my landlord and his partner that come out and drink with us a lot. I've got a lot of friends. All my friends have always been very supportive. Always.
>
> Interviewer: You say a lot. How many? I mean are there people that you would call up if you had a problem?
>
> Close, close friends, well, I can count them for you. I would say there's probably at least three or four close friends off the top of my head that I could contact if I had any problems or I needed anything. One of them, my best friend, she lives out-of-state, but if I ever needed her, all I have to do is call.

Andrew, an HIV-positive individual, explained how his friends pitched in to provide tangible support to both him and his HIV-negative partner, Matt, during a hospitalization. Andrew described feeling that his friends are supportive of him and Matt as a couple dealing with HIV, not simply himself as a person living with HIV. As Andrew stated:

> We both have, as I said, a number of friends who have been wonderful with us, and friends who I've made who have sort of adopted Matt, too, and they're always looking out for him. They step in and try to pick up some slack if there's really something big going on. Even if it's just to make dinner and bring it over. In fact, I remember there was one time last year when I had surgery and I was in the hospital for a couple days. A couple of our friends called to see if there was anything they could do. I said, 'Yeah, there is. You could help me and Matt by bringing us dinner so that he doesn't have to cook.' They brought dinner every night I was in the hospital. Things like that have been a great support to both of us.

In a similar way, Adam, an HIV-positive partner, discussed how helpful it can be to have a network of friends, especially other HIV-positive friends, with whom he can talk when he feels the need:

> Occasionally, friends that are HIV-positive will ask me how my results are, what's going on with it, and things like that. So as far as a support group, I do have some friends that would support me and that are in a similar predicament. But in recent months, I haven't been seeking a lot of information. Prior to that, when things were going bad as far as a skin condition I had and things like that, there is a couple friends that I would call and we'd talk about it. I'm really kind of a private person and so I'm not constantly calling them, you know, calling friends to ask for support.

George, who is HIV-positive, also underscored the importance of feeling connected to HIV-positive friends as he and his partner deal with HIV:

> There's several friends, some are couples and some are not, that are close to us.
>
> Interviewer: And is that important for your relationship, do you think?
>
> Yeah, I think so. Keeps you from killing yourself. No, you know, it's nice to have people around. Sometimes it's hard to talk to other people, and I don't know, it just feels better having people around every day. They're like me and him, and you can talk to them.
>
> Interviewer: Are any of your friends HIV-positive?
>
> Yeah. A couple of them. We kind of keep a check on each other. I'll call them, they'll call me. Like when I was sick with cancer and stuff, they called me a lot, wanted to make sure I was getting along all right and everything. And if one of the others, if somebody will flare up, I'd do the same thing. I think it makes you feel like somebody is around and cares.

Family support. Family member support for the couples in this sample appeared to be mixed. Several partners reported that support was lacking from family members, whereas others reported feeling satisfied with family support. Previous studies of individuals living with HIV have revealed that family members can be hesitant to provide support (Turner et al., 1994; Wrubel & Folkman, 1997). For example, Powell-Cope and Brown (1992) found that family members may wish to avoid taking on the stigma associated with HIV and AIDS. They also discovered that family members may have difficulty providing adequate support due to a lack of education about HIV or fear of infection. Biordi (1995) also has suggested that family members may resist the stress of becoming too closely involved in the lives of the chronically ill, which often results in social isolation of the ill person.

In this study, some family members were described as quite supportive, others quite avoidant. For example, Adam, an HIV-positive individual, detailed that his family seems to be in denial about his disease—wanting to believe it has gone into remission. As Adam explained:

> I've told quite a few friends. My family, they don't really discuss it. They acted like they were very interested in knowing, and they have offered to help, but they really haven't. I guess they feel that I'm in remission more or less. They haven't really offered that much.

Dennis, who is in an HIV-concordant relationship with Todd, explained that Todd does not have much support from his family due to the double stigma of AIDS and homosexuality, and possibly combined with a fear of infection:

> They know that he's gay and that he's positive. They kind of accept it, but they don't want to, you know, they don't really talk about it or want other gay people in their house. I don't know maybe they think they'll catch it or something, I don't know. So his family is kind of weird. He doesn't talk to them.

Several of the families of HIV-negative partners also seemed to avoid the issue of HIV or AIDS. Joe, an HIV-negative partner, stated, 'His family is somewhat supportive. My own family is a little different. They've been OK, but I think it's easiest for them if they don't think about it, so they don't think about it.' Similarly, Ed, who is HIV-positive, explained that his HIV-negative partner Larry's family is pleasant to him, but uninvolved:

> I think Larry's family is very big on not saying a lot. They're very nice. I mean if he gets a card or something, it's always to both of us now. But I don't know how much they know related to AIDS. We really don't have much contact with them.

Although some participants described a lack of family support, an important finding in this study was evidence of the presence of family support in comparison to the trend reported in past research of family rejecting family members with HIV or AIDS. Several participants stated that their family and their partner's family *do* attempt to provide support for both members of the couple as they cope with HIV or AIDS. Complete acceptance of HIV and the same-sex relationship, however, still was quite infrequent and placed couples under recurring strain in coping with different levels of family acceptance and rejection. Examples from participants describing experiences of family support included Joe, an HIV-negative partner, who explained that his partner Alex was quite hesitant to disclose his HIV status to his own family for fear of rejection. Joe asserted that despite lacking a complete understanding of HIV or AIDS, Alex's family turned out to be generally supportive once they found out about his HIV diagnosis:

> Yeah, his family is very, very close. Has been. And he was afraid to tell them at first primarily because his mother's a worrier. We knew that she would worry about it. I understood that. She lives way out in the country, and the whole gay thing and this whole AIDS thing, the AIDS thing would be really scary. I understood that, although I felt like he needed her support. So I didn't press him on telling her, although he was kind of getting my message. He wasn't going to tell them 'til he got real sick. But he finally did; he told his mother first, and she was very supportive, immediately. I was not in the room when he told her, but, no, there was never a drawing back and a disowning or 'I'm disappointed in you' kind of situation as we've seen with other people. It was basically, 'You're sick, and we need to pitch in and do what we can do to help you get better.'

In contrast, Peter, who is HIV-negative, explained that, except for his partner's mother, the rest of his partner's family is interpersonally pleasant, but avoids the issue of AIDS:

> He's got a great family. They're pretty much in denial about the whole thing, but they're very close. We were just down there for Easter. His family is great to me. They all know about the sickness and his mom calls a lot—once, twice every week to see how he's doing. And, I mean, he'll tell her when something happens also. He's pretty open with her about it. He has some of his medicine delivered down to her house when he knows he's not going to be at our house, the one that has to be frozen.

Gary, an HIV-negative partner, described the importance of his family's support because many of his friends have died from AIDS. He stated:

> My parents are a lot of help. We talk about it. They're open, we do talk about it. They're always there if I need to talk. Most of my friends that I would have talked to are dead.

Family members' willingness to accept the same-sex relationship also may be tied to their ability to provide illness-related social support to the couple (although a causal order cannot be established with these data). In an African American HIV-concordant couple, for example, Leon explained that his partner Reggie's family originally could not accept their relationship and tried to blame him for Reggie's HIV-positive status. Leon explained that Reggie's family became more supportive with time regarding HIV-related support, although they still are not comfortable with their gay relationship:

> Reggie's family? Everybody's supportive. They come by, they ask me questions because Reggie won't talk to them sometimes. And they're like, 'Is he doing this?' And I'm like, 'Yeah, he's doing this and this and this.' And they go, 'OK, just as long as you're watching.' I think that's really, really important for the person that has HIV to have people in their lives like their family that come together, and things like that. Because there's no sense in just trying to put blame. You can blame and blame and blame all you want, but you'll never know exactly where you got it from.

Dennis, who also is in a concordant relationship, explained that his family is emotionally supportive in times of health crisis, but, on a day-to-day basis, his partner Todd still provides most of his social support:

> My grandmother, my father, my sister and my cousins, my aunt, my two nieces, they're all real supportive, you know. I don't pick up the phone and say, 'Oh God, you know what?' But, like, when I was in the hospital, everybody was worried. I called them at home and said, 'It's really nothing serious.' I really didn't think it had that much to do with AIDS. It just was one of those things that happen. And so yeah, they're all supportive. But Todd on a day-to-day basis, he's real supportive. He's normally the one, he'll ask, 'Are you feeling OK? How was work?,' and things like that. So he is most supportive.

Andrew, another HIV-positive individual, recalled that initially he was hesitant to disclose his HIV status to his HIV-negative partner's family for fear of stigma. He explained, however, that his partner's family has turned out to be quite supportive in times of crisis:

> I didn't really want to worry his parents, that kind of thing. And so now that they know I'm HIV-positive, they've been really wonderful. They've helped out at different times, whenever we needed it. Sometimes they bring food for us. His dad came and picked me up from my doctor visit once. They've been really good about it.

Summary. Overall, relational partners provided the most support to both HIV-positive and HIV-negative partners, followed by close friends. However, contrary to past studies, which found that families frequently reject family members with HIV or AIDS, with a few exceptions, participants in this study generally reported feeling that their family members were somewhat supportive. This finding might indicate a slow shift toward increased HIV education and acceptance of family members with HIV or AIDS. The evidence of family support found in this sample also could be the result of the fairly long time since diagnosis (mean 6.5 years) of the persons living with HIV. Enough time may have passed for these family members to process and cope with the HIV-positive status of their family member, and, thus, enabled them to move toward providing increased support. Further research is needed to investigate the factors influencing HIV-related family social support provision over time.

Social Network Support as a Means of Relationship Maintenance

Research question two asked how social support affects relationship maintenance within gay male couples dealing with HIV In general, the use of social network support from friends and family was found to have an important impact on relationship maintenance in these couples. Evidence of the use of social networks in maintaining heterosexual couple relationships has been found in previous studies (e.g., Canary & Stafford, 1992; Haas & Stafford, 1998; Stafford et al., 2000), but married couples have viewed social networks as having a less influential role in maintaining their relationships than described by the gay male couples in the present study. In particular, these couples described how social networks affected a combination of HIV-related social support and social validation of their same-sex relationship.

Formal public validation of heterosexual couples most often takes the form of legal and/or religious marriage. Owing to the inability of gay and lesbian couples to obtain legal recognition of their relationship, more informal means of social recognition and validation often are sought as an important way to maintain these relationships (Haas & Stafford, 1998). For instance, some gay and lesbian couples increasingly are engaging in 'commitment ceremonies' as a more public means of seeking social validation of their relationship. Participants in this study also reported utilizing social networks to validate their relationship. For example, Ed, an HIV-positive individual, explained that, in addition to support regarding HIV, he also wants family network support for his gay relationship. He explained that he and his partner exchanged vows in a commitment ceremony, and that the attendance of his partner's family was very important to him. As Ed recalled:

> Last summer, Larry and I had a big wedding in the park. There were 20 people; Channel 6 and Channel 10 were there. It was really beautiful and wonderful, and every member of his family showed up, including his dad. Even though they came, they were constantly having to remind you that they accepted you. I'm not sure how they really feel, but at least they did it. So it was lovely to me.

Similarly, Jerry, who is HIV-positive, explained that his family showed support of his gay relationship with an ex-partner by attending a commitment ceremony. Since then, they have supported his latest relationship as well. Jerry suggested that this type of social network support is quite important to him:

> My other partner that I was telling you

> about, we had a wedding ceremony and they [his family] came to that and were very supportive. They've always been supportive through everything. Before that point, I had nobody and my mother knew that I was HIV-positive. She said if I ever got sick that I could come stay with them and she'd get me through it. And then I met Tom along the way. So, they're very, very supportive. We were just up there again last weekend because my one foster brother lives in Michigan and his wife's going to have a baby in June, so Mom threw them a shower and I hadn't seen them in eight years, so we drove up for that. So, they're very supportive in everything.

In addition, several participants explained that having a network of gay friends served both as social recognition of their relationship and as a connection to the support of a gay community. Social isolation is a frequent experience of persons living with HIV (Wrubel & Folkman, 1997) and having a network of gay friends was an important means of retaining social connections outside the relationship. Dave, an HIV-negative partner, recounted that he and his partner made a conscious effort to increase their gay social network to combat social isolation:

> I didn't have any access to the community. This was frightening, very frightening to me, and I certainly didn't know how I would possibly access that alone at this point in time. I don't just mean necessarily sexually, although that too, but just socially. Companionship. Our main sources of companionship have been each other. So that was pretty frightening. And I think he was frightened for me about that. But also to get us off of our butts, just trying to get out. So that was kind of a plan I made. Now, we go out a lot. We have a whole series of new acquaintances and developing some really decent friendships out of it, and exploring other people, and ourselves through other people, through how we interact with others. It's like a whole new thing. So in that respect, it's been really good for me, and us. So now I'm beginning to recognize there's a lot more. I keep saying, 'God, life is short. Get going.'

Gary, an HIV-negative partner, explained that he and his partner have many single gay friends and that he feels they look to his relationship as a model. He felt that this helped to provide support for their relationship:

> We have lots of single friends, not gay couples. I think they look up to us. If we can do it, then, you know, maybe they can. A lot of them have been together maybe six months, time-wise, and that's it. It does take a lot of work.

In a similar way, Daryl, an HIV-positive partner, explained that many of their gay friends are also single. He described how he and his partner make an effort to have parties and stay connected to this social network of friends; however, because many are single there is a tension related to being a couple in a group of single friends. As he explained:

> We have parties, like his 40th birthday's coming up. I've got something nice planned. I just had my 40th the other day, too. A real nice one for me. So we do a lot of things. We had a Super Bowl party. We have a Christmas party every year for our friends. Yeah, most of our friends are single. Half of them are HIV-positive, half of them are not. But they're all single, and they're all out at the bars five to seven days a week. And it's kind of hard for us to get along with them being a couple like we are, you know. The way they party so much, it's hard to get along with them. We see them when we want to.

Ed, an HIV-positive partner, pointed out that their network of friends had been seriously diminished due to AIDS-related deaths, increasing emotional strain for them as a couple. As Ed explained:

> We have good times with several friends going and coming. We've tried to stop going out to bars. We have very good friends. I was thinking about this today. We really don't have any AIDS friends anymore. They've died, which has been hard. Together, we've had to go through several people that we loved.

Several participants explained that partners, friends, family, and also health care workers combined to create a matrix of people that form a network of support. For example, Andrew, who is HIV-positive, stated:

> There's really no one person per se. With me, it's a combination, several pieces of the whole. Matt [his partner] certainly is a major part. A really good friend of mine, Janet, who helped me get my life back together, has adopted Matt, too, and my therapist who is also a part of it. They're the ones who have really helped me keep it together.

Jerry, an HIV-positive partner, described a similar combination of individuals making up his support system in addition to his HIV-negative partner Tom:

> Tom's the most supportive, you know. But my disability is a dual diagnosis because I have AIDS and severe depression combined with high anxiety. So I have to go to [a clinic] and I get my drugs through them for that. And I have a counselor down there, so I get it there. Then I have [a social worker] who is with [an AIDS service organization], and he's my case worker and everything, and he helps me get through it. Sometimes though he needs a push to get things done, so Tom calls and talks to him.

In general, participants described spending much of their time in quiet home life, watching television and just being together (again emphasizing the centrality of relational partners as a daily source of support). However, ties to social networks still were important. Brian, an HIV-negative partner, explained:

> Together, we sit at home and watch a lot of TV and movies. We'll go out for an occasional meal, have little parties for friends and that sort of thing. Last year or so, we've gotten into playing cards with another couple. Our landlord and his partner come up and we play various card games and dice and this sort of thing. So we're together sometimes, and sometimes we'll switch off partners and play against one another, board games, that sort of thing. So we do that together. Occasionally, we go to some dance performances.

Finally, William, an HIV-positive partner, said of he and his partner's social network interaction with friends:

> Our lives are pretty quiet. We do socialize a lot with friends and we go out occasionally. We do drink. No, I don't think we're drunks, but we go out and party and have a good time, dancing, etc. But mostly spending time with friends, dinners, and that sort of thing.

Summary. Overall, social support from networks was described as an important factor that helped to maintain the couple relationships in this study. Based on these couples' reports, social network support served both HIV-related illness support and relationship maintenance functions.

Implications of Social Support as Relationship Maintenance

In past research, the constructs of social support and relationship maintenance have been studied independently. The present research expands our understanding of how these constructs may function separately or interdependently in couples coping with chronic illness. The findings of this study examining the relationships of gay male couples dealing with HIV or AIDS provide initial evidence that the constructs of social support, caregiving, and relationship maintenance are likely interdependent for couples as they manage life with chronic illness. As the needs of illness-related support, caregiving, and relationship maintenance become integrated in daily life, many behaviors likely function to accomplish multiple goals (Miller, Cody, & McLaughlin, 1994). As chronic conditions persist, relational partners likely enact behaviors that meet multiple relational functions and goals simultaneously. In time, these behaviors begin to shape new relational definitions for partners.

Extending the work of Clark and Mills (1979), Coyne, Ellard, and Smith (1990) described the intimate dyadic relationship as a 'communal' one, meaning that behaviors are enacted and viewed on a global level rather than from a social exchange perspective. Thus, perhaps what helps to maintain couples dealing with HIV is their ability to care for one another while perceiving HIV to be yet another relational stressor, much the same as work-related stress, financial stress, family stress, and the like. Evidence from this study of a 'communal' perspective was seen in couples placing great importance on the reciprocity of social support. Much of the research on caregiving has been based on assumptions of a provider-receiver relationship. Cutrona, Suhr, and MacFarlene (1990) asserted that social support is a transactional communication process within relationships, and often is enacted through everyday routine talk (for a discussion of the role of everyday talk in relationships, see Duck, Rutt, Hurst, & Strejc, 1991). However, much of the HIV and AIDS social support literature has focused on HIV-positive individuals' receipt of social support. Couples in this study seemed to reject the notion that the HIV-positive partner wanted or needed a care 'giver.' Instead, similar to the findings of Hays, Chauncey, and Tobey (1990), persons living with HIV here reported relationships as more supportive when they were able to reciprocate support. The fact that HIV-partner's health conditions fluctuated between periods when symptoms interfered with day-to-day functioning and periods of relative 'good' health also seemed to prevent either partner from feeling that a caregiver relationship had been established. Overall, the HIV-positive partners in this study indicated they would be much less satisfied in a relationship in which they were the sole recipient of care or support.

Another important aspect that may influence the ability of these gay male relationships to deal with HIV is the flexibility and lack of sex-role assignments found within same-sex relationships (Kurdek, 1987, 1993; Kurdek & Schmitt, 1986a; Lynch & Reilly, 1985/86). Coyne and Delongis (1986) found that, in married couples where the wife had experienced a heart attack, she regained primary responsibility for household tasks shortly after returning home from the hospital, whereas male heart attack patients were relieved of any household responsibilities until full recovery. For the male couples in this study, the lack of sex-based task assignments allowed for flexibility and reciprocity of support, which may help prevent the type of stress overload often carried by one partner in an opposite-sex relationship.

References

Alonzo, A. A., & Reynolds, N. R. (1995). Stigma, HIV and AIDS: An exploration and elaboration of a stigma trajectory. *Social Science and Medicine, 41,* 303–315.

Attridge, M. (1994). Barriers to dissolution of romantic relationships. In D. J. Canary & L. Stafford (Eds.), *Communication and relational maintenance* (pp. 187–217). San Diego: Academic Press.

Barbee, A. P., Derlega, V. J., Sherburne, S. P., & Grimshaw, A. (1998). Helpful and unhelpful forms of social support for HIV-positive individuals. In V. J. Derlega & A. P. Barbee (Eds.), *HIV and social interaction* (pp. 83–105). Thousand Oaks, CA: Sage.

Baxter, L. A., & Dindia, K. (1990). Marital partners' perceptions of marital maintenance strategies. *Journal of Social and Personal Relationships, 7,* 187–208.

Berger, R. M. (1990). Men together: Understanding the gay couple. *Journal of Homosexuality, 19,* 31–49.

Biordi, D. (1995). Social isolation. In I. M. Lubkin (Ed.), *Chronic illness: Impact and interventions* (pp. 168–190). Boston: Jones and Bartlett.

Blumstein, P., & Schwartz, P. (1983). *American couples: Money, work, and sex.* New York: William Morrow.

Brashers, D. E., Neidig, J. L., Reynolds, N. R., & Haas, S. M. (1998). Uncertainty in illness across the HIV/AIDS trajectory. *Journal of the Association of Nurses in AIDS Care, 9,*66–77.

Brashers, D. E., Neidig, J., Cardillo, L., Dobbs, L., Russell, J. A., & Haas, S. M. (1999). 'In an important way I did die:' Uncertainty and revival in persons living with HIV and AIDS. *AIDS Care, 11,* 201, 220.

Brashers, D. E., Neidig, J. L., Haas, S., Dobbs, L. K., Cardillo, L. W., & Russell, J. A. (2000). Communication in the management of uncertainty: The case of persons living with HIV or AIDS. *Communication Monographs, 67,* 63–84.

Burnard, P. (1991). A method of analyzing interview transcripts in qualitative research. *Nurse Education Today, 11,* 461–466.

Canary, D. J., & Stafford, L. (1992). Relational maintenance strategies and equity in marriage. *Communication Monographs, 59,* 243–267.

Canary, D. J., & Stafford, L. (1994). Maintaining relationships through strategic and routine interaction. In D. J. Canary & L. Stafford (Eds.), *Communication and relationship maintenance* (pp. 3–22). New York: Academic Press.

Catania, J. A., Turner, H. A., Choi, K., & Coates, T. J. (1992). Coping with death anxiety: Help–seeking and social support among gay men with various HIV diagnoses. *AIDS, 6,* 999–1005.

Clark, M. S., & Mills, J. (1979). Interpersonal attraction in exchange and communal relationships. *Journal of Personality and Social Psychology, 37,* 12–24.

Clark, W. M., & Serovich, J. M. (1997). Twenty years and still in the dark? Content analysis of articles pertaining to gay, lesbian, and bisexual issues in marriage and family therapy journals. *Journal of Marital and Family Therapy, 23,* 239–253.

Corbin, J. M., & Strauss, A. (1988). *Unending work and care: Managing chronic illness at home,* San Francisco: Jossey-Bass.

Coyne, J. C., & Delongis, A. M. (1986). Going beyond social support: The role of social relationships in adaptation. *Journal of Consulting and Clinical Psychology, 54,* 454–460.

Coyne, J. C., Ellard, J. H., & Smith, D. A. (1990). Social support, interdependence, and the dilemmas of helping. In B. R. Sarason, I. G. Sarason, & G R. Pierce (Eds.), *Social support: An interactional view* (pp. 129–149). New York: Wiley.

Cutrona, C., & Suhr, J. (1994). Social support communication in the context of marriage: An analysis of couples' supportive interactions. In B. R. Burleson, T. L. Albrecht, & I. G. Sarason (Eds.), *Communication of social support: Messages, interactions, relationships, and community* (pp. 113–135). Thousand Oaks, CA: Sage.

Cutrona, C., & Suhr, J., & MacFarlene, R. (1990). Interpersonal transactions and the psychological sense of support. In S. Duck & R. Silver (Eds.), *Personal relationships and social support* (pp. 30–45). London: Sage.

Dakof, G. A., & Taylor, S. E. (1990). Victims' perceptions of social support: What is helpful from whom? *Journal of Personality and Social Psychology, 58,* 80–89.

Duck, S. W. (1994). Steady as (s)he goes: Relational maintenance as a shared meaning system. In D. J. Canary & L. Stafford (Eds.), *Communication and relationship maintenance* (pp. 45–60). New York: Academic Press.

Duck, S. W., Rutt, D. J., Hurst, M. H., & Strejc, H. (1991). Some evident truths about conversation in everyday relationships: All communications are not created equal. *Human Communication Research, 18,* 228–268.

Evans, D. L., Lesserman, J., Perkins, D. O., Stern, R. A., Murphy, C., Zheng, B., Gattes, D., Longmate, J. A., Silva, S. G., van der Horst, C. M., Hall, C. D., Folds, J. D., Golden, R. N., & Petitto, J. M. (1997). Severe life stress as a predictor of early disease progression in HIV infection. *American Journal of Psychiatry, 154,* 630–774.

Ferrari, J. R., McCown, W., & Pantano, J. (1993). Experiencing satisfaction and stress as an AIDS care provider: The AIDS caregiver scale. *Evaluations and Health Professions, 16,* 295–310.

Folkman, S., Chesney, M. A., Cooke, M., Boccellari, A., & Collette, L. (1994). Caregiver burden in HIV-positive and HIV-negative partners of men with AIDS. *Journal of Consulting and Clinical Psychology, 62,* 746–756.

Glaser, B., & Strauss, A. (1967). *The discovery of grounded theory.* Chicago: Adline, Atherton.

Goffman, E. (1963). *Stigma: Notes on the management of spoiled identity.* Englewood Cliffs, NJ: Prentice-Hall.

Gottlieb, B. H. (1981). Preventive interventions involving social networks and social support. In B. H. Gottlieb (Ed.), *Social networks and social support* (pp. 201–232). Beverly Hills, CA: Sage.

Greene, K., & Serovich, J. M. (1996). Appropriateness of disclosure of HIV testing information: The perspective of the PLWAs. *Journal of Applied Communication Research, 24,* 50–65.

Greif, G. L., & Porembski, E. (1988). AIDS and significant others: Findings from a preliminary exploration of needs. *Health and Social Work, 13,* 259–265.

Grieco, A. J., & Kowalski, W. (1987). The 'care partner.' In L. H. Bernstein, A. J. Grieco, & M. K. Dete (Eds.), *Primary care in the home* (pp. 71–82). Philadelphia: Lippincott.

Guba, E. G., & Lincoln, Y. S. (1989). *Fourth generation evaluation.* Newbury Park, CA: Sage.

Haas, S. M. (1999, June). *Exploring seropositive and seronegative partner motivations for relationship initiation in HIV-discordant and concordant couples.* Paper presented at the joint conference of the International Network on Personal Relationships and the International Society for the Study of Personal Relationships, Louisville, KY.

Haas, S. M., & Stafford, L. (1998). An initial examination of maintenance behaviors in gay and lesbian relationships. *Journal of Social and Personal Relationships, 15,* 846–855.

Hays, R. B., Chauncey, S., & Tobey, L. A. (1990). The social support networks of gay men with AIDS. *Journal of Community Psychology, 18,* 374–385.

Hays, R. B., McGee, R. H., & Chauncey, S. (1994). Identifying helpful and unhelpful behaviors of loved ones: The PWAs perspective. *AIDS Care, 6,* 379–392.

Hays, R. B., Turner, H., & Coates, T. J. (1992). Social support, AIDS-related symptoms, and depression among gay men. *Journal of Consulting and Clinical Psychology, 60,* 463–469.

Jacobson, D. E. (1986). Types and timing of social support. *Journal of Health and Social Behavior, 27,* 250–264.

Kalichman, S. C. (2000). Couples with HIV/AIDS. In K. B. Schmaling & T. Goldman Sher (Eds.), *The psychology of couples and illness: Theory, research, & practice* (pp. 171–190). Washington, DC: American Psychological Association.

Katz, A. (1996). Gaining a new perspective on life as a consequence of uncertainty in HIV infection. *Journal of Nurses in AIDS Care, 7,* 51–60.

Kennedy, S., Kiecolt-Glaser, J. K., & Glaser, R. (1990). Social support, stress, and the immune system. In B. R. Sarason, I. G. Sarason, & G. R. Pierce (Eds.), *Social support: An interactional view* (pp. 253–266). New York: Wiley.

Kessler, R. C., Foster, C., Joseph, J., Ostrow, D., Wortman, C., Phair, J., & Chmiel, J. (1991). Stressful life events and symptom onset in HIV infection. *American Journal of Psychiatry, 148,* 733–738.

Kimberly, J. A., & Serovich, J. M. (1996). Perceived social support among people living with HIV/AIDS. *The American Journal of Family Therapy, 24,* 41–53.

Kurdek, L. (1987). Sex-role self-schema and psychological adjustment in coupled homosexual and heterosexual men and women. *Sex Roles, 17,* 549–562.

Kurdek, L. (1993). The allocation of household labor in gay, lesbian, and heterosexual married couples. *Journal of Social Issues, 49*(3), 127–139.

Kurdek, L., & Schmitt, J. P. (1986a). Interaction of sex role self-concept with relationship quality and relationship beliefs in married, heterosexual cohabitating, gay, and lesbian couples. *Journal of Personality and Social Psychology, 51,* 365–370.

Kurdek, L., & Schmitt, J. P. (1986b). Relationship quality of partners in heterosexual married, heterosexual cohabitating, gay and lesbian couples. *Journal of Personality and Social Psychology, 57,* 711–720.

Leary, M. R., & Schreindorfer, L. S. (1998). The stigmatization of HIV and AIDS. In V. J. Derlega & A. P. Barbee (Eds.), *HIV and social interaction* (pp. 12–29). Thousand Oaks, CA: Sage.

Leserman, J., Petitto, J. M., Golden, R. N., Gaynes, B. N., Gu, H., Perkins, D. O., Silva, S. G., Folds, J. D., & Evans, D. L. (2000). Impact of stressful life events, depression, social support, coping, and Cortisol on progression to AIDS. *American Journal of Psychiatry, 157,* 1221–1228.

Lincoln, Y. S., & Guba, E. G. (1985). *Naturalistic inquiry.* Beverly Hills, CA: Sage.

Lowenthal, M., & Haven, C. (1968). Interaction and adaptation: Intimacy as a critical variable. *American Sociological Review, 33,* 20–30.

Lynch, J. M., & Reilly, M. E. (1985/86). Role relationships: Lesbian perspectives. *Journal of Homosexuality, 12*(2), 53–69.

Marecek, J., Finn, S. E., & Cardell, M. (1983). Gender roles in the relationships of lesbians and gay men. *Journal of Homosexuality, 8*(2), 45–50.

McLean, C., & Roberts, R. (1995). Sex, intimacy, and AIDS: Lessons in relationships from thirteen Australian gay men. *AIDS Patient Care, 9,* 166–171.

McWhirter, D. P., & Mattison, A. M. (1984). *The male couple: How relationships develop.* Englewood Cliffs, NJ: Prentice-Hall.

Mendola, M. (1980). *The Mendola report: A new look at gay couples.* New York: Crown.

Miller, L. C, Cody, M. J., & McLaughlin, M. L. (1994). Situations and goals as fundamental constructs in interpersonal communication research. In M. L. Knapp & G. R. Miller (Eds.), *Handbook of interpersonal communication* (2nd ed.; pp. 162–198). Thousand Oaks, CA: Sage.

Moore, J., Saul J., VanDevanter, N., Kennedy, C. A., Lesondak, L. M., & O'Brien, T. R. (1998). Factors influencing relationship quality of HIV-serodiscordant heterosexual couples. In V. J. Derlega & A. P. Barbee (Eds.), *HIV and social interaction* (pp. 165–192). Thousand Oaks, CA: Sage.

Nokes, K. M. (1991). Applying the chronic illness trajectory model to HIV/AIDS. *Scholarly Inquiry for Nursing Research: An International Journal, 5,* 197–204.

Ossana, S. M. (2000). Relationship and couples counseling. In R. M. Perez, K. A. DeBord, & K. J. Bieschke (Eds.), *Handbook of counseling and psychotherapy with lesbian, gay, and bisexual clients* (pp. 275–302). Washington, DC: American Psychological Association.

Ostrow, D. G., Monjan, A., Joseph, J., VanRaden, M., Fox, R., Kingsley, L., Dudley, J., & Phair, J. (1989). HIV-related symptoms and psychological functioning in a cohort of homosexual men. *American Journal of Psychiatry 146,* 737–742.

Pearlin, L. I. (1989). The sociological study of stress. *Journal of Health and Social Behavior, 30,* 241–256.

Pearlin, L. I., Semple, S., & Turner, H. (1988). Stress of AIDS caregiving: A preliminary overview of the issues. *Death Studies, 12,* 501–517.

Peplau, L. A. (1991). Lesbian and gay relationships. In J. C. Gonsiorek & J. D. Weinrich (Eds.), *Homosexuality: Research implications for public policy* (pp. 177–196). Newbury Park, CA: Sage.

Peplau, L. A., & Cochran, S. D. (1981). Value orientations in the intimate relationships of gay men. *Journal of Homosexuality, 6*(3), 1–19.

Peplau, L. A., & Cochran, S. D. (1990). A relational perspective on homosexuality. In D. P. McWhirter, S. A. Sanders, & J. M. Reinisch (Eds.), *Homosexuality/heterosexuality: Concepts of sexual orientation* (pp. 321–349). New York: Oxford University Press.

Powell-Cope, G. M. (1994). Family caregivers of people with AIDS: Negotiating partnerships with professional health care providers. *Nursing Research, 43,* 324–330.

Powell-Cope, G. M. (1995). The experiences of gay couples affected by HIV infection. *Qualitative Health Research, 5*(1), 36–62.

Powell-Cope, G. M. (1996). HIV disease symptom management in the context of committed relationships. *Journal of the Association of Nurses in AIDS Care, 7*(3), 19–28.

Powell–Cope, G. M., & Brown, M. A. (1992). Going public as an AIDS family caregiver. *Social Science and Medicine, 34,* 571–580.

Rabkin, J. G., Williams, J. B., Neugbauer, R., Remien, R. H., & Goetz, R. (1990). Maintenance of hope in HIV-spectrum homosexual men. *American Journal of Psychiatry, 147,* 1322–1326.

Rolland, J. S. (1994). In sickness and in health: The impact of illness on couples' relationships. *Journal of Marital and Family Therapy, 20,* 327–347.

Sarason, B. R., Shearin, E. N., Pierce, G., & Sarason, I. G. (1987). Interrelations among social support measures: Theoretical and practical implications. *Journal of Personality and Social Psychology, 52,* 813–832.

Shinn, M., Lehmann, S., & Wong, N. W. (1980). Social interaction and social support. *Journal of Social Issues, 40,* 55–76.

Stafford, L., & Canary, D. J. (1991). Maintenance strategies and romantic relationship type, gender, and relational characteristics. *Journal of Social and Personal Relationships, 8,* 217–242.

Stafford, L., Dainton, M., & Haas, S. M. (2000). Measuring routine and strategic relational maintenance: Scale revision, sex versus gender roles, and the prediction of relational characteristics. *Communication Monographs, 67,* 306–323.

Stern, A. P. (1980). Qualitative methods of analysis. *Image: Journal of Scholarly Nursing Research, 8,* 34–40.

Strauss, A. (1987). *Qualitative analysis for social scientists.* New York: Cambridge University Press.

Thibaut, J. W., & Kelly, H. H. (1959). *The social psychology of groups.* New York: Wiley. Reissued (1986). New Brunswick, NJ: Transaction Books.

Turner, H. A., Catania, J. A., & Gagnon, J. (1994). The prevalence of informal caregiving to persons with AIDS in the United States: Caregiver characteristics and their implications. *Social Science and Medicine, 38,* 1543–1552.

Turner, H. A., Hays, R. B., & Coates, T. J. (1993). Determinants of social support among gay men: The context of AIDS. *Journal of Health and Social Behavior, 34,* 37–53.

UNAIDS-The Joint United Nations Programme on HIV/AIDS. (2000). *Global AIDS epidemic update and country reports* [On-line]. Available (consulted June 2000): http://www.unaids.org/epidemic_update/report/index.html

van der Straten, A., Vernon, K. A., Knight, K. R., Gomez, C. A., & Padian, N. S. (1998). Managing HIV among serodiscordant heterosexual couples: Serostatus, stigma, and sex. *AIDS Care, 10,* 533–548.

Wethington, E., & Kessler, R. C. (1986). Perceived support, received support, and adjustment to stressful life events. *Journal of Health and Social Behavior, 27,* 78–89.

Wight, R. G., LeBlanc, J. A., & Aneshensel, C. S. (1995). Support service use by persons with AIDS and their caregivers. *AIDS Care, 7,* 509–520.

Wrubel, J., & Folkman, S. (1997). What informal caregivers actually do: The caregiving skills of partners of men with AIDS. *AIDS Care, 9,* 691–706.

Discussion Questions

1. What source of social support do you think you would turn to if facing a health issue? Why?
2. Would this source of support change depending on the health issue you faced?
3. Does being able to provide support for someone else depend on the type of illness he or she is facing? Explain your answer. ✦

Part VI

HEALTH PROMOTION

Chapter 19 Putting the Fear Back Into Fear Appeals

The Extended Parallel Process Model

Kim Witte

Health promotion and health campaigns are a major focus of health communication. Unlike the health-care provider-patient interactions, which are at the heart of the earlier parts of this volume, health promotion has its roots in classical persuasion theory and mass communication theory and practices. Health promotion, as much as patient-provider communication, has provided a way for communication scholars to take their work beyond the walls of academia and into the community to help address issues of health. While certainly many areas of communication have a history of being important outside of academia, perhaps no area as much as health communication has grown as rapidly or adopted the diversity of methods, theories, and traditions. Part VI consists of five exemplars of research on health promotion. Health promotion concerns the wide array of persuasive mechanisms used to encourage individuals to change a health behavior. Health promotion research often deals specifically with health campaigns, or mass mediated efforts to change behaviors through commercials, brochures, simulation games, and/or seminars. Taken together these chapters provide an array of the sorts of concerns and approaches that typify campaigns designed to promote good health or change health-related attitudes and behaviors. Each of them, in their own ways, sheds light on how the promotion campaigns of today are informed by communication theory and scholarship.

Part VI begins with Kim Witte's exemplar chapter, a classic piece that describes and reviews fear appeals as a device in the transformation of health behaviors and the advantages and disadvantages of fear-based approaches. Witte articulates an alternative theoretic approach to health campaigns. The author has streamlined the research on fear appeals and advocates a new model for understanding fear, threat, and efficacy. She argues that there are proper ways to induce behavior changes using fear; however, researchers must understand when and why fear appeals fail.

Related Topics: ethical issues, health campaigns, health-care behaviors, media

This is your brain
This is your brain on drugs
Any questions?

Persuasive strategies like this well-known drug-prevention commercial are known as "fear appeals." Fear appeals are persuasive messages designed to scare people by describing the terrible things that will happen to them if they do not do what the message recommends. For example, the creators of this drug-prevention commercial assume that people will avoid using drugs to keep their brains from "frying." While some studies substantiate the effectiveness of fear appeals (e.g., Beck, 1984; Insko, Arkoff, & Insko, 1965; Stainback & Rogers, 1983), others demonstrate their ineffectiveness (e.g., Janis & Feshbach, 1953; Kohn, Goodstadt, Cook, Sheppard, & Chan, 1982; Krisher, Darley, & Darley, 1973), and still others document mixed results (e.g., Hill & Gardner, 1980; Rogers & Mewborn, 1976). Overall, the empirical findings are disappointingly inconsistent, if not contradictory. There are at least three major reasons for the lack of convergence in fear appeal findings.

First, the interchangeable use of conceptually distinct terms has muddied the fear appeal waters considerably. For example, Sutton (1982) equated *threat* and *fear* in his

From "Putting the Fear Back Into Fear Appeals: The Extended Parallel Process Model," Kim Witte, 1992, *Communication Monographs*, Vol 59:4, pp. 329–349.

meta-analysis–even though (as will be argued later) fear and threat produce different outcomes. Terms such as fear, threat, and efficacy must be carefully defined and used in a consistent manner across studies if the literature is to be reconciled.

Second, current theoretical explanations overwhelmingly focus on processes associated with message acceptance and neglect processes associated with message rejection. To fully understand individuals' reactions to fear appeals, we need to understand when and why fear appeals fail, as well as when and why fear appeals work. The proposed theory suggests that fear arousal is the key to understanding message rejection processes. Because the role of fear in fear appeals has been essentially eliminated in current cognitive fear appeal theories (Dillard, 1992), one goal of the present work is to put the fear back into fear appeals.

Third, the interaction between threat and efficacy has not been consistently represented or addressed in fear appeal studies. Rogers and colleagues (e.g., Kleinot & Rogers, 1982; Rogers & Mewborn, 1976) have demonstrated that fear appeals with high levels of threat (e.g., "you are susceptible to the severe disease AIDS") and high levels of efficacy (e.g., "you are able to effectively and easily prevent AIDS by using condoms") produce message acceptance. In contrast, fear appeals with high levels of threat (e.g., "lung cancer is a severe disease that you are susceptible to because you smoke cigarettes") and low levels of efficacy (e.g., "it's unlikely that you'll be able to quit smoking cigarettes, and it's probably too late to prevent lung cancer anyway") result in message rejection. Yet, many researchers have failed to address or analyze the role of efficacy in their studies (e.g., Ben-Sira, 1981; Burnett, 1981; Burnett & Oliver, 1979; Kohn et al., 1982; Ramirez & Lasater, 1976, 1977). It will be argued that threat-by-efficacy interactions are the fundamental determinants of study outcomes. However, *knowing* that efficacy and threat are causal variables in study outcomes does not *explain why* they are causal variables. Thus, their theoretical functions will be explicated and expanded.

A theoretical approach that addresses these differences and explains the inconsistent empirical findings is needed. The theory presented in this paper evolves from earlier perspectives. The present work advances a theory based on Leventhal's (1970) danger control/fear control framework, and explains both successes and failures of fear appeals. Current theoretical approaches explain the danger control processes (Leventhal, 1970), or how people cognitively deal with a given danger or threat by changing their attitudes, intentions, or behaviors to prevent the threat from occurring (i.e., factors leading to message acceptance). But, current approaches virtually ignore the fear control processes (Leventhal, 1970), or how people deal with their fear by denying or defensively avoiding the threat (i.e., factors leading to message rejection). Elements of Rogers' (1975) original Protection Motivation Theory (PMT) are integrated into the proposed theory, because PMT explains the danger control processes that lead to message acceptance. However, neither Leventhal nor Rogers fully define or explain the fear control processes, or the factors leading to message rejection. Thus, the role of fear control processes must be clarified and expanded. Within the next few pages, key variables and processes will be defined and existing theoretical models will be reviewed.

Important Components of the Fear Appeal Process

Fear Appeals

Fear appeals (sometimes called threat appeals) can be defined in terms of their content, or by the reaction they engender from the audience (O'Keefe, 1990). For example, fear appeals usually contain "gruesome content" in the form of vivid language (e.g. "thick purulent, choking secretions welled into the tracheotomy wound," Leventhal, 1965), personalistic language (e.g., "smokers like you . . ."), or gory pictures (e.g., photographs of crash victims). Alternatively, fear appeals have been defined in terms of the amount of fear aroused and/or experienced by the audience (i.e., physiologically or psychologically). Reported or aroused fear is usually evaluated by a manipulation check, with a high fear appeal yielding significantly greater levels of reported or aroused fear than a low fear appeal.

O'Keefe (1990) makes an important distinction between the two definitions of fear appeals (i.e., message content vs. audience reactions) when he notes that messages with gruesome contents might not arouse fear, and fear might be aroused without grisly contents. However, the majority of fear appeal studies conducted have incorporated both definitions in their operationalizations of fear appeals—albeit informally. First, the majority of fear appeal studies include manipulation checks (the audience's response). Second, these same studies also describe the high fear appeal condition as one where the severe consequences of a threat are made applicable to the respondent—usually in the form of vivid and personalistic language with gruesome pictures or films. For example, when fear appeal researchers refer to a strong fear appeal condition, they usually mean that the message depicted a large threat and the receiver perceived a large threat (as assessed by the manipulation checks). Typically, fear appeals offer feasible recommendations that are presented as effective in averting the threat. Thus, the three central constructs in fear appeals are fear, threat, and efficacy.

Fear

Fear is a negatively-valenced emotion, accompanied by a high level of arousal, and is elicited by a threat that is perceived to be significant and personally relevant (Easterling & Leventhal, 1989; Lang, 1984; Ortony & Turner, 1990). Fear may be expressed physiologically (as arousal), through language behavior (verbal self-reports), or through overt acts (facial expressions) (Lang, 1984). In the fear appeal literature, fear has been operationalized as anxiety (i.e., self-rated feelings of anxiousness), physiological arousal (Mewborn & Rogers, 1979; Rogers & Deckner, 1975), responses to mood adjectives (e.g., frightened, anxious, nauseous), and ratings of concern or worry (Janis, 1967; Leventhal, 1970; Rogers, 1975, 1983; Sutton, 1982). Rogers (1983) has demonstrated that self-reported fear, as measured by mood adjectives (the most common measure of self-report fear in fear appeal studies), adequately captures our definition of fear, because of the correspondence between physiological arousal and self-ratings of mood adjectives. Specifically, Mewborn and Rogers (1979) found that a high fear film yielded higher self-ratings of fear, accelerated heart rate, and greater skin conductance, than a low fear film.[1] In fact, Rogers (1983) argues that "the verbal measure may be more sensitive than the physiological measures" because self-rated fear is more global in nature and more adequately reflects an overall emotional state, while physiological arousal fluctuates substantially during the presentation of a fear appeal (p. 164).

Threat

Threat is an external stimulus variable (e.g., an environmental or message cue) that exists whether a person knows it or not. If an individual holds a cognition that a threat exists, then he or she is *perceiving* a threat. Message characterizations of threat focus on the severity of the threat (e.g,. "AIDS leads to death") and on the targeted population's susceptibility to the threat (e.g.. "You're at-risk for AIDS because you share needles while using intravenous drugs") (Rogers, 1975, 1983). Correspondingly, *perceived severity* is an individual's beliefs about the seriousness of the threat, while *perceived susceptibility* is an individual's beliefs about his or her chances of experiencing the threat.

Efficacy

Efficacy also exists as an environmental or message cue and may lead to *perceived efficacy,* which refers to cognitions about efficacy. Message depictions of efficacy focus on the effectiveness of the recommended response (i.e., response efficacy) and on the targeted audience's ability to perform the recommended response (i.e., self-efficacy) (Rogers, 1975, 1983). Correspondingly, *perceived response efficacy* refers to an individual's beliefs as to whether a response effectively prevents the threat (e.g., "I believe condoms prevent HIV contraction"), and *perceived self-efficacy* refers to an individual's belief in his or her ability to perform the recommended response (e.g., "I think that I can easily use condoms to prevent HIV contraction") (Rogers, 1975, 1983).

Outcome Variables

The typical outcome in fear appeal research is *message acceptance,* defined as attitude, intention, or behavior change. Other outcomes less commonly assessed but equally important are defensive avoidance and reactance. *Defensive avoidance* is a motivated resistance to the message, such as denial or minimization of the threat. Individuals may defensively avoid a message by being inattentive to the communication (e.g., looking away from the message), or by suppressing any thoughts about the threat over the long term (Hovland, Janis, & Kelly, 1953; Janis & Feshbach, 1953; Janis & Mann, 1977). *Reactance* occurs when perceived freedom is reduced and an individual believes "that the communicator is trying to make him [or her] change" (Brehm, 1966, p. 94) (e.g., "I'll show them that they can't manipulate me, I'm going to smoke even more!").

A Brief History of Fear Appeal Theoretical Approaches

With these definitions in mind, previous theoretical approaches may now be reviewed. Following Dillard (1992), there are three major categories that correspond to three separate time periods in the evolution of fear appeal theories: (a) the drive models (Hovland et al., 1953; Janis, 1967; McGuire, 1968, 1969), (b) the parallel response model (Leventhal, 1970, 1971), and (c) the expectancy value theories (Rogers, 1975, 1983; Sutton, 1982).[2]

Drive Models

Two drive models were advanced in the 1950s and 1960s to explain individuals' reactions to fear appeals. The most prominent fear appeal model of this time period was Janis' (1967; Hovland et al., 1953) fear-as-acquired drive model. Janis (1967) proposed an inverted-U shaped relation between fear and message acceptance. He claimed that some fear arousal was needed to elicit a motivational drive state (i.e., create tension), but too much fear would result in maladaptive outcomes (e.g., defensive avoidance). Using a learning theory approach, Janis (1967) argued that the unpleasant tension caused by fear arousal motivated individuals to get rid of their fear. He said whatever *reduced* their fear—be it adaptive (e.g., behavior changes) or maladaptive (e.g., denial)— would be reinforced and become the preferred response to the threat.

McGuire (1968, 1969) also advanced an inverted-U explanation of fear appeals with his two-factor theory. McGuire (1968, 1969) argued that when fear acted as a *drive,* it motivated people to accept the message's recommendations. When fear acted as a *cue,* he said it elicited habitual responses that interfered with the acceptance or reception of the message. McGuire (1968, 1969) proposed that these two factors (i.e., cues and drives) combined to yield an overall inverted-U relationship between fear arousal and attitude change, where a moderate amount of fear arousal would produce the most attitude change.

Tests of these pioneering fear appeal theories have led to their rejection (see Beck & Frankel, 1981; Rogers, 1983; Sutton, 1982). No evidence has been offered to support McGuire's (1968, 1969) non-monotonic model (see Higbee, 1969). Janis' (1967) model has been similarly rejected. Specifically, the fear-as-acquired drive model's central hypothesis, that acceptance of the message occurred when fear was reduced, was not supported. Studies manipulating false physiological feedback found that increases in fear arousal were accompanied by increases in acceptance, independent of any fear "reduction" (Giesen & Hendrick, 1974; Hendrick, Giesen, & Borden, 1975; Rogers, 1983). In addition, Mewborn and Rogers (1979) found that only arousal, and not arousal reduction, affected intentions. Finally, Rogers and Deckner (1975) found that only cognitive appraisal of the threat and whether the response was seen as effective resulted in message acceptance. The empirical evidence has prompted researchers to reject the drive models as viable fear appeal explanations.

Parallel Response Model

Based on Hovland and Janis' (Hovland, et al., 1953; Janis, 1967) work, Leventhal (1970,

1971) developed the parallel response model (later called the parallel process model; Leventhal, Safer, & Panagis, 1983, p. 4), which began to focus more on cognitive processes, as opposed to emotional processes. Leventhal (1970) argued that protective adaptive behavior stemmed from attempts to control the danger or threat (cognitions), not from attempts to control die fear (emotions). Therefore, if people *thought* about the threatening message and developed strategies to avert the danger or threat (attitude, intention, or behavior changes), they were engaging in danger control processes. In contrast, if people focused on their feelings of fear, and tried to control their fear (e.g., denial), they were experiencing fear control processes.

Leventhal (1970) attempted to reconcile past literature with his model, but offered no evidence for its veracity with a single study. He made general statements about conditions leading to fear or danger control processes, but he failed to specify exactly when one process should dominate over another or what specific factors elicit the different processes. Thus, the main problem with the parallel response model is its lack of precision (Beck & Frankel, 1981; Rogers, 1975). Overall, however, the model offered a useful distinction between cognitive and emotional reactions to fear appeals.

Expectancy Value Theories

Further de-emphasizing the role of fear arousal in favor of cognition were Rogers' (1975, 1983) protection motivation theory (PMT) and Sutton's (1982) application of subjective expected utility (SEU) theory (Edwards, 1961) to fear appeals. In the latter. Sutton (1982) argued that decisions to accept a fear appeal's recommendations were a function of three variables: (a) the perceived utility of the threat; (b) the subjective probability that the threat will occur, given no changes in current behaviors; and (c) the subjective probability that the threat will occur if individuals make the recommended changes. To predict a person's decision to accept a fear appeal's recommendations, each subjective probability (i.e., "b" and "c" above) is multiplied by the utility. "According to the model, the individual will choose the alternative that has the higher SEU [subjective expected utility] value and hence, in this situation, the one that is associated with the *lower* subjective probability of occurrence of the unpleasant consequence" (Sutton, 1982, p. 326). Tests of this model were generally unsupportive (e.g., Sutton & Eiser, 1984; Sutton & Hallett, 1989). For example, Sutton and Eiser (1984) note "no evidence for the multiplicative combination of utilities and subjective probabilities" (p. 14).

Protection motivation theory. The theoretical framework for most fear appeal research since 1975 is Rogers' (1975, 1983) PMT. Rogers (1975,1983) advanced fear appeal research by specifying the message components and cognitive processes related to fear appeals. PMT focuses exclusively on Leventhal's (1970) danger control process (i.e., thoughts about the danger or threat and how to prevent it); fear control processes are not addressed. In PMT (Figure 19.1), four message components are proposed to cause corresponding cognitive mediation processes: (a) probability of oc-

Figure 19.1

Original Protection Motivation Theory, With Self-Efficacy Added

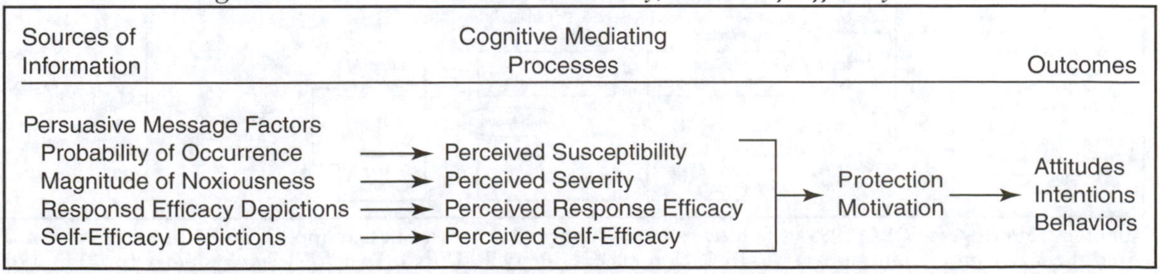

Sources of Information | Cognitive Mediating Processes | Outcomes

Persuasive Message Factors
Probability of Occurrence → Perceived Susceptibility
Magnitude of Noxiousness → Perceived Severity
Responsd Efficacy Depictions → Perceived Response Efficacy
Self-Efficacy Depictions → Perceived Self-Efficacy
→ Protection Motivation → Attitudes, Intentions, Behaviors

Adapted from Rogers (1975) and Maddux and Rogers (1983).

currence depictions in a message lead to perceived susceptibility; (b) magnitude of noxiousness in the appeal produces perceived severity; (c) descriptions of the effectiveness of the recommended response result in perceived response efficacy; and (d) characterizations of an individual's ability to perform the recommended response produce perceived self-efficacy. The first three components were outlined in Rogers' (1975) original description of PMT. Bandura's (1977) work on self-efficacy, and Beck and Frankel's (1981) delineation of personal versus response efficacy prompted Maddux and Rogers (1983) to add the last component (self-efficacy).[3]

These cognitive mediation processes are said to elicit protection motivation, the determinant of danger control actions. Protection motivation "is an intervening variable that has the typical characteristics of a motive: It arouses, sustains, and directs activity" (Rogers, 1975, p. 98) and it is operationalized as intentions (Rogers, 1983). When each of the four PMT variables is at a high level, then maximum protection motivation, and subsequent message acceptance, is proposed to occur. PMT studies have most consistently found two-way interactions between one of the threat variables (i.e., severity or susceptibility) and one of the efficacy variables (i.e., response efficacy or self-efficacy) (e.g., Kleinot & Rogers, 1982; Maddux & Rogers, 1983; Rogers & Mewborn, 1976). However, specific interactions between the four variables have proven difficult to predict (e.g., Rogers, 1985). For example, sometimes susceptibility interacts with response efficacy (Rogers & Mewborn, 1976, smoking experiment), while other times severity interacts with self-efficacy to influence behaviors (Wurtele & Maddux, 1987).

In a reformulation of PMT (Figure 19.2), Rogers (1983) extended the model into one that differentiates between maladaptive threat appraisal and adaptive coping appraisal processes. In the threat appraisal process, Rogers (1983) says people may continue to engage in maladaptive behaviors (e.g., unsafe sex) if the rewards of performing the maladaptive behavior (e.g., pleasure, social approval) are greater than the perceived severity of the danger (e.g., AIDS is fetal) and their perceived susceptibility to the danger (e.g., increased risk of HIV contraction). Thus, increases in rewards heighten the probability of a maladaptive response while increases in perceived threat (severity/susceptibility) decrease the probability of a maladaptive response (Prentice-Dunn & Rogers, 1986). For the coping appraisal, increases in perceived response/self-efficacy increase the likelihood of adaptive behavior while increases in response costs decrease the likelihood of adaptive behavior. For example, people may choose to perform the adaptive behavior (e.g., use condoms) if perceived response efficacy (e.g., "condoms are effective protectors against AIDS") and perceived self-efficacy (e.g., "I'm able to use condoms to effectively prevent AIDS") are greater than response costs (e.g., time, expense, difficulty). It is

Figure 19.2
The Current Formulation of Protection Motivation Theory

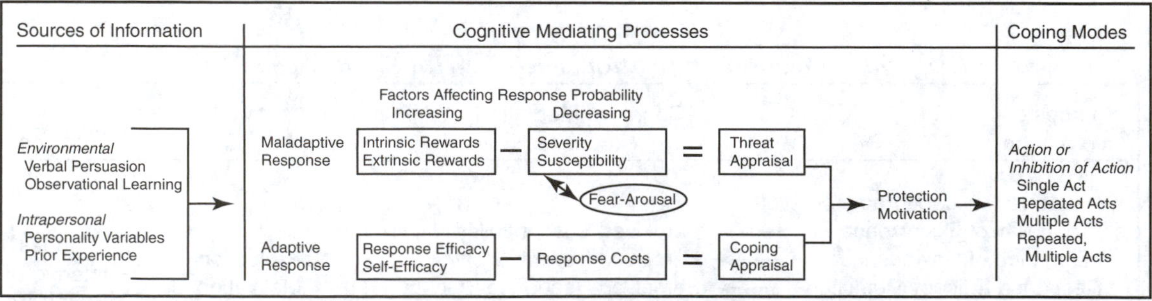

Adapted from Rogers, R.W. (1983). Cognitive and physiological processes in fear appeals and attitude change: A revised theory of protection motivation. In Cacioppo, J., & Petty, R. (Eds.), *Social Psychophysiology* (pp. 153–176). Copyright by Guilford Press, New York. Reprinted with permission.

important to note that in both original and current PMT, fear is given a backseat role. Specifically, fear is predicted to "only indirectly" affect message acceptance "through the appraisal of severity" (Rogers, 1983, p. 169). Rogers and colleagues have produced some support for this proposition (e.g., Rippetoe & Rogers, 1987; Rogers & Mewborn, 1976).

Analysis of the current PMT model. There are two key problems with the current PMT model (Figure 19.2). First, empirical inconsistencies exist between what the revised model predicts (Figure 19.2), and what is found empirically. For instance, Figure 19.2 shows that factors *increasing* the likelihood of an adaptive response are greater response/self-efficacy beliefs coupled with fewer response costs, and "factors *decreasing* the probability of the occurrence of the maladaptive response (i.e., punishers) are the severity of the threat and the expectancy of being exposed to the threat" coupled with reduced intrinsic/extrinsic rewards (Rogers, 1983, p. 169, italics added). Thus, according to Figure 19.2, *increases* in perceptions of susceptibility/severity (with few rewards) should *decrease the likelihood of a maladaptive response, even if efficacy is held constant at a line level* (as long as efficacy is greater than response costs).

However, the empirical literature indicates the opposite of this derived prediction. Namely, if perceived efficacy is low, then increases in perceived threat result in *increases* in maladaptive behaviors (e.g., Kleinot & Rogers, 1982; Rogers & Mewborn, 1976; Witte, 1992). Indeed, Rogers (1983) writes that if perceived efficacy is low, increases in perceived threat will "either have no effect or a boomerang effect" (p. 170). But, the formal model (i.e., Figure 19.2) suggests exactly the opposite. In short, it is not possible to derive nor explain boomerang predictions from the revised graphic PMT model.

Second, logical flaws exist between the proposed relations of some of the PMT variables. For example, even though Rogers (1983) proposes a multiplicative relationship between threat appraisal and coping appraisal, the PMT does not provide explicit mechanisms to explain how threat appraisal (i.e., rewards minus severity/susceptibility) and coping appraisal (i.e., efficacy minus costs) *work together* to influence protection motivation and subsequent behavior. How does the combination of these separate appraisal processes elicit protection motivation and behaviors? Rogers (1983) does specify what will happen in one situation. Namely, if both threat appraisal and coping appraisal are high, then there should be decreases in maladaptive behaviors, and increases in adaptive behaviors (maximum protection motivation) (Rogers, 1983, p. 171). This scenario is logically consistent in that increases in adaptive behaviors (e.g., increased safer sex practices) coupled with decreases in maladaptive behaviors (e.g., decreased unsafe sex practices) should yield congruent responses—safer sex practices. However, the following scenario, which is derived from the revised PMT model, lacks logical consistency. According to Figure 19.2, if coping appraisal is high (greater efficacy over costs) there should be increases in adaptive behaviors (e.g., quitting cigarette smoking), and if threat appraisal is low (greater rewards over severity/susceptibility) there should be no changes in maladaptive behaviors (e.g., continuing cigarette smoking). Logically, however, how can one quit smoking cigarettes (increase adaptive behaviors) while at the same time continue smoking cigarettes (no change in maladaptive behaviors)?

In sum, the current PMT model (a) yields derived predictions that are inconsistent with the empirical data, and (b) does not explain why or how an interaction between threat appraisal and coping appraisal occurs, or how the interaction is related to protection motivation and subsequent behaviors. In contrast, the original PMT (with self-efficacy added), does an excellent job explaining factors leading to message acceptance. In addition, the original PMT model does not suffer from the logical and empirical inconsistencies of the revised model. However, both PMT models fail to explain the specific factors leading to message rejection.

The Lost Role of Fear in Fear Appeals

As one examines the evolutionary development of fear appeal theories, it is striking to note the declining role of fear. Dillard (1992) noted that in the drive models, "fear was at the center of the theoretical stage" (p. 13). However, as the cognitive revolution in psychology took hold, the importance of fear faded so much that by the time PMT and Sutton's SEU model gained popularity: "Fear was virtually excluded from the study of fear appeals. In the most recent investigations based strongly on the cognitive perspective, fear has been treated as a control variable (e.g., Sutton & Eiser, 1984; Wolf, Gregory, & Stephan, 1986), if it is measured at all (e.g., Rogers, 1985; Self & Rogers, 1990)" (Dillard, 1992, p. 13). The following analysis argues that fear should play a central role in theoretical explanations.

Development of the Extended Parallel Process Model

The inconsistencies in the empirical literature indicate that the fear appeal puzzle has yet to be solved. The overemphasis on cognitions in current theories, coupled with the relative neglect of emotions, are potential reasons for the lack of convergent findings. Few theoretical leaps have been made since Rogers (1975, 1983) published PMT. The theory proposed here, called the Extended Parallel Process Model (EPPM), uses Leventhal's (1970) parallel process model as the overall framework (hence, the *extended* parallel process model) to differentiate between two processes, danger control and fear control. Beck and Frankel (1981) noted that the parallel process model is the most broad of the fear appeal theories and although virtually untestable, offers a nice framework in which to further theorize. Rogers (1975) did just this when he defined and clarified the danger control processes in his original PMT (Figure 19.1). However, current theories fail to explain why fear appeals are rejected.

The EPPM picks up where the original PMT left off. Specifically, the EPPM adopts the original PMTs explanation of danger control processes that lead to message acceptance (one side of the parallel process model), and defines and expands the fear control processes which lead to message rejection (the other side of the parallel process model). To give readers a basic understanding of the theory as a whole, an overview will be given first, followed by a detailed explication.

Overview of the EPPM

As an overview, consider what happens when a person is presented with a fear appeal depicting the components of threat (i.e., severity and susceptibility), and the components of efficacy (i.e., response efficacy and self-efficacy) (Figure 19.3). A fear appeal initiates two appraisals in the cognitive encoder (i.e., individual).[4] First, persons appraise the perceived threat of the hazard. If the appraisal of threat results in moderate to high perceived threat, then fear is elicited (Easterling & Leventhal, 1989; Lang, 1984) and people are motivated to begin the second appraisal, which is an evaluation of the efficacy of the recommended response. When the threat is perceived as low (i.e., trivial or irrelevant), there is no motivation to process the message further; efficacy is not evaluated and there is no response to the fear appeal.

When both perceived threat and perceived efficacy are high, danger control processes are initiated. When people fear an applicable and significant threat, *and* when they perceive a response that would feasibly and effectively avert the threat, they are motivated to control the danger (protection motivation) by thinking of strategies to avert the threat (adaptive outcomes). When danger control processes are dominating, *individuals respond to the danger, not to their fear.* Conversely, when perceived threat is high, but perceived efficacy is low, fear control processes are initiated. The fear originally evoked by the personally relevant and significant threat becomes intensified when individuals believe they are unable to effectively deter the threat. Thus, they become motivated to cope with their fear (defensive motivation) by engaging in maladaptive responses (e.g., denial). When fear control processes are dominating, *individuals respond to their fear, not to the danger.*

Fear may contribute to the motivation to process a message *if* it is cognitively appraised (see feedback loop in Figure 19.3). That is, thinking about the threatening mes-

Figure 19.3
The Extended Parallel Process Model (EPPM)

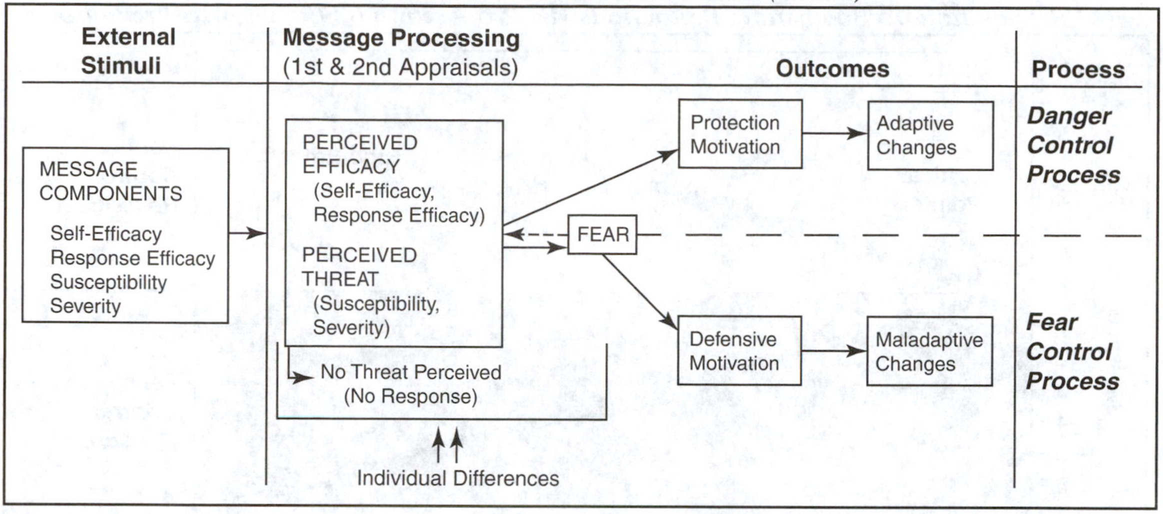

sage may first contribute to the experience of fear, and experiencing fear may then cause a person to upgrade his or her estimates of the threat. Fear causes maladaptive responses, and may indirectly influence adaptive responses, as mediated by perceived threat. In short, *perceived threat determines the degree or intensity of the reaction to the message, while perceived efficacy determines the nature of the reaction* (i.e., which process is initiated—danger control or fear control) (cf. Lazarus, 1991a, 1991b, 1991c; Lazarus & Folkman, 1984).

Individual differences influence the appraisal of threat and efficacy. Each person evaluates the components of a message in relation to his or her prior experiences, culture, and personality characteristics. Thus, the same fear appeal may produce different perceptions in different people, thereby influencing subsequent outcomes. For example, if one individual perceives high threat and low efficacy from a message, and the other individual perceives high threat and high efficacy from the same message, then the former would be expected to engage in fear control processes, while the latter would be expected to engage in danger control processes.

Detailed Explication of the EPPM

The EPPM proposes that threat initiates and motivates message processing because the greater the threat, the greater the fear aroused, the more attention-getting the message (through depictions of the significance of the severity), and the more involving the message (through depictions of susceptibility). (Many researchers have noted the crucial role of involvement in persuasion, e.g., Johnson & Eagly, 1989; Petty & Cacioppo, 1986.) If perceptions of threat are low, then people are not motivated to continue message processing, because the threat is perceived as either irrelevant or trivial.

> *Proposition 1. When perceived threat is low, regardless of perceived efficacy level, there will be no further processing of the message.*

Thus, there is no response to the fear appeal because the message is not processed any further. Figure 19.4 illustrates that when perceptions of threat are low, there is little or no message acceptance in both efficacy conditions. Witte (1991) found the least amount of attitude, intention, and behavior change in the low threat condition, regardless of efficacy level.

Once a threat has been determined to exist by a person, efficacy is evaluated. Perceived efficacy is the crucial variable that determines which parallel process will dom-

Figure 19.4
Hypothetical Results Patterns of the Different Parallel Processes (A) Proposition 4's Boomerang Predictions (B) Proposition 6's Curvilinear Predictions

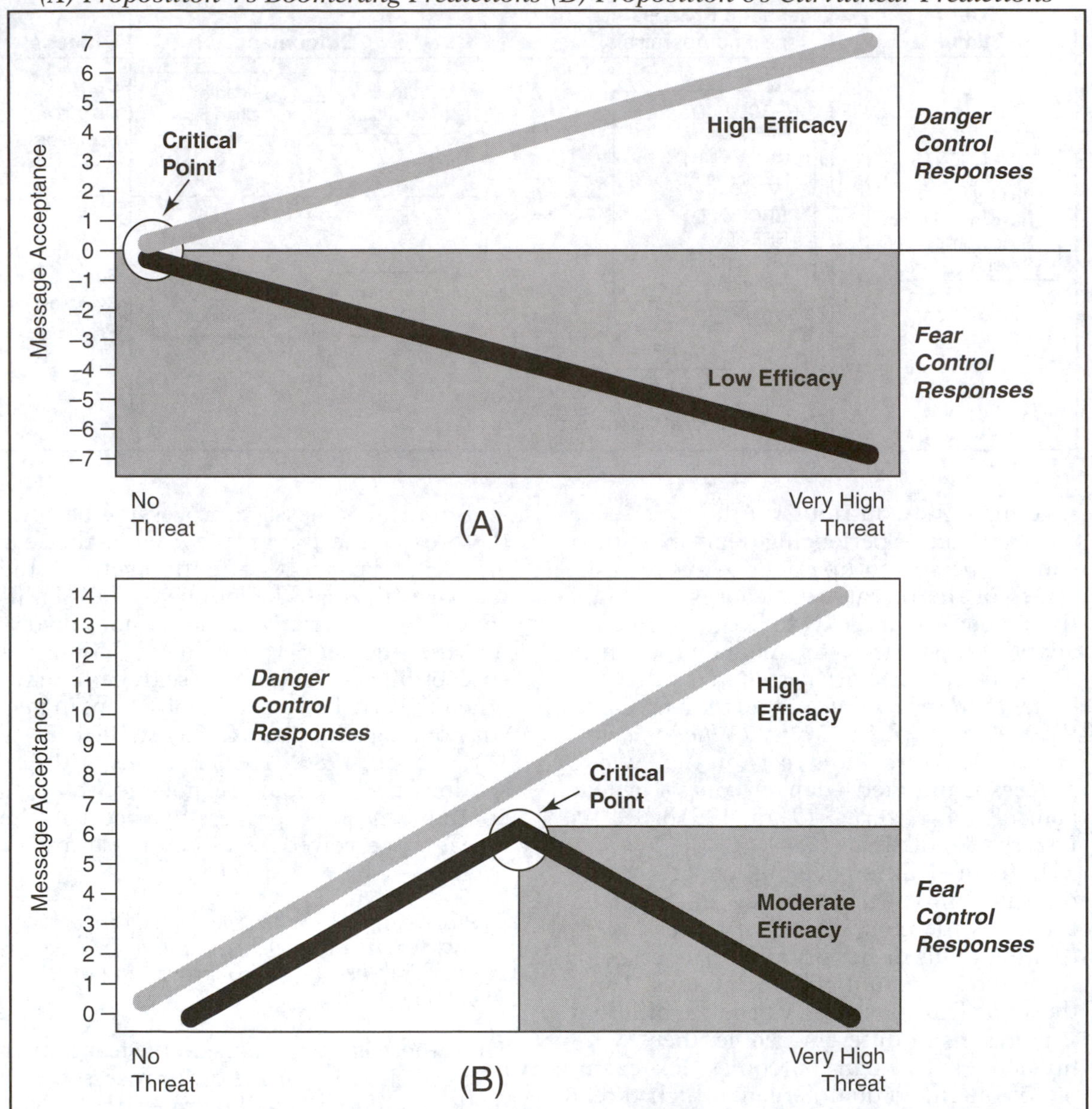

inate. Thus, perceived efficacy interacts with perceived threat to influence individuals' responses to fear appeals (Job, 1988; Rogers, 1975, 1983). Much accumulated evidence demonstrates the robust interaction between at least one perceived threat dimension (i.e., susceptibility or severity) and one perceived efficacy dimension (i.e., response efficacy or self-efficacy) (e.g., Beck & Lund, 1981; Kleinot & Rogers, 1982; Maddux & Rogers, 1983; Mulilis & Lippa, 1990; Rogers & Mewborn, 1976; Witte, 1991; Wurtele & Maddux, 1987). However, many studies not addressing this construct have yielded conflicting findings (e.g., Kohn et al., 1982; Krisher, Darley, & Darley, 1973).

The EPPM proposes that the lack of attention to the efficacy construct is the key reason for the inconsistency. For instance, regardless of whether the efficacy construct is explicitly addressed in a fear appeal study, every fear appeal message has an inherent level of efficacy that may inadvertently influence study outcomes. For example, the efficacy construct was not addressed in the following two studies, which had very different outcomes. Ramirez and Lasater (1976) found positive linear effects in their fear appeal study, where each message had a whole section on response and self-efficacy (e.g., the message "illustrated the correct use of a dental kit containing a toothbrush, disclosing wafers, fluoride dentrifice, and dental floss" [p. 812]). In contrast, boomerang results emerged in Kohn et al.'s (1982) study on drinking and driving, where apparently no explicit recommendation was given to avert the threat. Therefore, positive linear findings should be found in studies with strong efficacy depictions, and boomerang findings should be found in studies with weak or missing efficacy depictions. Overall, the KPPM claims that perceived efficacy determines whether danger control processes or fear control processes are initiated, and perceived threat determines the intensity of these responses.

Danger control processes. Danger control processes are primarily cognitive processes where individuals evaluate their susceptibility to the threat, the severity of the threat, their ability to perform the recommended response (perceived self-efficacy), and the effectiveness of the recommended response (perceived response efficacy). Danger control cognitions are deliberate and complex in nature—changing behavior requires intentional and volitional thought (Bargh, 1989; Lazarus, 1991a, 1991b). Danger control processes appear to work as Rogers (1975) specified in his original PMT (with self-efficacy added). That is, when perceived efficacy (i.e., perceived response efficacy and perceived self-efficacy) and perceived threat (i.e., comprised of perceived severity and perceived susceptibility) are both high, protection motivation is elicited, and individuals make adaptive changes (see Figure 19.4).

> *Proposition 2. As perceived threat increases when perceived efficacy is high, so will message acceptance.*

People (a) realize they are at risk for a severe danger and become motivated to protect themselves (high threat), (b) they believe they can prevent the danger (high efficacy), and (c) they deliberately and cognitively confront the danger (e.g., "When I'm with my boyfriend next time, I'm going to talk to him about using condoms"). Many investigators have found that fear appeals with high levels of perceived threat (e.g., "I am susceptible to heart attacks because I have elevated cholesterol") *and* high levels of perceived efficacy (e.g., "I am able to change my diet, which will effectively decrease my cholesterol") produce message acceptance (e.g., Kleinot & Rogers, 1982; Maddux & Rogers, 1983; Rogers & Mewborn, 1976; Witte, 1992). The cognitions occurring in the danger control processes stimulate adaptive actions such as attitude, intention, or behavior changes that control the danger.

> *Proposition 3. Cognitions about threat and efficacy cause attitude, intention, or behavior changes (i.e., adaptive responses).*

Fear control processes. Fear control processes are defined as primarily emotional processes where people respond to and cope with their fear, not to the danger. Fear control processes are more automatic and involuntary in nature and may occur outside our conscious awareness (Bargh, 1989; Lazarus, 1991a). Automatic or unconscious information processing is characterized by at least two conditions: (a) individuals are unaware of when or "how such processing occurs," and (b) individuals are "unable to inhibit or control these processes once they have begun" (Branscombe, 1987, p. 15). If one's well-being is threatened by a perceived unavoidable threat, then unconscious or automatic defense mechanisms may be activated to protect the individual from further distress (Lazarus, 1991a). For example, some have argued that there is "full semantic identification [of information] prior to conscious perception" (Erdelyi, 1974, p. 18). Furthermore, perceptual defense research has demonstrated that if too much "anxiety is evoked at an early stage, further recognition processes are impeded and the later stages may never emerge" (Gleitman, 1981, p. 481). While some fear may be aroused from the initial appraisal of threat, it is the heightened and intensified fear resulting from the perception of low efficacy/high threat together that automatically activates defensive motivation and results in maladaptive outcomes (see bottom portion of Figure 19.4a).

> *Proposition 4. As perceived threat increases when perceived efficacy is low, people will do the opposite of what is advocated (boomerang).*

To control the overwhelming fear stemming from a high perceived threat/low perceived efficacy situation, people either consciously or unconsciously deny the threat or react against the message (e.g., "you can't believe all of those studies anyway, they're just trying to manipulate us"), and do even more of the forbidden behavior to reduce fear or anxiety (e.g., increase cigarette smoking, misuse alcohol). Implicit support for proposition 4 can be found in studies demonstrating that high perceived threat (e.g., "I am susceptible to heart attacks because I have elevated cholesterol") coupled with low perceived efficacy (e.g., "there's no way I can change my diet, and even if I did, my cholesterol reading probably wouldn't change anyway") results in message rejection and boomerang responses (e.g., Kleinot & Rogers, 1982; Rippetoe & Rogers, 1987; Rogers & Mewborn, 1976; Witte, 1992).

The critical point. As long as perceptions of efficacy are greater than perceptions of threat (e.g., "I know that AIDS is a terrible threat, but I can protect myself by using condoms correctly"), danger control processes will dominate and the message will be accepted. However, at some *critical point,* where persons perceive that they cannot prevent a serious threat from occurring, either because the response is perceived as ineffective or they believe they are incapable of performing the recommendation (e.g., "AIDS is terrible and easy to get; I don't think I can do anything to prevent contraction"), fear control responses will begin to dominate. Thus, (a) the critical point occurs when perceived threat exceeds perceived efficacy (see Figures 19.4a and 19.4b), and (b) this critical point is where fear control processes begin to dominate over danger control processes.

Overall, fear control responses (defensive avoidance, perceived manipulation) would be expected to interfere with danger control responses (attitude, intention, behavior change). If people are thinking of ways to change their behaviors, they are not defensively avoiding the threat. Conversely, if persons are defensively avoiding the threat, they are not thinking of ways to protect themselves.

> *Proposition 5. Maladaptive responses will be inversely related to adaptive responses.*

In addition, when perceived efficacy is at a moderate level, the critical point may not occur immediately, but at some moderate level of threat. For example, when perceived efficacy is at a moderate level, people may initially believe that they can prevent the threat. But as the threat increases in magnitude and relevance, individuals may begin to give up any hopes of averting the threat. Thus:

> *Proposition 6. As perceived threat increases when perceived efficacy is moderate, will first increase, and then decrease, resulting in an inverted U-shape function.*

Figure 19.4 depicts possible results patterns. In both Figures 19.4a and 19.4b, the critical point (where perceived threat exceeds perceived efficacy) is never reached in the high efficacy condition, so message acceptance is positive and linear (proposition 2). However, in the low efficacy condition, the critical point occurs immediately (Figure 19.4a; proposition 4). In the moderate efficacy condition, the critical point is reached at a moderate level of threat (Figure 19.4b; proposition 6). Up to the critical point, danger control responses would be expected to prevail. Once the critical point is reached, however, fear control processes would be expected to dominate. The area encompassing fear control responses (the shaded area) is dependent on where the critical point is located. The propositions offer specific guidelines for prediction. In general, the point that perceived threat surpasses perceived efficacy (i.e., the critical point) is likely to be dependent on a variety of factors including the study topic or individual differences.

The role of fear. Discussions about fear have been noticeably absent from recent fear appeal theories. As stated previously, fear is aroused when a significant and relevant threat has been perceived (Easterling & Leventhal, 1989). The EPPM proposes that message threat causes an appraisal of a threat, and the appraisal of a threat causes fear (i.e., message threat → perceived threat → fear). Perceptions of efficacy determine what happens when fear is aroused. If efficacy is believed to be low, fear is increased further. Defensive motivation will be elicited due to the overwhelming fear generated by this high perceived threat/low perceived efficacy condition, and maladaptive responses will ensue (again, it is probable that this occurs automatically, without conscious awareness). Thus, fear is a direct cause of maladaptive responses (i.e., message threat → perceived threat → fear → maladaptive outcomes). Empirical support for this proposition is offered in Rippetoe and Rogers (1987), where fear was found to directly increase avoidance coping patterns.

> *Proposition 7. Fear causes maladaptive responses.*

If efficacy is perceived as high, aroused fear will be cognitively assessed and will influence perceptions of threat (i.e., a nonrecursive relationship), thereby *indirectly* influencing adaptive outcomes (i.e., message threat → perceived threat → fear → increased perceived threat → adaptive outcomes). That is, a message leads to the appraisal of a threat, which causes fear. If perceived efficacy is greater than perceived threat, fear will be cognitively appraised as a situational cue, and will lead an individual to upgrade his or her estimate of the threat (i.e., increased perceived threat). Janis and Mann (1977) note that "every physical symptom a person notices in himself [or herself] constitutes a warning signal" (p. 66). For example, a person might process a fear appeal in the following manner (O'Keefe, 1990): (a) "I'm now aware of the consequences of cigarette smoking" (cognitive representation of the threat); (b) "And, this scares me—my heart is racing" (fear arousal; cognitive appraisal of the fear); (c) "Gee, the consequences of cigarette smoking are probably worse than I thought" (further cognitions about the threat); and (d) "I'm going to think of ways to quit smoking" (adaptive response). This proposition is empirically plausible in that Rogers and Mewborn (1976) found that fear affected perceived severity (a cognition about threat), which in turn affected intentions (an adaptive outcome), but fear arousal did not predict intentions directly. Therefore:

> *Proposition 8. When perceived efficacy is high, fear indirectly influences adaptive outcomes, as mediated by perceived threat.*

In addition, the relation between perceived threat and fear is proposed to be nonrecursive (i.e., bidirectional) when efficacy beliefs outweigh threat beliefs (see Figure 19.3, feedback loop).

> *Proposition 9. When perceived efficacy is high, there is a reciprocal relationship between perceived threat and fear.*

An analysis of empirical findings with these propositions in mind helps to reconcile some of the literature. For example, the studies measuring or inducing actual physiological arousal found no direct relation between fear arousal and adaptive outcomes (Mewborn & Rogers, 1979; Rogers & Deckner, 1975).

However, fear induced through *false* feedback techniques did change attitudes (Giesen & Hendrick, 1974; Hendrick, Giesen, & Borden, 1975). Thus, when fear was cognitively appraised (i.e., people were told through false feedback that they were aroused), it contributed to message acceptance.

Boster and Mongeau's (1984; Mongeau, 1991) meta-analysis of fear appeals also offers support for the proposed indirect relationship between fear and adaptive outcomes. Boster and Mongeau (1984) reported that the correlation between fear arousal and attitudes was $r = .21$, and the relation between fear arousal and behavior was $r = .10$. They suggested that one reason for these modest correlations was that the fear manipulations were too weak to properly induce a range of fear arousal. Alternatively, the EPPM suggests that fear and attitudes/behaviors are modestly correlated because an underlying variable, perceived threat, explains the relationship between them. For example, the EPPM (Figure 19.3) posits the following relationships when perceived efficacy is high: Message threat → perceived threat → fear → increased perceived threat → adaptive outcomes. Thus, a simplified EPPM path model, illustrating the indirect relationship between fear and adaptive outcomes, as mediated by perceived threat when perceived efficacy is high, would be depicted as fear (X) → perceived threat (Y) → adaptive outcomes (Z).

Kenny and colleagues (Baron & Kenny, 1986; Judd & Kenny, 1981) provide three criteria tor establishing the existence of a mediational relationship: (a) X and Y must be correlated (fear and perceived threat); (b) X and Z must be correlated (fear and attitudes/behaviors); and (c) if one correlates X and Z, while controlling for Y (removing Y's influence), then the relationship between X and Z should disappear if Y is a mediator. The literature indicates that all three criteria have been met in terms of the indirect influence of fear on adaptive outcomes, as mediated by perceived threat. First, Rippetoe and Rogers (1987) showed that fear and perceived threat are associated. Second, Boster and Mongeau's (1984) meta-analysis demonstrated that fear is related to adaptive outcomes (i.e., attitudes and behaviors). Third, a study by Rogers and Mewborn (1976) showed that the relationship between fear and intentions vanished when controlling for perceived threat. Thus, Boster and Mongeau (1984) may have discovered positive correlations between fear and attitudes/behaviors, because these variables are indirectly related, as mediated by perceived threat when perceived efficacy is high. Overall, fear does not directly cause adaptive changes, but fear can influence adaptive changes when it is mediated by perceived threat in high perceived efficacy conditions.[5]

One final comment about the role of fear and cognitions is in order. It is important to note that one can experience tear in danger control processes, and one can have thoughts in fear control processes—although fear is not necessary for danger control processes and cognitions are not necessary for fear control processes. However, the explicit relationships are specified as:

Proposition 10. Cognitions about efficacy are unrelated to maladaptive responses

Because perceived threat causes fear.

Proposition 11. Cognitions about threat are indirectly related to maladaptive responses.

Individual differences. Individual differences are likely to influence the appraisals of threat and efficacy, which will then affect the critical point at which individuals begin to cope with fear, instead of danger. Research has indicated that people who are high anxious, lack coping skills, have low self-esteem, or feel highly vulnerable to the threat are more likely to engage in maladaptive responses (i.e., fear control processes) when faced with a strong fear appeal than those who are not anxious, have high self-esteem, or do not feel vulnerable to the threat (e.g., Boster & Mongeau, 1984; Dabbs & Leventhal, 1966; Hale & Mongeau, 1991; Janis & Feshbach, 1954; Kornzweig, 1967; Leventhal & Trembly, 1968; Leventhal & Watts, 1966; Niles, 1964; Rosen, Terry, & Leventhal, 1982). In addition, people who can be classified as repressors, poor copers, or avoiders, tend to reject strong fear appeals, while those who are sensitizers or good copers tend to accept strong fear appeals (e.g., Dziokonski & Weber, 1977; Goldstein, 1959; Hill & Gardner, 1980; Self & Rogers, 1990). Thus, according to the EPPM, low self-esteem persons may appraise a message recommendation to be unfeasible and ineffective, while high self-esteem persons might appraise the same message recommendation as being effective and easy to do. As perceived threat increases, low self-esteem persons might be more likely to engage in fear control processes because the high perceived threat/low perceived efficacy condition has been met, while high self-esteem persons might be more likely to engage in danger control processes because they perceive both efficacy and threat as high. In summary, dispositional characteristics are posited to affect the appraisal of threat or efficacy and thereby influence the subsequent initiation of danger control or fear control processes.

Conclusion

The EPPM expands on previous approaches in three ways: (a) it explains why fear appeals fail; (b) it re-incorporates fear as a central variable; and (c) it specifies the relationship between threat and efficacy in prepositional forms. It is believed that the reconceptualized and expanded version of Leventhal's (1970) parallel process model offers a better and more precise explanation of fear appeal message processing than Rogers' PMT or Leventhal's parallel process model by themselves. In short, the EPPM consolidates earlier theoretical views by arguing that fear leads to message rejection (as Janis, 1967, argued) and cognitions (i.e., perceived threat and efficacy) lead to message acceptance (as Leventhal, 1970, and Rogers, 1975, 1983, suggest).

The original PMTs explication of danger control processes is diagrammed in the top portion of the EPPM (Figure 19.3). That is, message threat results in the cognitive mediators of perceived threat (beliefs about severity and susceptibility) and perceived efficacy (beliefs about response efficacy and self-efficacy), which elicit protection motivation, and adaptive responses, if both threat and efficacy are perceived as high. However, the EPPM departs from PMT after this point. Unlike PMT, the EPPM specifies the variables and processes leading to maladaptive responses, which PMT does not do. Specifically, the EPPM argues that high fear, first caused by high perceived threat, and then intensified by low perceived efficacy, elicits defensive motivation, which induces maladaptive outcomes. The EPPM demonstrates that fear directly causes maladaptive responses, but that fear can be indirectly related to adaptive responses, as long as it is cognitively appraised. In sum, threat determines the degree or intensity of the response, while efficacy determines the nature of the response.

Overall, fear appeals have great potential for stimulating behavioral change—if used correctly. The principles set forth in the present work are offered as guidelines for their effective use. These ideas now await empirical testing.

Endnotes

1. It is important to note that Mewborn and Rogers (1979) were more interested in the *pattern* of findings for physiological arousal and self-rated fear (e.g., the high fear condition yields a consistent pattern which is different from the low fear condition), than in the correlation between the two, which was actually quite modest.
2. While not a fear appeal theory, per se, one additional theoretical approach to fear appeals is language expectancy theory (Burgoon, 1990; Burgoon & Miller, 1985; Miller, 1963). Burgoon and Miller (1985) outlined research showing that expectations may have been negatively violated and persuasiveness inhibited when strong fear appeals were used by low credibility speakers (Hewgill & Miller, 1965; Miller & Hewgill, 1966). In contrast, they noted that strong fear appeals were successful when given by high credibility speakers, who presumably did not negatively violate expectations because they were allowed greater latitude in their language choices. Few fear appeal researchers have considered the potentially important role of expectancy violations in their research.
3. Readers will notice similarities between the PMT and the health belief model (Janz & Becker, 1984; Rosenstock, 1974). Prentice-Dunn and Rogers (1986) discuss the differences between the two.
4. Knowledge and appraisal are both forms of cognition. Knowledge consists of attributions and "what a person believes about the way the world works in general and in a specific context," while appraisal "is an evaluation of the personal significance of what is happening" (Lazarus, 1991a, p. 154). Cognitive appraisal can, and often does, occur automatically, involuntarily, effortlessly, and outside our awareness (Bargh, 1989; Langer, 1989; Lazarus, 1991a). See Buck (1984) and Zajonc (1980, 1984) for additional views.
5. An alternative explanation for the relationship between fear. perceived threat, and adaptive outcomes is that fear may be spuriously related to adaptive outcomes, simply because it also is related to perceived threat. Unfortunately, with current statistical methods, "the mediated and spurious relation-

ship are indistinguishable and thus are tested for in the same manner . . . thus, distinguishing these two models from one another must be done on the basis of *substantive or theoretical reasons*" (Levine & Cruz, in press). One study did find a direct path from fear to intention based on the subjective expected utility (SEl) model, but this was based on a path analysis that did not include the perceived threat construct or the variables of perceived susceptibility or perceived severity (Sutton & Eiser, 1984). Thus, the model may have had a very poor fit (no model fit estimates were given) because it was missing important constructs. The EPPM would suggest that if perceived threat were included in this model, then the relation between fear and intentions would be mediated by perceived threat.

References

Bandura, A. (1977). Self-efficacy: Toward a unifying theory of behavioral change. *Psychological Review, 84,*191–215.

Bargh, J. A. (1989). Conditional automaticity: Varieties of automatic influence in social perception and cognition. In J. S. Uleman & J. A. Bargh (Eds.). *Unintended thought* (pp. 3–51). New York: Guilford Press.

Baron, R. M., & Kenny, D. A. (1986). The moderator-mediator variable distinction in social psychological research: Conceptual, strategic, and statistical considerations. *Journal of Personality and Social Psychology, 6,* 1175–1182.

Beck, K. H. (1984). The effects of risk probability, outcome severity, efficacy of protection and access to protection on decision making: A further test of Protection Motivation Theory. *Social Behavior and Personality, 12,* 121–125.

Beck, K. H., & Frankel, A. (1981). A conceptualization of threat communications and protective health behavior. *Social Psychology Quarterly, 44,* 204–217.

Beck, K. H., & Lund, A. K. (1981). The effects of health threat seriousness and personal efficacy upon intentions and behavior. *Journal of Applied Social Psychology, 11,* 401–405.

Ben-Sira, Z. (1981). Latent fear-arousing potential of fear-moderating and fear-neutral health promoting information. *Social Science and Medicine, 15e,* 105–112.

Boster, F. J., & Mongeau, P. (1984). Fear-arousing persuasive messages. In R. N. Bostrom & B. H. Westley (Eds.), *Communication yearbook 8* (pp. 330–375). Newbury Park. CA: Sage.

Branscombe, N. R. (1987). Conscious and unconscious processing of cognitive and affective information. In K. Fiedler & J. Forgas (Eds.), *Affect, cognition, and social behavior* (pp. 3–24). Toronto: CJ Hogrefe.

Brehm, J. W. (1966). *A theory of reactance.* New York: Academic Press.

Buck, R. F. (1984). *The communication of emotion.* New York: Guilford Press.

Burgoon, M. (1990). Language and influence. In H. Giles & W. P. Robinson (Eds.), *Handbook of language and social psychology* (pp. 51–72). New York: John Wiley & Sons.

Burgoon, M., & Miller, G. R. (1985). An expectancy interpretation of language and persuasion. In H. Giles & R. St. Clair (Eds.), *Recent advance in language, communication, and social psychology* (pp. 199–229). London: Eribaum.

Burnett, J. J. (1981). Internal-external focus of control as a moderator of fear appeals. *Journal of Applied Psychology, 66,* 390–393.

Burnett, J. J., & Oliver, R. L. (1979). Fear appeal effects in the field: A segmentation approach. *Journal of Marketing Research, 16,* 181–190.

Dabbs, J. M., & Leventhal, H. (1966). Effects of varying the recommendations in a fear-arousing communication. *Journal of Personality and Social Psychology, 4,* 525–531.

Dillard, J. P. (1992). *Rethinking the study of fear appeals.* Manuscript under review.

Dziokonski, W., & Weber, S. J. (1977). Repression-sensitization, perceived vulnerability, and the fear appeal communication. *The Journal of Social Psychology, 102,* 105–112.

Easterling, D. V., & Leventhal, H. (1989). Contribution of concrete cognition to emotion: Neutral symptoms as elicitors of worry about cancer. *Journal of Applied Psychology, 74,* 787–796.

Edwards, W. (1961). Behavioral decision theory. *Annual Review of Psychology, 12,* 473–498.

Erdelyi, M. H. (1974). A new look at the new look: Perceptual defense and vigilance. *Psychological Review, 81,* 1–25.

Giesen, M. F., & Hendrick, C. (1974). Effects of false positive and negative arousal feedback on persuasion. *Journal of Personality and Social Psychology, 4,* 449–457.

Gleitman, H. (1981). *Psychology.* NY: W.W. Norton.

Goldstein, M. J. (1959). The relationship between coping and avoiding behavior and response to fear-arousing propaganda. *Journal of Abnormal and Social Psychology, 58,* 247–252.

Hale, J., & Mongeau, P. (1991, May). *Testing a causal model of the persuasive impact of fear appeals.* Paper presented at the annual meeting of the International Communication Association, Chicago.

Hendrick, C., Giesen, M., & Borden, R. (1975). False physiological feedback and persuasion: Effect of fear arousal vs. fear reduction on attitude change. *Journal of Personality, 43,* 196–214.

Hewgill, M. A., & Miller, G. R. (1965). Source credibility and response to fear-arousing communications. *Speech Monographs, 32,* 95–101.

Higbee, K. L. (1969). Fifteen years of fear arousal: Research on threat appeals 1955–1968. *Psychological Bulletin, 72,* 426–444.

Hill, D., & Gardner, G. (1980). Repression-sensitization and yielding to threatening health communications. *Australian Journal of Psychology, 32,* 183–193.

Hovland, C., Janis, I., & Kelly, H. (1953). Communication and persuasion. New Haven, CT: Yale University Press.

Insko, C. A., Arkoff, A., & Insko, V. M. (1965). Effects of high and low fear-arousing communications upon opinions toward smoking. *Journal of Experimental Social Psychology, 1,* 256–266.

Janis, I. L. (1967). Effects of fear arousal on attitude change: Recent developments in theory and experimental research. In L. Berkowitz (Ed.), *Advances in experimental social psychology* (Vol. 3, pp. 166–225). New York: Academic Press.

Janis, I. L., & Feshbach, S. (1953). Effects of fear-arousing communications. *The Journal of Abnormal and Social Psychology, 48,* 78–92.

Janis, I. L., & Feshbach, S. (1954). Personality differences associated with responsiveness to fear-arousing communications. *Journal of Personality, 231,* 154–166.

Janis, I. L., & Mann, L. (1977). *Decision-making: A psychological analysis of conflict, choke, and commitment.* New York: Free Press.

Janz, N. K., & Becker, M. H. (1984). The health belief model: A decade later. *Health Education Quarterly, 11,* 1–47.

Job, R. F. S. (1988). Effective and ineffective use of fear in health promotion campaigns. *American Journal of Public Health, 78,* 165–167.

Johnson, B., & Eagly, A. (1989). Effects of involvement on persuasion: A meta-analysis. *Psychological Bulletin, 106,* 290–314.

Judd, C. M., & Kenny, D. A. (1981). Process analysis: Estimating mediation in evaluation research. *Evaluation Research, 5,* 602–619.

Kleinot, M. C., & Rogers, R. W. (1982). Identifying effective components of alcohol misuse prevention programs, *Journal of Studies on Alcohol, 43,* 802–811.

Kohn, P. M., Goodstadt, M. S., Cook, G. M., Sheppard, M., & Chan, G. (1982). Ineffectiveness of threat appeals about drinking and driving. *Accident Analysis and Prevention, 14,* 457–464.

Kornzweig, N. D. (1967). *Behavior change as a function of fear arousal and personality.* Unpublished doctoral dissertation, Yale University.

Krisher, H. P., III, Darley, S. A., & Darley, J. M. (1973). Fear-provoking recommendations, intentions to take preventive actions, and actual preventive actions. *Journal of Personality and Social Psychology, 26,* 301—308.

Lang, P. J. (1984). Cognition in emotion: Concept and action. In C.V. Izard. J. Kagan, & R.B. Zajone (Eds.), *Emotions, cognition, and behavior* (pp. 192–226). Cambridge: Cambridge University Press.

Langer, E. J. (1989). *Mindfulness.* Reading. MA: Addison-Wesley.

Lazarus, R. S. (1991a). Cognition and motivation in emotion. *American Psychologist, 46,* 352–367.

Lazarus, R. S. (1991b). Progress on a cognitive-motivational-relational theorv of emotion. *American Psychologist, 46,* 819–834.

Lazarus, R. S. (1991c). *Emotion and adaptation.* NY: Oxford University Press.

Lazarus, R. S., & Folkman, S. (1984). *Stress, appraisal, and coping.* New York: Springer-Verlag.

Leventhal, H. (1965). *"Tetanus" messages.* American Documentation Institute, #9011.

Leventhal, H. (1970). Findings and theory in the study of fear communications. In L. Berkowitz (Ed.). *Advances in experimental social psychology* (Vol. 5. pp. 119–186). New York: Academic Press.

Leventhal, H. (1971). Fear appeals and persuasion: The differentiation of a motivational construct. *American Journal of Public Health, 61,* 1208–1224.

Leventhal, H., Safer, M. A., & Panagis, D. M. (1983). The impact of communications on the self-regulation of health beliefs, decisions, and behavior. *Health Education Quarterly, 10,* 3–29.

Leventhal, H., & Trembly, G. (1968). Negative emotions and persuasion. *Journal of Personality, 16,* 154–168.

Leventhal, H., & Watts, J. (1966). Sources of resistance to fear-arousing communications on smoking and lung cancer. *Journal of Personality, 34,* 155–175.

Levine, T., & Cruz, M. (in press). Detecting and assessing statistical interactions with multiple regression. *Communication Research Reports.*

Maddux, J. E., & Rogers, R. W. (1983). Protection motivation and self-efficacy: A revised theory of fear appeals and attitude change. *Journal of Experimental Social Psychology, 19,* 469–479.

McGuire, W. J. (1968). Personality and susceptibility to social influence. In E. Borgatta & W. Lambert (Eds.), *Handbook of personality theory and research* (pp. 1130–1187). Chicago: Rand McNally.

McGuire, W. J. (1969). The nature of attitudes and attitude change. In G. Undzey & E. Aronson (Eds.). *The handbook of social psychology* (Vol. 3, pp. 136–314). Reading, MA: Addison-Wesley.

Mewborn, C. R., & Rogers, R. W. (1979). Effects of threatening and reassuring components of fear appeals on physiological and verbal measures of emotion and attitudes. *Journal of Experimental Social Psychology, 15,* 242–253.

Miller, G. R. (1963). Studies on the use ot tear appeals: A summary and analysis. *Central States Speech Journal, 14,* 117–125.

Miller, G. R., & Hewgill, M. A. (1966). Some recent research on fear-arousing message appeals. *Speech Monographs, 33,* 377–391.

Mongeau, P. (1991, February). *Fear-arousing persuasive messages: A metaanalysis revisited.* Paper presented at the annual meeting of the Western States Communication Association, Phoenix, AZ.

Mulilis, J. P., & Lippa, R. (1990). Behavioral change in earthquake preparedness due to negative threat appeals: A test of protection motivation theory. *Journal of Applied Social Psychology, 20,* 619–638.

Niles, P. (1964). *The relationship of susceptibility and anxiety to acceptance of fear-arousing communications.* Unpublished doctoral dissertation, Yale University.

O'Keefe, D. J. (1990). *Persuasion: Theory and research.* Newbury Park. CA: Sage.

Ortony, A., & Turner. P. J. (1990). What's bask about bask emotions? *Psychological Review, 97,* 315–331.

Petty, R., & Cacioppo, J. T. (1986). *Communication and persuasion: Central and peripheral routes to attitude change.* New York: Springer-Verlag.

Prentice-Dunn, S., & Rogers, R. W. (1986). Protection motivation theory and preventive health: Beyond the health belief model. *Health Education Research, 1,* 153–161.

Ramirez, A., & Lasater, T. L. (1976). Attitudinal and behavioral reactions to fear-arousing communications. *Psychological Reports, 38,* 811–818.

Ramirez, A., & Lasater, T. L. (1977). Ethnicity of communicator, self-esteem, and reactions to fear-arousing communications. *Psychological Reports, 38,* 79–91.

Rippetoe, P. A., & Rogers, R. W. (1987). Effects of components of protection-motivation theory on adaptive and maladaptive coping with a health threat. *Journal of Personality and Social Psychology, 52,* 596–604.

Rogers, R. W. (1975). A protection motivation theory of fear appeals and attitude change. *Journal of Psychology, 91,* 93–114.

Rogers, R. W. (1983). Cognitive and physiological processes in fear appeals and attitude change: A revised theory of protection motivation. In J. Cacioppo & R. Petty (Eds.), *Social psychophysiology* (pp. 153–176). New York: Guilford.

Rogers, R. W. (1985). Attitude change and information integration in fear appeals. *Psychological Reports,56,* 179–182.

Rogers, R. W., & Deckner, C. W. (1975). Effects of fear appeals and physiological arousal upon emotion, attitudes, and cigarette smoking. *Journal of Personality and Social Psychology, 32,* 222–230.

Rogers, R. W., & Mewborn, C. R. (1976). Fear appeals and attitude change: Effects of a threat's noxiousness, probability of occurrence, and the efficacy of the coping responses. *Journal of Personality and Social Psychology, 34,* 54–61.

Rosen, T. J., Terry, N. S., & Leventhal, H. (1982). The role of esteem and coping in response to a threat communication. *Journal of Research in Personality, 16,* 90–107.

Rosenstock, I. M. (1974). The health belief model and preventive health behavior. *Health Education Monographs, 2,* 354–586.

Self, C. A., & Rogers, R. W. (1990). Coping with threats to health: Effects of persuasive appeals on depressed, normal, and antisocial personalities. *Journal of Behavioral Medicine, 13,* 545–357.

Stainback, R. & Rogers, R. W. (1985). Identifying effective components of alcohol abuse prevention programs: Effects of fear appeals, message style, and source expertise. *International Journal of the Addictions, 18,* 595–405.

Sutton, S. R. (1982). Fear-arousing communications: A critical examination of theory and research. In J.R. Eiser (Ed.), *Social psychology and behavioral medicine* (pp. 305–557). London: Wiley.

Sutton, S. R., & Eiser, J. R. (1984). The effects of fear-arousing communications on cigarette smoking: An expectancy-value approach. *Journal of Behavioral Medicine, 7,* 15–55.

Sutton, S. R., & Hallett, R. (1989). Understanding seat-belt intentions and behavior: A decision-making approach. *Journal of Applied Social Psychology, 19,* 1310–1325.

Witte, K. (1991). *Preventing AIDS through persuasive communications: Fear appeals and preventive-action efficacy.* Unpublished doctoral dissertation, University of California, Irvine.

Witte, K. (1992). The role of threat and efficacy in AIDS prevention. *International Quarterly of Community Health Education, 12,* 225–249.

Wolf, S., Gregory, W. L., & Stephan, W. G. (1986). Protection motivation theory: Prediction of intentions to engage in anti-nuclear war behaviors. *Journal of Applied Social Psychology, 16,* 510–321.

Wurtele, S. K., & Maddux, J. E. (1987). Relative contributions of protection motivation theory components in predicting exercise intentions and behavior. *Health Psychology, 6,* 455–466.

Zajonc, R. B. (1980). Feeling and thinking: Preferences need no inferences. *American Psychologist, 33,*151–175.

Zajonc, R. B. (1984). On the primacy of affect. *American Psychologist,* 39, 117–123.

Discussion Questions

1. How are fear, threat, and efficacy related in Witte's model?
2. What are some memorable health campaigns in which fear appeals have been used effectively?
3. What are the situations in which fear appeals would not be useful and might even be harmful? ✦

Chapter 20
A Case Against 'Binge' as the Term of Choice

Convincing College Students to Personalize Messages About Dangerous Drinking

Linda C. Lederman,
Lea P. Stewart,
Fern Walter Goodhart,
and Lisa Laitman

In Chapter 20, Linda C. Lederman, Lea P. Stewart, Fern Goodhart, and Lisa Laitman present their decade-long research from Rutgers University. From this research, they created a persuasive strategy and designed and eventually implemented a successful campaign to reduce dangerous drinking. The chapter focuses on the ways students talk about drinking in their own words. It is an exemplar of the application of audience analysis prior to the construction of any health campaign. Promotion and prevention campaigns present communication scholars with key challenges concerning persuasive and relational messages, the social construction of reality, and health outcomes. This chapter focuses on the words chosen to construct a health campaign designed to prevent dangerous college drinking. In this campaign specifically, health messages are used to raise awareness, correct misperceptions, and help students learn more about the culture of college drinking.

Related Topics: alcohol prevention, college drinking, culture, ethical issues, groups, health campaigns, health-care behaviors, media, qualitative methods

From "A Case Against 'Binge' as the Term of Choice: Convincing College Students to Personalize Messages About Dangerous Drinking," Linda C. Lederman, Lea P. Stewart, Fern Walter Goodhart, and Lisa Laitman, 2003, *Journal of Health Communication*, Vol. 8:1, pp. 70–91.

The most recent literature on the prevention of problematic drinking on the college campus includes a growing controversy about approaches to the reduction of college drinking. On the one hand, there is an increasing body of literature reporting success in driving down drinking on college campuses using social norms-based approaches (Haines, 1996; Jeffrey & Negro, 1996; Lederman, Stewart, Barr, Powell, Goodhart, & Laitman, 2000; Perkins & Wechsler, 1996). Advocates of social norms-based approaches claim that students operate under the misperception that everyone on campus drinks excessively (Butler, 1993; Burns, Ballou, & Lederman, 1991; Jeffrey & Negro, 1996). Social norms strategies target these misperceptions by providing students with actual norms, reporting that this approach both changes perceptions and drives down actual drinking. On the other hand, some well established researchers report finding increased college drinking and refute social norms campaigns as an unsubstantiated and perhaps harmful fad (Wechsler, Lee, Kuo & Lee, 2000).

These contradictory findings make it unclear as to whether the inaccurate perception that most students drink excessively is shared by the majority of students as the advocates of social norms approaches claim or merely found among sub-groups as articulated by Keeling (2000). Nonetheless, strong evidence exists that in one way or another many college students (and their parents and teachers) do share the perception that excessive college drinking is a cultural norm (Butler, 1993) and that this perception is consistently re-created and/or reinforced by the media (including college newspapers with ads for "All You Can Drink" and "Happy Hours"), major advertising that targets students (e.g., beer companies with Spring Break Drinking Campaigns), and even students' own interpersonal experience (e.g., sharing war stories about the "night before"; attending fraternity parties and other social events that encourage alcohol abuse) (Cohen & Lederman, 1998; Haines, 1996; Lederman, 1993; Perkins & Wechsler, 1996).

Despite these differences regarding the effectiveness of social norming, there is certainly no disagreement that college campuses are plagued by drinking and drinking-related problems. Furthermore, there can be little disagreement that many of the college students who drink do so in ways that are much more problematic than they themselves comprehend. Wechsler, Lee, Kuo, & Lee (2000) report that binge drinkers consistently perceive the norm of heavy drinking as higher than it actually is. In another recent study, researchers at Rutgers found that 92% of students did not think of themselves as binge drinkers, even though 35% of these students drank at levels that researchers use to operationalize binge drinking (Lederman et al., 2000). And as early as 1989, Burns and Goodstadt found students reporting that they didn't think drinking was a problem. "Problem drinking?" asked one student in an interview by Burns and Goodstadt (1989), "I drink. I get drunk. I fall down. No problem."

While the literature focuses on arguments about strategies to reduce problematic drinking-related behaviors among college students, little attention is currently being paid to the words used to conceptualize students' drinking behavior. Since individual behaviors are based on constructs that are developed in a social context, it is important to use language that accurately reflects the interpretive schemes that college students have developed (Delia, 1987; Littlejohn, 1996). By using language that is outside the interpretive schemes of college students, health educators and researchers may be unwittingly contributing to a failure among students to identify their drinking as problematic. One way in which this is very likely happening is in using the word "binge" to describe drinking on the campus.

What's in a Word? Binge Drinking

"Binge drinking" is the newest phrase used to describe college drinking that is problematic (Meilman, Cashin, McKillip, & Presley, 1998; Presley, Meilman, & Cashin, 1998; Thombs, Mahoney, & Olds, 1998; Wechsler, 1996; Wechsler, Fulop, Padilla, Lee, & Patrick, 1997). The drinking-related phenomenon that the word is used to describe is five or more drinks in a setting for a male and four or more for a female. Previously the same drinking behavior was referred to in the literature as "at risk drinking" (Burns & Goodstadt, 1989; Carey, 1995a; Pasavac, 1993; Perkins, 1992). None of these terms are the words that students themselves use to describe their own drinking. In fact, a study at a major Midwestern university found that calling drinking "risky" was appealing to students; that these students liked to think of themselves as risk-takers (Workman, 1998). Milgram and Anderson (2000) argue that binge actually refers to a situation in which an individual consumes alcohol to the point of intoxication over a long period of time (e.g., two or three days. Furthermore they point out, when "binge" is used to refer to a set number of drinks, it fails to take into account what the person is drinking, how large the drinks are, and how much the person weighs (p. 9).

If students do not relate to the word "binge" as a descriptor of their behaviors, if that word has very different meanings and connotations for them than five or more drinks at a time, health educators and researchers may be making it simply too easy for most students to dismiss reports of binge drinking as what "happens to other people" and to view binges as more extreme behaviors than those with which they can identify.

The problem, then, is what do we do to raise students' consciousness and to make them aware of the dangers associated with drinking more than three drinks during a given time period. The purpose of this paper is to address this challenge. It will suggest that one of the ways to help students personalize messages about drinking is to change the use of the word "binge" to a term that more appropriately describes their behavior. It will also suggest that it is necessary to examine how students themselves think to find an alternative word that expresses the concern that anyone ought to have if drinking more than four (women) or five (men) drinks. In order to do this, the paper will review what we have learned about students at our own university, how they themselves think about drinking, and how we are using what we have learned *from them* to frame our own language, and our decision to use the term "dangerous drinking" to replace "binge drinking."

How College Students Think About Drinking

Students themselves know a great deal about drinking on campus—whether they drink or do not drink, and whether or not researchers and educators accept the social norms advocates' assertion that students misperceive the norms in terms of how much people drink. Drinking and/or observations of others' drinking-related behaviors are part of what students on the campus experience as part of their college life. This is clear in several ways. First, data collected in surveys across the country support this contention. Through the analysis of the data gathered through survey research, students' knowledge of drinking on the campus as well as their own self-reported drinking-related behaviors, attitudes, and perceptions is evident (Butler, 1993; Carey, 1995b; Harper et al., 1999; Klein, 1992; Marshall, Scherer, & Real, 1998; Nezlek, Pilkington, & Bilbro, 1994; Rabow & Duncan-Schill, 1995; Thombs, Wolcott, & Farkash, 1997; Wechsler, 1996, 2000). At Rutgers University, random surveys of students also indicated the familiarity of students with drinking-related issues (Burns & Goodstadt, 1989; Burns, Ballou, & Lederman, 1991; Lederman, 1993). While data were being collected at Rutgers using these random surveys, qualitative research was undertaken using individual and group interviews in order to gather more insight and triangulate the data collection (Burns & Goodstadt, 1989; Cohen & Lederman, 1998). In addition to providing insights as to what students do and how they think, these qualitative studies provided insights into why students behave as they do and why they think the way they think. For more than a decade since the end of the 1980s, this triangulated approach has continued at Rutgers. Taken together, researchers at Rutgers have learned a great deal about what college students know or think they know about drinking (Lederman et al., 2001).

One thing that has been learned from these studies is that college students who drink do not usually characterize their drinking as problematic. Many of them don't think that five or more drinks is too much to drink, and most don't believe that they have a problem with drinking unless they drink every day (Butler, 1993; Haines, 1996; Lederman & Stewart, 1998; Lederman et al., 2001; Perkins, 1994; Schall, Kemeny, & Maltzman, 1992; Senchak, Leonard, & Greene, 1998; Wechsler, Lee, Kuo, & Lee, 2000). Many of them think that no matter how much they drink that there are others who drink more (Berkowitz & Perkins, 1986; Burns, Ballou, & Lederman, 1991; Butler, 1993; Cohen & Lederman, 1998; Lederman et al., 1999). Many also think that binges are things that happen to others, not to them. In a recent study at Rutgers University, Lederman et al. (2001) report finding that among students who drink 5 or more drinks, 78.8% disagree with the statement—"Do you consider yourself a binge drinker?" in contrast with the 35.8% who drank dangerously during their last episode of drinking.

Furthermore, in explaining binge drinking as five or more drinks for a male and four or more drinks for a female, researchers may have created a way of looking at drinking that is simply foreign to most students. Burns, Ballou, and Lederman (1991) interviewed students and found that they had a list of terms they used that described how they felt and when they had enough. "When I get the spins, I stop" was typical of the kinds of measures students reported. Nowhere was there any mention of quantity as a measure. Lederman et al. (1998) in following up Burns, Ballou, and Lederman's qualitative data found in a random survey of Rutgers University students that 71% of responses indicated that students measured their drinking by behavioral consequences, such as how they felt, instead of by the number of set drinks they drank.

While Wechsler, Lee, Kuo & Lee (2000)

report that the students they label as binge drinkers have a self-serving reason for their differences with the research definition of binge drinking, they do not take into account any of the real differences in the associative meanings, the connotations of the word, "binge," to these drinkers.

If students do not think there is a problem with their drinking behavior there is little hope that they will be motivated to change that behavior. It seems important, then, to look at the subject of college drinking through the eyes of college students (Burns, Ballou, & Lederman, 1991; Klein, 1992; Lederman et al., 1999; Rapaport, Minelli, Angera, & Thayer, 1999). If we want to do more to change their behaviors, we have to attempt to understand their drinking and their drinking-related behaviors through their own eyes. It is by understanding their attitudes and behaviors through their own ways of seeing that we can become more effective in framing what we say to them about their drinking and in creating ways of communicating with them that will resonate with them.

Talking to Students at Rutgers

Rutgers University is a site for on-going qualitative data collection designed to find out what students themselves think. At Rutgers University we have attempted to understand drinking through the eyes of students by engaging in on-going qualitative data collection alongside the quantitative surveys we administer regularly. As noted in the previous section, our qualitative research began more than a decade ago through the work of an interdisciplinary team led by David Burns (Burns, Ballou, & Lederman, 1991; Burns & Goodstadt, 1989).

For more than ten years, researchers at Rutgers University who had initially conducted campus-wide random surveys followed by focus group and individual interviews found qualitative evidence of a widely held misperception of drinking norms (Burns & Goodstadt, 1989; Lederman, 1993; Lederman & Stewart, 1998). Beginning in 1989, a comprehensive quantitative study was undertaken with two major goals: (1) to develop an understanding of students', parents', administrators' and faculty's perceptions of the nature, extent, and origins of students' problems, and (2) to develop effective communicative interventions based on this research. At the same time, a series of 16 focus groups was conducted to determine the "why" behind the behaviors of college drinking (Burns & Goodstadt, 1989; Burns, Ballou, & Lederman, 1991; Lederman, 1993).

In these interviews, students were gathered and asked about their social life on campus and the role of drinking in that social life. Groups were selected through a screening interview that determined if they met the selection criteria. The selection criteria for group members were age, gender, and risk level. Groups were conducted by professional group moderators (male for men, female for women) using a Focus Group Guide created by a team of researchers including alcohol prevention specialists, communication faculty, and health educators. The Focus Group Guide began with individual written responses that were then shared, followed by a semi-structured discussion. All groups were tape-recorded, and transcripts were created.

In order to maximize openness and honesty among group members, participants were informed at the outset of the interviews that their identities would be kept in confidence. To accomplish this, specific names were removed from the summary transcripts of the tapes. Transcripts were analyzed using a constant comparison method (Strauss & Corbin, 1998) to identify themes. These themes were the basis for the findings from the focus group interviews. In addition, a series of individual interviews and modified focus group meetings was conducted to gather further information. The modified focus group meeting technique (Lederman, 1990) is an in-depth data collection technique in which a trained moderator elicits thick data from homogenous groups of carefully selected and screened participants (Calder, 1977; Herndon, 2001).

The use of the focus group interview was continued periodically between 1995 and 2000 using the same methodology and focusing more on the role of alcohol and the language in which students talked about it, following up on a baseline survey from 1998 (Lederman et al., 1998). In 1998, data gathered from these interviews was one of the bases used by the Rutgers team to develop the Personal Report of Student Perception (Lederman et al., 1998) , a survey instrument randomly administered on the campus in the spring of 1998 and 2000. The PRSP was developed using questions previously incorporated in the 1987 Rutgers Student Alcohol and Drug Survey, relevant questions selected from the CORE (Southern Illinois University) survey, and questions developed to assess students' communication of alcohol-related norms developed from qualitative interviews.

In order to institutionalize the line of inquiry that has been carried on in recent years by the authors as an on-going collaborative entity, The Center for Communication and Health Issues (CHI) was founded on the belief that communication is an integral part of the relationally-based nature of health issues. [In the last three years CHI's work has been funded by the United States Department of Education Safe and Drug Free Schools Program ($240,000; $98,000), the New Jersey Higher Education Consortium on Alcohol and Other Drug Prevention ($15,000; $15,000; $15,000), the U.S. Department of Justice ($400,000); the Rutgers University Health Services ($10,000), Rutgers University Department of Communication ($5,000) and the Communities Against Tobacco Coalition of the National Council on Alcoholism and Drug Dependence (NCADD) ($10,000).]

With its funding, CHI has engaged in ongoing qualitative research into drinking practices on the campus, and also created and administered a survey instrument, the Personal Report of Student Perceptions (PRSP) (1998, 2000), designed and administered intercept interview survey instruments (1998, 1999, 2000, 2001, 2002), developed various curriculum infusion projects and, most importantly, in terms of understanding students, CHI has developed the Socially Situated Experiential Learning Model (SSEL) (Lederman & Stewart, 1998). The model identifies the conceptual bases that can be used to understand the socially situated nature of college drinking. It relies most heavily on *experiential learning theory,* which argues that learning is cyclical. A person has an experience, reflects on that experience, draws some conclusions about the lessons to be drawn from that experience, and then uses those lessons as part of his or her basis for reactions to future experiences (Kolb, 1984; Lederman, 1992). In terms of college drinking, for example, Burns and Goodstadt (1989) and Burns, Ballou, and Lederman (1991) report that students who engage in risky sexual behavior while drinking do not perceive themselves as outcasts in their social circles since in their everyday "experience" their behaviors are the norm as they perceive them. Cohen and Lederman (1998) found that students valued their own first hand experiences as ways of learning how to drink, unaware of or unconcerned by the potentially life-threatening consequences of learning by trial and error. Experiential learning theory would suggest that it is important to look at the reflection that students do about their drinking and the conclusions to which it leads them. If they interpret fellow students' reactions to heavy drinking, for example, as making them seem socially attractive, then they may have "learned from the experience" to drink heavily.

The SSEL model provides the conceptual base upon which CHI approaches learning about drinking on the campus and creating interventions to address drinking-related issues and students' drinking-related experiences. One such intervention, "Imagine That!" (Lederman, 1992), is a game about drinking-related decisions and dating that is currently in use at more than 250 institutions across the U.S. and in Canada. The purpose of these interventions is to insert other ways of interpreting experiences into the learning cycles of students.

Based on the years of work at Rutgers, CHI has come to learn a great deal about students, their drinking and their thinking, and how and why they interpret their experiences as they do. It is what we have learned that forms the basis for our argument against using "binge" as the word of choice to describe drinking practices of students. Students themselves know much about their drinking and have much to learn. We need to review what they know, and what we have learned from them, as the basis for providing an alternative word to "binge" that is meaningful for both the academic community and the subjects of their studies—the students themselves.

What DO Students Think Is Problem Drinking

As early as the focus group interviews and survey in 1989, which have been described in the previous section, researchers at Rutgers and elsewhere (Burns & Goodstadt, 1989; Burns, Ballou, & Lederman, 1991; Cohen & Lederman, 1998; Klein, 1992) were conducting focus group research to understand the "why" behind the numbers reported in quantitative studies of drinking on the campus. As Cohen and Lederman (1998) report, students have their own way of thinking about drinking, and their own ways of explaining what drinking does for them, and why drinking is part of the learning experience during the college years. From the interviews at Rutgers which have been conducted over a period of more than 10 years, we have learned about students' perceptions of the role alcohol plays in their lives and their own sense of the problems and consequences associated with drinking.

In one of the early series of the Rutgers focus group interviews, a team of researchers at Rutgers University led by David Burns found that students thought that alcohol functioned as a social facilitator by making it possible for students under the influence to initiate relationships or have interactions they might not normally have (Burns, Ballou, & Lederman, 1991). Alcohol was reported by many of the students interviewed as helping them to overcome shyness and in doing so allowing those students who were too shy or feeling isolated, lonely, or alienated from their peers to make connections with others. Said one female undergraduate: "It is a social medium to help people relax and relate with each other."

Students expressed this perception of alcohol by referring to it as a social "glue" (Burns, Ballou, & Lederman, 1991). They reported thinking that alcohol bonds them together in situations that are normally more private or isolated. For example, many students reported over-consuming alcohol and vomiting at the end of the night. When they are not doing this in full view of others in the common bathrooms, they reported making sure to tell their roommates and neighbors about it the next day.

In interviews conducted both for the 1989 study (Burns, Ballou, & Lederman, 1991) and in 1997 (Cohen & Lederman, 1998), students reported alcohol was an inducement to bonding because it forced students to depend on their friends. Interviewees described that often a student gets too drunk and needs, literally, to be taken care of, e.g., carried home, given a garbage can to throw up in, or extracted from a sexually threatening situation. In an interview conducted by Lederman for the study with Cohen (Cohen & Lederman, 1998), one female student reported that she knew that "Beth was my best friend, when she held my hair back from my face when I was throwing up into the toilet."

It was not unusual either, to have students report that they or others use alcohol to excuse "wild" behavior or sexual behavior that they might not otherwise admit to having engaged in. Reported one male undergraduate: "So Gina says she was with Tony last night cause she was buzzed. And last week she said the same thing when she hooked up with some other guy named Tom. It's just an excuse, she just likes to do it."

Said another undergraduate in another interview:

> . . . you have a couple of extra drinks and you can be an asshole, you can be obnoxious, you can try to blame it the next day on being drunk. That is another thing, a lot of people use it as an excuse to act wild, as long as they supposedly had a couple of drinks they can get away with it.

In sum, these qualitative reports express that students themselves have first hand experience with drinking and drinking-related behaviors either themselves or as witnesses to others. This makes them think that they know a great deal about alcohol. And in some ways they do. Certainly what these interviews provide is some insight into the role they think that alcohol plays for them in their social lives. If this is what they think alcohol does for them in terms of positive social experiences, it is easier to understand why they'd be reluctant to give it up, or to being told that there is something wrong with their drinking behavior.

Clearly not all students on any campus make these same attributions to alcohol. It is well known, however, that those who drink the most tend to make the most positive attributions to alcohol (Burns & Goodstadt, 1989; Prendergast, 1994). Since it is those people, and the people influenced by their behaviors, that we most want to reach with prevention campaigns, we need to know that this is what they may be thinking.

This is not to say that students are blind to problem drinking. To the contrary, they have their own ways of thinking about problem drinking. In the most recent random mailed surveys at Rutgers University (1998, 2000), students reported that they thought that frequency rather than quantity was the measure of someone having a problem with alcohol. A drink a day would be seen to these students as more problematic than eight drinks on one occasion once a semester. Students do not think that drinking until they get "buzzed," "plastered," or "out of it" is a problem (Lederman, 1993).

In the earlier focus group studies done at Rutgers, Burns, Ballou, and Lederman (1991) found that students classify problem drinking into four broad categories. The first category of problem drinking the students labeled as "Drinking Until You Are Out of Control." This was described by them in the series of sixteen focus group interviews described in the sections above as when there is an inability to stop or a loss of control/ when there is too much emphasis placed upon alcohol in your life and you are giving up everything to drink/if you can't say no/if you can't go through a "dry" weekend.

The second category of problem drinking reported from the sixteen focus group interviews was based on "Frequency." This was described as when the number of times a person drinks during a given period of time is "excessive." It was talked about when the person drinks every night. It was also described as when a person drinks all the time or when a person is perceived as drinking continuously. The third category of problem drinking was focused on people whose behavior was "Hurtful to Themselves or Others." This was described as the instance in which drinking causes behavior which is physically, emotionally, or academically hurtful to the person or to others.

Finally, students described another category of problem drinking. This was called the "Motivation or Attitude Problem." A person's attitude toward alcohol can be a "tipoff" to a problem with it, i.e., if someone is drinking just to drink, it is a problem. If someone is drinking to relax or reduce stress, it is not a problem. Students said that even if they were drinking a whole case of beer to reduce the stress, it isn't a problem. The problem had to do with the motivation. This category is independent of quantity and reliant upon motivation. Said one interviewee: "It's why you drink. If it's cause you want to get messed up that's a problem. Not like when you want to just let it all hang out after exams."

What was conspicuously absent from this list generated from the students during these interviews was any mention at all of quantity. This same finding occurred in later studies conducted at Rutgers and reported by Lederman (1993) and Cohen and Lederman (1998). The quantity of alcohol consumed didn't seem to affect what students defined as a problem, hence the students did not pay attention to limiting the amount they drank. Instead, they spoke of limits in terms of impaired judgment and the resultant negative consequences or illness. They were also not fundamentally disturbed by the frequency of vomiting. This is understandable in light of the students' perceptions of bonding around dealing with the consequences of drinking too much. In an interesting triangulation of the data, the most recent survey at Rutgers indicates that students were more concerned with frequency than quantity (Lederman, Stewart, Kennedy, et al., 2001).

There is more that we know about how students think about drinking. Students, even heavy drinking students, are aware of the consequences, or at least some of them, of heavy drinking. The most consequential of these are seen as relational consequences: getting taken advantage of (sexually or socially), getting into sexually intimate relationships too quickly, embarrassing oneself, or getting into situations that are violent.

These are not only consequences that appear on the police rosters or campus police data sheets, but also things that students themselves report in one-to-one and focus group interviews (Burns, Ballou, & Lederman, 1991; Cohen & Lederman, 1998; Harper et al., 1999). While students report personal and physical consequences, e.g., vomiting, passing out, hangovers/headaches, these are not as significant to them unless they affect their relationships with others. Furthermore, students reported that they thought that they simply had to learn about drinking from their own experiences (Burns, Ballou, & Lederman, 1991; Cohen & Lederman, 1998; Lederman et al., 1999). When asked who had taught them to drink in these ways, again and again students explained that they simply had to learn through experience what they personally could and could not do. They had to learn for themselves their own limits/capacity (Cohen & Lederman, 1998). For instance, in the original interviews conducted by the Burns team in 1991, a student reported: "The first time I got drunk I puked and I got really sick and ugly. I realized that drinking a lot is not a whole lot of fun."

Drinking and learning to handle it was seen as a rite of passage into adulthood. It was about testing limits and learning from those experiments. As a student working on a research report exclaimed when talking about first year students: "Those cheesy freshman girls. It embarrasses me to realize that two years ago I was one of them."

In interviewing students, Cohen and Lederman (1998) found that students did not want to interfere in what they perceived to be other students' rights to learn from their own experiences. In more recent interviews with undergraduates, those who drink heavily find themselves skeptical that they are in the minority, since they surround themselves with others who drink like them.

Implications

In sum, what the above discussion indicates is that it is important to re-examine the basis on which we are trying to get information from students about their drinking and the ways in which we use the terms we select to indicate drinking-related problems. The problem of drinking on campus is complex, so, too, must be the answers and approaches. Multiple approaches to dealing with this problem, which includes evaluation research for all of them, and continuous assessment of our effectiveness, are necessary but not sufficient. In addition, it is important to look at the language being used to convey to students what is problematic about excessive college drinking. To the extent that there is much that is known about our primary audience, college students, and the ways in which they think, there is a solid basis for making decisions about the word to choose to indicate problematic drinking. There are two very different but important drawbacks to the word "binge" as the word of choice. The word "binge" is inflammatory. On the one hand, it creates an image far worse than what is happening and, on the other hand, it is easy to deny, seeing it as what happens to others. What is an alternative? We suggest the term "dangerous drinking" as an alternative.

Dangerous Drinking: Advantages of the Term

As an alternative to the term "binge drinking," we advocate "dangerous drinking." It is a term that has several advantages. First, it is a term that came from students themselves. When a group of student leaders at Rutgers University was asked by a university-wide blue ribbon committee to identify what term, if any, they thought they could identify with more than binge drinking, they suggested "dangerous drinking." They rejected "binge drinking" because they thought that students didn't identify with it. They rejected "high risk drinking" because they thought that some students thought that high risk was "cool." They rejected "responsible drinking" because they did not like the value judgment in it, pointing out to the committee that those members of the community who had alcoholism were the drinkers who would be labeled irresponsible and that that seemed to them to be blaming the victim of a disease. "Dangerous drinking" was a term they liked because they saw that it had differential application the way that "responsible drinking" does but without the value judgment. Instead they saw the term "dangerous drinking" as putting the focus where it should be—on outcomes.

The term "dangerous drinking" places the focus on the type of drinking that needs to be addressed, that which is dangerous, in an arena that perhaps most students and adults can agree. Instead of having the situation where students are almost always at odds with adults, we may have more agreement of what is a problem if we were both discussing drinking that is a problem. If a male student has 5–6 drinks during a party that starts at 11 pm and ends at 4 am, consumes food and spaces his drinks out over this period, this is not necessarily problem drinking. Yet if a student has too much to drink in a short amount of time and needs to be taken to the hospital with alcohol poisoning, this should be defined as dangerous drinking. Yet the definition of "binge drinking" does not include time or consequence as a factor, an issue that is often raised by students.

Conclusion: It's Not What You Call It—Entirely

The use of the term "dangerous drinking" grows out of what we have learned from employing this approach to our research at Rutgers. It is our term of choice based on what we have learned about students from students.

While using the term "dangerous drinking" does resonate with students, it does not solve the controversy over social norms approaches. It does grow out of a socially situated approach to college drinking, Lederman and Stewart's (1998) Socially Situated Experiential Learning Model. Fundamentally the approach argues that what students know about drinking they learn in their social interactions with one another. It is an approach that focuses on understanding students' thinking in order to try to change their drinking.

Given that we know that the people who need to be reached the most are those students who are the least likely to want to learn that their drinking is problematic, the words we choose to describe their drinking need to be carefully thought out. The word "binge" lets them off the hook; it is easy for them to think of binges as something that other people do, to associate it with alcoholics, and to think of alcoholism as something to avoid rather than as a disease. For many students, the word "alcoholic" still carries with it the stigma that many health educators try to eliminate. For many students, despite the fact that their families may contain people suffering from alcoholism, the word alcoholic is a put down, and so long as they don't have to use that word to describe themselves, they think they have no problems with alcohol. This means, of course, that when they go out to party and get "smashed" they may be ignorant of the real dangers associated with what they are doing; dangers that go beyond what they know about drinking and problems associated with drinking. If we want to alert them, first we have to get their attention. The word "binge" doesn't do it. Let's see if "dangerous drinking" can be a better way to get them to be more able to reflect upon their own drinking-related choices.

References

Berkowitz, A. D., & Perkins, H. W. (1986). Problem drinking among college students: A review of recent literature. *Journal of American College Health, 35,* 21–28.

Burns, D., Ballou, J., & Lederman, L. (1991). *Perceptions of alcohol use and policy on the college campus: Preventing alcohol/drug abuse at Rutgers University.* Unpublished. U.S. Department of Education Fund for the Improvement of Post Secondary Education (FIPSE) conference paper.

Burns, D., & Goodstadt, M. (1989). *Alcohol use on the Rutgers University campus: A study of various communities.* Unpublished. U.S. Department of Education Fund for the Improvement of Post Secondary Education (FIPSE) conference paper.

Butler, E. R. (1993). Alcohol use by college students: A rite of passage ritual. *NASPA Journal, 31* (1), 48–55.

Calder, B. (1977). Focus groups and the nature of qualitative marketing research. *Journal of Marketing Research, 14,* 353–364.

Carey, K. B. (1995a). Alcohol-related expectancies predict quantity and frequency of heavy drinking among college students. *Psychology of Addictive Behaviors, 9*(4), 236–241.

Carey, K. B. (1995b). Heavy drinking contexts and indices of problem drinking among college students. *Journal of Studies on Alcohol, 56,* 287–292.

Cohen, D., & Lederman, L. (1998). Navigating the freedom of college life: Students talk about alcohol, gender, and sex. In N. Roth & L. Fuller (Eds.), *Women and AIDS: Negotiating safer practices, care, and representation* (pp. 101–126). New York: Haworth Press.

Delia, J. G. (1987). Interpersonal cognition, message goals, and organization of communication: Recent constructivist research. In D. L. Kincaid (Ed.), *Communication theory: Eastern and western perspectives* (pp. 255–274). San Diego, CA: Academic Press.

Haines, M. P. (1996). *A social norms approach to preventing binge drinking at colleges and universities.* U.S. Department of Education (Publication No. ED/OPE/96–18): Education Development Center, Inc.

Harper, N. L., Lederman, L., Stewart, L., Yee, M., Kennedy, L., Galen, L., et al. (1999). A study of drinking among Grand Valley State University and Rutgers University students: Preliminary results of the personal report of student perceptions (PRSP). *Communication and Health Issues Research Series: Report #7.* New Brunswick, NJ: Center for Communication and Health Issues, Rutgers University.

Herndon, S. L. (2001). Using focus group interviews for preliminary investigation. In S. L. Herndon & G. L. Kreps (Eds.), *Qualitative research: Applications in organizational life* (pp. 63–72).Cresskill, NJ: Hampton Press.

Jeffrey, L. R., & Negro, P. (1996). *Contemporary trends in alcohol and other drug use by college students in New Jersey.* Unpublished. New Jersey Higher Education Consortium on Alcohol and Other Drug Prevention and Education.

Keeling, R. (2000). The political, social, and public health problems of binge drinking in college. *Journal of American College Health, 48,* 243–246.

Klein, H. (1992). Self-reported reasons for why college students drink. *Journal of Alcohol and Drug Education, 37*(2), 14–28.

Kolb, D. (1984). *Experiential learning: Experience as a source of learning.* Englewood Cliffs, NJ: Prentice-Hall.

Lederman, L. C. (1990). Assessing educational effectiveness: The focus group interview as a technique for data collection. *Communication Education, 39,* 117–127.

Lederman, L. C. (1992). *IMAGINE THAT! A simulation of drinking and decision-making.* New Brunswick, NJ: Rutgers University Health Education Services.

Lederman, L. C. (1993). Friends don't let friends beer goggle: A case study in the use and abuse of alcohol and communication among college students. In E. B. Ray (Ed.), *Case studies in health communication* (pp. 161–174). Hillsdale, NJ: Lawrence Erlbaum.

Lederman, L. C., & Stewart, L. P. (1998). Addressing the culture of college drinking through correcting misperceptions: Using experiential learning theory and Gilligan's work. *Communication and Health Issues Research Series: Report #4.* New Brunswick, NJ: Center for Communication and Health Issues, Rutgers University.

Lederman, L. C., Stewart, L. P., Barr, S., Powell, R., Laitman, L., & Goodhart, F. (1999). Reconceptualizing college drinking as socially situated experiential learning. *Communication and Health Issues Research Series: Report #5.* New Brunswick, NJ: Center for Communication and Health Issues, Rutgers University.

Lederman, L. C., Stewart, L. P., Kennedy, L., Donovan, B., Powell, R., Goodhart, F., et al. (2001). Using qualitative and quantitative methods to triangulate the research process: The role of communication in perpetuating the myth of dangerous drinking as the norm on college campuses. In S. L. Herndon & G. L. Kreps (Eds.), *Qualitative research: Applications in organizational communication,* 2nd ed. (pp. 251–268). Cresskill, NJ: Hampton Press.

Lederman, L. C., Stewart, L. P., Kennedy, L., Powell, R., & Goodhart, F. (1998). Self report of student perceptions: An alcohol awareness measure. *Communication and Health Issues Research Series: Report #2.* New Brunswick, NJ: Center for Communication and Health Issues, Rutgers University.

Lederman, L. C., Stewart, L. P., Barr, S. L., Powell, R., Goodhart, F., & Laitman, L. (2000). The role of communication theory and experiential learning in addressing dangerous drinking on the college campus. In L. C. Lederman & W. D. Gibson (Eds.), *Communication theory: A casebook approach* (pp. 325–335). Dubuque, IA: Kendall Hunt.

Littlejohn, S. W. (1996). *Theories of human communication,* 5th ed. Belmont, CA: Wadsworth.

Marshall, A., Scherer, C. W., & Real, K. (1998). The relationship between students' social networks and engaging in risky behaviors: The college tradition of "Drink 'til You Drop." *Journal of Health Communication,* 11(2), 34–41.

Meilman, P. W., Cashin, J. R., McKillip, J. R., & Presley, C. A. (1998). Understanding the three national databases on collegiate alcohol and drug use. *Journal of American College Health, 46* (4), 168.

Milgram, G. G., & Anderson, D. S. (2000). *Action planner: Steps for developing a comprehensive campus alcohol abuse prevention program.* Fairfax, VA: George Mason University.

Nezlek, J. B., Pilkington, C. J., & Bilbro, K. G. (1994). Moderation in excess: Binge drinking and social interaction among college students. *Journal of Studies on Alcohol, 55,* 342–351.

Pasavac, E. J. (1993). College students' views and excessive drinking and the university role. *Journal of Drug Education, 23*(3), 237–245.

Perkins, W. H. (1992). Gender patterns in consequences of collegiate alcohol abuse: A 10-year study of trends in an undergraduate population. *Journal of Studies on Alcohol, 53,* 458–462.

Perkins, W. H. (1994). Confronting misperceptions of peer drug use norms among college students: An alternative approach for alcohol and other drug education programs. In L. Grow (Ed.), *FIPSE drug prevention programs in higher education training institute manual,* 4th. Ed., Washington, D.C. Fund for the Improvement of Post Secondary Education. Washington, D.C.: U.S. Department of Education.

Perkins, W. H., & Wechsler, H. (1996). Variation in perceived college drinking norms and its impact on alcohol abuse: A nationwide study. *Journal of Drug Issues, 26*(A), 961–974.

Prendergast, M. L. (1994). Substance use and abuse among college students: A review of recent literature. *College Health, 43,* n.p.

Presley, C. A., Meilman, P. W., & Cashin, J. R. (1998). Weapon carrying and substance abuse among college students. *Journal of American College Health, 46*(1), 16.

Rabow, J., & Duncan-Schill, M. (1995). Drinking among college students. *Journal of Alcohol and Drug Education,* 40(3), 52–64.

Rapaport, R. J., Minelli, M. J., Angera, J. J., & Thayer, J. E. (1999). Using focus groups to quickly assess students' opinions about alcohol issues and programs. *Journal of College Student Development, 40*(3), 311–314.

Schall, M., Kemeny, A., & Maltzman, I. (1992). Factors associated with alcohol use in university students. *Journal of Studies on Alcohol, 53*(2), 122–136.

Senchak, M., Leonard, K. E., & Greene, B. W. (1998). Alcohol use among college students as a function of their typical social drinking context. *Psychology of Addictive Behaviors, 12*(1), 62–70.

Strauss, A. L., & Corbin, J. M. (1998). *Basics of qualitative research: Techniques and procedures for developing grounded theory.* Thousand Oaks, CA: Sage.

Thombs, D. L., Mahoney, C., & Olds, R. S. (1998). Application of a bogus testing procedure to determine college students' utilization of genetic screening for alcoholism. *Journal of American College Health, 47*(3), 106.

Thombs, D. L., Wolcott, B. J., & Farkash, L. G. E. (1997). Social context, perceived norms, and drinking behavior in young people. *Journal of Substance Abuse, 9,* 257–267.

Wechsler, H. (1996, July/August). Alcohol and the American college campus: A report from the Harvard School of Public Health. *Change,* pp. 20–25.

Wechsler, H., Davenport, A., Dowdall, G., Mooykens, B., & Castillo, S. (1994). Health and behavioral consequences of binge drinking in college. *Journal of the American Medical Association, 272*(21), 1672–1677.

Wechsler, H., Dowdall, G., Maenner, G., Gledhill-Hoyt, J., & Lee, H. (1998). Changes in binge drinking and related problems among American college students between 1993 and 1997. Results of the Harvard School of Public Health College Alcohol Study. *Journal of American College Health, 47,* 2, 57-68.

Wechsler, H., Fulop, M., Padilla, A., Lee, H., & Patrick, K. (1997). Binge drinking among college students: A comparison of California with other states. *Journal of American College Health, 45*(6), 273.

Wechsler, H., & Kuo, M. (2000). College students define binge drinking and estimate its prevalence: Results of a national survey. *Journal of American College Health, 49,* 57-64.

Wechsler, H., Lee, J. E., Kuo, M., & Lee, H. (2000). College binge drinking in the 1990s: A continuing problem: Results of the Harvard School of Public Health 1999 College Alcohol Study. *Journal of American College Health, 48,* 199–211.

Wechsler, H., Moeykens, B., Davenport, A., Castillo, S., & Hansen, J. (1995). The adverse impact of heavy episodic drinking on other college students. *Journal of Alcohol Studies on Alcohol, 56*(6), 628–634.

Workman, T. A. (1998). *Constructions from within the collegiate drinking culture: An analysis of fraternity drinking stories.* Paper presented at the annual meeting of the National Communication Association, New York, NY.

Discussion Questions

1. What is the difference between "binge" drinking and "dangerous" drinking? What is the importance of distinguishing between these two terms?
2. What are the benefits and drawbacks of using focus groups as a method of research, particularly for research on health-related issues?
3. How does the culture and campaign at Rutgers relate to your own college campus? Would a similar campaign work on other college campuses where dangerous drinking might be a problem? ✦

Chapter 21
Use of Inoculation to Promote Resistance in Smoking Initiation Among Adolescents

Michael Pfau, Steve Von Bockern, and Jong Geun Kang

Chapter 21 addresses another health issue that lends itself to a health promotion campaign: nicotine use. The chapter draws upon inoculation theory as a strategy to prevent children from beginning to smoke. The inoculation model tries to prevent individuals from making a behavior change from a healthy state (e.g., non-smoker) to a less healthy state (e.g., smoker). Once again we see the ways in which communication theory informs effective ways to try to promote healthier choices in a target population. Individuals acquire a number of healthy and unhealthy habits at a young age. As health messages move from a curative focus to a preventative one, strategies like inoculation have proven most beneficial for reaching adolescents with low self-esteem, which is a group that happens to be the most at-risk to start smoking.

Related Topics: culture, health campaigns, health-care behaviors, media, quantitative methods

From "Use of Inoculation to Promote Resistance in Smoking Initiation Among Adolescents," Michael Pfau, Steve Von Bockern, and Jong Geun Kang, 1992, *Communication Monographs*, Vol. 59:3, pp. 213–230.

Despite the mounting evidence about the dangers of cigarette smoking, the U.S. Surgeon General (Department of Health and Human Services, 1989) estimates that more than 3,000 teenagers join the ranks of regular smokers each day, and that as a result millions will die of smoking-related illnesses in their later years. More than half of all people who become regular smokers acquire their habit prior to starting high school (McAlister, Perry, & Maccoby, 1979), a tendency that has intensified because smoking onset is occurring at younger ages among more recent birth cohorts (DHHS, 1989). The health consequences of this trend are particularly grave since "mortality rates for smoking-related diseases are higher for smokers with younger ages of initiation" (DHHS, 1989, p. 298).

As a result, experts maintain that smoking preventative strategies must target young adolescents in order to have any potential for success (Chassin, Cony, Presson, Olshavsky, Bensenberg, & Sherman, 1981; Elder & Stern, 1986; Johnson, 1982; Killen, 1985). Hamburg maintains that the critical period for preventative efforts is the year of "transition from elementary to secondary school," reasoning that this transition "produces far-reaching physiological upheavals . . ." in young adolescents, rendering them particularly vulnerable to smoking onset (1979, p. 1031).

In response, preventative efforts are aimed increasingly at younger adolescents. Such efforts should be viewed as part of a gradual shift in the emphasis of the health care system from a curative to a more preventative focus (Einsiedel & Cochrane, 1988), and are reinforced by research that has affirmed the high cost and low efficacy of cessation approaches (Hunt, Barnett, & Branch, 1971).

Research also indicates that, while younger children often possess strong attitudes opposing smoking, these attitudes are particularly vulnerable during early adolescence. During this critical period, adolescents begin to manifest indifference to the health consequences of smoking (Rokeach, 1987) at the same time that they are increasingly vulnerable to the influence of peer pressure (Bewley & Bland, 1977; Evans & Raines, 1982;

Flay, d'Avernas, Best, Kersell, & Ryan, 1983; Foon, 1986; Friedman, Lichtenstein, & Biglan, 1985; Goldberg & Garn, 1982; Gottlieb & Baker, 1986; McAlister et al., 1979; O'Rourke, O'Byrne, & Wilson-Davis, 1983; Pechacek & McAlister, 1980: Pederson & Lefcoe, 1982; Salomon, Stein, Eisenberg, & Klein, 1984).

These research findings suggest two important implications for preventative strategies. First, they should target younger adolescents at the point of their transition from elementary to secondary school (sixth or seventh graders) (Chassin et al., 1981; Elder & Stern, 1986; Hamburg, 1979; Johnson, 1982; Killen, 1985; McAlister et al., 1979; Urberg & Robbins, 1984). Second, they should attempt to instill resistance to attitude slippage and change in those who oppose smoking (Bernstein & McAlister, 1976).

Inoculating Against Smoking Initiation

This investigation examined the potential of the inoculation approach to confer resistance to cigarette smoking onset among younger adolescents. Whereas most strategies of persuasion seek attitude formation or change, the inoculation approach seeks to strengthen existing attitudes against change (Miller & Burgoon, 1973). The inoculation approach is appropriate in this context because, while adolescents enter the transition from primary to secondary school with negative attitudes toward smoking, these attitudes soften throughout the year (Elder & Stern, 1986; Evans & Raines, 1982; Hamburg, 1979; Johnson, 1982; Killen, 1985).

The Inoculation Model

McGuire provided the theoretical rationale and the initial research base for the inoculation construct (Anderson & McGuire, 1965; McGuire, 1961a, 1961b, 1962, 1964; McGuire & Papageorgis, 1961, 1962; Papageorgis & McGuire, 1961). Inoculation employs threat, operationalized as the warning of impending persuasive challenge to attitudes, along with refutational preemption. The threat component is designed to trigger the receiver's motivation to strengthen arguments supporting attitudes, thereby conferring resistance to subsequent challenges (Anderson & McGuire, 1965; McGuire, 1964, 1970; Papageorgis & McGuire, 1961). As a result, inoculation does more than simply preempt the content of specific arguments that the receiver might encounter. Through the use of threat, inoculation confers a broad blanket of protection against all potential challenges, a claim supported by extant research (McGuire, 1961a, 1962, 1970; Papageorgis & McGuire, 1961; Pfau & Burgoon, 1988; Pfau, Kenski, Niu, & Sorenson, 1990).

Although much of the early research on inoculation focused on validation of the construct in laboratory conditions, recent studies have examined inoculation in field settings, supporting the viability of inoculation as a strategy to foster resistance in voters against the persuasiveness of political attack messages (Pfau & Burgoon, 1988; Pfau et al., 1990), and also to promote resistance in consumers against the persuasiveness of comparative advertising messages for high-involving products (Pfau, 1992).

Application to Smoking Prevention

Because research on smoking initiation identifies peer pressure as the most powerful predictor of adolescent smoking (Gordon, 1986; McCaul, Glasgow, O'Neill, Freeborn, & Rump, 1982; Mettlin, 1976), a number of studies have used peer-led social inoculation strategies to promote resistance to adolescent smoking. These approaches have achieved considerable success in preventing (or delaying) the onset of smoking among junior-high school students (Evans, Rozelle, Maxwell, Raines, Dill, Guthrie, Henderson, & Hill, 1981; Hansen, Malotte, & Fielding, 1988; Murray, Richards, Luepker, & Johnson, 1987; Perry, 1987; Perry, Killen, & Slinkard, 1980), and to some degree among high school students (Johnson, Hansen, Collins, & Graham, 1986).

Despite these successes, however, the issue of whether it is possible to inoculate adolescents against initiation of smoking is far from resolved. Although these research efforts claim to use social inoculation, past studies foiled to operationalize threat, the feature that distinguishes inoculation from other approaches. The threat component of the inoculation approach is the integral element, because it triggers an internal process in receivers that motivates them to bolster their attitudes, thus making them resistant to subsequent counterarguments (McGuire, 1962).

In addition, these studies relied on various combinations of methods, including: videos, slide shows, school-wide campaigns, peer modeling, teacher-led discussions, and so forth. It is the extensiveness of these efforts that makes replication both costly and difficult, and consequently, renders social inoculation less useful to health educators. As Foon (1986, p. 1025) queries: "If these programs are working, what special features are working and how? Unfortunately, this question has not been assessed in the literature to date."

The problem is compounded by the fact that so many of the social inoculation studies were flawed methodologically, failing to employ proper randomization, often using entire schools as the basis for treatment implementation, and then conducting the data analysis on individual subjects (Best, Thomson, Sand, Smith, & Brown, 1988; Biglan & Ary, 1985; Cook, 1985; Flay, 1985; Flay et al., 1983; McCaul & Glasgow, 1985). Flay concludes his syntheses of the extant research, observing that: ". . . we really know very little at this time about which of these program components are necessary for program effectiveness or how other components . . . might or might not add to program effectiveness" (1985, p. 378).

The single component that can be replicated easily, namely videos, has not achieved much success in past social inoculation campaigns. Murray, Davis-Hearn, Goldman, Pirie, and Luepker (1988) stressed the difficulties in operationalizing the social influence model, particularly the video component. Also, Evans, Rozelle, and Mittlemark (1978), who compared the effectiveness of psychological monitoring as opposed to inoculative films in preventing the onset of adolescent smoking, reported monitoring to be more effective. The videos alone produced relatively weak effects. In both cases, researchers placed the blame for their null findings on failings in operationalization, and not inherent limitations in the medium.

McGuire's theoretical rationale suggests that an inoculation approach should promote resistance to smoking onset among younger adolescents who reach the critical threshold of transition from elementary to secondary school with attitudes opposed to smoking intact. The key may lie in effective operationalization of the inoculation model, particularly the threatening component, which past studies failed to accomplish. McGuire's theoretical logic both accounts for the failings in past social inoculation studies and supports the prediction that:

> *H1:* For adolescents who receive an inoculation pretreatment, as compared to those who do not, inoculation pretreatments promote resistance to smoking initiation.

Beyond the relative effectiveness of refutational-same and novel pretreatments, there has been very little emphasis in the inoculation literature on the effectiveness of the construct at multiple time periods. McGuire (1962) and Pryor and Steinfatt (1978) reported that inoculation diminishes over time, although Pfau and Burgoon (1988) qualified this finding, indicating that, whereas the impact of inoculation on receiver attitudes decays significantly over a period of two lo three weeks, the impact on behavioral intention carries greater persistence.

Because the impact of inoculation pretreatments, like any message stimulus, will deteriorate over time, it makes intuitive sense that reinforcement messages should strengthen resistance. However, there has been very little emphasis in the inoculation literature on reinforcement. In original laboratory research of the inoculation model, McGuire (1961b) indicated that "double defenses" provided a significant boost against refutation-same counterarguments, while Tannenbaum, Macaulay, and Norris (1966) found that "concept boost" messages offered a slight increase in resistance. However, in a field study dealing with inoculation and political persuasion, Pfau et al. (1990) reported that the administration of reinforcement messages tailed to boost initial resistance. The authors explained that an inoculative stimulus "carries considerable persistence" (p. 38), thus not requiring reinforcement quite so soon following the administration of the original pretreatment. Thus, the limited research suggests that reinforcement may boost inoculation, but that issues concerning the timing of the administration of reinforcing materials remain unresolved.

Since the effectiveness of an inoculation stimulus depends on threatening and refutational content, and because of evidence indicating inoculation decays over time (McGuire, 1962; Pfau & Burgoon, 1988; Pryor & Steinfatt, 1978), reinforcement materials should boost the effectiveness of the initial pretreatments. It is thus predicted that:

> *H2:* For adolescents who receive inoculation plus follow up reinforcement pretreatments, compared to those who receive only inoculation, reinforcement pretreatments confer added resistance to smoking initiation.

Relevant Receiver Factors

One of the most important unresolved questions concerns the possible interaction of inoculation and relevant receiver factors (Flay, 1985). Botvin (1982, p. 143) criticizes smoking research for a tendency "to underestimate or ignore the role of individual characteristics, particularly personality" in the prevention of adolescent smoking, arguing that such factors may "attenuate" or "potentiate" program effectiveness. Best et al. (1988) concur, maintaining that a common failing of extant research on smoking prevention is that it ignores other relevant factors:

> The need for research that addresses the interactions among program content, client characteristics, provider variables, and setting is well established. . . . Nevertheless, . . . smoking prevention researchers have focused very heavily on program content considerations, and paid virtually no attention to the other potentially equally powerful, and conceptually critical, determinants of program impact (p. 165).

Self-Esteem. One of these "powerful, conceptually critical" factors is self-esteem. Rosenberg (1965) and Coopersmith (1967) define self-esteem as an attitude toward oneself indicating the extent that an individual ". . . believes himself to be capable, significant, successful and worthy" (Coopersmith, 1967, p.5).

Self-esteem is particularly relevant to smoking onset among adolescents because of the powerful role that peer pressure plays in smoking initiation, as was documented previously. Self-esteem affects the adolescent's susceptibility to peer pressure. As Coopersmith (1967) notes, "Experimental studies indicate that a person with low self-esteem is less capable of resisting pressure to conform" (p. 4). Not surprisingly, research on smoking onset among adolescents shows that smokers "manifest diminished self-esteem" (Elder & Stern, 1986, p. 183; Foon, 1986; Harken, 1987). Best et al. (1988, p. 165) posit that, "Self-esteem may mediate the effects of social environment," which is the "single most important determinant of smoking onset" (p. 164).

Elder and Stern (1986) speculated that social inoculation may vary in effectiveness based on adolescent self-esteem levels. The question is how. In synthesizing early persuasion research, McGuire (1969, p. 250–251) explained conflicting findings about the relationship between self-esteem and persuasibility in terms of an "inverted-U relationship," such that as self-esteem rises, persuasibility increases, up to a point, beyond which increases in self-esteem reduce persuasibility. In a subsequent synthesis of research involving self-esteem and resistance to persuasion, Miller, Burgoon, and Burgoon (1984, p. 447) concluded that, with relatively simple messages, persons who are higher in self-esteem are more resistant to persuasion, although this is not true with more complex messages.

These explanations are supported by the smoking initiation research, which indicates that low self-esteem adolescents are most vulnerable to peer pressure, and thus to smoking initiation. For the same reason, low self-esteem adolescents should be more susceptible to inoculation. Furthermore, because the inoculation pretreatments in this investigation were designed for consumption by young adolescents, they featured relatively simple messages, providing an additional argument for greater susceptibility to inoculation. Thus, this investigation predicts that inoculation pretreatments are effective primarily with low self-esteem adolescents.

> *H3:* For adolescents who receive an inoculation pretreatment, as compared to those who do not, inoculation pretreatments are more effective in conferring resistance to smoking onset among those with low self-esteem.

Gender. Another receiver factor examined extensively in persuasion is gender. Early research clearly indicated that women are more persuasible than men (Cronkhite, 1969; McGuire, 1969). Although this claim was questioned in two extensive secondary reviews a decade later (see Eagly, 1978, and Maccoby & Jacklin, 1974), three meta-analyses generally supported the previous position that females are more persuasible (Becker, 1986; Cooper, 1979; Eagly & Carli, 1981). Eagly (1987) provides a social role explanation as to why women are more persuasible than men. She argues that societal role emphasis results in "stereotypic sex differences" in which women are more communal, therefore more person oriented, whereas men are more agentic, therefore more assertive and controlling, making women more persuasible (1987).

Gender appears particularly relevant in smoking prevention because of the early evidence that it interacts with pretreatment effectiveness and program approach. Alexander et al. (1983) and Hansen et al. (1988) indicated that prevention is more effective among female students. Additional studies suggest that gender interacts with approach, such that a social consequences approach is effective only for female students (Barton, Chassin, Presson, & Sherman, 1982; O'Neill, Glasgow, & McCaul, 1983).

> *H4:* For adolescents who receive an inoculation pretreatment, as compared to those who do not, inoculation pretreatments are more effective in conferring resistance to smoking onset among females as opposed to males.

Method

Subjects

The study involved all seventh grade students in all junior high schools in Sioux Falls, SD (N = 1,047).

Independent Variables and Procedures

This investigation employed a 2 × 3 × 2 factorial design. Independent variables were experimental condition (inoculation and control), student self-esteem (low, moderate, and high), and gender (female and male). Experimental condition was modified slightly as inoculation, inoculation-plus-reinforcement.

Effectiveness of the pretreatments in conferring resistance to the onset of smoking was assessed by comparing the attitudes of students who received an inoculation pretreatment versus those who received no pretreatment, the latter serving as controls in the investigation. Those students assigned as controls simply participated in the assessments conducted during the study.

Procedures

Students were surveyed during the week of September 10–14, 1990, to gather basic demographic information, measure self-esteem, and determine attitudes about smoking. The results of the initial surveys identified 68 students as past or present regular smokers (6.5%).[1] Smokers and nonsmokers were treated alike in terms of subsequent administration of the study. However, because inoculation is a strategy designed to promote resistance to attitude change, not to change attitudes, the regular smokers were not included in statistical analyses, leaving 979 subjects at the start of the study. Of these, 31 failed to complete one or more of the subsequent assessments, leaving 948 subjects who completed all phases of the study.

After the administration of the pretreatment survey, all students were grouped according to their health class and then assigned intact to one of three inoculation conditions or to the control condition.

The study featured three inoculation conditions in order to assess the relative efficacy of specific inoculation approaches:

peer-led, featuring a young adolescent spokesperson; adult-led, employing an adult spokesperson; and reinforcement, a booster session, depicting interaction of peer and adult spokespersons, administered to a portion of those subjects who had previously received either the peer- or adult-led inoculation pretreatment. The combined adult and peer approach used for the reinforcement condition was designed to provide a unique format, yet maintain continuity with the initial inoculation materials.

All seventh-grade students in the four junior high schools are randomly assigned to a health class. The 38 health class sections were randomly assigned to one of the conditions, as follows: inoculation, 18; inoculation-plus-reinforcement, 10; and control, 10. The health classes employ a common seventh-grade curriculum which includes a single unit of instruction on tobacco, alcohol, and drug use, administered during the second semester.

Students in health classes assigned to one of the treatment conditions were shown an inoculation video during the week of October 1–5. Students in the 10 health class sections assigned to the treatment condition, but also the reinforcement phase of the investigation, were shown a reinforcement video during the week of November 26–30. The teachers were instructed not to comment on or in any way discuss the videos with their students.

All students were periodically assessed to monitor their attitudes and behavioral disposition toward smoking. Results reported in this manuscript are based on February 1991 data, gathered approximately 19 weeks following administration of the inoculation pretreatments and 10 weeks after administration of reinforcement materials, and on May 1991 data, gathered 33 weeks after administration of the initial inoculation pretreatments, and 25 weeks following administration of reinforcing materials.

Inoculation Videos

Inoculation was manipulated in the study via three 12–15-minute professionally produced videotapes. Two videos were designed to inoculate students against initiation of smoking, and included threat plus refutational preemption. In the threatening component of the videos, students were cautioned that, in spite of their attitudes opposing smoking, as a result of significant peer pressure in the seventh grade, many of them would become uncertain about smoking, and some would change their minds and try smoking. In the refutational preemption component, specific challenges to their attitudes were raised (e.g., smoking is socially "cool"; experimental smoking won't result in regular smoking; smoking won't affect me), and then refuted. The third video was designed to reinforce the initial pretreatment, using the threat plus refutational preemption approach described above.

Existing video materials available for use in junior high health education classes were previewed prior to preparation of the three videos. Scripts were written for each of the videos and actors hired to perform them. The three videos contained both visual footage and musical material that were designed to complement the respective verbal messages. The videos were previewed by health educators prior to their actual use in the study. They judged the videos to be appropriate for the target audience, highly credible, and potentially effective in combating smoking initiation.

Dependent Variables and Manipulation Checks

All of the instruments employed in this investigation, with the exception of likelihood of smoking, a one-item measure, were evaluated for reliability using Cronbach's (1951) coefficient alpha.

The threat of the inoculation pretreatments, which served as a manipulation check, was gauged using five 7-interval semantic differential items, used previously by Pfau et al. (1990) and Pfau (1992). The items included safe/dangerous, not risky/risky, unintimidating/intimidating, nonthreatening/threatening, and unharmful/harmful. The threat manipulation was administered immediately following viewing of the inoculation videos. The coefficient alpha reliability was .92.

Self-esteem was assessed using ten 7-interval Likert scales, adapted from the general self-esteem component of the Coopersmith

Self-Esteem Inventory (SEI), considered to be the most widely employed measure of self-esteem (Johnson, Redfield, Miller, & Simpson, 1983). The measure, which asks subjects to indicate the degree of truth in such descriptive statements as "Most people like me," "I am an intelligent person" etc., is similar to one employed in past smoking prevention research (see Botvin, Renick, & Baker, 1983). Reliability was .83. Average self-esteem scores were subsequently trichotomized as low, moderate, and high, using clear break points in the data to generate three groups of about the same size. Scores of less than 4.4 on the 7-point continuum were classified as low; those from 4.4 to 6.0 as moderate; and scores of 6.1 or more as high.

Two measures were used to assess attitude toward smoking. Six 7-interval semantic differential scales used previously in studies by Burgoon, Cohen, Miller, and Montgomery (1978), Miller and Burgoon (1979), Pfau and Burgoon (1988), Pfau (1990), and Pfau et al. (1990) measured students' attitudes toward smoking and attitudes toward other adolescents who smoke. The scale items included favorable/unfavorable, acceptable/unacceptable, positive/negative, right/wrong, wise/foolish, and good/bad. The reliabilities were .91 for attitude toward smoking, and .92 for attitude toward smokers.

Behavioral disposition toward smoking was assessed using a one-item 0–100 probability scale in response to the statement: "I will smoke cigarettes." The likelihood of resisting smoking was measured using three 0–100 probability scales in response to the following items: "When friends my age ask me to smoke cigarettes with them, I will say 'no'"; "I will tell my friends who smoke cigarettes that their smoking bothers me"; and, "I will tell members of my family who smoke that their smoking bothers me." Reliability was .65.

Results

Because the dependent measures were highly intercorrelated (in February, the average r was .52, and the range .34; in May, the average r was .54, and the range .30), multivariate analysis of variance, using the Wilk's lambda test, was conducted in order to determine significant omnibus effects, followed by univariate tests. Subsequent analyses consisted of tests of simple effects, if needed, and examination of means for all hypothesized effects using Dunn's multiple comparison procedure (Kirk, 1982).

Manipulation Checks

Two manipulation checks were employed as a prerequisite to subsequent analyses of hypotheses. The first manipulation check was designed to assess the presence of sufficient threat levels among the inoculated subjects. Threat is an integral component of inoculation since it triggers an internal process in receivers that motivates them to bolster their attitudes, thus making them resistant to change (McGuire, 1962).

One-way MANOVAs assessing threat levels among nonsmokers on the four dependent variables produced a main effect for threat in February, F (8,1946) = 5.36, $p <$ .001, $R^2 = .04$. The subsequent planned comparisons revealed maximum resistance among subjects experiencing high as opposed to either low or moderate threat on attitude toward smoking, F (1,976) = 14.18, $p < .001$, $\eta^2 = .03$, attitude toward smokers, F (1,976) = 28.83, $p < .001$, $\eta^2 = .03$, the likelihood of smoking, F (1,976) = 7.27, $p < .01$, $\eta^2 = .01$, and chance of resisting smoking, F (1,976) = 3.76, $p < .05$, one-tailed, $\eta^2 = .01$. Analysis of May data also produced a main effect for threat, F (8,1946) = 4.25, $P < .01$, $R^2 = .03$. The planned comparisons again revealed maximum resistance among subjects experiencing high as opposed to either low or moderate threat on attitude toward smoking, F (1,976) = 12.93, $p < .001$, $\eta^2 = .02$, attitude toward smokers, F (1,976) = 8.54, $p < .01$, $\eta^2 = .01$, the likelihood of smoking, F (1,976) = 6.51, $p < .05$, $\eta^2 = .01$, and chance of resisting smoking, F (1,976) = 12.05, $p <$ .001, $\eta^2 = .01$. One-way MANOVAs also were computed to assess threat levels for smokers. The results on the February and May data indicated no main effects.

The second manipulation check was designed to determine the appropriateness of an inoculation, as opposed to a persuasion, model. An examination of nonsmokers' and smokers' responses on dependent variables, first during middle September, prior to the administration of any of the pretreatments, and then again in February and May, confirms the appropriateness of the inoculation model. The September, February, and May scores for nonsmokers, those assigned to the inoculation and the control conditions, are reported in Table 21.1.

First, the September data reveal sharp contrasts in smokers' and nonsmokers' attitudes concerning smoking. A one-way MANOVA comparing smokers' and nonsmokers' September responses revealed significant differences, F (4,1042) = 78.38, $p <$ .001, R^2 = .23. Subsequent univariate tests indicated differences on attitude toward smoking, F (1,1045) = 173.85, p .001, η^2 = .17 (smokers M = 3.04, nonsmokers M = 1.52), attitude toward smokers, F (1,1045) = 143.54, $p <$ .001, η^2 = .14 (smokers M = 3.70, nonsmokers M = 1.92), the likelihood of smoking, F (1,1045) = 187.57. $p <$ .001, η^2 = .18 (smokers M = 37.64, nonsmokers M = 4.67), and chance of resisting smoking, F (1,1045) = 123.33, $p <$ .001, η^2 .12 (smokers M = 29.23, nonsmokers M = 68.69). These results confirm that nonsmokers commence the transition from primary to secondary school with strong attitudes opposing smoking.

Second, the data reveal the vulnerability of nonsmokers' attitudes toward smoking during the transition year from primary to secondary school. Mixed design MANOVAs (inoculation versus control across September, February, and May scores) were computed on each of the four dependent variables. The results indicated no main effect for experimental condition, but did reveal main effects involving time on the measures attitude toward smoking, F (2,945) = 120.85. $p <$ .001, R^2 = .20, attitude toward smokers, F (2,945) = 112.40, $p <$ .001, R^2 =. 19, and likelihood of smoking, F (2,942) = 37.12, $p <$ .001, R^2 = .07. Subsequent univariate tests indicated significant differences between September and February scores on attitude toward smoking, F (1,946) = 133.65, $p <$ .001, η^2 = .14, attitude

Table 21.1
Summary of the Experimental Condition Means Across Time for All Nonsmoking Adolescents

	Time and Experimental Condition					
	September		*February*		*May*	
Dependent Measure	*Control*	*Inoculation*	*Control*	*Inoculation*	*Control*	*Inoculation*
Attitude toward Smoking						
Mean	1.54	1.52	2.02	1.95	2.22	2.16
	(*n* = 222)	(*n* = 726)	(*n* = 222)	(*n* = 726)	(*n* = 222)	(*n* = 726)
SD	1.01	0.89	1.24	1.09	1.24	1.17
Attitude toward Smokers						
Mean	1.97	1.90	2.38	2.30	2.76	2.64
	(*n* = 222)	(*n* = 726)	(*n* = 222)	(*n* = 726)	(*n* = 222)	(*n* = 726)
SD	1.24	1.18	1.41	1.31	1.38	1.33
Likelihood of Smoking						
Mean	3.73	4.97	7.16	7.18	14.09	14.17
	(*n* = 222)	(*n* = 723)	(*n* = 222)	(*n* = 723)	(*n* = 222)	(*n* = 723)
SD	16.03	17.60	20.56	19.97	28.57	29.14
Chance of Resisting Smoking						
Mean	69.29	68.82	67.02	68.26	66.22	67.22
	(*n* = 222)	(*n* = 726)	(*n* = 222)	(*n* = 726)	(*n* = 222)	(*n* = 726)
SD	29.25	28.60	29.95	27.58	28.88	27.45

Note: The ratings of attitude toward smoking and attitude toward smokers are based on seven-point scales. The assessment of the likelihood of smoking is based on a 100-point probability scale. The lower the rating or assessment, the more resistant to smoking onset. Measurement of the chance of resisting smoking also is based on 100-point probability scales. In this case, however, the higher the assessment, the more resistant to smoking onset.

toward smokers, F (1,946) = 78.44, $p < .001$, $\eta^2 = .08$, and likelihood of smoking, F (1,943) = 11.48, $p < .001$, $\eta^2 = .01$, as well as differences between February and May scores on attitude toward smoking, F (1.946) = 133.08, $p < .001$, $\eta^2 = .14$, attitude toward smokers, F (1,946) =172.90, $p = .001$, $\eta^2 = .18$, and likelihood of smoking, F (1,943) = 65.25. $p < .001$, $\eta^2 =.07$.

Thus, the results indicate that, while nonsmokers begin the transition year from primary to middle or junior high school with negative attitudes toward smoking, those attitudes are vulnerable to slippage throughout the year. These outcomes, which have been supported in past research (Elder & Stern, 1986; Evans & Raines, 1982; Hamburg, 1979; Johnson, 1982; Killen, 1985), offer support for the appropriateness of the inoculation model.

Hypotheses

Hypotheses 1, 3, and 4 were examined using a 2 (experimental condition) × 3 (ordinalized self-esteem) × 2 (gender) factorial MANOVA design conducted on the February and May measures of the four dependent variables. The results suggest qualified support for Hypothesis 1 that inoculation promotes resistance to smoking initiation and strong support for Hypothesis 3 that inoculation is more effective for low self-esteem adolescents. The results revealed no support for Hypothesis 4 that inoculation is more effective with females.[2]

The omnibus MANOVAs revealed a consistent pattern of results on the dependent variables. They indicated no main effects for either pretreatment approach or gender. However, they did reveal a main effect for receiver self-esteem in February, F (8,1866) = 7.63, $p < .001$, $R^2 = .06$, with univariate tests indicating effects on attitude toward smoking, F (2,936) = 20.88, $p < .001$, $\eta^2 = .04$, attitude toward smokers, F (2,936) = 16.56, $p < .001$, $\eta^2 = .04$, likelihood of smoking, F (2,936) = 13.45, $p < .001$, $\eta^2 = .03$, and chance of resisting smoking, F (2,936) = 19.83, $p < .001$, $\eta^2 = .04$; and in May, F (8,1866) = 6.14, $p < .01$, $R^2 = .05$, with subsequent univariate tests indicating significant effects for attitude toward smoking, F (2,936) = 13.15, $p < .001$, $\eta^2 = .03$, attitude toward smokers, F (2,936) = 15.50, $p < .001$, $\eta^2 = .03$, likelihood of smoking, F (2,936)= 17.09, $p < .001$, $\eta^2 = .04$, and chance of resisting smoking, F (2,936) = 12.96, $p < .001$, $\eta^2 = .03$.

Planned comparisons were then computed assessing low versus moderate and high self-esteem subjects. As expected, the results indicated that low self-esteem adolescents were more susceptible to smoking initiation. As Table 21.2 reveals, in February, low self-esteem adolescents possessed more positive attitudes toward smoking, F (1,936) = 25.4l, $p < .001$, $\eta^2 = .03$, more positive attitudes toward smokers, F (1,936) = 20.67, $p < .001$, $\eta^2 = .02$, greater likelihood of smoking, F (1,936) = 24.20, $p < .001$, $\eta^2 = .03$, and less chance of resisting smoking, F (1,936) = 30.16, $p < .001$, $\eta^2 = .03$. In May, low self-esteem subjects manifested more positive attitudes toward smoking, F (1,936) = 17.01, $p < .001$, $\eta^2 = .02$, more positive attitudes toward smokers, F (1,936) = 22.27, $p < .001$, $\eta^2 = .02$, a greater likelihood of smoking, F (1,936) = 26.86, $p < .01$, $\eta^2 = .03$, and less chance of resisting smoking, F (1,936) = 16.40, $p < .001$, $\eta^2 = .02$.

However, the omnibus MANOVAs revealed two-way interactions which override the main effect findings for self-esteem. Results indicated two-way interactions involving experimental condition and self-esteem in February, F (8,1866) = 3.30, $p < .01$, $R^2 = .03$, and May, F (8,1866) = 1.88, $p < .05$, one-tailed, $R^2 = .02$. The subsequent univariate tests confirmed interaction effects on the February measures on attitude toward smoking, F (2,936) = 5.30, $p < .01$, $\eta^2 = .02$, attitude toward smokers, F (2,936) = 6.20, $p < .01$, $\eta^2 = .01$, and chance of resisting smoking, F (2,936) = 5.37, $p < .01$, $\eta^2 = .01$, and on the May measures of attitude toward smoking, F (2,936) = 5.13, $p < .01$, $\eta^2 = .01$, attitude toward smokers, F (2,936) = 2.80, p likelihood of smoking, F (2,936) = 4.23, $p < .05$, $\eta^2 = .01$. These interaction means are depicted in Table 21.3.

Tests of simple effects were computed for the experimental condition means across low, moderate, and high self-esteem as a prerequisite to further analyses. The one-way MANOVAs revealed a consistent pattern with significant differences in pretreat-

Table 21.2
Summary of the Self-Esteem Means Among Nonsmoking Adolescents

	Time and Self-Esteem Rating					
	February			May		
Dependent Measure	Low (n = 285)	Moderate (n = 315)	High (n = 348)	Low (n = 285)	Moderate (n = 315)	High (n = 348)
Attitude toward Smoking						
Mean	2.23[a]	1.89	1.82	2.39[a]	2.17	1.99
SD	1.23	1.03	1.10	1.23	1.18	1.16
Attitude toward Smokers						
Mean	2.62[a]	2.20	2.18	2.96[a]	2.66	2.45
SD	1.41	1.23	1.35	1.39	1.35	1.31
Likelihood of Smoking						
Mean	12.06[a]	4.92	5.06	21.34[b]	11.28	10.86
SD	25.78	16.80	16.80	34.52	25.57	26.33
Chance of Resisting Smoking						
Mean	61.15[a]	67.29	74.18	61.56[a]	65.52	72.76
SD	29.50	27.19	25.85	28.18	27.99	26.08

[a]significant at $p < .001$
[b]significant at $p < .01$
Note: The ratings of attitude toward smoking and attitude toward smokers are based on seven-point scales. The assessment of thee likelihood of smoking is based on a 100-point probability scale. The lower the rating or assessment, the more resistant to smoking onset. Measurement of the chance of resisting smoking also is based on 100-point probability scales. In this case, however, the higher the assessment, the more resistant to smoking onset.

ment approach, but only among subjects with low self-esteem.

In February, the results indicated significant differences in the experimental condition means only among low self-esteem subjects, F (4,933) = 5.06, $p < .01$, $R^2 = .02$. Univariate tests indicated differences on attitude toward smoking, F (1,936) = 18.02, $p < .001$, $\eta^2 = .02$, attitude toward smokers, F (1,936) = 12.16, $p < .001$, $\eta^2 = .01$, and the chance of resisting smoking, <1,936> = 8.45, $p < .01$, $\eta^2 = .01$.

Subsequent planned comparisons revealed that, for adolescents possessing low self-esteem, the inoculation pretreatments both contributed to less positive attitudes toward smoking, F (1,936)= 17.17, $p < .001$, $\eta^2 = .03$, and smokers, F (1,936) – 11.54, $p < .001$, $\eta^2 = .01$, and increased the chance of resisting smoking, F (1,936) = 9.66, $p < .01$, $\eta^2 = .01$.

In May, the results also revealed differences only among subjects of low self-esteem, F (4,933) = 2.66, $p < .05$, $R^2 = .01$. Subsequent univariate tests indicated differences on attitude toward smoking, F (1,936) = 9.94, $p < .01$, $\eta^2 = .01$, attitude toward smokers, F (1,936) = 7.07, $p < .01$, $\eta^2 = .01$, and the likelihood of smoking, F (1,936) = 5.77, $p < .05$, $\eta^2 = .01$. Planned comparisons indicated that, for those subjects possessing low self-esteem, inoculation pretreatments contributed to less positive attitudes toward smoking F (1,936) = 9.80, $p < .01$. $\eta^2 = .02$, and smokers, F (1,936) = 6.82, $p < .05$. $\eta^2 = .01$, and reduced the likelihood of smoking, F (1,936) = 6.28, $p < .05$. $\eta^2 = .01$.

Hypothesis 2 posited that inoculation-plus-reinforcement is more effective than inoculation alone in conferring resistance to smoking onset. The experimental condition was reconfigured as inoculation, inoculation-plus-reinforcement. and control, and 3 (experimental condition) × 3 (self-esteem) × 2 (gender) MANOVAs were computed involving the four dependent measures in February and May to examine this prediction. The results at both times indicated no main effects for experimental condition or gender, main effects for self-esteem, and two-way interactions involving experimental condition and self-esteem. Subsequent univariate tests, tests of simple effects, and planned comparisons revealed the same

Table 21.3
Summary of the Experimental Condition Means Among Low Self-Esteem Adolescents

	Time and Experimental Condition			
	February		May	
Dependent Measure	Control (n = 64)	Inoculation (n = 221)	Control (n = 64)	Inoculation (n = 221)
Attitude toward Smoking				
Mean	2.74	2.08[a]	2.79	2.27[b]
SD	1.46	1.13	1.36	1.14
Attitude toward Smokers				
Mean	3.11	2.48[a]	3.34	2.85[c]
SD	1.59	1.33	1.49	1.29
Likelihood of Smoking				
Mean	15.33	11.12	29.20	19.07[c]
SD	29.84	24.91	37.82	33.37
Chance of Resisting Smoking				
Mean	51.82	63.85[b]	55.85	63.21
SD	30.34	28.81	31.02	27.29

[a]significant at $p < .001$.
[b]significant at $p < .01$.
[c]significant at $p < .05$.
Note: The ratings of attitude toward smoking and attitude toward smokers are based on seven-point scales. The assessment of the likelihood of smoking is based on a 100-point probability scale. The lower the rating or assessment, the more resistant to smoking onset. Measurement of the chance of resisting smoking also is based on 100-point probability scales. In this case, however, the higher the assessment, the more resistant to smoking onset.

pattern of means as were reported previously. However, no additional boost was found for inoculation-plus-reinforcement.

Finally, one-way MANOVAs were conducted on the treatment and control subjects across instructor and then section in February and May to determine whether either factor was responsible for the mean differences reported above. The results revealed no significant differences involving the control subjects, based either on instructor or section, and no differences involving the treatment subjects based on section.

The results revealed no differences involving the treatment subjects for instructor in February, but did indicate differences in May involving two of the nine teachers. Because differences in instructor did not appear until the May assessment, the most plausible explanation is that the May result stemmed from varying effectiveness of the two instructors in leaching the unit dealing with cigarette, alcohol, and drug use, which occurred during the second semester, and not from intrinsic differences in the two subject groups.

Discussion

The results of this investigation confirm the importance of the transition year from primary to middle or junior high school in combating smoking initiation. The results indicate that those adolescents who have not yet succumbed to smoking onset commence the transition year from primary to secondary school with strong negative attitudes toward smoking. The results also reveal that these attitudes experience significant slippage throughout this transition year because of both physiological and psychological upheavals which render many adolescents vulnerable to peer pressures, and thus smoking initiation (Chassin et al., 1981; Elder & Stern, 1986; Evans & Raines, 1982; Hamburg, 1979; Johnson, 1982; Killen, 1985; McAlister et al., 1979).

However, the results of this study suggest that inoculation carries potential to arrest attitude slippage, thereby promoting resistance to smoking initiation, but only among low self-esteem adolescents. Among low self-esteem adolescents, the inoculation pretreatment videos were effective, initially in maintaining less positive attitudes toward smoking and greater chance of overtly resisting smoking, and subsequently in reducing the likelihood of smoking.

These findings offer additional support for the viability of McGuire's inoculation model in general, and its application to still another field context. They also provide further support for research indicating that intervention targeting adolescents during the transition from elementary to secondary school can prevent (or significantly delay) the onset of cigarette smoking (Evans et al., 1981; Hansen et al., 1988; Murray et al., 1987; Perry, 1987; Perry et al., 1980).

The pattern of results suggests important insights about the potential of inoculation in smoking prevention. Past studies had employed a smorgasbord of methods under the umbrella heading of social inoculation, including videos, slide shows, school-wide campaigns, peer modeling, teacher- and peer-led discussions, and others. Many operationalized social inoculation absent the integral threatening component, which serves as the motivational catalyst for resistance (McGuire, 1962; Papageorgis & McGuire, 1961), thus raising the distinct possibility that one or more features of these interventions other than the preemptive component was actually responsible for their results. Concerns such as these have led scholars to question the value of social inoculation in smoking prevention (Flay, 1985; Foon, 1986; McCaul & Glasgow, 1985).

The one method of such studies that can be operationalized to insure replication in subsequent uses is videos, which were employed as the vehicle for inoculation in this investigation. However, past research has failed to demonstrate the efficacy of videos (Evans et al., 1978; Murray et al., 1988), perhaps because they failed to operationalize threat, or because they failed to anticipate an interaction of treatment efficacy and receiver characteristics. However, the results of this study suggest that inoculation via video can promote resistance to adolescent smoking initiation, thereby providing a simple and relatively inexpensive tool to aid health educators in their efforts.

The results, indicating that inoculation fosters resistance to smoking, but only among adolescents of low self-esteem, is particularly important. First, this finding helps explain the conflicting failings of past research about social inoculation and smoking. Best et al. (1988), Botvin (1982), and Flay (1985) have criticized past social inoculation research for virtually ignoring those relevant individual characteristics that should affect program effectiveness. The interaction finding of this study is instructive in this regard. Since the results revealed no main effect for inoculation, if this investigation had foiled to include self-esteem as a potential interactant, the results would have reaffirmed the general ineffectiveness of inoculation in smoking prevention, consistent with past research.

Second, the pattern of results provides guidance for those practitioners involved in smoking prevention programs, stressing the need to design and target approaches according to adolescent self-esteem levels. The results of this study indicate that low self-esteem adolescents are most at risk to smoking initiation, confirming the previous findings of Best et al. (1988), Elder and Stern (1986), Harken (1987), and others. Thus, the finding of this investigation that inoculation promotes resistance to smoking initiation, but only for low self-esteem adolescents, suggests a very specific, but important, role for this approach in future campaigns against adolescent smoking.

Finally, the results revealed no significant difference in the effectiveness of inoculation based on receiver gender, and no additional boost for reinforcement. One possible explanation for the null finding regarding gender stems from social role theory, posited as the explanation for differences in persuasibility. If gender differences are the result of unique social roles, the resulting differences between females and males should be less established in the young adolescents employed in this study than in adults.

The failure to find a booster effect for the reinforcement materials is disappointing. The initial inoculative materials, however, maintained their effects over a period of 33 weeks. This fact provides further evidence that an inoculative stimulus carries considerable persistence (Pfau & Burgoon, 1988; Pfau et al., 1990, p. 38). Clearly reinforcement is not required quite so soon following inoculation. If the reinforcement materials were administered later, perhaps at the start of the following semester, they might have proven to be more effective.

An additional caveat must be posited concerning the small effect sizes for the inoculation findings, ranging from one to three percent. Such effect sizes are meaningful in the context of this study. Because only a small proportion of seventh grade students join the ranks of smokers during the course of the year (Centers for Disease Control, 1991), the inoculative materials would not be expected to account for large effect sizes. Another way to characterize the significance of effects that is much more revealing in this context is to convert η^2 to *r,* and then directly compare the effectiveness of treatment (.50 + *r*/2) and control (.50 – *r*/2) conditions using the binomial effect-size display (BESD) (Rosenthal & Rosnow, 1984). BESD reveals considerable difference in smoking initiation rates of low self-esteem subjects depending on whether or not they were exposed to inoculative pretreatments: in February ranging from 41% (exposed) to 58% (not exposed) on attitude toward smoking, and 45% to 55% on attitude toward smokers and chance of resisting smoking; and in May ranging from 43% to 57% on attitude toward smoking, and 45% to 55% on attitude toward smokers and likelihood of smoking. The BESD method illustrates the practical meaning of these results. The inoculation pretreatments, in instilling more negative attitudes toward smoking in up to 17% of younger adolescents and discouraging 10% of them from smoking onset, can make an important contribution to efforts to combat adolescent smoking.

Endnotes

1. This study identified 6.5% of entering seventh grade students as regular smokers, higher than national norms. The Centers for Disease Control (1991) indicates that 2.4% of 12-year-olds and 5.2% of 13-year-olds smoke during a 30-day period. Because the inoculation approach seeks to promote resistance to initiation of smoking, the questionnaire item used to identify regular smokers was phrased to include past and present smokers. This nuance in wording is the most likely explanation tor the higher incidence of smokers in the study population.
2. This investigation also tested for differences in the relative effectiveness of adult- and peer-led inoculation approaches. Peer- and adult-led program providers were employed in the early social inoculation efforts to reduce the initiation of adolescent smoking. Subsequent research concerning the relative superiority of the two approaches was equivocal (Best et al., 1988). Results of this study indicated that both inoculation approaches were effective in fostering resistance to smoking initiation, but only among low self-esteem adolescents. However, the results failed to reveal any significant differences between the two approaches.

References

Alexander, H. M., Callcott, R., Dobson, A. J., Hardes, G. R., Lloyd, D. M., O'Connell, D. L.,& Leeder, S. R.(1983). Cigarette smoking and drug use in school children: IV—Factors associated with changes in smoking behavior. *International Journal of Epidemiology, 12,* 59–66.

Anderson, L. R., & McGuire, W. J. (1965). Prior reassurance of group consensus as a factor in producing resistance to persuasion. *Sociometry, 28,* 44–56.

Barton, J., Chassin, L., Presson, C. C., & Sherman, S. J. (1982). Social image factors as motivators of smoking initiation in early and middle adolescence. *Child Development, 53,* 1499–1511.

Becker, B. J. (1986). Influence again: Another look at studies of gender differences in social influence. In J. S. Hyde & M. C. Linn (Eds.). *The psychology of gender: Advances through meta-analysis* (pp. 178–209). Baltimore, MD: Johns Hopkins University Press.

Bernstein, D. A., & McAlister, A. L. (1976). The modification of smoking behavior. *Addictive Behaviors, 1,* 89–102.

Best, J. A., Thomson, S. J., Sand, S. M., Smith, E. A., & Brown, K. S. (1988). Preventing cigarette smoking among school children. *Annual Review of Public Health, 9,* 161–201.

Bewley, B. R., & Bland, J. M. (1977). Academic performance and social factors related to cigarette smoking by school children. *British*

Journal of Preventative and Social Medicine, 31, 18–24.

Biglan, A., & Ary, D. V. (1985). Methodological issues in research on smoking prevention. In C. S. Bell & R. Barnes (Eds.), *Prevention research: Deterring drug abuse among children and adolescents* (pp. 170–195). Rockville, MD: National Institute on Drug Abuse.

Botvin, G. J. (1982). Broadening the focus of smoking prevention strategies. In T. J. Coates, A. C. Petersen, & C. Perry (Eds.), Promoting adolescent health: A dialogue on research and practice (pp. 157–147). New York: Academic Press.

Botvin, G. J., Renick, N. L., & Baker, E. (1983). The effects of scheduling format and booster sessions on a broad-spectrum psychosocial approach to smoking prevention. *Journal of Behavioral Medicine, 6,* 359–579.

Burgoon, M., Cohen, M., Miller, M. D., & Montgomery, C. L. (1978). An empirical test of a model of resistance to persuasion. *Human Communication Research, 5,* 27–39.

Centers for Disease Control (1991). Cigarette smoking among youth—United States, 1989. *Morbidity and Mortality Weekly Report, 41,* 712–715.

Chassin, L. T., Cony. E., Presson, C. C., Olshavsky, R. W., Bensenberg, M., & Sherman, S. J. (1981). Predicting adolescents' intentions to smoke cigarettes. *Journal of Health and Social Behavior, 22,* 445–455.

Cook, T. D. (1985). Priorities in research in smoking prevention, in C. S. Bell & R. Battjes (Eds.). *Prevention research: Deterring drug abuse among children and adolescents* (pp. 196–220). Rockville, MD: National Institute on Drug Abuse.

Cooper, H. M. (1979). Statistically combining independent studies: A meta-analysis of sex differences in conformity research. *Journal of Personality and Social Psychology,* 131–146.

Coopersmith, S. (1967). *The antecedents of self-esteem.* San Francisco: W. H. Freeman & Company.

Cronbach, L. J.(195l). Coefficient alpha and the internal structure of tests. *Psychometrika, 16,* 297–334.

Cronkhite, G. (1969). *Persuasion: Speech and behavioral change.* New York: The Bobbs-Merrill Company, Inc.

Department of Health and Human Services (1989). *1989 Surgeon General's report Reducing the health consequences of smoking: 25 years of progress* (DHHS Publication No. CDC 9-8411). Washington, DC: U.S. Government Printing Office.

Eagly, A. H. (1978). Sex differences in influenceability. *Psychological Bulletin, 85,* 86–116.

Eagly, A. H. (1987). *Sex differences in social behavior: A social-role interpretation.* Hillsdale, NJ: Lawrence Eribaum Associates.

Eagly, A. H., & Carli, L. L. (1981). Sex of researchers and sex-typed communications as determinants of sex differences in influenceability: A meta-analysis of social influence studies. *Psychological Bulletin, 90,* 1–20.

Einsiedel, E. F., & Cochrane, K. (1988, June). *Using social marketing and theoretical perspectives for health campaigns to adolescents.* Paper presented at the annual meeting of the International Communication Association, New Orleans, LA.

Elder, J. P., & Stern, R. A. (1986). The ABCs of adolescent smoking prevention: An environment and skills model. *Health Education Quarterly, 13,* 181–191.

Evans, R. I., & Raines, B. E. (1982). Control and prevention of smoking in adolescents: A psychosocial perspective. In T. J. Coates, A. C. Petersen, & C. Perry (Eds.), *Promoting adolescent health: A dialogue an research and practice* (pp. 101–136). New York: Academic Press.

Evans, R. I., Rozelle, R. M., Maxwell, S. E., Raines, B. E., Dill, C. A., Guthrie, T. J., Henderson, A. H., & Hill, P. C. (1981). Social modeling films to deter smoking in adolescents: Results of a three-year field investigation. *Journal of Applied Psychology, 66,* 399–414.

Evans, R. I., Rozelle, R. M., & Mittlemark, M. B. (1978). Deterring the onset of smoking in children. *Journal of Applied Social Psychology, 8,* 126–135.

Flay, B. R. (1985). Prosocial approaches to smoking prevention: A review of findings. *Health Psychology, 4,* 449–488.

Flay, B. R., d'Avernas, R. J., Best, J. A., Kersell, M. W., & Ryan, K. B. (1983). Cigarette smoking: Why young people do it and ways of preventing it. In P. J. McGrath & P. Firestone (Eds.), *Pediatric and adolescent behavioral medicine* (pp. 132–183). New York: Springer.

Foon, A. E. (1986). Smoking prevention programs for adolescents: The value of social psychological approaches. *The International Journal of the Addictions, 21,* 1017–1029.

Friedman, L. S., Lichtenstein, E., & Biglan, A. (1985). Smoking onset among teens: An empirical analysis of initial situations. *Addictive Behaviors, 10,* 1–13.

Goldberg, M. E., & Garn, G. J. (1982). Increasing the involvement of teenage cigarette smokers in antismoking campaigns, *Journal of Communication, 32* (1), 75–86.

Gordon, N. P. (1986). Never smokers, triers and

current smokers: Three distinct target groups for school-based antismoking programs. *Health Education Quarterly, 13,* 163–179.

Gottlieb, N., & Baker, J. (1986). The relative influence of health beliefs, parental and peer behaviors and exercise program participation on smoking, alcohol use and physical activity. *Social Science and Medicine, 22,* 915–927.

Hamburg, D. A. (1979). Disease prevention: The challenge of the future. *American Journal of Public Health, 69,* 1026–1033.

Hansen, W. B., Malotte, C. K., & Fielding, J. E. (1988). Evaluation of a tobacco and alcohol abuse prevention curriculum for adolescents. *Health Education Quarterly. 15,* 93–114.

Harken, L. S. (1987). The prevention of adolescent smoking: A public health priority. *Evaluation & the Health Professions, 10,* 373–393.

Hunt, W., Barnett, L., & Branch, L. G. (1971). Relapse rates in addiction programs. *Journal of Clinical Psychology, 27,*455–456.

Johnson, B. W., Redfield, D. L., Miller, R. I., & Simpson, R. E. (1983). The Coopersmith self-esteem inventory: A construct validation study. *Educational and Psychological Measurement, 43,* 907–913.

Johnson, C. A. (1982). Untested and erroneous assumptions underlying antismoking programs. In T. J. Coates, A. C. Petersen, & C. Perry (Eds.), *Promoting adolescent health: A dialogue on research and practice* (pp. 149–165). New York: Academic Press.

Johnson, C. A., Hansen, W. B., Collins, L. M., & Graham, J. W. (1986). High-school smoking prevention: Results of a three-year longitudinal study. *Journal of Behavioral Medicine, 9,* 439–452.

Killen, J. D. (1985). Prevention of adolescent tobacco smoking: The social pressure resistance training approach. *Journal of Child Psychology and Psychiatry, 26,* 7–15.

Kirk, R. E. (1982). *Experimental design: Procedures for the behavioral sciences* (2nd ed.). Belmont, CA: Brooks/Cole.

Maccoby, E. E., & Jacklin, C. N. (1974). *The psychology of sex differences*. Palo Alto, CA: Stanford University Press.

McAlister, A. L., Perry, C., & Maccoby, N. (1979). Adolescent smoking: Onset and prevention. *Pediatrics, 63,* 650–658.

McCaul, K. D., & Glasgow, R. E. (1985). Preventing adolescent smoking: What we have learned about treatment construct validity? *Health Psychology, 4,* 361–387.

McCaul, K. D., Glasgow, R., O'Neill, H. K., Freeborn, V., & Rump, B. S. (1982). Predicting adolescent smoking. *The Journal of School Health, 52*(6), 342–346.

McGuire, W. J. (1961a). The effectiveness of supportive and refutational defenses in immunizing and restoring beliefs against persuasion. *Sociometry, 24,* 184–197.

McGuire, W. J. (1961b). Resistance to persuasion conferred by active and passive prior refutation of the same and alternative counterarguments, *Journal of Abnormal and Social Psychology, 63,* 326–332.

McGuire, W. J. (1962). Persistence of the resistance to persuasion induced by various types of prior belief defenses. *Journal of Abnormal and Social Psychology, 64,* 241 –248

McGuire, W. J. (1964). Inducing resistance to persuasion. Some contemporary approaches. In L. Berkowitz (Ed.), *Advances in experimental social psychology* (Vol. 1, pp. 191–229). New York: Academic Press.

McGuire, W. J. (1969). The nature of attitudes and attitude change. In G. Lindzey & E. Aronson (Eds.). *The handbook of social psychology* (2nd ed., Vol. 3, pp. 136–514). Reading, MA: Addison-Wesley.

McGuire, W. J. (1970, February). A vaccine for brainwash. *Psychology Today, 3,* 36–39, 63–64.

McGuire, W. J., & Papageorgis, D. (1961). The relative efficacy of various types of prior belief-defense in producing immunity against persuasion. *Journal of Abnormal and Social Psychology, 62,* 327–337.

McGuire, W. J., & Papageorgis, D. (1962). Effectiveness of forewarning in developing resistance to persuasion. *Public Opinion Quarterly, 26,* 24–34.

Mettlin, C. (1976). Peer and other influences on smoking behavior. *The Journal of School Health, 46,* 529–536.

Miller, G. R., & Burgoon, M. (1973). *New techniques of persuasion*. New York: Harper & Row.

Miller, G. R., Burgoon, M., & Burgoon, J. K. (1984). The functions of human communication in changing attitudes and gaining compliance. In C. C. Arnold & J. W. Bowers (Eds.), *Handbook of rhetorical and communication theory* (pp. 400–474). Boston: Allyn and Bacon, Inc.

Miller, M. D., & Burgoon, M. (1979). The relationship between violations of expectations and the induction of resistance to persuasion. *Human Communication Research, 5,* 301–313.

Murray, D. M., Davis-Hearn, M., Goldman, A. I., Pirie, P., & Luepker, R. V. (1988). Four- and five-year follow-up results from four seventh-grade smoking prevention strategies. *Journal of Behavioral Medicine, 11,* 395–105.

Murray, D. M., Richards, P. S., Luepker, R. V., & Johnson, G. A. (1987). The prevention of cigarette smoking in children: Two- and three-year follow-up comparisons of four prevention strategies. *Journal of Behavioral Medicine, 10,* 595–611.

O'Neill, H. K., Glasgow, R. E., & McCaul, K. D. (1983). Component analysis in smoking prevention research: Effects of social consequences information. *Addictive Behaviors, 8,* 419–423.

O'Rourke, A. H., O'Byrne. D. J., & Wilson-Davis, K. (1983). Smoking among schoolchildren. *Journal of the Royal College of General Practitioners, 33,* 569–572.

Papageorgis, D., & McGuire, W. J. (1961). The generality of immunity to persuasion produced by pre-exposure to weakened counterarguments. *Journal of Abnormal and Social Psychology, 62,* 475–481.

Pechacek, T. F., & McAlister, A. K. (1980). Strategies for the modification of smoking behavior: Treatment and prevention. In T. Gerguson (Ed.). *The comprehensive handbook of behavioral medicine* (Vol. 3, pp. 257–298). New York: Spectrum Publications, Inc.

Pederson, L. L., & Lefcoe, N. M. (1982). Multivariate analysis of variables related to cigarette smoking among children in grades four to six. *Canadian Journal of Public Health, 73,* 172–175.

Perry, C. L. (1987). Results of prevention programs with adolescents. *Drug and Alcohol Dependence, 20,* 13–19.

Perry, C. L., Killen, J., & Slinkard, L. A. (1980). Peer teaching and smoking prevention among junior high students. *Adolescence, 40,* 275–281.

Pfau, M. (1990). A channel approach to television influence. *Journal of Broadcasting & Electronic Media, 14,* 1–20.

Pfau, M. (1992). The potential of inoculation in promoting resistance to the effectiveness of comparative advertising messages. *Communication Quarterly, 40,* 26–44.

Pfau, M., & Burgoon, M. (1988). Inoculation in political campaign communication. *Human Communication Research, 15,* 91–111.

Pfau, M., Kenski, H. C., Niu, M., & Sorenson, J. (1990). Efficacy of inoculation strategies in promoting resistance to political attack messages: Application to direct mail. *Communication Monographs, 57,* 1–12.

Pryor, B., & Steinfatt, T. M. (1978). The effects of initial belief level on inoculation theory and its proposed mechanisms. *Human Communication Research, 4,* 217–230.

Rokeach, M. (1987). *Health values.* Paper presented to the Institution for Health Promotion and Disease Prevention, Pasadena, CA.

Rosenberg, M. (1965). *Society and adolescent self-image.* Princeton, NJ: Princeton University Press.

Rosenthal, R., & Rosnow, R. L. (1984). *Essentials of behavioral research: Methods and data analysis.* New York: McGraw-Hill.

Salomon, G., Stein, Y., Eisenberg, S., & Klein, L. (1984). Adolescent smokers and nonsmokers: Profiles and their changing structure. *Preventative Medicine, 13,* 446–461.

Tannenbaum, P. H., Macaulay, J. R., & Norris, E. L. (1966). Principle of congruity and reduction in persuasion. *Journal of Personality and Social Psychology, 2,* 225–238.

Urberg, K., & Robbins, R. (1984). Perceived vulnerability in adolescents to the health consequences of cigarette smoking. *Preventative Medicine, 13,* 367–376.

Discussion Questions

1. What do successful inoculation strategies look like? To what other contexts might inoculation strategies apply?
2. What are some consequences of moving from a public health agenda that focuses on curing disease to one that focuses on preventing disease?
3. If our public health agenda is truly focused on preventing disease, why does the public continue to underfund health and physical education programs for children? What more can be done to make children more health literate so that they can engage in better preventative practices? ✦

Chapter 22
'I'm Not a Druggie'
Adolescents' Ethnicity and (Erroneous) Beliefs About Drug Use Norms

Michelle Miller-Day and Jacqueline M. Barnett

Chapter 22 addresses the need for better drug-prevention health campaigns by examining ethnic identity and the perception of cultural norms that may be linked to drug use and the attitudes and beliefs about it. Again, the chapter reminds us that communication theory and practices have application to yet another important and complex health issue. The authors interviewed both African American and non-Hispanic white adolescents to learn more about the youths' personal and ethnic identities, their own drug use behavior, and their perceptions of drugs and drug use. Ethnic identity and the perception of cultural norms may be linked to drug use and attitudes and beliefs about drug use, so there is a need for increased health campaign prevention efforts.

Related Topics: culture, drug use, health campaigns, health-care behaviors, qualitative methods

A 12-year-old boy who was interviewed for a previous study (Miller, 1999) exclaimed to the interviewer, "I'm Black so it is more important for me not to use drugs!" This exclamation brought the constructs of ethnicity and attitudes toward drug use into sharp juxtaposition. After the discussion with this youth and several similar conversations with other young Black adolescents over the years, we discovered that ethnic identity may play a role in adolescent choices to use or not use illicit drugs. Even so, few researchers have examined ways in which youths' perceptions of their ethnic or cultural identity shape their drug use behavior. Therefore, an initial purpose of this study was to explore both Black and non-Hispanic White youths' self-systems of personal and ethnic identity in relation to their attitudes about drug use.

Cross-Cultural Differences in Drug Use

Substance abusers face substantial health risks; reports over the past 2 decades have established that adolescent drug use is a major public health issue (Centers for Disease Control and Prevention [CDCP], 1995; Wallace, Bachman, O'Malley, & Johnston, 1995). These reports are based on large national samples designed to provide direct cross-cultural comparisons across ethnic groups. These studies have repeatedly reported that Black youth in Grades 8 to 12 use fewer drugs (e.g., alcohol, tobacco, marijuana, cocaine) than non-Hispanic Whites (see reports by Bachman et al., 1991; CDCP, 1995; Substance Abuse and Mental Health Services Administration [SAMHSA], 2001; Wallace et al, 1995). Allen and Page (1994) focused specifically on Black and non-Hispanic White adolescents in their research and found Blacks of both genders were significantly less likely than non-Hispanic White[1] males and females to report that they drink alcohol; get drunk; smoke cigarettes; and use smokeless tobacco, hallucinogens, and sedatives. The National Household Survey on Drug Abuse (NHSDA) serves as the primary source of information on the prevalence, patterns, and consequences of drug and alcohol use and abuse in the general U.S. civilian noninstitutionalized population ages 12 and older. This survey obtains drug use data from approximately 70,000 persons per year. In

From " 'I'm Not a Druggie': Adolescents' Ethnicity and (Erroneous) Beliefs About Drug Use Norms," Michelle Miller-Day and Jacqueline M. Barnett, 2004, *Health Communication*, Vol. 16:2, pp. 207–288.

both the 1999 and the 2000 data sets, the NHSDA reported a continued disparity among ethnic groups in drug use prevalence (SAMHSA, 2001). The 2000 findings indicate that Whites were more likely than any other race-ethnicity group to report current use of alcohol in 2000. An estimated 50.7% of Whites ages 12 and older reported using alcohol in the past month compared with 33.7% of Blacks. In addition, among youth ages 12 to 17, 18.4% of White youth reported frequent use of alcohol and 12% of those participated in "binge" drinking, compared with 8.8% of Black youth reporting frequent alcohol use and 4% participating in binge drinking. In the 2000 survey, as observed in prior years, the level of alcohol use was strongly associated with illicit drug use. Among the 12.6 million heavy drinkers ages 12 and older, 30.0% were current illicit drug users. The percentages of individuals reporting lifetime illicit drug use (e.g., marijuana, cocaine, heroin, inhalants) revealed that 41.7% of Whites had used illicit drugs compared with 36.6% of Black respondents. Further, percentages of those youth ages 12 to 17 reporting lifetime use of cigarettes in 2000 revealed that 40.3% of the White youth compared with 27.5% of the Black youth had smoked cigarettes.

Over and over again, the prevalence statistics suggested lower drug usage rates among young Blacks when compared with young Whites. Scholars such as Bass (1993); Belgrave, Brome, and Hampton (2000); Blackwell (1991); and Brook, Whiteman, Balka, Thet Win, and Gursin (1998) have suggested that disparities in drug use prevalence rates might best be understood by attending to ethnic identity and cultural values in each ethnic group. That is, the cultural values specific to particular ethnic groups may provide a vantage point from which to view a more accurate interpretation of ethnic differences in drug use behavior. Unfortunately, the cultural approach to understanding adolescent drug use patterns has been neglected (Belgrave et al., 2000; Botvin, Schinke, & Orlandi, 1995; Miller, Alberts, Hecht, Trost, & Krizek, 2000).

Cultural Approach to Understanding Ethnic Differences in Drug Use

Scholars who have reviewed prevention approaches over the past decade, such as Belgrave et al. (2000); Burlew, Neely, Johnson, and Hucks (2000); and Myers, Newcomb, Richardson, and Alvy (1997) have argued for programming that is specifically targeted to cultural ideals and norms. A cultural approach to adolescent drug use behavior entails investigating and describing a culture's normative beliefs and the perceptions of cultural members (i.e., members of a particular ethnic culture) toward those beliefs as tied to cultural practices. Arguments for this framework suggest that drug prevention information presented in ways that are meaningful and culturally relevant to the targeted population is more likely to be retained and used than information presented in ways that do not reflect group values or norms (Belgrave et al., 2000).

Implicit in the cultural approach is the assumption that both Black and White individuals identify with a particular ethnic culture. Ethnic cultural identification entails a sense of belonging to a particular group to the extent that one labels oneself as belonging to this group, thereby shaping attitudes toward the membership group (Phinney & Chavira, 1992). Therefore, to assess beliefs about cultural norms, a person's sense of identification with that particular ethnic culture must also be examined. Belgrave and her colleagues have provided a body of evidence that indicates ethnic identity may be a significant predictor of drug use and of drug attitudes (Belgrave et al., 2000; Townsend & Belgrave, 2000). These researchers have focused mainly on the experiences of Black youth and have posited that youth who possess a positive and clear ethnic identity are better able to resist and/or delay drug initiation than are youth who do not possess a clear or positive ethnic identity (Belgrave et al., 2000; Belgrave, Townsend, Cherry, & Cunningham, 1997). Yet, little cross-cultural research has been conducted in this area. If youths' self-conceptualization or perception of self serves to guide behavior, then ethnic identity should function similarly across cultures. However, Townsend and Belgrave suggested that ethnic identity may function differently across ethnic cultures and most powerfully within Black cultures. They proposed that Black children derive much of their sense of personal self from the collective or group cultural norms they perceive—the self as an extension of the collective. They pointed out that Azibo (1996) articulated this view with the phrase, "I am because we are" (p. 212).

Surprisingly, there has been little to no qualitative exploration of perceptions of drug use norms within distinct ethnic groups. The previous research points to two assumptions: that adolescents' perceptions of self may guide their drug use attitudes and behavior, and that for Black adolescents, ethnic identification with the Black culture and perceptions of ethnic cultural norms may affect attitudes and drug use behaviors. Yet, because there is so little research in this area, a grounded investigation of these assumptions is needed.

Thus, this study was designed as a cultural approach to understanding adolescent drug use behavior, providing a description of ethnic identity and perceived cultural norms among a sample of Black and White youth. In addition, this investigation explores patterns in the reported normative beliefs both within and across ethnic groups and then links those patterns with youths' drug behaviors.

Ethnic Identity

Rotheram-Borus and Wyche (1994) argued that ethnicity and race are often confused. "Race," they claimed, involves narrow definitions based on physical characteristics (such as skin color) that cannot be changed; however, ethnicity refers to "identification . . . with a larger social group on the basis of common ancestry, race, religion, language, or national origin" (p. 63). Ethnic identity, in particular, refers to a sense of collective identity based on one's perception that he or she shares a common heritage with a particular ethnic group (Helms, 1990). Moreover, ethnic identity is a central domain within personal identity development for adolescents (Archer, 1994; Aries, 1998; Phinney & Chavira, 1992; Rotheram-Borus & Wyche, 1994) and one that may be more salient to Blacks than to Whites (Helms, 1990; Phinney & Alipuria, 1990; Stiffman & Davis, 1990).

Gaines, Marelich, Bledsloe, and Steers (1997) found that in the United States, persons of color had higher levels of race consciousness and had a stronger sense of ethnic identity than did Whites. Ethnicity is defined not only by race but by patterns of behavior linked to an ethnic group. Ethnic identity therefore includes multiple aspects of attachment to one's heritage, including participation in the culture and its traditions (Clark, 1982; Keefe & Padilla, 1987; Phinney & Chavira, 1992).

Researchers such as Guerra, Huesmann, and Hanish (1995) have suggested that when ethnic group members articulate their normative beliefs, cultural values will become evident. Additional studies by Huselid and Cooper (1992) and Ramirez, Chalela, and Presswood (2000) and culturally sensitive prevention work (see, e.g., Miller et al., 2000) suggest that one's personal norms for behavior (e.g., "I should not accept drug offers") are tied inextricably to one's perception of how others in one's cultural group "normally" behave.

Norms

Adolescent drug use norms are viewed most often as adolescents' perceptions about the prevalence of drug use among peers and friends (Hansen, 1991). Cialdini, Kallgren, and Reno (1990), however, took a more detailed approach to normative beliefs and behaviors in their norms focus theory. According to this theory, a *norm* is broadly defined as an individual's behaviors as motivated by some guideline or standard. The norm focus theory distinguishes among three types of normative messages: injunctive, descriptive, and personal. *Injunctive norms* describe what people ought to do; these norms are approval oriented and externally imposed by others (e.g., the society at large, parents, and peers). Injunctive norms may also motivate behavior by providing messages that promise either rewards or punishments (sanctions). An example would be the following typical edict from parents and authorities: "Drugs are bad; don't do them. If you do drugs you will be punished." *Descriptive norms* describe what people do most often. These messages provide frequency information about the behavior of important reference figures or groups and motivate behavior by providing information about what will be most effective and adaptive in a particular situation. Finally, *personal norms* are internalized values and expectations for one's own behavior, regardless of external rewards or evidence. Students express personal norms when they declare, "[Irrespective of what others do, or what I'm told I should do] I'm not the type of person who does drugs" (Miller et al., 2000, p. 13).

Research involving norm focus theory indicates that two or more conflicting norms may operate in any given situation, blurring what is appropriate behavior (Cialdini et al., 1990). According to Miller et al. (2000), distinguishing among injunctive, descriptive, and personal norms acknowledges the complexity of normative processes and emphasizes their unique contribution to motivating behavior. Consequently, if researchers want to understand adolescents from the adolescents' own perspectives and understand how drug use fits or does not fit into that individual identity it is necessary to understand more fully the normative messages perceived by the adolescent.

Because the purpose of this study is to provide a descriptive account of adolescents' culturally specific normative beliefs about ethnicity and alcohol, tobacco, and other drug use, we queried both Black and White youth about their identity and about their normative beliefs and behaviors regarding alcohol, tobacco, and other drug use: In addition, when examining the data, we asked, "What patterns of normative beliefs and behaviors regarding alcohol, tobacco, and other drug use emerge within and across both ethnic groups?"

Method

Participants and Research Sites

Participants were recruited using a stratified purposeful sample (Taylor & Bogdan, 1984) in which volunteers were selected from classrooms in two inner-city schools, two inner-city churches, and two inner-city community centers within a 10-mile (approximately 16-km) radius of one another in the mid-South. In this particular U.S. urban area, Blacks composed 53% of the overall population, Whites composed 46% of the population, and other ethnic groups composed the remaining 1%. After institutional review board approval to conduct this research was secured, a list of all schools, churches, and community centers within a 10-mile (approximately 16-km) radius of a downtown urban center was compiled. Two organizations were randomly selected from each list (e.g., two churches, two schools). The first author had conducted research in the community previously, and so she contacted each organization, secured permission to recruit participants, and solicited participation in person at the various organizations.

The authors and their staff of ethnically diverse undergraduate assistants solicited participants by describing the project and asking for student participation. These presentations occurred during the course of the school day in an English class required of all students. The staff at the churches and community centers provided the same description of the project and recruited a sample of teens interested in participating in the interviews. Consent forms were provided to those students who expressed interest; they were asked to present the form to a parent, so the parent could read the information about the project and sign the form. As part of a larger project designed to elicit descriptions of adolescents' drug offers and refusal strategies, 12 participants were randomly selected from each of the six sites from those students who returned the signed consent forms to their teachers or leaders (n = 72). We ultimately discarded 5 of these (because of low-quality recording of the recorded data) for a total number of 67 participants.[2]

There were 22 participants from the schools, 22 participants from the churches, and 23 participants from the community center sites. Ninety percent of the participants were age 16 or younger, with a mean age of 13 years. Sixty-three percent were

Black ($n = 42$), and 37% were non-Hispanic White ($n = 25$). In addition, 46% of the sample was male ($n = 31$), and 54% of the sample was female ($n = 36$). Interviewees were paid $5 and were offered coupons for free food at a local yogurt store and/or McDonald's restaurant.

The Interview

Because paper-and-pencil surveys have had limited success in data-gathering activities among Black youth because of their general mistrust of written approaches to data collection (Bass, 1993), face-to-face semistructured interviews with White and Black interviewers were conducted to ascertain the youths' attitudes about alcohol and other drugs, their drug-related behaviors, and perceptions of their personal identity. Four undergraduate interviewers attended two 4-hr sessions for training in general interviewing techniques and cultural sensitivity (Session 1) and inflow to conduct the actual project interview (Session 2). The principal investigator of this project provided general instructions, written protocols, and role playing to the interviewers-in-training and offered individual instruction on a case-by-case basis. The first author and the four trained interviewers conducted the interviews based on a semistructured interview schedule with open-ended questions similar to those used in the Hecht, Trost, Bator, and MacKinnon (1997) study.

The interviews began with a short introductory period followed by a discussion of consent. Each youth was informed that he or she could refuse to answer questions, responses were confidential, and he or she could terminate the interview at any time. Students were also informed that the interview was being audio-taped. In addition to written consent, each youth provided verbal consent that was audio-taped. Because this study was part of a larger study on drug offers and refusals, all respondents were asked to provide narrative accounts of any drug offers made in the previous 2 years and their choices to refuse or accept the offer. After the participants discussed these offers, they were asked if they had accepted or refused the offers and were asked details about their responses. The interview schedule was designed to move from discussion of drug resistance behavior to adolescents' attitudes and normative beliefs about alcohol, tobacco, and other drugs. After addressing the issues of drug offers, interviewers were directed to elicit descriptions of ethnic or cultural identity. Not wanting to guide the participants directly into talk about ethnicity and culture, interviewers began with general questions about personal identity. Participants were directed to "talk a little bit about yourself" and were asked, "If someone asked you to describe yourself, and asked 'Who are you?' and we don't mean, your name, what would you say?"

This choice to avoid direct questions about ethnicity in the first round of description was guided by past research that suggested ethnicity might be more salient for Black youth than for White youth (e.g., Jackson, 1999); we attempted to see if this was the case in this sample. Interviewers were instructed to take note of the presence or absence of comments pertaining to ethnicity in each adolescent's description of self. Then, only after the adolescent described his or her "self" was ethnicity specifically introduced. Each participant was asked to "Tell me a bit about how important your ethnicity (e.g., being Black or White) is to who you are as a person." In response to this question, participants would self-identify with a particular ethnic group.

Normative beliefs were elicited via a series of generally framed questions. On the basis of a decade's worth of research by the first author, it was expected that personal normative beliefs would emerge in the participants' descriptions of their resistance episodes. Questions such as "Why did you resist or accept the drug offer?" generated discussion of personal norms and standards regarding drug use (e.g., "I didn't want it because I just don't do that, I don't think it's right"). These questions also elicited stories about injunctions that motivated their behavior to accept or reject the offer (e.g., "I told him no and explained that my mom said never to even try it once"), yet additional questioning such as "What kinds of messages do you receive about the benefits or risks of alcohol, tobacco, pot, or other drugs?" was added to further probe the issue of messages conveying injunctive norms.

Descriptive norms were investigated by asking participants the following: "What are your ideas about your peers' alcohol, tobacco, or other drug use? Do you think more than half or less than half of the kids in your class have used drugs like these? Have you experimented with drugs?" In addition, ethnically based descriptive norms were investigated by asking participants the following: "Do you think your ethnic group uses alcohol and other drugs more than, less than, or about the same as other ethnic groups? Why do you think that?" And "How important a role has your ethnicity played in shaping your attitudes toward alcohol, tobacco, or other drug use?" Probes were used to follow up on the participants' responses to gather additional description. In addition, as the interviewing process proceeded, responses from previous interviews were used to guide the discussion and serve as possible prompts. For example, in an interview during the 1st week of the interviewing period, a non-drug user emphasized her pride in the fact that people just "know" not to offer her drugs. This was integrated into subsequent interviews with other youth to further explore this issue of pride in nonuse and identity.

Each interview was taped using a cassette recorder with a multidirectional microphone placed on a table in front of and in full view of the adolescent. The interviews were 30 to 60 min long and generated an average of 10 pages of transcribed data.

Analysis of Interview Data

Interview data were entered into the qualitative analysis software program NVIVO. This is an upgraded version of NUD*IST that stands for Non-numerical, Unstructured Data: Indexing, Searching and Theorizing (Fielding & Lee, 1998). This analysis tool indexes and manages textual and nontextual documents, provides tools to examine intersections of ideas, and supports theoretical development (Fielding & Lee, 1998). NVIVO provided a means of storing the transcribed data and facilitated the process of coding and developing categories.

After the data were imported into the software program, they were analyzed using the general techniques of constant comparison. Data units (i.e., participant comments) were categorized, defined, and explained, with each subsequent unit compared to the previous unit to assess whether it fit conceptually with the other coded units. If the coded unit fit with the others, it expanded understanding of that conceptual category. If it did not fit conceptually with the existing categories, new categories were developed (Leichtentritt & Rettig, 1999). The data were coded into two domains of responses: ethnic identity and perceptions of drug use norms. Each domain included categories and subcategories. For example, the domain address "perceptions of drug use norms/descriptive norms/ethnic group" indicates that at this location units coded into the domain "perceptions of drug use norms" would be found in the category of "descriptive norms" contained in the subcategory of "ethnic group " The two overarching domains were the most parsimonious descriptive organization for these data given the goals of the study.

Next, each interview transcript was assigned two differed attributes of interest to this study—whether the respondent was Black or White (ethnicity) and whether the respondent was not offered, accepted, or refused a drug offer (response to offer). These attributes were "attached" to each coded unit. The following example illustrates this process.

1. The comment "I think Blacks drink more alcohol than other ethnic groups" was coded into the category "perceptions of drug use norms/descriptive norms" because the comment (the unit of data) addressed a perception of a descriptive drug use norm.[3]

2. The comment came from a Black youth and/therefore was assigned the attribute "Ethnicity/Black."

3. The comment came from a youth who had accepted the discussed drug offer and therefore was assigned the attribute "Response to offer/accepted."

4. Once these attributes were assigned, we could specifically examine the responses about perceptions of drug use

norms by the Black youth who had accepted drug offers.

5. In NVIVO we conducted a search for all units coded into the "perceptions of drug use norms" with attributes of "Black," and "accepted drug offer" and then examined all those units coded within this category.
6. Next, when we were ready to compare and contrast coded data across categories, we could conduct other searches such as cross-tabulations of "perceptions of drug use norms" with "Black" and "rejected [drug offer]," or "perceptions of drug use norms" with "White" and "accepted [drug offer]." The results of these searches enabled us to examine the data within each category and across categories by ethnicity and response to drug offers.

Results

The participants in this study displayed a willingness to share their attitudes about and experiences with alcohol, tobacco, and other drugs. These responses suggest how these particular youth consider drugs and drug use in their own lives. Seventy-three percent of the teens from the churches, 64% of the teens from schools, and 83% of the teens from the community centers had received at least one offer of an illicit substance (e.g., alcohol, tobacco, or other drug) within the previous 2 months (n = 49).

How each adolescent felt about drugs, drug use, and normative expectations regarding substance use, however, played out in a variety of ways in the lives of these particular participants. Although space does not allow everyone's story to be told, conveying a few "typical" stories may help illustrate what averages and percentages cannot.

Personal Identity

Among the respondents there was no confusion or hesitation when claiming an ethnicity; however, politically correct or not, most adolescents defined themselves as either Black or White rather than using the classifications "African American" or "European American." When asked about their personal identity, these adolescents described themselves in varied fashions, some with embarrassed restraint and some with confident swagger. Generally, these youth had not given much thought to "who they are" or had little experience in articulating their personal identity.

Once these youth began talking, however, mention of personality traits, skills, and the importance of being physically similar to or different from others emerged as central to these respondents' articulated constructions of self. Descriptions of self included descriptors such as "nice," "good," "very caring," "friendly," "kid," with a "decent personality," and these adolescents universally complimented themselves on either athletic ability (e.g., "I can play basketball pretty good," "Most people say I'm a good athlete") or academic skill (e.g., "I get good grades," "I'm good at school"). Ethnic differences across the youths' responses surfaced when respondents began engaging in social comparisons. The White youth in this study were much more focused than the Black youth in pointing out their similarities and differences from their peers (e.g., "I'm just like all the other kids"), and physical appearance played a much larger role in the White youths' accounts with confessions of "[I don't like] my physical appearance—my big thighs," "I wish I looked better," "I don't like the way I look," "I don't like having glasses," but "I like my hair mostly" and "[I like] that I'm tall and built."

In contrast, the Black youth in this study shared very few concerns about their physical traits: "I love myself" and "I can't think of anything [I don't like about myself]." In addition, rather than emphasizing their perceived similarity to others, Black respondents tended to emphasize pride in their perceived uniqueness: "My vocabulary is more advanced than theirs." "I'm different. I go to church." "I am different. I don't try to act like nobody. I don't try to be like nobody. I just want to be me." And "People my age do drugs; I don't do drugs."

Ethnic Identity

Without prompting, the initial descriptions of self rarely included any mention of ethnicity. Only 6% of the overall sample (n = 4) mentioned their ethnicity as a salient component of their construction of self without specific prodding about ethnic identity. Yet, when asked, "Tell me a bit about how important your ethnicity (i.e., being Black or White) is to who you are as a person," many of the Black adolescents expressed that ethnicity was central to personal identity (64%). Twenty percent of the White adolescents revealed opinions such as the following: "Sometimes [race] is [important], and sometimes it isn't. I'm proud of the color I am. But that really doesn't mean that much to me. If I was Black, I'd still have pride." In contrast, 20% of the Whites had not previously considered the centrality of ethnicity to their definitions of self and had no opinion to express on this matter, and 60% indicated that ethnicity was not important to who they are as a person.

Most of the Black respondents perceived ethnicity as central to their identity, but the degree of salience apparently varied. Some Black youth expressed strong identification with their Black heritage as illustrated by the following comments: "My race is very important to me." "I'm proud to be Black." "I try to be Black. I learn how we got here and our history." And "[My race is] very important because a long time ago Blacks didn't have any rights to vote or do anything." Further

> It's real important to me. Because a lot of people I know—their relatives—they live in really bad areas, and that's where most Blacks I know live. I feel really privileged that my mom and dad work so hard so we can live in a nice neighborhood. I know a lot of people don't have that. It's very important to me, because back then, people used to be slaves. Their history may have something where I can learn stuff. I want to know more about my people.

Other Black respondents, in comparison, did not articulate such a strong identification with ethnicity. One of these youth said the following: "Race is not a big thing to me. It doesn't affect me much." Yet this claim was immediately called into question when the same respondent recounted the following experience:

> It is just like me being a Black and the schooling thing. They don't expect me to excel because of the color of my skin. Certain things I do, they don't expect me to do them because of the color of my skin. Certain things I participate in . . . they say most [youth] my age have had babies or stuff like that. It is because of my race, I am held back by things I'm expected to do. In school I have to work harder just because of the color of my skin.

Even when ethnicity was not perceived as central to personal identity, the issue of the salience of skin color for these youth became apparent. One youth mentioned, "color of my skin" three times (see the preceding paragraph) and continued to refer to skin color throughout the interview (e.g., "[I'm] not too dark complected," "I am light-skinned," and "I am bright-skinned"). Moreover, commonalities running throughout the composite narratives of Black respondents were references to "my people" and the use of the possessive pronoun *my* as a way to associate self with the entire Black population and culture. This reference was absent from White responses, even when White respondents were probed specifically for perceptions of ethnic identity. The majority of the Black youth tended to associate strongly with their cultural group through possessive pronoun usage.

Generally, the Black adolescents' narratives revealed personal identities emphasizing uniqueness, differentiating themselves from others in their peer culture, yet situating themselves firmly within an ethnic culture. When they expanded beyond personal identity to discuss ethnic identity, for some, a palpable pride in ethnic heritage was revealed. However, for other Black youth, a dialectical tension surfaced between negotiating a unique personal identity within a commonly shared cultural identity. Within this tension these youth struggled to differentiate at an individual level while retaining identification with other members at the cultural level. In sharp contrast, the narratives of the White youth did not reveal this tension between differentiation at the individual level and identification at the cultural group level. They expressed connection to others at the level of an individual but articulated very little conscious connection between themselves and members of a more inclusive cultural group. This finding supports the claims of cultural identity theorists who assert that cultural membership may function more powerfully among Blacks than other ethnic groups. However, the dialectical tension of managing differentiation (at the individual level) and simultaneously sustaining identification (at the cultural level) is an unexamined contradiction. This contradiction is formed when the adolescent engages in the management of these two interrelated but opposing factors.

Drug Use Norms

Injunctive norms. Injunctive norms describe society's prescriptive (e.g., what one should not do) and prescriptive (e.g., what one should do) messages regarding teen drug use. The responses of these youth, irrespective of ethnicity, suggested they were well aware of underlying injunctive societal norms about not using drugs. All youth made it clear that they were being bombarded with social norm messages warning them of the dangerous nature of drugs. Some value-laden messages were as follows: "They (my parents) don't want us to be bad people." "I've been taught well by my parents." "My parents think [drugs] are bad and people shouldn't do it." "They (my parents) say it's not good for me." "I have been brought up in a good family." "I've been taught well by my parents. They taught me to choose my friends well." Other messages were a little more dramatic: "My parents don't want us to be bad people. They want us to have good lives. They don't want us to grow up and be some kind of psychopath."

Some injunctive norms that reportedly emanated from parental sources were reinforced via threats: "They (my parents) say you better not drink alcohol or nothing," and "She (my mom) would probably throw me out of the house; my dad would probably kill me or something." Some included prescriptive advice on how to handle drug offers: "My mom was telling me that drugs were bad. And if someone tries to get me to do drugs, I should just turn around, say no, or tell them to leave me alone."

One youth's perception of society's message to young people was reflected in this statement: "They say it (drugs) ain't right and we shouldn't do it." But all the adolescents were quick to point out contradictions such as, "[Some athletes] be celebrating when they win basketball, and that has alcohol in it." Yet most felt that celebrities did not use drugs because drugs would hinder their performance as illustrated in these comments: "[Sports heroes] wouldn't be there if they used drugs when they were younger." "They all look pretty healthy and they don't seem like they'd want to [do drugs]." "Some people who drink alcohol or use drugs don't get all the opportunities like singing and acting. They aren't healthy, so they can't act." And "If [the girls in Destiny's Child did drugs], they wouldn't be where they are now."

Despite these perceived injunctive norms, some of these youth reported personal norms condoning drug use. Regardless of gender, the respondents who reported they were users of alcohol or other illicit drugs, despite an awareness of injunctive norms against use, indicated they had personal norms that favored drug use. The other youth were similarly aware of societal norms for adolescent nonuse of illicit substances yet reported nonuse of illicit substances, described personal norms against use, and articulated a strong nonuse identity.

Personal norms. When recruiting participants for this study, one Black adolescent pointed out to the recruiter, "I'm not a druggie, I don't have nothin' to say about using (drugs). I just walk away from it." Personal norms refer to what an adolescent believes he or she "should" do.

Many of the teens had received an offer(s) of alcohol, tobacco, or other drugs within the previous 2 months, but the experiences differed across users and non-users. Nonusers articulated clear anti-drug use identities with statements such as the following: "I don't act like I take drugs. It makes me feel good that I don't use drugs." "[My peers] know me well enough to know that I am not that kind of person. I wouldn't take drugs if they asked me" "[Drugs] have no place in my life." "I am the type that wouldn't [do drugs.] I don't hang out with people that do drugs." And "People know not to offer me that." One youth indicated "being good" was a reason not to do drugs, adding this: "Drugs mess up your mind. And you won't be a good person to be around. No one will want to be around you." One youth emphasized this with the following exclamation: "Drugs are wrong. You're not supposed to do that. You can't have no job. I think about what they say every day." One respondent perceived support from a network of friends and shared the following: "We all say drugs are bad. They make you do stupid things. Alcohol does the same thing. We try to get [other friends who are using a drug] off it and stuff."

Those who admitted to accepting drug offers attempted to justify their behaviors, possibly to save face (Goffman, 1955, 1959). That is, youth who admitted to drug use may have wanted the interviewer to view them favorably—for example: "I don't drink to where I get to the point [of drunkenness]. I just drink a little bit." One youth admitted to alcohol and marijuana use but insisted, "I mean, I don't really take drugs." Another echoed this by claiming "I still use [alcohol and marijuana]" but "can turn down drugs [anytime I want]" and that drug use played no part in his identity construction, because—he asserted—"I can change."

One of the speculations that guided this study was that social practices specific to one's cultural group (adolescent culture and/or ethnic culture) would shape individual practices. The following section illustrates how these youth perceived the social practices of both peers and other members of their identified ethnic culture.

Descriptive norms. Descriptive norms describe perceptions of what "most" people do, and most of the youth in this study perceived that more than half of their peers had experimented with alcohol, tobacco, or other drugs. According to one adolescent, "Most, if not all, of kids my age have at least tried drinking or smoking." These youth were also careful to link peer drug use with context, noting places where drug and alcohol use was common: "I don't hang out at arcades or anything like that (because drugs are there)." "[They do drugs] on their free time. At the river they do it." And some attributed drug use to the users' living environment: "All of them that do [drugs] . . . they come from the Projects. You know, the Projects. They got all that stuff going around there."

Despite the perception that "most" of their peers had experimented with drug use, drug users did not believe they received pressure from their peers to engage in personal drug use. As a matter of fact, because they perceived use as normative among peers, they indicated no conflict in their personal beliefs that drugs, particularly alcohol, were "cool" and "harmless." A distinction between "soft" drugs such as alcohol and marijuana and "hard" drugs such cocaine and inhalants appeared to be the locus of what was considered "drug use" in the minds of some of these youth.

The most interesting difference that emerged in the stories of the Black respondents was that "Blacks do more drugs than other races." The Whites generally did not perceive drug use to be normative among other Whites. When asked if members of their own race used more, less, or about the same amount of drugs as other races, 64% of all Black youth reported their race used more.[4] This may be compared with the 12% of the White youth who reported that their race used more drugs. Of interest, all of the Black youth who reported actual drug use also perceived greater drug use among Blacks than among other ethnic groups. However, these same youth did not perceive ethnic identity as being particularly salient to their construction of self.

Most adolescents who rejected offers of drugs were aware of societal norms against adolescent substance use, described personal norms in opposition to illicit drug use, and articulated a strong nonuse identity. For the Black youth in the latter group, the perception of cultural norms included a belief that most peers experimented with drugs and that Blacks participated in drug use more than other ethnic groups. However, for these Black youth, it was precisely their strong personal identity as a nonuser in combination with a belief that ethnicity is important that apparently motivated them to assert a positive drug-free identity as a representative of their cultural group, to contradict the perception of what is normative and assert their "unique" identity—that is, be a nonuser. Although 10% of the White youth who rejected drug offers perceived Whites to use more drugs than other ethnic groups, very few held that perception (*n* = 2). Generally, the White respondents believed that no particular ethnic group used more or fewer drugs than other groups. For these adolescents, ethnicity had little relevance to their nonuse identity. Table 22.1 illustrates the general patterns of responses across the three different types of norms.

Discussion

The purpose of this study was to provide a descriptive account of Black and White adolescents' identity and normative beliefs about ethnicity and alcohol, tobacco, and other drug use. When we compared responses within each case and then across cases, an intriguing picture emerged.

Most of the youth in this study had not given much thought to how to define their personal identity. Yet when challenged to do so, White youth tended to emphasize within-group similarities to their peers, whereas Black respondents were more likely to ignore similarities and emphasize their uniqueness or differences from school-aged peers. The dichotomy between similarity and difference appeared to present an awkward dialectic for some of the Black youth. Many seemed to struggle with managing differentiation from peers at an individual level while simultaneously not differentiating from, but sustaining identification with, members of their larger ethnic cultural group. A creative tension arose between the need to construct a separate personal identity and the need for communion and belonging within a larger cultural membership. This duality between individuality and collectivity has not been explored in the literature. Certainly it needs to be studied more fully in order to better understand Black adolescent identity development, especially in light of the growing literature supporting identity as a significant predictor of drug use and of drug attitudes for Black adolescents (Belgrave et al., 2000; Townsend & Belgrave, 2000). We argue that Hecht, Collier, and Ribeau's (1993) communication theory of identity development might be useful when investigating Black youths' identity development and drug use.

Hecht et al. (1993) provided the initial foundation of a theory of identity, and then Hecht (1993) gave a more thorough explanation of this theory that argues identity is inherently a communicative process and that message exchange serves to create and express identities. Four frames of identity are characterized in this theory—personal, enacted, relational, and communal—with the theoretical propositions based on the inherent tension and juxtaposition of these

Table 22.1
General Patterns of Responses Across Youth

	Black Youth		White Youth	
Type of Norms	*Use ATOD (n = 7), 16%*	*Do Not Use ATOD (n = 35), 83%*	*Use ATOD (n = 6), 24%*	*Do Not Use ATOD (n = 19), 76%*
Injunctive	Don't use drugs	Don't use drugs	Don't use drugs	Don't use drugs
Personal	Drug use is acceptable, especially the use of alcohol	Drug use is unacceptable	Drug use is acceptable, especially the use of alcohol	Drug use is unacceptable
Descriptive peer	86% perceived at least half or "most" of their peers had used drugs (*n* = 6)	43% perceived at least half or "most" of their peers had used drugs (*n* = 15)	100% perceived at least half or most of their peers had used drugs (*n* = 6)	10% perceived at least half or "most" of their peers had used drugs (*n* = 2)
Descriptive peer	100% perceived Blacks use more drugs than other ethnic groups (*n* = 7)	51% perceived Blacks use more drugs than other ethnic groups (*n* = 18)	33% perceived Whites use more drugs than other ethnic groups (*n* = 2)	10% perceived Whites use more drugs than other ethnic (*n* = 2)

Note: ATOD = alcohol, tobacco, and other drugs. The total sample of Black participants was 42; the total sample of White participants was 25.

frames within any identity. According to this theory, identities are personal (self-constructs), enacted (through social and symbolic behavior), relational (emerge out of interaction and relationship with others who provide symbolic information), and communal (community as the locus of identity with jointly held constructions). Accordingly, frames are not isolated from each other; instead, they may (and should) be examined in combination. Hecht further argued that an understanding of ethnic identity requires examination of the interpenetration of these frames. The data from the present study provide grounded evidence of the juxtaposition of communal and personal frames for Black adolescents. Further investigation into this juxtaposition is warranted with a possible addition of looking at the enactment of Black youth identity within American culture and how these youth are constructing a sense of self through social symbols.

In contrast, few of the White youth perceived ethnic identity as a salient construct to their developing sense of self. This finding may not be surprising when one considers that minority groups typically have a heightened awareness of their minority status. According to Jackson (1999), there is an historical lack of ethnic, identity among Whites. Of interest, though, the Anglo youth who perceived ethnic identity as salient to their sense of self also tended to be those who admitted to alcohol, tobacco, and other drug use as well as personal norms favorable to drug use. Indeed, the White adolescents who reported drug use professed a desire to be similar to others and considered ethnicity important to their developing sense of self. A closer look at the perceived drug-use norms, to understand this pattern, is warranted.

Normative beliefs about alcohol, tobacco and other drug use were broken down into three different types of norms: injunctive, personal, and descriptive (see Table 22.1). All respondents reported receiving clear societal messages from teachers, media, and parents that adolescent drug use was "bad." Yet, many adolescents questioned the negative casting of alcohol as a drug. To these youth, alcohol was not a drug (e.g., "Drugs are bad and alcohol is not—it is harmless"). Most youth reported clearly defined personal norms against drug use. For some youth, though, despite powerful injunctive norms against use, personal norms favorable to drug use still emerged in their talk. When accompanied by descriptive peer norms of drug use (e.g., "Most of my peers experiment with or use drugs"), personal norms appeared to be reinforced, thus overriding injunctive norms perceived in their social world.

Descriptive peer norms of use and experimentation were consistently important across all respondents—users and nonusers. However, an important contribution to our understanding is the identification of ethnic differences in the perception of cultural norms among ethnic group members. It is notable that 59% of the Black youth in this study and 16% of all White youth reported their ethnic group (i.e., the one they self-identified with) as using more drugs than other ethnic groups. Of even more interest is that 100% of the Black youth who reportedly used alcohol, tobacco, or other drugs also perceived their race as using more drugs than other races. Perhaps, for Black youth, messages that members of their ethnic group used "more" drugs than other ethnic groups, along with perceptions that most of their peers used drugs, may—in combination—have been more powerful than societal injunctive norms against use.

The perception among many Black youth that their ethnic group uses more drugs than other ethnic groups should concern scholars because it contradicts actual patterns of use in the United States as reported in drug use prevalence studies. These studies report that when population differences are controlled for, Blacks use fewer drugs than other ethnic groups (Bachman et al., 1991; CDCP, 1995; Johnston & Larison, 1995; Wallace, Bachman, O'Malley, & Johnston, 1995). Perhaps a goal of public health officials should be to closely examine culturally specific normative messages that may provide cultural enactments of Black identity. Then, perhaps, a cultural norms campaign should be developed to increase awareness of lower usage rates among Black populations in an attempt to alter normative impressions among youth that Blacks use more drugs than other ethnic groups. After all, as Helms (1990) suggested, it is the perception of what people believe, feel, and think about their ethnic group that has implications for intrapersonal and interpersonal functioning. Clearly, the messages these youth are receiving about cultural norms within their ethnic group are shaping their perceptions about normative alcohol, tobacco, and other drug use behavior. One youth indicated that it is precisely because ethnicity was important to identity that she made a conscious choice to contradict the negative perceptions of Blacks. As she said, "The negative press, you just gotta beat it." Many of the Black youth who refused drug offers suggested that the way to establish oneself as unique is to establish a non-drug use identity.

These results shed light on identity, ethnicity, and drug use norms for 67 adolescents in an urban mid-South community. We suggest that prevention researchers and health care providers consider different alcohol, tobacco, and other drug prevention strategies that are sensitive to actual and perceived cultural differences among ethnic groups. Youth may benefit from receiving messages that accurately represent social and cultural norms in order to dispel erroneous perceptions of normative behavior. Clinicians could assess youths' perceptions of normative behavior and then clarify misperceptions and dispel misinformation. A social norms approach to alcohol prevention has been implemented on college campuses with much success (Keeling, 2000). In this approach a "social marketing program [is] designed to promote better or healthier decisions" (Keeling, 2001, p. 53). The emphasis of this approach, historically, has unfortunately been limited to crafting messages addressing descriptive norms of peer use. Several articles in the *Journal of College Health* have reported social norms programs focusing almost solely on peer norms (e.g., see Perkins, Meilman, Leichliter, Cashin, & Presley, 1999; Werch, Pappas, Carlson, & DiClemente, 2000). To our knowledge, descriptive ethnic group norms have not been addressed in current social norm campaigns. A cultural norms approach to prevention is also responsive to Bass (1993) and Blackwell's (1991) suggestion that scholars must begin to account for differences in cultural values if they are to address ethnic differences in drug use.

This study is descriptive and generative in nature, and we do not seek to claim generalizability of the findings to all Black and White youth. In fact, we do recognize that there is variety within any ethnic grouping. However, patterns were discovered in these data, and these descriptions may be usefully transferred to other youths' experiences in order to improve scholars' understanding of the ways in which ethnicity and (erroneous) beliefs about norms may shape adolescent drug use behavior. Currently, very little information is available that applies normative theories and ethnicity to adolescent outcomes. This study speculates that norms focus theory might serve to provide a foundation for an applied cultural norms approach to drug prevention with ethnically diverse populations. This approach could complement the social norms approaches that currently focus only on perceptions of peer use.

In addition, the findings in this study suggest that face-to-face interviewing techniques may be helpful in supplementing our existing drug use prevalence data and in gathering increasingly valid data from Black youth. Although these findings are exploratory, they nonetheless have implications for future research on adolescent drug use norms, identity, and ethnicity, as well as implications for drug use prevention efforts.

Lastly, although normative beliefs may shape adolescent drug use behaviors, a plethora of additional factors could shape drug use behaviors. This study was not designed to address factors beyond ethnic identity and normative beliefs regarding drug use, yet its findings do answer the call of scholars who recommend increased scholarly attention to the role of ethnicity and culture in substance use and abuse (Bass, 1993; Blackwell, 1991; Botvin et al., 1995). This study contributes a detailed description of the ways in which perceptions of norms may shape adolescent decisions to engage in drug use, and it provides direction to prevention and health communication scholars who wish to further investigate the role of ethnically based social norms on adolescent drug use.

Notes

1. The term *White* replaces the more cumbersome term *non-Hispanic White* from this point forward.
2. Two tapes were unintelligible because of extraneous noise present outside the interview space. Three tapes were damaged by a malfunctioning tape recorder.
3. Had the comment been "My teachers tell me I shouldn't drink alcohol because I could get addicted," then it would be coded as "perceptions of drug use norms/injunctive norm."
4. All respondents were asked and answered this question.

References

Allen, O. & Page, R. M. (1994). Variance in substance use between rural Black and White Mississippi high school students. *Adolescence, 29,* 401–424.

Archer, S. (Ed.). (1994). *Interventions for adolescent identity development*. Thousand Oaks, CA: Sage.

Aries, E. (1998). Race and gender as components of the working self-concept. *Journal of Psychology, 138,* 277–290.

Azibo, D. A. (1996). *African psychology in historical perspective and related commentary.* Trenton, NJ: African World Press.

Bachman, J. G., Wallace, J. M., Jr., O'Malley, P. M., Johnston, L. D., Kurth, C. L., & Neighbors, H. W. (1991). Racial/ethnic differences in smoking, drinking, and illicit drug use among American high school seniors, 1976–1989. *American Journal of Public Health, 81,* 372–377.

Bass, L. (1993). Stereotype or reality: Another look at alcohol and drug use among Black children. *Public Health Reports Annual, 108,* 78–85.

Belgrave, F. Z., Brome, D. R., & Hampton, C. (2000). The contribution of Africentric values and racial identity to the prediction of drug knowledge, attitudes, and use among African American youth. *Journal of Black Psychology, 26,* 386–401.

Belgrave, F. Z., Townsend, T. G., Cherry, V. R., & Cunningham, D. M. (1997). The influence of an Africentric worldview and demographic variables on drug knowledge, attitudes, and use among African American youth. *Journal of Community Psychology, 25,* 421–433:

Blackwell, R. (1991). *The Black community.* New York: HarperCollins.

Botvin, G. J., Schinke, S., & Orlandi, M. A. (Eds.). (1995). *Drug abuse prevention with multiethnic youth.* Thousand Oaks, CA: Sage.

Brook, J. S. Whiteman, M., Balka, E. B., Thet Win, P., & Gursin, M. D. (1998). Drug use among Puerto Ricans: Ethnic identity as a protective factor. *Hispanic Journal of Behavioral Sciences, 20,* 241–254.

Burlew, K., Neely, D., Johnson, C. & Hucks, T C. (2000). Drug attitudes, racial identity, and alcohol use among African American adolescents. *Journal of Black Psychology, 26,* 402–420.

Centers for Disease Control and Prevention. (1995). *1993 youth risk behavior surveillance system.* Atlanta, GA: U.S. Department of Health and Human Services.

Cialdini, R., Kallgren, C. & Reno, R. (1990). A focus theory on normative conduct: Recycling the concept of norms of reduced littering in public places. *Journal of Personality and Social Psychology, 58,* 1015–1026.

Clark, M. L. (1982). Racial group concept and self-esteem in Black children. *Journal of Black Psychology, 81*, 75–88.

Fielding, N. G., & Lee, R. M. (1998). *Computer analysis and qualitative research.* Thousand Oaks, CA: Sage.

Gaines, S. O., Marelich, W. D., Bledsloe, K. L., & Steers, N. (1997). Links between race/ethnicity and cultural values as mediated by racial/ethnic identity and moderated by gender. *Journal of Personality and Social Psychology, 72,* 1460–1476.

Goffman, E. (1955). On face-work: An analysis of ritual elements in social interaction. *Psychiatry, 18,* 213–231.

Goffman, E. (1959). *Presentation of self in everyday life.* New York: Doubleday.

Guerra, N. G., Huesmann, L. R., & Hanish, L. (1995). The role of normative beliefs in children's social behavior. In N. Eisenberg (Ed.), *Social development review of personality and social psychology* (pp. 140–158). Thousand Oaks, CA: Sage.

Hansen, W. B. (1991). School-based substance abuse prevention: A review of the state of the art in curriculum, 1980–1990. *Health Education Research, 7,* 403–430.

Hecht, M. L. (1993). A research odyssey: Toward the development of a communication theory of identity. *Communication Monographs, 60,* 76–82.

Hecht, M. L., Collier, M. J., & Ribeau, S. (1993). *African American communication: Ethnic identity and cultural interpretations*. Newbury Park, CA: Sage.

Hecht, M. L., Trost, M. R., Bator, R. J., & Mac-

Kinnon, D. (1997). Ethnicity and sex similarities and differences in drug resistance. *Journal of Applied Communication Research, 25,* 75–97.

Helms, J. E. (1990). *Black and White racial identity: Theory, research, and practice.* New York: Greenwood.

Huselid, R. E. & Cooper, M. L. (1992). Gender norms as mediators of sex differences in adolescent alcohol use and abuse. *Journal of Health and Social Behavior, 33,* 348–362.

Jackson, R. L. (1999). *The negotiation of cultural identity: Perceptions of European Americans and African Americans.* Westport, CT: Praeger.

Johnston, R. A., & Larison, C. (1995). *Prevalence of substance use among racial and ethnic subgroups in the United States 1991–1993* (NIH Publication No. 95–0002). Rockville, MD: Substance Abuse and Mental Health Services Administration.

Keefe, S., & Padilla, A. (1987). *Chicano ethnicity.* Albuquerque: University of New Mexico Press.

Keeling, R. P. (2000). Social norms research in college health. *Journal of American College Health, 49,* 53–65.

Leichtentritt, R. D., & Rettig, K. D. (1999). My parent's dignified death is different from mine: Moral problem solving about euthanasia. *Journal of Social & Personal Relationships, 16,* 385–406.

Miller, M. A. (1999). The social process of drug resistance in a relational context. *Communication Studies, 49,* 358–375.

Miller, M., Alberts, J. K., Hecht, M. L., Trost, M., & Krizek, R. L. (2000). *Adolescent relationships and drug use.* Mahwah, NJ: Lawrence Erlbaum Associates, Inc.

Myers, H., Newcomb, M. D., Richardson, M. A., & Alvy, K. T. (1997). Parental and family risk factors for substance use in inner-city African American children and adolescents. *Journal of Psychopathology and Behavioral Assessment, 19,* 109–131.

Perkins, H. W., Meilman, P. W., Leichliter, J. S., Cashin, J. R., & Presley, C. A. (1999). Misperceptions of the norms for the frequency of alcohol and other drug use on college campuses. *Journal of American College Health, 47,* 253–258.

Phinney, J. S., & Alipuria, L. L. (1990). Ethnic identity in college students from four ethnic groups. *Journal of Adolescence, 13,* 171—183.

Phinney, J. S., & Chavira, V. (1992). Ethnic identity and self-esteem: An exploratory longitudinal study. *Journal of Adolescence, 15,* 211–281.

Ramirez, A. G., Chalela, P., & Presswood, D. T. (2000). Developing a theory-based anti-drug communication campaign for Hispanic children and parents. *Journal of Public Health Management and Practice, 6,* 72–80.

Rotheram-Borus, M. J., & Wyche, K. F. (1994). Ethnic differences in identity development in the United States. In S. Archer (Ed.), *Interventions for adolescent identity development* (pp. 62–83). Thousand Oaks, CA: Sage.

Stiffman, A. R., & Davis, L. E. (1990). *Ethnic issues in adolescent mental health.* Newbury Park, CA: Sage.

Substance Abuse and Mental Health Services Administration. (2001). *Summary of findings from the 2000 National Household Survey on Drug Abuse* (NHSDA Series H–13, DHHS Publication No. [SMA] 01–3549). Rockville, MD: Office of Applied Studies.

Taylor, S. J., & Bogdan, R. (1984). *Introduction to qualitative research methods.* New York: Wiley.

Townsend, T. G., & Belgrave, F. Z. (2000). The impact of personal identity and racial identity on drug attitudes and use among African American children. *Journal of Black Psychology, 26,* 421–436.

Wallace, J. M., Jr., Bachman, J. G., O'Malley, P. M., & Johnston, L. D. (1995). Racial/ethnic differences in adolescent drug use: Exploring possible explanations. In G. Botvin, S. Schinke, & M. Orlandi (Eds.), *Drug abuse prevention with multi-ethnic youth* (pp. 59–80). Thousand Oaks, CA: Sage.

Werch, C. E., Pappas, D. M., Carlson, J. M., & DiClemente, C. C. (2000). Results of a social norm intervention to prevent binge drinking among first-year residential college students. *Journal of American College Health, 49,* 85–92.

Discussion Questions

1. How do you think ethnicity affects other health behaviors beyond drug and alcohol use?
2. The authors suggest that a cultural norms campaign should be developed to increase awareness of lower usage rates among African American populations. What would a campaign like this look like?
3. This chapter suggests that health-care providers and prevention researchers consider prevention strategies that are sensitive to perceived and actual cultural differences, and that youth particularly may benefit from this approach. Do you think older adults would benefit as much from this strategy? Explain your answer. ✦

Chapter 23 Ethical Dilemmas in Health Campaigns

Nurit Guttman

The final chapter in Part VI outlines several ethical considerations that are relevant to the design and implementation of any health promotion. The author focuses on four main areas including strategies and content of health-communication campaign messages, inadvertent adverse outcomes from campaign activities, power and control, and social values. This thoughtful chapter provides another dimension to health promotion for communication researchers: an awareness of the power of the strategies that are used to influence attitudes and behaviors and the inherent responsibilities implied by the knowledge of what moves people in the direction of change. Health campaigns involve ethical concerns and dilemmas throughout the entire process of design, implementation, and evaluation. Examples are given from national and community-based health communication interventions to illustrate these considerations. Considering ethical issues involved in health promotion research has many implications for both health researchers and the community.

Related Topics: culture, ethical issues, groups, health campaigns, health-care behaviors, media, organizations

The design and implementation of public health campaigns invariably raise ethical dilemmas. These ethical dilemmas, however, are often invisible. Certain health-related topics such as abortion or euthanasia stir heated public debates abounding with ethical concerns, some of which are also conspicuous in HTV-related campaigns (e.g., Fortin, 1991; Kleining, 1990; Manuel et al., 1991; Mariner, 1995). These topics are characterized as relatively more glamorous (Barry, 1982). In contrast, in other intervention areas such as the prevention of cancer or heart disease, ethical issues, although inextricably linked to intervention goals and strategies (Doxiadis, 1987; McLeroy, Gottlieb, & Burdine, 1987; Ratzan, 1994; Rogers, 1994; Salmon, 1989; Witte, 1994), are less visible, tend to be discussed in limited contexts, and lack conceptual frameworks (Salmon, 1992).[1] Because such campaigns typically employ persuasive strategies aimed at influencing people to adopt or avoid certain practices, the argument can be made that they are also inundated with ethical concerns (Burdine, McLeroy, & Gottlieb, 1987; Eisenberg, 1987; Faden, 1982, 1987; Griming, 1989; Salmon, 1989; Winett, King, & Altman, 1989; Witte, 1994), many of which are similar to concerns typically raised in biomedical contexts (Gillon, 1990). Furthermore, although health campaigns are presumably for the good of the target populations (Rogers, 1994), benefits from their outcomes might not be distributed equally across target populations. In fact, critics argue that well-meaning messages might cause particular members of the population inadvertent harm (Barsky, 1988; Becker, 1993; Wang, 1992). In addition, because health campaigns increasingly adopt sophisticated social marketing techniques, this enhanced ability to persuade and enable practitioners to design and implement more effective interventions raises concerns regarding the extent to which campaigns might engage in unethical manipulation (Faden, 1987). We need to be reminded, say ethicists, that "[a] preventive health campaign is a marketing effort, subject to all the risks of motivational marketing hyperbole, demagoguery, or preying upon fears and prejudices" (Goodman & Goodman, 1986, p. 29). Making ethical concerns more explicit and examining them more systematically in health campaigns is an important but often neglected process in research and

From "Ethical Dilemmas in Health Campaigns," Nurit Guttman, 1997 *Health Communication*, Vol. 9:2, pp. 155–190.

practice, though it can be seen as crucial to their analysis, design, and evaluation.[2]

This article provides a conceptual approach for identifying ethical issues in health campaigns by presenting 13 dilemmas associated with four major areas: (1) intervention strategies, (2) inadvertent harm, (3) power and control, and (4) social values. The framework presented in this article draws on Brown and Singhal's (1990) discussion of ethical dilemmas in the use of television programs to promote social issues that they refer to as prosocial television. Brown and Singhal underscored the importance of considering four types of dilemmas: dilemmas regarding the content of messages and the promotion of equality among viewers—included here in the area of strategies; dilemmas related to unintended effects, expanded here to include the area of social values; and dilemmas related to the use of the media for development—included here in the area of strategies.[3]

The framework also draws on Forester's (1989, 1993) adaptation of Habermas' (1979) work to the context of planning. Forester (1993) suggested that planners, or in this context the designers of health campaigns, make normative claims that relate to Habermas' three processes of social reproduction: cultural, in which views are elaborated and shaped; social integration, in which norms, rules, and obligations are shaped or reinforced; and socialization in which social identities and expressions of self are influenced. Planned social interventions, in which we can include health campaigns, are communicative processes. Their potential impact, following Forester's framework, raises concerns regarding possible distortions in (a) the truth of the messages, which can affect people's beliefs about the issue and can be related to ethical concerns about strategies and values or cultural reproduction; (b) the legitimacy of the norms invoked, which might affect people's consent and can be related to ethical concerns about power and control, or the reproduction process of social integration; (c) expressiveness, which might affect perceptions of relationships or identity and can be related to ethical concerns about inadvertent outcomes such as privileging, labeling and culpability, or the reproductive process of socialization; and (d) framing, through the selection or prioritization of issues, which can be related to ethical concerns regarding social values and ideologies.

The ethical concerns discussed in this article also draw from the bioethics literature, specifically ethical principles such as respect for autonomy and justice or fairness, and from a feminist emphasis on the ethic of care.

Dilemmas Concerning Campaign Strategies

Choosing to use specific campaign strategies elicits implicit moral judgments. The first two dilemmas (Persuasion and Coercion) raise concerns regarding manipulation and infringement of people's personal autonomy for the sake of doing good (beneficence), or for the sake of ensuring the effectiveness of the campaign. The first dilemma focuses on the use of persuasive appeals and the second on restrictive strategies. Both raise ethical concerns regarding rights of the individual. The third dilemma (Targeting), which addresses mainly (risk) group or societal level issues, raises ethical concerns related to targeting. These concerns tend to be discussed in the context of ethical principles of justice or fairness, or from a feminist perspective of caring. The fourth dilemma (Harm Reduction) is whether it is justified to use strategies that support behaviors seen as socially deviant, immoral, or harmful, because they might prevent further harm to target populations. The ethical issues it raises are related both to pragmatic societal-level concerns such as preventing the spread of infection and individual-level concerns such as doing good.

Persuasion Dilemma

To what extent is it justified to use persuasive strategies to reach the intended health-promoting effects of the campaign, even if the use of such strategies might infringe on individuals' rights?

This dilemma is often shared, though less often acknowledged, by many, if not all, public communication campaigns (Witte, 1994). Because public health campaign goals typically aim to influence target populations' beliefs or behaviors, usually persuasive and social marketing strategies are employed (Elder, Hovell, Lasater, Wells, & Carleton, 1985; Evans, 1988; Fine, 1981; Lefebvre & Flora, 1988; Jaccard, Turrisi, & Wan, 1990; Manoff, 1985; Rogers & Storey, 1987; Scherer & Juanillo, 1992).[4] The ultimate goal of these intervention strategies, Witte (1994) pointed out, is to get people to practice what the campaign sponsors believe are health-promoting behaviors. Health promoters, in their efforts to do good and to convince the public of the benefits of adopting particular behaviors or of avoiding others, might use persuasive strategies to arouse anxieties or fears and facilitate persuasion. Faden and Faden (1982) stated that although campaigners might argue that their efforts are restricted to information and skill building, we might ask whether it is "possible to distinguish a purely informational or educative effort from a persuasive appeal in the context of a communicative program?" (p. 10). This raises concerns regarding the use of manipulative or persuasive tactics, which by definition, infringe on individuals' rights for autonomy or self-determination. Faden and Faden added that campaigns have tended to be designed to promote predetermined behavioral changes through specially constructed persuasive appeals. This raises concerns regarding paternalism or the notion that certain experts or professionals know what is best for particular members of society or the public as a whole.

Although these concerns traditionally are raised in the practitioner-patient context (e.g., Bok, 1978; Childress, 1982; Veatch, 1980), they are also highly relevant in the campaign context because campaigns are a purposeful effort to get people to adopt health-related practices that are perceived as beneficial to them or help them avoid potential harm (Beauchamp, 1988; Campbell, 1990; Doxiadis, 1987; Faden, 1987; Pinet, 1987). According to the principle of respect for autonomy, health promoters should honor the self-respect and dignity of each individual as an autonomous, free actor. The underlying assumption is that all competent individuals have an intrinsic right to make decisions for themselves on any matter affecting them, at least so far as such decisions do not bring harm to another party (Hiller, 1987), and that only the individual knows and is interested in his or her own well-being (Mill, 1978).

The use of persuasive appeals also raises concerns regarding the extent to which they distort or manipulate information to persuade target populations (as elaborated by Forester, 1993) or the extent to which such manipulative strategies can undermine the development of connectedness, responsiveness, and a sense of caring, that are important components in an ethic of care (Baier, 1993). Similarly, this raises concerns regarding legitimacy and control, because persuasive messages inherently aim to limit people's choices and to control their perceptions to facilitate the adoption of the recommended behaviors (Faden & Faden, 1982, in their discussion of Mendelsohn's perspective). As Salmon (1989) reminded us, "at the center of this conflict is the fundamental tension between social control and individual freedoms. Social marketing efforts, by definition, employ mechanisms of social control" (p. 19).[5] Inherent in the design and implementation of health campaigns is, therefore, a tension between competing values of autonomy and values of doing good, or of effectiveness or utility.

Witte (1994) maintained that health communication researchers and practitioners are adept at using persuasive strategies (e.g., how much and which type of information to use about a certain topic, how to order it) to manipulate people's perceptions. Consequently, we face dilemmas regarding whether the use of manipulative and persuasive strategies is justified to achieve certain goals, and to what extent health promoters should model their persuasive messages on advertising or marketing techniques, even when these tactics are viewed as the most promising venues for affecting attitudes and behaviors.[6] Highly persuasive appeals such as emotion-, fear-, and guilt-raising messages tend to be justified on the basis of utility, especially when they are based on research on target audience members' perceptions[7] regarding what types of messages would "work" for them. The latter was used to justify the use of fear-arousal messages in television public service announcements (PSAs) produced by the National High Blood Pressure Education Program (NHBPEP).[8] The use of persuasive strategies in the context of advertising has been criticized as being potentially unethical because of its potential use of manipulative, misleading, or deceptive messages, concerns that are compounded because advertising campaigns tend to target populations that are particularly vulnerable. This critique can be applied to public campaigns as well (Pollay, 1989). A recent example is the use of what critics maintain were inflated statistics by the American Cancer Society (ACS) in its efforts to persuade more women to engage in preventive behaviors. A message, critics say, that might unduly terrify some women but is justified by ACS as an effective means to get women to adopt preventive measures (Blakeslee, 1992). In contrast, Salmon (1992), reported that practitioners in the National AIDS Information and Education Programs (NAIEP), a government-sponsored public health agency, decided to give prominence to the principle of what they considered *do no harm* and to avoid messages that could potentially frighten target populations.[9] A different approach was revealed in a surprising announcement made by an advisory panel to the National Cancer Institute that it recommends the Institute should only provide scientific data and should not engage in persuasive appeals to get women to get mammograms at a certain age, but instead let the public draw its own conclusions (Kolata, October 22, 1993). This raises ethical concerns as well: to what extent are health promoters obligated to use persuasive strategies if they believe these strategies are the most effective method to achieve the goals of the campaign and to fulfill their mandate of maximizing the health of the target population?[10]

Coercion Dilemma

To what extent is it justified to promote restrictive policies or regulations on individuals' behavior to achieve the health goals of the campaign?

The use of coercion poses the same types of concerns raised regarding persuasion:

> Questions about the morality of coercion, manipulation, deception, persuasion, and other methods of inducing change typically involve a conflict between the values of individual freedom and self-determination, on one hand, and such values as social welfare, economic progress, or equal opportunity, on the other hand. (Warwick & Kelman, 1973, p. 380)

One of the arguments in support of regulative strategies is that they are relatively effective in promoting desired outcomes. As McKinlay (1975) stated: "One stroke of effective health legislation is equal to many separate health intervention endeavors and the cumulative efforts of innumerable health workers over long periods of time" (p. 13). For example, legislation for smoke-free environments is seen as having a larger impact on smoking behavior of large numbers of people than educational programs (Glantz, 1996). Similarly, engineering-type solutions can also be seen as relatively effective strategies (Brown, 1991). For example, redesigning roadways and improving the safety-engineering of cars has been shown to significantly reduce automobile accidents and fatalities, independently of the actions of the drivers, and changing lunch menus of schools or work organization has been shown to affect the food consumption of the students or workers in these organizations (Ellison, Capper, Goldberg, Witschi, & Stare, 1989; Glanz & Mullis, 1988). Similarly, it could be argued that regulation of the food industry and restrictions on food production could increase the likelihood that consumers would buy foods relatively low in saturated fats and free of contaminants, making their food consumption healthier. Adopting this position and justifying it by such claims can be seen as applying the principle of utility or the obligation to maximize the greatest utility from the health promotion efforts to the greatest number of people or the public as a whole (Hiller, 1987). The emphasis, however, on principles of utility or promoting the public good raises concerns regarding the ethical principle of individual autonomy-the right not to be restricted in personal choices.

An important justification for the use of restrictive strategies is based on the assumption that individuals' choices are, in fact, not autonomous, and influenced by powerful social and market conditions. People in our society, explain proponents of regulative strategies, are surrounded by persuasive antihealth messages and an antihealth environment and therefore, do not "freely" choose unhealthy behaviors. This, they say, justifies the use of prohealth persuasive or coercive strategies or of policies to restrict the freedom of groups or of marketers of certain products (Pinet, 1987). An example of this approach are efforts to restrict the placement of cigarette vending machines, a strategy that has been shown to be effective in curtailing cigarette sales, especially among children and adolescents (Feighery, Altaian, & Shaffer, 1991). Another example of government policies to promote health through restricting public access to a product is the Japanese government's ban of birth control pills. This regulation has been adopted in part to promote the use of condoms and justified in part by being perceived as a way to curb the spread of HIV infection (Jitsukawa & Djerassi, 1994; Weisman, 1992).

Coercive approaches are clearly fraught with ethical concerns, including the infringement on individuals' free choice and the free-marketplace enterprise, which are prominent values in American society. Market autonomy, according to its proponents, is the optimal method for the distribution of goods and for balancing economic contribution and economic rewards, and restricting it would impose restrictions on individuals' choices, and thus impinge on individual autonomy as well (Garret, Baillie, & Garret, 1989). Critics maintain, however, that the marketplace, does not provide free choices for individuals or communities because other socioeconomic factors influence the distribution of goods, services and wealth (Beauchamp, 1987; Bellah, Madsen, Sullivan, Swidler, & Tipton, 1985, 1991). Beauchamp (1987), in support of regulative strategies, argued that relative to other intervention approaches, enforcement strategies enhance the public good on the societal level while minimally intruding on individuals, because they mainly place controls on the marketplace. Instead of posing restrictions on personal liberty, he explained, by controlling potential hazards through a collective action and sharing the burdens of protection, intervention policies can foster a sense of community responsibility for the welfare of its members. Even if one adopts these justifications, we are still left with questions regarding the extent to which individuals should be restricted from engaging in practices perceived risky from a health-promotion perspective, but nevertheless desired by some. A crucial concern here is the issue of boundaries: *when* should society intervene? Does society have an obligation to intervene when the individual's well-being is threatened by their own action (Pinet, 1987; Wikler, 1987), or should it intervene only when a person presents a danger to others (e.g., as in the case of communicable diseases)?

Regulative strategies might also be applied to channels for the dissemination of campaign messages. Because broadcast media, although it might be considered a public good, is licensed to commercial or not-for-profit organizations, the question is to what extent should health campaigns be able to use these media as dissemination channels: should commercial media be regulated to support the messages of health campaigns (Packer & Kauffman, 1990), or should campaigns be able to use tax money ("sin taxes") to pay for their advertisements?[11]

Targeting Dilemmas

Who should be targeted by the campaign? Should the campaign devote its resources to target populations believed to be particularly needy, or should those who are more likely to adopt its recommendations be targeted?

The issue of targeting evokes a host of ethical concerns. These include concerns of equally reaching different segments of the population, or who should be targeted by the campaign's activities and messages. A second concern is whether campaigns might in fact serve to widen the gap between those who have more opportunities and those who have fewer[12] and whether the issues they emphasize are more relevant to certain cultural groups than to others. Similarly, concerns can be raised regarding the extent to which campaigns address issues important to groups with special needs and the extent to which campaigns provide a forum for diverse perspectives on how to address the problem and solutions. These concerns represent tensions between principles of justice and utility. According to the latter, one is obliged to maximize the greatest utility from the health promotion efforts (Hiller, 1987). However, when campaign budgets are limited, should only those who are most likely to adopt the recommended practices be targeted? In contrast, should the campaign target those seen as having the greatest need, but least likely to be affected by the campaign (Des Jarlais, Padian, & Winkestein, 1994; White & Maloney, 1990)?

Many health campaigns target populations that are considered underserved. The problem with this approach, suggest critics, is that to address inequalities in healthcare one must face inequalities in other areas of life as well. Thus, despite sincere efforts, if campaigns do not address structural or socioeconomic factors, disadvantaged target groups who might not have sufficient opportunities to adopt their health-related recommendations are not likely to do so. Consequently, campaigns' messages and activities tend to have only a minimum of the desired effects, and the intervention approaches they utilize can be deemed ineffective or a waste of precious public resources.[13]

Ethical concerns can also be raised regarding the adoption of a population approach[14] in which campaigns target relatively large segments of the population. The premise of the population approach is that small changes (e.g., in blood cholesterol levels or systolic blood pressure) in large populations produce relatively large changes in overall morbidity and mortality, and this serves as the main rationale for many campaigns. However, this type of broad impact might not affect certain subgroups, who might be particularly in need of an intervention, and from the individual's perspective, it might bring little benefit As Geoffrey Rose (1985), a noted epidemiologist and proponent of the population approach suggested, this tension illustrates the Prevention Paradox—an intervention strategy that "brings much benefit to the population [but] offers little (at least on the short term) to each participating individual" (p. 38). An alternative targeting approach is to focus on those at high risk, and aim to make significant changes in the health-related behavior of a relatively small number of individuals. The dilemma is therefore whether the campaign should target those who seem to be most in need but are relatively few in number, or whether it should devote its limited resources to reaching as many people as possible, thus resulting in increasing the health of the population as a whole.[15]

The final ethical concern regarding targeting relates to campaigns often serving as social experiments for policy makers or researchers. Policy makers want to know *what works* or which types of interventions can be considered as effective. Consequently, campaigns often are designed as clinical trials and utilize designs in which some populations are not targeted and are not provided with resources or activities believed to potentially benefit them. This raises the same kind of ethical concerns raised in the context of clinical trials: is it ethical to deny certain people a treatment that might benefit them for the sake of proving the efficacy of the intervention strategy?[16]

Harm Reduction Dilemma

To what extent should a campaign engage in strategies that support behaviors that are not socially approved, or might be seen by some as immoral, to prevent further harm to certain populations?

On what grounds is it justified to provide people who use injection drugs with syringes or to train them on how to clean injection needles for the purpose of avoiding HIV infection? Should adolescents be provided with contraceptive devices and education on sexual practices that are less likely to transmit infections even if their parents or their community believes that premarital sexual activity is immoral? Should campaigns promote the legalization of nonmedical use of illicit drugs? Should campaigns promote a message that an effective way to avoid automobile accidents is to have designated drivers that take turns refraining from excessive alcohol consumption?[17] Campaigns that adopt strategies that would answer these questions in the affirmative often base their justification (though not always explicitly or consciously) on a harm-reduction justification. The harm reduction perspective was articulated in England in the mid-1980s and has gained momentum in Europe and Australia as a response to the urgency of preventing the spread of HIV infection in the area of injection drug use. Its proponents say that although it raises ethical concerns such as sanctioning behaviors seen as immoral or harmful to the individual, harm-reduction strategies can in fact be justified on both moral and practical grounds. Syringe-exchange programs, for example, can be justified on the basis of several ethical approaches that for the purpose here are characterized as the following: (a) doing good, because protecting individuals from the adverse effects of HIV infection; (b) utility, because findings on the reduction of HIV infection among users of injection drugs who participate in syringe exchange programs indicate that they are also more likely to enroll in drug-rehabilitation programs; (c) justice, because there are limited rehabilitation programs and opportunities for those who use injection drugs; (d) public good, because the users of drugs are an integral part of the community and protecting the health of the community requires protecting the health of drug users; and (e) caring, because those who use injection drugs should be seen as people who need help and connectedness.

Critics of harm-reduction strategies, however, might believe their use reinforces immoral or harmful behaviors (e.g., sexual behavior or drug abuse), but these views are contested by others who propose that such programs do not increase and might actually decrease the risk-promoting behavior.

Dilemmas Concerning Inadvertent Harm

Although well-meaning, and usually with distinct health-promoting objectives (Rogers, 1994), health campaigns might contribute to unintended outcomes that can be considered detrimental for individuals or society. The dilemmas specified later concern three types of outcomes that might contribute to potential harm:

1. labeling or stigmatizing individuals,
2. denying the less privileged pleasures they can afford,
3. unfairly placing the responsibility and blame on individuals or groups.

Labeling Dilemma

By telling people they have a certain medical condition that puts them at risk, to what extent does the campaign label them as *ill?* To what extent does the campaign stigmatize certain individuals by portraying the health-related conditions they have as undesirable or bad?

The principle of do no harm or *nonmaleficence* is the obligation to bring no harm to one's client (Hiller, 1987). The Labeling Dilemma evokes two interrelated concerns regarding causing potential harm to direct and indirect target populations. The first is to what extent it increases people's level of anxiety or worry by assigning them to the role of a person who is ill (Barsky, 1988). Campaigners' goals on one hand are to encourage target populations to participate in screening activities and to identify those who are considered to be at risk for a particular disease to manage or prevent it. On the other hand, these interventions serve to frame particular medical conditions, such as high blood pressure or high level of blood cholesterol, as diseases and to label individuals as *patients* (Guttmacher, Teitelman, Chapin, Garbowski, & Schnall, 1981; Moore, 1989). This labeling might actually cause them harm (Barsky, 1988; Bloom & Monterossa, 1981).The second concern is to what extent the intervention contributes to the stigmatization of people who already possess the medical condition or attributes alluded to by the intervention as something that should be avoided or is greatly socially undesirable (e.g., having to use a wheelchair; see Wang, 1992).

Individuals identified as having certain risk factors find themselves in a peculiar variation of the Parsonian sick role (Parsons, 1958): they have officially become patients, however, they are not truly sick at the present, only at risk, and therefore are not eligible for the privileges associated with the sick role. They are, however, characterized as *needing help* or in a new variation of the at-risk role (McLeroy et al., 1987), which obligates them to accept help from those considered experts, and to cooperate actively with the agency or professional that proffers the helping service. Labeled individuals are thus placed in the role of being obliged to follow a therapeutic regimen and to continuously worry about their health. This raises ethical concerns regarding the extent to which social interventions affect people's sense of identity (Forester, 1993). Barsky (1988), a physician, observed high levels of anxiety in many of his patients, whom he labeled the *worried well.*

The dilemma is how to advise individuals that they might be at risk for potentially detrimental health complications without labeling them or others, thus contributing to their anxiety and affecting their well-being or sense of identity adversely (MacDonald, Sackett, Haynes, & Taylor, 1984; Milne, Logan, & Lanagan, 1984). Similarly, ethical concerns about what has been characterized as spoiling people's identity or stigmatizing them are raised when campaign messages use fear-raising appeals that present a negative image of those who are in that situation already, for example, individuals who are infected with HIV (e.g., Herek & Capitanio, 1993) or people with disabilities. Wang (1992) argued that campaign messages against drunk driving or those promoting the use of seatbelts that focus on the horror of being confined to a wheelchair were perceived by individuals with mobility disabilities as devaluing them and attacking their self-esteem and dignity.

Depriving Dilemma

To what extent might campaigns, while pointing out risks associated with certain behaviors or practices, in fact serve to deprive people of pleasures?

Health campaigns that aim to change certain practices they believe put people at risk for disease or injury might inadvertently cause harm. Typical *risky pleasures* are often relatively inexpensive in terms of money and mental or physical effort and more accessible to people with less income. Individuals with greater means and resources can find it easier to refrain from practices considered risky than those with less means. The quality of life of the latter may in fact suffer from what critics have labeled "forceful, evangelistic health propaganda" (Strasser, Jeanneret, & Raymond, 1987, p. 190). Denying people inexpensive pleasures without providing them with alternative ones poses an ethical dilemma because the health campaign, although trying to do good, might actually harm those who can not avail themselves of more costly alternatives. Similarly, certain practices, such as smoking, that are deemed unhealthy might serve people in disadvantaged situations as their only means of perceived control. For example, bans on smoking in hospitals have raised an outcry among advocates of individuals with mental health problems. They argue that expecting mental health patients "to kick the habit when they're going into the hospital, which is an awful event to begin with, is really cruelty to the n'th degree" and that "having a cigarette is a patient's one pleasure, the one opportunity for personal autonomy" (Foderaro, 1994, p. 44). Similarly, campaigns, by characterizing certain foods or practices as unhealthy might deprive members of particular cultural communities of activities that have special cultural significance. Thus, practitioners or researchers engaged in the design and implementation of health campaigns should examine the extent to which the practices, foods, substances or products they ask their target populations to relinquish might deny them important rewards that cannot be readily substituted (e.g., because of economic or social circumstances or special cultural meanings). This represents tension between principles of doing good and doing no harm, as well as concerns for justice and caring.

Culpability Dilemmas

Three major concerns related to the emphasis on personal responsibility in campaigns are outlined next:

- To what extent should an individual be

responsible for the behavior of significant others?

- To what extent should the individual be responsible for ill-health outcomes associated with his or her behaviors?
- To what extent should certain *risky* behaviors be socially approved and socially desired whereas others disapproved of, thus identifying those who practice them as irresponsible?

The first dilemma concerns the extent to which one is responsible for the behavior of others. Campaigns often have messages that appeal to significant others to ensure the person who is seen as being at risk will adopt the recommended practices.[18] Although these campaigns intend to do good by using what they consider effective persuasive messages, they might do harm by implicitly blaming the significant other when the behavior of the person who is seen at risk does not adopt the recommendations.

With growing emphasis on individuals' *lifestyle* behaviors as prominent risk factors for ill-health, personal responsibility has become a highly visible theme in many health campaigns (McLeroy et al, 1987). Campaign messages often urge individuals to take responsibility for their own health and to adopt health-promoting behaviors. The emphasis on individual responsibility presumably is based on the assumption that particular health-related behaviors are freely chosen or at least under the voluntary control of the individual. Those who fail to adopt practices promoted as health-protective, by implication, can be characterized as irresponsible. Target populations, however, might not adopt recommended practices because of the constraints imposed by economic or sociocultural circumstances and therefore should not be held accountable for not adopting the health-promoting practices.

The issue of accountability or personal responsibility underscores one of the most widely discussed ethical issues in the context of health promotion—victim blaming (e.g., Beauchamp, 1987; Crawford, 1977; Eisenberg; 1987; Faden, 1987; Marantz, 1990; Ryan, 1976)—locating the causes of social problems within the individual rather than in social and environmental forces. On one hand, because individuals are seen as autonomous and able to make voluntary decisions regarding their behaviors—especially those characterized as related to lifestyle—the responsibility for modifying their behavior is seen as primarily their own. On the other hand, many who do not adopt health-promoting behaviors, because of their social or economic circumstance, are viewed as particularly vulnerable to antihealth influences. This argument adds complexity to the issue of personal responsibility or culpability: when is the person's behavior voluntary and when is it affected by powerful cultural or institutional factors (McLeroy et al., 1987)?

The question of how to determine what is voluntary leads us to another dilemma associated with responsibility: should one be free to choose whether to adopt or not to adopt practices that might lead to illness or disability? Furthermore, who should be responsible for adverse outcomes that result from people taking risks with their health? Some claim that people who take risks with their health impose burdens on others and society as a whole, especially when the public needs to take care of them or pay for their healthcare or disability (McLeroy et al., 1987; Veatch, 1980). This points to tensions between ethical principles of personal autonomy and the public good, and raises the following questions: should health campaigns promote messages that suggest that individuals should be liable for increased costs they might place on the medical care system, under the assumption that their voluntary acts may cause injury to others? Should people who do not adopt what are considered responsible practices be charged with higher health insurance premiums, or be denied all or part of their insurance claims if they do not, for example, use seatbelts? (Beauchamp, 1987).

A contentious issue is which behaviors can be characterized as truly voluntary, for which one can or cannot be held culpable. The latter would exempt one from full responsibility for adverse health outcomes (Veatch, 1980). This leads to the dilemma concerning the extent to which certain risk-taking behaviors are socially desired or sanctioned: should certain injury-prone behaviors be approved of as socially desirable (e.g., sports or dangerous occupations) whereas others not, and what are the moral criteria for making such distinctions? Should individuals who engaged in socially non-approved health-related risks be blamed for their injury or disease, whereas others, whose behaviors might lead to the same kind of consequences, should be seen as heroes (Keeney, 1994)?

Campaign messages raise ethical concerns, suggested a bioethicist,[19] if they frame the individual's behavior as a sufficient condition for causing the potential harmful outcome. Although most messages do not explicitly state that individuals' behaviors are the only cause for ill-health, people who are increasingly bombarded with messages on personal responsibility and the notion that certain practices will result in adverse outcomes might interpret them as such.[20] For example, in a series of *Health Notes* in a kit for professionals produced by NHLBI and reproduced by local campaigns, messages typically state that "It's Up to You: High blood pressure can be controlled, but you are the *only* person who can control it" (emphasis added).[21] The methods specified are weight control, limited salt intake, avoidance of alcohol, exercise, and compliance with a medication regimen that are, by implication, presented as the main and presumably only (sufficient) means to avoid getting a stroke. Similarly, a television PSA produced by NHBPEP solemnly tells viewers that individuals who did not take their high blood pressure medication appropriately died, leaving their families behind. Clearly these messages imply nonadherence caused their death.

Findings from a focus group conducted by a local campaign studied by Guttman indicate that respondents tended to blame themselves or their *weak character* for not adopting the recommended medical regimens. These respondents did not consider socioeconomic factors that might impinge on adopting a healthier lifestyle. This echoes concerns regarding blaming the victim[22] and justice or fairness, because health promoters have the obligation to treat their target population fairly in terms of burdens (e.g., risks, costs) and benefits (Hiller, 1987).[23] Ethical concerns regarding justice include the following: Does the campaign provide all members of the population with reasonable opportunities to pursue the goals emphasized in the campaign (Daniels, 1985)? What are reasonable opportunities and who should decide on the definition? The issue of equal opportunity was raised by focus group members in a community program studied by Guttman. Campaign messages that emphasized choice and responsibility to prevent heart disease (originally produced by NHLBI) were contested by members of a focus group. The messages state that one's "choice begins at the grocery store." Members of a focus group felt that consumption choices of members of the target community were limited because they were restricted by the relatively high-priced and low-quality produce available to them at the only grocery store in walking distance (the population that uses the store does not usually have easy access to other options).[24]

Daniels (1985) explained that having an opportunity does not necessarily mean individuals can purchase what they would like to, but it does mean they should be provided with equal opportunity to purchase nutritious foods seen as necessary to maintain good health. This raises concerns regarding principles of justice, as indicated by epidemiological studies: decreases in morbidity and mortality from heart disease are usually more prevalent in the more affluent population, because they are more likely to adopt healthier lifestyle behavioral modifications (e.g., Blane, 1995; Thomas, 1990; Whitehead, 1992; Williams, 1990; Winkleby, 1994).[25]

An additional concern is the extent to which the emphasis on an individualistically oriented conception of personal responsibility raises people's expectations from the healthcare system as a whole. This issue is discussed in the next dilemma concerning the promise of good health.

Dilemmas Concerning Power and Control

Embedded in interventions are issues of power and control that also raise concerns regarding inadvertent outcomes. These can be related to concerns about justice mainly on a societal level. Three dilemmas are presented here:

1. Are certain stakeholders likely to benefit more than others from the campaign?
2. Are certain stakeholders likely to be exploited to achieve the goals of the sponsors of the campaign?
3. Do health campaigns serve as a means of social or organizational control?

Privileging Dilemma

When focusing on specific health problems or particular ways to address them, to what extent does the campaign privilege certain stakeholders or ideologies?

By focusing on particular medical conditions, interventions, by definition, prioritize these conditions and privilege certain individuals or social institutions over others. This privileging can include those who have this particular medical condition, the agencies and professionals who specialize in treating it, and pharmaceutical companies whose products have been developed to treat it. Clearly this raises ethical concerns regarding who (both purposefully and inadvertently) is privileged by a certain campaign, and what the implications to society as a whole are. Many commercial enterprises can profit from campaign efforts by increasing markets for their products or services (Freimuth, Hammond, & Stein, 1988; Wang, 1992), and often, as illustrated in the case of the National High Blood Pressure Education Programs and the National Cholesterol Education Programs, campaigns tend to support the authority of biomedical professionals by urging the public to "see their doctor." In fact, one of the criteria for the success of these campaigns is the increase in the number of visits to physicians.

Labeling a particular physical condition as a medical condition or a disease has serious political, economic and social consequences and privileges the medical establishment. Once a condition or behavior is defined as a matter of health and disease, the medical profession is thereby licensed to diagnose, treat, control, or intervene. The mere act of characterizing a certain level of blood cholesterol as an important medical condition, and having the detection and treatment of this condition promoted through a campaign, potentially results in placing a large number of individuals in the social position of patients, and in the creation or enhancement of a whole industry of screening and monitoring paraphernalia. It might also privilege particular food products recommended by the campaign. This raises ethical concerns regarding the extent to which one condition should be prioritized over others, and the extent to which particular stakeholders' perspectives and interests are given more prominence.

A related concern is to what extent a campaign prioritizes particular social values and beliefs over others. Values related to individual responsibility (or individualism), individual-level solutions, and market autonomy are often emphasized in health campaigns. This emphasis is likely to reproduce values that are dominant in American culture, which include individualism (Bellah et al., 1991), a distrust in government intervention, a preference for private solutions to social problems, a standard of abundance as a normal state of affairs, and the power of technology (Priester, 1992a). To what extent does a campaign, whether intentionally or not, contribute to sustaining or reproducing certain beliefs and the social and cultural institutions that support them?

Another concern is the extent to which campaigns privilege particular agencies or groups by collaborating with them or providing them with resources or legitimacy. Campaigns tend to work with groups in the target community that are established and already have resources, thus emphasizing principles of utility. Critics maintain this can help perpetuate the power of these groups while depriving less-established or nonmainstream organizations of potential resources and legitimization. Although campaigns might attempt to involve individuals and groups from a wide spectrum, constituencies who are given priority are most likely to be established agencies and groups that already have considerable resources and networks, or are predisposed to the topic of the intervention. Consequently, they are less likely to address the needs and concerns of those who are unaffiliated and who are relatively marginalized. As a result, the latter are least likely to be given the opportunities to get involved in policy-making processes related to an intervention that aims to affect their lives (Wallace-Brodeur, 1990). Finally, an additional concern is the extent to which certain groups or organizations are more privileged by being able to produce (persuasive) information and get it disseminated (Rakow, 1989). To what extent, we need to ask, do particular organizations or groups have more access to information that will support their claims regarding which health issues should be focused on, or which strategies should be adopted?

Exploitation Dilemma

When involving community or other voluntary organizations in a health campaign, whereas on one hand this might support values of participation and empowerment, to what extent does it serve to exploit these organizations?

More and more campaigns, including those sponsored by the federal government, follow a model of using local agencies or organizations to implement much of the intervention process. This raises ethical concerns regarding the extent to which campaigns create expectations that voluntary groups will carry out functions that should be served through public services. National and state-level initiatives, for example, rely on local screening activities that take place through the collaboration of local agencies and voluntary groups to achieve the programs' official goals. These programs' long-term goals are to institutionalize these types of activities so that local organizations can continue to carry them on in the future without sponsorship or funding. Capek (1992) and Green (1989) noted that there is a potentially problematic aspect related to the goal of institutionalization—having community organizations eventually take over the mission of the (funded) intervention program—especially if that mission entails service delivery. Green (1989) said that community organizations "should not have to function as a permanent substitute for federal agencies, particularly because their tax dollars fund the regulatory structure. They themselves do not have the financial means to sustain such an effort, and their involvement in competition for scarce funds is frequently disempowering" (p. 743).

On one hand, local involvement promotes democratic goals. On the other hand, concerns can be raised regarding the extent to which the involvement of the group or agency in the intervention serves this group or the community it represents in the long run. Are organizations that become involved being exploited by the program because it might not serve their interests in the long run? In addition, are its constituents given the opportunity to decide on the goals and priorities of the intervention? This also raises concerns regarding the extent to which particular organizations should be obligated to participate in the campaign. Should organizations be seen as having obligations for community members' health? Similarly, should organizations that choose not to be involved be sanctioned?

Control Dilemma

To what extent might organizations use health-promoting programs to increase their management or control organizational members?

Organizations increasingly offer wellness and health promotion programs. The provision of such programs often indicates the success of health campaigns. Obviously, worksite disease-prevention activities, as part of a health campaign, have numerous advantages. Worksite interventions can provide campaigners with access to particular groups and workers with opportunities or even often tangible incentives to participate in health-promoting activities.[26] Justification for these activities relates mostly to principles of doing good (for the employees) and utility (e.g., by increasing productivity, decreasing absenteeism, and enhancing the organization's image). Nevertheless, numerous ethical concerns regarding the worksite as a place to promote health have been raised (e.g., Hollander & Hale, 1987; Roman & Blum, 1987). One of the major concerns is the extent to which involvement with employee health gives the work organization a mandate to literally pry into what until now had been considered employees' private affairs.

With health linked to lifestyle, organizations can engage—in the name of concern for their employees' health—in activities to find out what their employees do on and off the job. They can use this information to justify managerial decisions that are not necessarily for employees' benefit. Similarly, management can make presumably health-related demands on employees that are not directly linked to their work (Conrad & Chapman Walsh, 1992; Feingold, 1994). The *new health ethic* might serve, say these critics, as a new vehicle for enhancing worker discipline, screening for undesired workers, or foster uncritical loyalty to the company. Ethical concerns related to autonomy, privacy, and justice can be raised in this context, specifically the following: To what extent are individuals discriminated against because they are characterized as a potential liability to the organization (Feingold, 1994)?

Furthermore, wellness and health promotion programs typically construct disease etiology in terms of individual behavior and individual responsibility for being healthy, and they adopt a biomedical framework for assessing risk and risk factors (Alexander, 1988). Alternative conceptualization of risk factors for illness include social and institutional factors such as the extent to which workers have latitude for decision making on the job (e.g., Karasek & Theorell, 1990). This raises concerns regarding the extent to which it is justified for health campaigns to emphasize one particular version of health-risk etiology, and what possible implications are—an issue raised in the dilemmas related to social values discussed next.

Dilemmas Concerning Social Values

Do health campaigns serve to turn health into an ideal? Do health campaigns contribute to making health a *super value* that should be vigorously pursued? Do campaigns imply that *good health* should be a reward for *good people?* These are some of the concerns that are raised with the growing emphasis on health in public campaigns. Planners of campaigns, argued Pollay (1989), need to consider how their campaigns contribute to cultural changes such as the reinforcement or transformation of specific values or ideologies. Over time, he suggested, campaigns as an aggregate, even if they do not change individuals' behaviors, produce cultural changes. The three dilemmas reflect these concerns, while focusing on issues characterized as distraction, promises, and health as a value.

Distraction Dilemma

By emphasizing the importance of certain health-related issues in personal, organizational, and societal agendas, to what extent does this emphasis serve to distract people from important social issues?

Having health-related issues capture such a prominent position on the personal and public agenda serve, suggest critics, to distract individuals and society from other, more significant problems, such as economic equity or environmental hazards.[27] As communicative action, health campaigns can be seen as framing issues and selectively drawing attention to them, although deemphasizing others, thus making the issues promoted by the intervention seem more important. Communicative practice, argued Forester (1993) cannot be seen as simply an enactment of goals but as the "practical communicative organizing (or disorganizing) of others' attention to relevant and significant issues at hand" (p. 5). Pollay (1989) reiterated this argument: "Campaigns also serve to set agendas, direct people's attention and order people's priorities. Health programs aimed at making individuals more responsible for their diets may also direct attention away from government and industry policies putting pollutants, toxic waste and carcinogens into the ecology and food chain" (p. 190). These assertions are supported by research findings from the agenda-setting perspective, according to which substance abuse prevention campaigns have been found to influence public perceptions on the importance of these issues (Shoemaker, 1989). Health campaigns can serve to prioritize or frame certain issues as important, and they raise concerns regarding the extent to which the campaign serves to become a distraction from important social issues that face individuals and society as a whole. Bellah et al. (1985, 1991) expressed this concern when they described social institutions as on one hand forms of paying attention to particular issues, but on the other hand as socially organized forms of distractions. The process of distraction is significant because of its impact on the functioning of a democratic society: "One way of defining democracy would be to call it a political system in which people actively attend to what is significant" (Bellah et al., 1991, p. 273).

Campaigns, particularly those that employ social marketing approaches that tend to emphasize and affirm mainly individual-level solutions, similarly raise the following concerns: to what extent do campaigns affect public perceptions and emphasize individual-level solutions as the main course of action, at the expense of other approaches (e.g., organizational or societal)? To what extent does the campaign promote only a lifestyle-modification agenda and not present the public with alternative perspectives (Farrant & Russell, 1987).[28] These might include messages on how health risks of the public are intricately vested in competing interests of powerful organizations such as the food and tobacco industry, government interests, or those of the medical profession.[29]

Green and Kreuter (1991) distinguished between a reductionist and expansionist approach to health interventions. In the former, health is identified from broader social issues; in the latter, the specific health issue of the intervention, which is often assigned to the practitioner as its sole mission, can serve as a basis for consideration of a broader range of social issues. But this is not easily accomplished. As a campaign practitioner emphatically explained in an interview, he did not see his role as a social change agent in the sense of trying to change structural factors. "If I would have wanted to do that [social change], I would have gone to be a social worker," he said. Another campaign practitioner lamented in an interview that neither she nor the other staff members in their program were trained in community development, and she felt they lacked skills and resources to develop programs to address community-level or structural factors.

Clearly the issue of affirming multiple types of causation of health and illness poses challenges to communication researchers and practitioners: What is the ethical mandate of the researchers or practitioners? Are they mandated to emphasize only the types of messages that are directly related to the specific domain of behavior change of the intervention, thus possibility distracting their attention from other causes? Are they obligated to provide messages on sociocultural or other factors and ways to assess and address them?

Promises Dilemma

Do health campaigns that urge people to adopt particular practices and behaviors and say that by doing so the person will be healthier, in fact make promises that might not be beneficial to the public?

Campaigns tend to emphasize good health as a reward for adopting what is considered a responsible lifestyle. Their messages often promise individuals that if they adopt recommended regimes or act responsibly, they will be rewarded with good health. This, maintain critics, reinforces the notion of individual needs as the basis for healthcare, and is problematic not only from a practical perspective, but a moral one as well. Callahan (1990) and others (e.g., Barsky, 1988) argued that a major challenge facing the healthcare system is the escalating expectations of the public regarding medicine and healthcare. Two related premises and promises that underlie the current healthcare system are flawed, suggested Callahan (1990). The first is that healthcare should emphasize meeting individual needs, and the second is that this can be done economically and in an efficient manner. From a practical perspective, it is argued, the more individuals' expectations are raised, the more they will increase their demands from the health care system, which in turn will increase demands for expensive procedures and services for an ever-increasing range of what can be considered medically related (Gaylin, 1993). According to Callahan (1990), there is a direct conflict between preferences of the individual, whom he suggests, given the choice, will tend to demand the most expensive and comprehensive health care possible, and the limited resources of society. The problems of the high cost of healthcare today, suggest critics, are rooted in medicine's successes that have increased demands for its services, which society cannot afford (Gaylin, 1993).

The ethical concerns raised in this context mainly relate to doing harm (by raising expectations that cannot be met), and the public good (an overtaxed and costly healthcare system), deemphasizing caring and connectedness to others and relationships (Nodding, 1984). Another concern relates to justice. There is a growing gap in use of healthcare between those who have easy access to medical services and those who do not (Gold & Franks, 1990; Thomas, 1990). On one hand, individuals who have the opportunity to adopt recommended health-promoting regimens have raised expectations, and will increasingly see medicine as an unlimited social good. On the other hand, those who have fewer opportunitics to adopt health promoting regimens might be made to feel inadequate, guilty, or hopeless. In addition, with more and more personal and social issues (e.g., infertility) seen as potentially solved by medical technology—and therefore within the domain of medical care—it can be argued that those who have more opportunities will be tempted to demand even more medical services. These demands, it is suggested, will increase the cost of the health care system to society, beyond any cost-saving measures that are proposed by health insurance policies (Gaylin, 1993). Those who have fewer opportunities will be less likely to utilize current resources, which can adversely affect their health status (Gold & Franks, 1990; Thomas, 1990). This corresponds to the communication studies concerned with the knowledge-gap (Dervin, 1980; Olien et al., 1983; Rakow, 1989), and raises ethical concerns regarding what one considers a just and fair society. The promises that cannot be fulfilled lead to the final dilemma presented in this articler—the implications of emphasizing the importance of health to such an extent that it becomes an important value.

Health as a Value Dilemma

By making health an important social value that should be pursued by the public, does the campaign promote a certain moralism that might not be compatible with other values?

Broadening the definition of health and expectations from medicine raises additional concerns. Do campaigns, by emphasizing the importance of health and a healthy lifestyle, contribute to health becoming an ultimate-value or a morality? (Gillick, 1984).[30] What are the implications of promoting health as a value (see Rokeach, 1979) for people's perception of self and others, or their sense of identity? Might an emphasis on health serve to promote values of individualism at the expense of values of connectedness and caring? For example, slogans such as "It won't happen to me," "It's your health," "Take care of yourself," reflect an emphasis on individualism and a separation between those who value health, and those who do not (Burns, 1992).[31] Campaigns for AIDS prevention tend to emphasize the enhancement use of *negotiation skills* for achieving sexual partners' compliance in adopting safer-sex practices (e.g., Fisher & Misovich, 1990; Franzini, Sideman, Dexter, & Elder, 1990). The word *negotiations*, though, connotes an interchange that emphasizes personal interests, similar to a marketplace transaction (Burns, 1992), one that is personal health, rather than values that emphasize relationships or caring. Critics of the emphasis on negotiation do not propose that interventions should not help people enhance their communication skills with sexual partners to prevent potential harm. They are, however, concerned that this type of emphasis can put women and members of particular cultures, who tend to greatly value caring and relationships, in a double bind (Lyman & Engstrom, 1992; Scott & Mercer, 1994).

A related concern is the extent to which the promotion of health as a value by campaigns contributes to the medicalization of life (Fox, 1977) and, using Habermas' terms, to the colonization of human experience (Habermas, 1979). Callahan (1990) argued that with health increasingly being viewed as an important value, definitions of what is a *good life* become dependent on medical criteria. Barsky (1988), a physician who became concerned with people's growing obsession with health when he saw many of his patients become what he calls the *worried well* made a similar point: "The point is that the pursuit of health can be paradoxical. Secure well-being and self-confident vitality grows out of an acceptance of our frailties and our limits and our mortality as much as they can result from our trying to cure every affliction, to evade every disease and to relieve every symptom" (pp. xi–xii). Callahan (1990) emphatically added:

> Health sought for its own sake, or because of the jobs or profits it produces, leads to a kind of personal and social madness. One can never get enough or be too safe. We will spend too much on health, be in a state of constant anxiety about mortality, and be endlessly distracted from thinking about more important purposes and goals of life. (p. 113)

To this, Becker (1986) in an article tided "The Tyranny of Health Promotion" added a warning that health has become a "New Morality"[32] and that

> health promotion, as currently practiced, fosters a dehumanizing self-concern that substitutes personal health goals for more important, humane, societal goals. It is a new religion, in which we worship ourselves, attribute good health to our devoutness, and view illness as just punishment for those who have not yet seen the Way. (p. 20)

Health, noted Crawford (1994), becomes a metaphor for self-control, self-discipline, self-denial, and will power. It becomes a moral discourse and "an opportunity to reaffirm the values by which self is distinguished from other" (p. 1353). Viewing health as an ultimate value might harm those who, according to these criteria, are not healthy, by making them feel punished or unworthy. This also raises concerns about the extent to which the value of health is shared across different cultural groups.

An additional concern is the trend to broaden the definition of health into a construct of all-inclusive wellness that encompasses physiological, psychological, and social factors including character traits, personal appearance, criminal activities, moods, and desires. These might serve to medicalize human existence. Increasingly, human experiences of life, birth, pain, death, coping, and joy are defined as health-related, and people, it is suggested, tend to lose the capacity to live and cope without medical definitions (Fitzgerald, 1994).[33] Ethical concerns, in other words, focus on the extent to which health campaigns serve to *colonize* or medicalize human experiences, foster dependency on medical institutions, or deemphasize people's cultural arid spiritual well-being.

Conclusions

Health campaigns, as other social interventions, can be seen as communicative action, which involves making claims in four dimensions: (a) shaping people's sense of truth, which affects their beliefs about, for example, what is illness, and which activities are considered health-promoting or responsible; (b) establishing legitimacy, which might affect their consent, for example by giving authority to certain institutions to label people as sick and make decisions about priorities and allocations of resources; (c) the use of expressiveness, which gains people's trust or affects their sense of identity, for example by using persuasive strategies or by identifying certain people as being at risk; and (d) by framing issues in certain ways, which affects people's comprehension or perceptions of priorities, for example, that certain health conditions should be pursued mainly through education, rather than through institutional or structural changes.

The 13 dilemmas outlined in this article can help ask questions about each of these four areas of concern and articulate the embedded ethical issues—the research, analysis, design, implementation, and evaluation. These dilemmas can provide a conceptual approach, which can help scholars and practitioners identify more clearly ethical concerns related to health campaigns.

The consideration of ethical issues in health intervention research has important implications for the development of both theory and practice. Campaigns, as prevention activities, are seen as important means to control cost or address issues of justice. Yet, as economists have pointed out, prevention activities are not necessarily cost-effective (Russell, 1986, 1987) and therefore need to be based on moral justifications. The analysis, design, and evaluation of health campaigns should not depend on cost-benefit indicators or efficiency criteria. Instead, ethical concerns and social values can provide morally and socially acceptable justifications for adopting certain health-promotion goals and strategies or evaluation criteria (Priester, 1992b). For this purpose, we need to further conceptual approaches to enable scholars, practitioners, policy makers, and the public to assess and make decisions on priorities and strategies in health promotion.[34]

This poses three challenges for scholars and practitioners. The first challenge is to define what constitutes *health,* or *good health.*[35] Does health constitute a summary of medical definitions or should we adopt the World Health Organization's encompassing definition that includes societal and economic factors? The second challenge is to develop theoretical frameworks to identify social processes that contribute to particular definitions of health and good health in society, and to make more explicit which stakeholders' definitions tend to prevail. Dilemmas concerning inadvertent outcomes can be incorporated as part of the research agenda, both regarding the design and evaluation of campaigns.

The third challenge is to decide which questions and research agendas should be pursued to help ensure that communication campaigns promote notions of health, and personal and social responsibility that are compatible with social values and meet acceptable moral criteria. This can help serve as a basis for the design and evaluation of campaigns, as well as a deeper theoretical understanding of the social processes involved in setting their priorities and constructing their goals.

Acknowledgments

This article was supported in part by Grant 1 T32 PE10011-01 from the Division of Medicine of the Health Resources and Services Administration (HRSA). Its contents are solely the responsibility of the author and do not necessarily represent the views of HRSA.

Earlier versions of this article were presented at the 1994 Communication Ethics Conference in Michigan, the 1995 International Communication Association's Annual Convention in Albuquerque, Mew Mexico, and the 1995 American Public Health Association's Annual Meeting in San Diego, California.

My sincere thanks to Robert Like, Charles T. Salmon and to the anonymous reviewer for their thoughtful comments and suggestions. Special thanks also to Rebecca Spoerri for editorial comments.

Endnotes

1. Interest in ethical issues in the healthcare context is increasing, which is evident in the inclusion of ethics in health professionals training, in the growth of the number of books on bioethics, the creation of ethics committees in hospitals, and in recent editions of health communication books (e.g., Kreps & Thornton, 1992; Northouse & Northouse, 1992; Thornton and Kreps, 1993).
2. For example, which goals should be pursued, how to achieve these goals, what are indicators of desired outcomes, and how to assess the extent to which these outcomes serve to enhance the health of the population (see Salmon, 1989).
3. Stuart Nagel (1983) presented ethical dilemmas in policy evaluation. Some of the dilemmas he outlined share the same concerns raised in this article. The nine dilemmas he discussed concern policy optimization, sensitivity analysis, partisanship, unforeseen consequences, equity, efficient research, research sharing, research validity, and handling official wrongdoing.
4. For example, the National Cholesterol Education Program's (NCEP) 1992 Communication Strategy document stated that it "is not enough to create messages based on scientific consensus—it is critical to provide messages that the audience will understand, that they will care about, and that they can act upon. To accomplish this, the NHLBI's public education efforts have successfully employed the principles of social marketing" (p.8).

5. See also a discussion by Laczniak, Lusch, and Murphy (1979) on ethical issues in social marketing.
6. Clearly not all health promoters believe these are the most effective techniques. See a critique by Wallack (1989).
7. A popular approach is the use of focus groups.
8. See Arkin(1992).
9. In this case, though, the planners, according to Salmon and Kroger, might have also assumed that fear appeals might be ineffective. The use of fear appeals, however, has been endorsed as effective, for example by the National Heart, Lung and Blood Institute's National High Blood Pressure Education Program in its 1993 communication strategy plans.
10. Citing Woods, Davis, and Wesover (1991), Ratzan and his colleagues (1994) gave an example how in the development of public service announcements (PSAs) in its "America Responds to AIDS" (ART A) campaign, the Centers of Disease Control and Prevention (CDC) decided to adopt nonoffensive language. The result, suggested these researchers, was that audiences were provided with a muddled message.
11. For a recent treatment of the ethical issues regarding the use of "sin taxes" see Kahn (1994).
12. This is further developed in the dilemmas concerning inadvertent outcomes.
13. In fact, it might even cause inadvertent harm, as discussed later in the Culpability Dilemmas that discuss the notion of blaming the victim.
14. This approach is mentioned in many official NCEP and NHBPEP documents, and detailed in NCEP's (1991) report. For a detailed epidemiological rationale, see Rose (1981,1985).
15. Nagel (1983), in the context of policy analysis, described a similar dilemma he called the Equity Dilemma that refers to a frequent conflict between policy goals of efficiency and equity.
16. Everett Rogers gave an example in the 1993 conference of the International Communication Association of how practitioners and researchers decided to forego an experimental design of interventions for smoking prevention among children and youth after they got requests to implement their program in communities that were supposed to provide a control.
17. The Designated Driver campaign typically has not been framed as following a harm reduction approach but it can be seen as such because its messages essentially condone, or at least do not aim to change, excessive alcohol consumption (by those who are not designated to drive). An implicit underlying assumption is that although interventions cannot change people's alcohol consumption behavior, at least health promoters can try to prevent accidents. This approach raises additional concerns regarding the framing of the issue of alcohol consumption discussed in the Distractions Dilemma later.
18. 18NHBPEP Communication Strategy (Draft, 1993. p. 24). Examples of messages are: "Husband: Darling, did you take your high blood pressure medicine today?; Daughter: Mom, I made Dad's favorite dish for dinner: macaroni and cheese. Mother: Did you remember to use the skim milk and low-fat cheese? Daughter: I sure did." (*NHLBI Kit '90;* pp. 19–20).
19. This was suggested by Dan Wilder, a bioethicist, in a personal communication.
20. As previously mentioned, NHLBI PSAs present individuals who did not follow their medical regimen, had a stroke, and consequently are dependent on others, or even ruined their retirement plans. This can be seen as falling within the category of one's (irresponsible) behavior being a necessary cause for their condition, as well as the implication that they were not behaving responsibly toward their loved ones.
21. These are found in *NHLBI Kit '90*. A typical message in this type of campaign is "It's your life, it's your move." This message is from NHBPEP's public service announcements (PSAs). Other types of messages in campaigns are "You can Lower Your Blood Cholesterol: It's up to you. All it takes are some simple diet changes," or "You are in control." These messages imply that one's behavior change is sufficient to influence one's health, which, as discussed next, puts the main burden on the person.
22. For example, in a report of a focus group from one of the local heart disease prevention programs reviewed by Guttman, participants, who were all from a lower socioeconomic background, described themselves as being "weak" (of character) or having "lack of willpower" to explain why they do not consume only low-fat foods to prevent potential health complications. The focus group report concluded that the par-

ticipants generally did not perceive themselves as mentally tough or competent to put up with sacrifice, pain, or suffering. Their discussion contained many statements of low self-worth. This observation suggests that they blame themselves for not adopting the recommended health-promoting behaviors, and feel guilty about it.

23. There are different theories of justice and perspectives on how costs and benefits should be distributed. One perspective emphasizes the notion of having equal availability of the health promotion resources to everyone (i.e., following egalitarian principles), whereas others allocate resources according to those perceived as bearing the greatest need, in an attempt to balance the principle of equity with people's inequalities regarding personal abilities and circumstances (Garret et al., 1989).

24. The National Cholesterol Education Program's (1991) report found that foods particularly sensitive to income level are meats, fresh fruit, and vegetables, which are seen as important to a nutritious diet. It also reported that the consumption of low-fat milk and whole-grain bread is positively related to income, possibly reflecting the growing concern regarding health in the higher socioeconomic groups. According to this report, the use of fresh vegetables, fruits, and juices decreases as household size increases, and intake of vitamins C and Be is inversely related to household size, as expected from lower income elasticity for fresh fruits and vegetables in larger households. Educational levels can also influence food consumption, where higher educational level is associated with consumption of fruits and milk, and lower consumption of "convenience" foods.

25. Daniels (1985) presented a framework often cited in the bioethics literature for the analysis of justice in the context of health care. He argued that justice is based on providing access or opportunity to resources that allow individuals to provide for their necessary needs, but not necessarily their preferences. Once individuals have access to resources or opportunities, they can make their own choices regarding the type of risks they want to take. Daniels also argued that for a prevention activity to meet claims for justice it needs to provide equal opportunities to prevent individuals from being exposed to risks. Prevention efforts that provide opportunities only for people with greater socioeconomic status, such as the promotion of nutritious foods that are only available at higher prices, can be seen as not meeting this criterion of justice.

26. Incentives such as competition and prizes were used successfully in one of the local programs studied. Feingold (1994) reported *disincentives* posed by Hershey Foods Corporation to its employees: They must pay an extra $30 a month if they have high blood pressure and $10 if they do not exercise.

27. Pollay (1989) made a similar point in his discussion of distractions in the context of advertising: "Promoting the trivial is criticized as wasteful or indulgent, distracting resources from more substantial needs" (p. 187). Pollay, though, suggested that in the case of public information campaigns "the criticism of triviality is less germane than in the case of product advertising" (p. 187). The authors cited in this article (e.g., Forester, Bellah and his colleagues, Barsky) might disagree with this comment.

28. See Milio (1981) for a detailed discussion. Farrant and Russell (1987) described in detail how health promotion materials for the prevention of heart disease were developed in Great Britain, which excluded the discussion of how social factors can contribute to this disease.

29. For an argument on why the socio-political-economic factors of the etiology of illnesses should be raised in the context of the medical practitioner-patient encounter, see Waitzkin (1989, 1991). This criticism can be aimed also at the campaigns that promote the Designated Driver, a topic discussed in the dilemma of harm reduction. The campaign on this topic can be seen as framing the issue of drunk driving as logistical—people need to make sure that the person who is supposed to drive is not intoxicated. The issue is not framed as a cultural and normative issue.

30. Rather than as a means to another end, or as an instrumental value, as explained by Green and Kreuter (1991).

31. See Tesh's (1988) discussion on ideologies and values in health interventions.

32. See also Fitzgerald (1994) and Gillick (1984).

33. See Illich (1975), Zola (1975), and Fox (1977) for a critique of medicalization.

34. Garland and Hasnain (1990) reported on activities in which they engaged the public in discussions of ethical issues for the purpose

of developing and adopting healthcare policy in Oregon.

35. Callahan (1990), for example, criticized the World Health Organization's definition of health as encompassing too much. This poses particular challenges to communication scholars: how should health be viewed from a communication perspective? (See Zook, 1994, on a discussion in the provider-patient context).

References

Alexander, J. (1988). The ideological construction of risk: An analysis of corporate health promotion programs in the 1980s. *Social Science and Medicine, 26*(5), 559–567.

Arkin, E. B. (1992). *Analysis of high blood pressure and cholesterol target audience and message test reports,* 1978–1991. Manuscript submitted for publication.

Baier, A. C. (1993). What do women want in moral theory? In M. J. Larrabee (Ed.). *An ethic of care: Feminist and interdisciplinary perspectives.* New York: Routledge.

Barry, V. (1982). *Moral aspects of health care.* Belmont, CA: Wadsworth.

Barsky, A. J. (1988). *Worried sick: Our troubled quest for wellness.* Boston: Little, Brown.

Becker, M. H. (1993). A medical sociologist looks at health promotion. *Journal of Health and Social Behavior, 34,* 1–6.

Becker, M. H. (1986). The tyranny of health. *Public Health Reviews, 14,* 15–25.

Beauchamp, D. E. (1987). Life-style, public health and paternalism. In S. Doxiadis (Ed.), *Ethical dilemmas in health promotion* (pp. 69–81). New York: Wiley.

Beauchamp, D. E. (1988). *The health of the republic: Epidemics, medicine, and moralism as challenges to democracy.* Philadelphia: Temple University Press.

Bellah, R. N., Madsen, R., Sullivan, W. M., Swidler, A., & Tipton, S. M. (1985). *Habits of the heart: Individualism and commitment in American life.* Berkeley: University of California Press.

Bellah, R. N., Madsen, R., Sullivan, W. M., Swidler, A., & Tipton, S. M. (1991). *The good society.* New York: Knopf.

Blakeslee, S. (1992, March 15). *Faulty math heightens fears of breast cancer.* The *New York Times.*

Blane, D. (1995). Editorial: Social determinants of health—socioeconomic status, social class, and ethnicity. *American Journal of Public Health, 85,* 903–905.

Bloom, J. R., & Monterossa, S. (1981). Hypertension labeling and sense of well-being. *American Journal of Public Health, 71,* 1228–1232.

Bok, S. (1978). *Lying: Moral choice in public and private life.* New York: Harper & Row.

Brown, W. J. (1991). An AIDS prevention campaign: Effects on attitudes, beliefs, and communication behavior. *American Behavioral Scientist, 34,* 666–678.

Brown, W. J., & Singhal, A. (1990). Ethical dilemmas of prosocial television. *Communication Quarterly, 38,* 268–280.

Burdine, J. N., McLeroy, K, B., & Gottlieb, N. H. (1987). Ethical dilemmas in health promotion: An introduction. *Health Education Quarterly, 14,* 7–9.

Burns, W. D. (1992, July). *Connections and connectedness: Ideas of the self and their relationship to achieving our "Common Health."* Remarks presented at the New Jersey Collegiate Summer Institute for Health in Education and the New Jersey Peer Education Institute, Rutgers University, New Brunswick, NJ.

Callahan, D. (1990). *What kind of life: The limits of medical progress.* New York: Simon & Schuster.

Campbell, A. V. (1990). Education for indoctrination? The issue of autonomy in health education? In S. Doxiadis (Ed.), *Ethics in health education* (pp. 15–27). New York: Wiley.

Capek, S. (1992). Environmental justice, regulation, and the local community. *International Journal of Health Services, 22,* 729–746.

Childress, J. F. (1981). *Priorities in biomedical ethics.* Philadelphia: Westminister Press.

Childress, J. F. (1982). *Who shall decide? Paternalism in health care.* New York: Oxford University Press.

Conrad, P., & Chapman Walsh, D. (1992). The new corporate health ethic: Lifestyle and the social control of work. *International Health Services, 22,* 69–111.

Crawford, R. (1977). You are dangerous to your health: The ideology and politics of victim blaming. *International Journal of Health Services, 7,* 663–680.

Crawford, R. (1994). The boundaries of the self and the unhealthy other: Reflections on health, culture and AIDS. *Social Science and Medicine, 38,* 1347–1356.

Daniels, N. (1985). *Just health care.* New York: Cambridge University Press.

Dervin, B. (1980). Communication gaps and inequalities: Moving toward a reconceptualization. In B. Dervin & M. Voigt (Eds.), *Progress in communication science* (Vol. 2). Norwood, NJ: Ablex.

Des Jarlais, D. C, Padian, N. S., & Winkestein, W.

(1994). Targeted HIV-prevention programs. *New England Journal of Medicine, 331,* 1451–1453.

Doxiadis, S. (1987). Conclusions. In S. Doxiadis, (Ed.), *Ethical dilemmas in health promotion* (pp. 225–229). New York: Wiley.

Eisenberg, L. (1987). Value conflict in social policies for promoting health. In S. Doxiadis, (Ed.), *Ethical dilemmas in health promotion* (pp. 99–116). New York: Wiley.

Elder, J. P., Hovell, M. F., Lasater, T. M., Wells, B. L., & Carleton, R. A. (1985). Applications of behavior modification to community health education: The case of heart disease prevention. *Health Education Quarterly, 12,* 151–168.

Ellison, R. C, Capper, A. L., Goldberg, R. J., Witschi, J. G, & Stare, F. J. (1989). The environmental component: Changing school food service to promote cardiovascular health. *Health Education Quarterly, 16,* 285–297.

Evans, R. I. (1988). Health promotion: Science or ideology? *Health Psychology, 7*(3), 203–219.

Faden, R. R., & Faden, A. I. (1982). The ethics of health education as public health policy. In B. P. Mathews (Ed.), *The practice of health education* (pp. 5–23). Oakland, CA: Society for Public Health Education (Reprinted from *Health Education Monographs, 6,* 180–197).

Faden, R.R. (1987). Ethical issues in government sponsored public health campaigns. *Health Education Quarterly, 14,* 227–237.

Farrant, W., & Russell, J. (1987). *The politics of health information: "Beating heart disease" as a case study of Health Education Council publications* (Bedford Way Paper No. 28). London: Kegan Paul.

Feighery, E., Altaian, D. G., & Shaffer, G. (1991). The effects of combining education and enforcement to reduce tobacco sales to minors. *Journal of the American Medical Association, 266,* 3168–3171.

Feingold, E. (1994). Your privacy or your health. *The Nation's Health, 24,* 2.

Fine, S. H. (1981). *The marketing of ideas and social issues.* New York: Praeger.

Fisher, J. D., & Misovich, S. J. (1990). Evolution of college students' AIDS-related behavioral responses, attitudes, knowledge and fear. *AIDS Education and Prevention 2,* 322–337.

Fitzgerald, F. T. (1994). The tyranny of health. *New England Journal of Medicine, 331,* 196–198.

Foderaro, L. W. (1994, February 19). Battling demons and nicotine: Hospitals' smoking bans are new anxiety for mentally ill. *The New York Times,* pp. 44,48.

Forester, J. (1989). *Planning in the face of power.* Berkeley: University of California Press.

Forester, J. (1993). *Critical theory, public policy, and planning practice: Toward a critical pragmatism.* Albany: State University of New York.

Fortin, A. J. (1991). Ethics, culture, and medical power: AIDS research in the third world. *AIDS and Public Policy Journal, 6,* 15–24.

Fox, R. C. (1977). The medicalization and demedicalization of American society. In J. H. Knowles (Ed.), *Doing better and feeling worse: Health in the United States* (pp. 9–22). New York: Norton.

Franzini, L. R., Sideman, L. M., Dexter, K. E., & Elder, J. P. (1990). Promoting AIDS risk reduction via behavioral training. *AIDS Education and Prevention, 2,* 313–321.

Freimuth, V. S., Hammond, S. L., & Stein, J. A. (1988). Health advertising: Prevention for profit. *American Journal of Public Health, 78,* 557–561.

Garland, M. J., & Hasnain, R. (1990). Health care in common: Setting priorities in Oregon. *Hastings Center Report, 20*(5), 16–18.

Garret, T. M., Baillie, H. W., & Garret, R. M. (1989). *Health care ethics: Principles and problems.* Englewood Cliffs, NJ: Prentice Hall.

Gaylin, W. (1993, September 15). The health plan misses the point. *The New York Times,* p. A27.

Gillick, M. R. (1984). Health promotion, jogging, and the pursuit of the moral life. *Journal of Health Politics, Policy and Law, 9,* 369–387.

Gillon, R. (1990). Health education: The ambiguity of the medical role. In S. Doxiadis (Ed.), *Ethics in Health Education* (pp. 29–41). New York: Wiley.

Glantz, S. A. (1996). Preventing tobacco use—the youth access trap. *American Journal of Public Health, 86,* 156–157.

Glanz, K., & Mullis, R. M. (1988). Environmental interventions to promote health eating: A review of model, programs, and evidence. *Health Education Quarterly, 15,* 395–415.

Gold, M., & Franks, P. (1990). The social origin of cardiovascular risk: An investigation in a rural community. *International Journal of Health Services, 20,* 405–416.

Goodman, L. E., & Goodman, M. J. (1986). Prevention: How misuse of a concept undercuts its worth. *Hastings Center Report, 16,* 26–38.

Green, L. W. (1989). Comment: Is institutionalization the proper goal of grantmaking? *American Journal of Health Promotion, 5,* 44.

Green, L. W., & Kreuter, M. W. (1991). *Health promotion planning: An educational and environmental approach* (2nd ed.). Mountain View, CA: Mayfield Publishing.

Griming, J. E. (1989). Publics, audiences and market segments: Segmentation principles for campaigns. In C. T. Salmon, (Ed.), *Infor-*

mation campaigns: Balancing social values and social change (pp.199–228). Newbury Park, CA: Sage.

Guttmacher, S., Teitelman, M., Chapin, G., Garbowski, G., & Schnall, P. (1981). Ethics and preventive medicine: The case of borderline hypertension. *Hastings Center Report, 11,* 12–14.

Habermas, J. (1979). *Communication and the evolution of society.* Boston: Beacon Press.

Herek, G. M., & Capitanio, J. P. (1993). Public reactions to AIDS in the United States: A second decade of stigma. *American Journal of Public Health, 83,* 574–577.

Hiller, M. D. (1987). Ethics and health education: Issues in theory and practice. In P. M. Lazes, L. H. Kaplan, & K. A. Gordon (Eds.), *The handbook of health education* (2nd ed., pp. 87–107). Rockville, MD: Aspen Publishers.

Hollander, R. B., & Hale, J. F. (1987). Worksite health promotion programs: Ethical issues. *American Journal of Health Promotion, 2,* 37–43.

Illich, I. (1975). *Medical nemesis.* London: Calder & Boyars.

Jaccard, J., Turrisi, R., & Wan, C K. (1990). Implications of behavioral decision theory and social marketing for designing social action programs. In J. Edwards, R. S. Tindale, L. Heath, & E. J. Posavac (Eds.), *Social influence processes and prevention* (pp. 103–142). New York: Plenum.

Jitsukawa, M., & Djerassi, C. (1994). Birth control in Japan: Realities and prognosis. *Science, 265,* 1048–1051.

Kahn, J. P. (1994). Sin taxes as a mechanism of health finance: Moral and policy considerations. In J. F. Humber & R. F. Almeder (Eds.), *Biomedical ethics review* (pp. 179–202). Totowa, NJ: Harmon Press.

Karasek, R., & Theorell, T. (1990). *Healthy work: Stress, productivity, and the reconstruction of working life.* New York: Basic Books.

Keeney, R. L. (1994). Decisions about life–threatening risks. *New England Journal of Medicine, 557*(3), 193–196.

Kleining, J. (1990). The ethical challenge of AIDS to traditional liberal values. *AIDS and Public Policy Journal, 5*(1), 42–44.

Kolata, G. (October 22, 1993). Panel tells cancer institute to stop giving advice on mammograms. *The New York Times.*

Kreps, G. L., & Thornton, B. C. (1992). *Health communication: Theory and practice* (2nd ed.). Prospect Heights, IL: Waverland Press.

Laczniak, G. R., Lusch, R. F., & Murphy, P. E. (1979). Social marketing: Its ethical dimensions. *Journal of Marketing, 43,* 29–36.

Lefebvre, R. C, & Flora, J. A. (1988). Social marketing and public health intervention. *Health Education Quarterly, 15,* 299–315.

Lyman, C. & Engstrom, L. (1992). HIV and sexual health education for women. In R. P. Keeling (Ed.), *Effective AIDS education on campus* (pp. 23–37). San Francisco: Jossey-Bass.

MacDonald, L. A., Sacket, D. L., Haynes, R. B., & Taylor, D. W. (1984). Labelling in hypertension: A review of the behavioral and psychological consequences. *Journal of Chronic Disease, 376,* 933–942.

Manoff, R. K. (1985). *Social marketing: New imperative for public health.* New York: Praeger.

Manuel, C., Enel, P., Chanel, J., Reviron, D., Larher, M. P., Auquier, P., & San Marco, J. L. (1991). Ethics and AIDS: The protection of society versus the protection of individual rights. *AIDS and Public Policy Journal, 6,* 31–35.

Marantz, P. R. (1990). Blaming the victim: The negative consequence of preventive medicine. *American Journal of Public Health, 80,* 1186–1187.

Mariner, W. K. (1995). AIDS phobia, public health warnings, and lawsuits: Determining harm or rewarding ignorance? *American Journal of Public Health, 85,* 1562–1586).

McKinlay, J. B. (1975). A case for refocusing upstream: The political economy of illness. In A. J. Enelow & J. B. Henderson (Eds.), *Applying behavioral science to cardiovascular risk* (pp. 7–17). Washington, DC: American Heart Association.

McLeroy, K. R., Gottlieb, N. H., & Burdine, J. N. (1987). The business of health promotion: Ethical issues and professional responsibilities. *Health Education Quarterly, 14,* 91–109.

Milio, N. (1981). *Promoting health through public policy.* Philadelphia: F. A. Davis.

Mill, J. S. (1978). *On liberty.* Indianapolis, IN: Hackett Publishing.

Milne, B. J., Logan, A. G., & Lanagan, P. T. (1984). Alterations in health perception and life-style in treated hypertensives. *Journal of Chronic Disease, 38,* 37–45.

Moore, T. J. (1989). *Heartfailure: A critical inquiry into American medicine and the revolution in heart care.* New York: Simon & Schuster.

Nagel, S. S. (1983). Ethical dilemmas in policy evaluation. In W. N. Dunn (Ed.), *Values, ethics, and the practice of policy analysis* (pp. 65–85). Lexington, MA: Lexington Books.

National Cholesterol Education Program (1991). *Report of the expert panel on population strategies for blood cholesterol reduction* (NIH Publication No. 90–3046).

National Cholesterol Education Program (1992). *A communications strategy for public educa-*

tion for the National Cholesterol Education Program. Unpublished manuscript.

Nodding, N. (1984). *Caring: A feminine approach to ethics and moral education.* Berkeley: University of California Press.

Northouse, P. G., & Northouse, L. L. (1992). *Health communication: Strategies for health professionals* (2nd ed.). Norwalk, CT: Appleton & Lange.

Olien, C. N., Donohue, G. A., & Tichenor, P. J. (1983). Structure, communication and social power: Evolution of the knowledge gap hypothesis. In E. Wartella, D. C. Whitney, & S. Windahl (Eds.), *Mass Communication Review Yearbook,* Vol 4. Beverly Hills, CA: Sage.

Packer, C. & Kauffman, S. (1990). Reregulation of commercial television: Implications for coverage of AIDS. *AIDS and Public Policy, 5,* 82–87.

Parsons, T. (1958). Definitions of health and illness in the light of American values and social structure. In E. G. Jaco (Ed.), *Patients, physicians and illness.* Glencoe, IL: Free Press.

Pinet, G. (1987). Health legislation, prevention and ethics. In S. Doxiadis (Ed.), *Ethical dilemmas in health promotion* (pp. 83–97). New York: Wiley.

Pollay, R. W. (1989). Campaigns, change and culture: On the polluting potential of persuasion. In C. T. Salmon (Ed.), *Information campaigns: Balancing social values and social change* (pp. 185–196). Newbury Park, CA: Sage.

Priester, R. (1992a). *Taking values seriously: A values framework for the U.S. health care system.* Minneapolis: The Center for Biomedical Ethics, University of Minnesota.

Priester, R. (1992b). A values framework for health system reform. *Health Affairs, 11,* 84–107.

Rakow, L. F. (1989). Information and power: Toward a critical theory of information campaigns. In C. T. Salmon (Ed.), *Information campaigns: Balancing social values and social change* (pp. 164–184). Newbury Park, CA: Sage.

Ratzan, S. R. (1994). Editor's introduction: Communication—the key to a healthier tomorrow. *American Behavioral Scientist, 38*(2), 202–207.

Ratzan, S. R., Payne, G., & Massett, H. A. (1994). Effective health message design. *American Behavioral Scientist, 38*(2), 294–309.

Rogers, E., & Storey, J. D. (1987). Communication campaigns. In C. R. Berger & S. H. Chaffee (Eds.), *Handbook of communication science* (pp. 817–846). Beverly Hills, CA: Sage.

Rogers, E. M. (1994). The field of health communication today. *American Behavioral Scientist, 38,* 208–214.

Rokeach, M. (1979). Value theory and communication research: Review and commentary. In D. Nimmo (Ed,), *Communication yearbook 3,* (pp. 7–28). New Brunswick, NJ: Transaction.

Roman, P. M., & Blum, T. C. (1987). Ethics in worksite health programming: Who is served? *Health Education Quarterly, 14,* 57–70.

Rose, G. (1981). Strategy of prevention: Lessons from cardiovascular disease. *British Medical Journal, 282,* 1847–1851.

Rose, G. (1985). Sick individuals and sick populations. *International Journal of Epidemiology, 14,* 32–38.

Russell, L. B. (1986). *Is prevention better than cure?* Washington, DC: The Brookings Institution.

Russell, L. B. (1987). *Evaluating preventive care: Report on a workshop.* Washington, DC: The Brookings Institution.

Ryan, W. (1976). *Blaming the victim.* New York: Random House.

Salmon, C. T. (1989). Campaigns for social "improvement": An overview of values, rationales and impacts. In C. T. Salmon (Ed.), *Information campaigns: Balancing social values and social change* (pp. 19–53). Newbury Park, CA: Sage.

Salmon, C. T. (1992). Bridging theory "of" and theory "for" communication campaigns: An essay on ideology and public policy. In S. A. Deetz (Ed.), *Communication yearbook 15* (pp. 346–358). Newbury Park, CA: Sage.

Scherer, C. W., & Juanillo, N. K. (1992). Bridging theory and praxis: Reexamining public health communication. In S. A. Deetz (Ed.), *Communication yearbook 15* (pp. 312–345). Newbury Park, CA: Sage.

Scott, S. J., & Mercer, M. A. (1994). Understanding cultural obstacles to HIV/AIDS prevention in Africa. *AIDS Education and Prevention, 6,* 81–89.

Shoemaker, P. J. (1989). Introduction. In P. J. Shoemaker (Ed.), *Communication campaigns about drugs: Government, media and the public* (pp. 1–5). Hillsdale, NJ: Lawrence Erlbaum Associates, Inc.

Strasser, T., Jeanneret, O., & Raymond, L. (1987). Ethical aspects of prevention trials. In S. Doxiadis (Ed.), *Ethical dilemmas in health promotion* (pp. 183–193). New York: Wiley.

Tesh, S. N. (1988). *Hidden arguments: Political ideology and disease prevention policy.* New Brunswick, NJ: Rutgers University Press.

Thomas, S. B. (1990). Community health advocacy for racial and ethnic minorities in the United States: Issues and challenges for health education. *Health Education Quarterly, 17,* 13–19.

Thornton, B. C., & Kreps, G. L. (1993). *Perspec-*

tives on health communication. Prospect Heights, IL: Waverland Press.

Veatch, R. M. (1980). Voluntary risks to health: The ethical issues. *Journal of the American Medical Association, 243,* 50–55.

Waitzkin, H. (1989). A critical theory of medical discourse: Ideology, social control, and the processing of social context in medical encounters. *Journal of Health and Social Behavior, 30,* 220–239.

Waitzkin, H. (1991). *The politics of medical encounters; How patients and doctors deal with social problems.* New Haven, CT: Yale University Press.

Wallace-Brodeur. (1990). Community values in Vermont health planning. *Hastings Center Report, 20*(5), 18–19.

Wallack, L. M. (1989). Mass communication and health promotion: A critical perspective. In R. E. Rice & C. K. Atkin (Eds.), *Public communication campaigns* (2nd ed., pp. 353–367). Newbury Park, CA: Sage.

Wang, C. (1992). Culture, meaning and disability: Injury prevention campaigns and the production of stigma. *Social Science and Medicine, 55*(9), 1093–1102.

Warwick, D. P., & Kelman, H. C. (1973). Ethical issues in social intervention. In G. Zaltman, (Ed.), *Processes and phenomena of social change* (pp. 377–417). New York: Wiley.

Weisman, S. R. (1992, March 19). Japan keeps ban on birth control pill. *The New York Times,* p. A3.

White, M. S., & Maloney, S. K. (1990). Promoting healthy diets and active lives to hard-to-reach groups: Market research study. *Public Health Reports,* 105, 224–231.

Whitehead, M. (1992). The concepts and principles of equity and health. *International Journal of Health Services, 22,* 429–445.

Wikler, D. (1987). Who should be blamed for becoming sick? *Health Education Quarterly, 14,* 11–25.

Williams, D. (1990). Socioeconomic differences in health. *Social Psychology Quarterly, 55* (2), 81–99.

Williams, G. (1984). Health promotion—caring concern or slick salesmanship? *Journal of Medical Ethics, 10,* 191–195.

Winett, R. A., King, A., & Altman, D. G. (1989). *Health psychology and public health: An integrative approach.* New York: Pergamon.

Winkleby, M. A. (1994). The future of community-based cardiovascular disease intervention studies. *American Journal of Public Health, 84,* 1369–1372.

Witte, K. (1994). The manipulative nature of health communication research: Ethical issues and guidelines. *American Behavioral Scientist, 38,* 285–293.

Woods, D. R., Davis, D., & Wesover, B. J. (1991). "America responds to AIDS": Its content, development process, and outcome. *Public Health Reports, 106,* 616–662.

Zola, I. K. (1975). In the name of health and illness: On some socio-political consequences of medical influence. *Social Science and Medicine, 9,* 83–87.

Zook, E. G. (1994). Embodied health and constitutive communication: Toward an authentic conceptualization of health communication. In S. A. Deetz (Ed.), *Communication yearbook 17* (pp. 344–377). Newbury Park, CA: Sage.

Discussion Questions

1. Identify a current health campaign in your community. In your opinion, is this campaign ethical? Why or why not?
2. Suppose that you have been hired to work on a "stop smoking" health campaign. Your new boss wants you to find an underage child to pose for an advertisement to illustrate that children do have access to cigarettes. Why would this be unethical? How would you tell your boss how you feel?
3. Which of the 13 ethical dilemmas are the most important to consider? Why? ✦

Part VII

MEDIA LITERACY AND HEALTH ISSUES

Chapter 24
Television Viewers' Ideal Body Proportions

The Case of the Curvaceously Thin Woman

Kristen Harrison

Part VII is the final section of this anthology. The chapters address issues about the role of media literacy and health. As the technologies of the twenty-first century permit access to health information that was once impossible, increased responsibility is placed on the Internet and the mass media to create an understanding of its impact on health information. Organizational communication has long carried the maxim that information is power. Information retrieved through the media requires that the user of that information be literate in the ways in which the medium selects and shapes the information. Many of the mass media require knowledge of the roles of the various gatekeepers and how the information that finds its way to the media is shaped by them. But the Internet is a medium that requires yet another kind of literacy. The Internet user needs to always be cognizant of the fact that the value of information to which it allows access is always determined by the source of the information. No medium before the Internet has been so thoroughly capable of separating the source from the information. Literacy with any medium, Internet or other, requires awareness of the ways in which that particular medium is the channel, and often shaper, of the information it can provide.

The first chapter in Part VII examines how exposure to mediated images of men and women has an influence on how people perceive the size and weight of their own bodies. Kristen Harrison illustrates ideal-body media and the relationship to risky health practices like plastic surgery or extreme dieting. Specifically, she argues that viewing television images of thin-ideal bodies shapes how both men and women evaluate female figures.

Related Topics: body image, culture, ethical issues, media, quantitative methods

~~34~~ 36–24–36

WonderBra advertisement

The ideal American woman is not only thin, she is thin with specific bust, waist, and hip proportions that, if we are to believe the makers of the WonderBra, need correction if they stray from their ideal dimensions by as little as 2 in. It is outside the scope of this paper to explore the origin of the 36–24–36-in. ideal female body, but it bears mentioning that this particular configuration is not as balanced as it may appear because it represents a woman who, by garment industry standards, simultaneously wears a size 4 (hips), a size 2 (waist), and a size 10 (bust). She represents a sexual ideal, a fantasy, a nonrealistic woman who is nonetheless used by real women as a point of comparison in their efforts to "improve" their bodies. Given the discrepancy between the upper and lower halves of this ideal, women's efforts to mold their bodies to these proportions must include not only dieting to whittle down the lower bodily stratum, but creative methods of simultaneously maintaining an average-sized upper stratum. At the same time that the prevalence of eating disorders is at an all-time high (Gleaves, Miller, Williams, & Summers, 2000), more and more women are turning to breast-reduction surgery, breast augmentation surgery, and lipoplasty (also known as liposuction) to reconfigure their bodies.

Studies of young adults' perceptions of the ideal female figure suggest that a slim body with comparatively large breasts indeed sets the standard. Jourard and Secord

From "Television Viewers' Ideal Body Proportions: The Case of the Curvaceously Thin Woman," Kristen Harrison, 2003, *Sex Roles*, Vol. 28:5-6, pp. 255–264.

(1955) reported that a sample of women rated their ideal waist and hips as significantly smaller than their actual waist and hips; in contrast, they rated their ideal bust as larger. There is a cap to the "largeness" of the ideal bust, however. Koff and Benavage (1998) found that among European American and Asian American women, both large and small bustedness were associated with lower breast size satisfaction than was medium bustedness.

Mass Media and the Thin Ideal

Where do young people learn about the skinny-yet-medium-busted ideal? Most are likely to have learned about this body ideal through the mass media.

Television programs such as *Baywatch* and Comedy Central's *The Man Show* are just two of the many outlets that broadcast or illustrate body ideals. A number of important studies (e.g., Harrison & Cantor, 1997; Stice, Schupak-Neuberg, Shaw, & Stein, 1994) have shown that exposure to ideal-body media is linked to the drive for thinness among women and the preference, among men, for thinness in women.

Content analyses of television and magazines show that thinness has become the norm, and the most desirable or successful female characters and media personalities are typically thin. Silverstein, Perdue, Peterson, and Kelly (1986) reported that the body shape standard on television is slimmer for women than for men. In their study, two independent coders rated 69% of female characters, but only 17% of male characters, as conspicuously thin. Thinness is portrayed as the female ideal not only through depictions of thinness as attractive and virtuous but also through depictions of fatness as disgusting and worthy of ridicule. Fouts and Burggraf (1999, 2000) analyzed television situation comedies and found that thinner female characters received more positive comments from male characters than did heavier female characters, whereas heavier female characters received more *negative* comments from male characters than did thinner characters.

Further, results of both surveys and experiments show that exposure to media images of the female body ideal is linked among female audience members to the desire to be slimmer. Harrison and Cantor (1997) measured thin-ideal television and magazine exposure and thinness-favoring attitudes and behaviors. They reported that exposure to thin-ideal media images predicted college women's tendency to idealize thinness. This relationship remained even when selective exposure to thin-ideal media (based on interest in fitness and dieting as media topics) was controlled. Moreover, McCreary and Sadava (1999) reported a positive correlation between television viewing and young women's and men's belief that they were overweight, regardless of their actual weight.

Cause-and-effect relationships are best demonstrated within experimental research, and there is plenty of experimental research on the effects of thin-ideal media images on young women's physical self-perceptions. Irving (1990) reported that undergraduate women exposed to slides of thin models reported poorer subsequent physical self-evaluations. Stice and Shaw (1994) found that exposure to photos of thin models increased negative mood and body dissatisfaction among female undergraduates. These findings have been replicated for a number of dependent measures, including increased preoccupation with thinness (Turner, Hamilton, Jacobs, Angood, & Dwyer, 1997) and poorer body image (Cattarin, Thompson, Thomas, & Williams, 2000). Women are not the only ones who respond this way to images of female attractiveness. Kenrick and Gutierres (1980) found that exposure to attractive actresses (relative to controls) led men to rate an average-looking woman as less attractive, which supports the hypothesis that exposure to highly idealized images produces a contrast effect that works against the average woman.

Finally, the way young women perceive their bodies to begin with can moderate the effects of thin-ideal media on their physical self-evaluations. Henderson-King and Henderson-King (1997) found that participant weight functioned as a moderator of the effects of exposure to slides that depict ideal-body advertising images. Relative to participants in a control condition composed of advertisements with nonhuman images, female undergraduates in the ideal-body condition reported more negative physical self-evaluations if they were heavier, whereas those ideal-body condition participants who were thinner actually felt better about themselves after exposure. This finding speaks to the need to factor body mass and perceived body size into analyses of the relationship between ideal-body media exposure and body cognitions.

Importance of Studying the Curvaceously Thin Ideal

A focus on the ideal female body as merely thin paints an incomplete picture, however. The size 10–2–4 standard of female beauty suggests that the female body ideal is in fact "curvaceously thin," in that her lower half is proportionately thin compared to her upper half. Although she possesses an extremely small waist and narrow hips, she possesses an average bustline. To complement the studies of thinness in the mass media, a unique series of studies has focused on specific icons of American female beauty whose body measurements were public and therefore available for analysis. These are *Playboy* magazine centerfold models and Miss America pageant contestants. In the first of these studies, Garner, Garfinkel, Schwartz, and Thompson (1980) reported a significant decrease in the body measurements and weights of centerfold models and pageant contestants between 1959 and 1978. Wiseman, Gray, Mosimann, and Ahrens (1992) updated this study by documenting a continued decline in centerfold models' and pageant contestants' weights between 1979 and 1988. More recently, Spitzer, Henderson, and Zivian (1999) analyzed the body mass indices (BMIs or weight-to-height ratios) of centerfold models and pageant contestants, and found that the body sizes of pageant winners continued to decrease through the 1990s, whereas centerfold models remained below average in weight.

The only researchers to report actual bust, waist, and hip measurements (rather than BMIs or ratios) were Garner et al. (1980). They reported average bust, waist, and hip measurements for *Playboy* centerfold models of 90.8, 58.6, and 89.3 cm, respectively, very close to the 36-24-36-in. ideal. This ideal represents a woman with bust-to-waist and hip-to-waist ratios of 1.5; and three other studies have documented media ideals that are close to this ratio. Silverstein, Perdue, Peterson, and Kelly (1986) reported bust-to-waist ratios that varied over time, but centered around 1.5. Moreover, Silverstein, Perdue, Peterson, Vogel, and Fantini (1986) showed that the bust-to-waist ratio of models depicted in popular women's magazines changed over time from as little as 1.1 to over 2.0, but they also centered around 1.5. More recently, Barber (1998) reported similar variation in the bust-to-waist ratios of Miss America pageant winners, *Vogue* models, and *Playboy* centerfold models, but again, these ratios centered around 1.5. Thus, the curvaceously thin female figure, which consists of a small waist and hips coupled with a medium bust, appears to have dominated portrayals of the ideal female, both historically and recently.

What is curious about this ideal figure is its unusual fat distribution. Breasts are composed mainly of fat, not glandular tissue (Sherwood, 1993). Because breast fat is positively correlated with total body fat (Katch et al., 1980), it is impossible to lose body fat without reducing breast size. Thus, women who wish to meet the skinny-yet-busty body ideal generally cannot do so through diet and exercise alone. The demands of meeting this ideal put women at risk for doing "double damage" to their bodies, through extreme dieting or disordered eating to reduce the lower half and surgery or the use of potentially dangerous drugs or herbal treatments to maintain or increase the upper half. It is therefore important to understand not only what drives women and men to embrace this ideal, but also what body-alteration methods they would approve of in the name of obtaining it.

The Cultivation Approach

Although the curvaceously thin female body ideal seems to be widely embraced, it has not yet been empirically linked with media exposure. That was the purpose of this study. According to cultivation theory (Gerbner, Gross, Morgan, & Signorielli, 1994), television exposure "cultivates" beliefs, attitudes, and ideals about the real world that match the media-depicted world. According to this theory, the real-world perceptions of heavier media users should correspond more closely with the media-depicted world than should the perceptions of lighter media users. Predictions that can be derived from cultivation theory are typically straightforward: Media exposure will be positively correlated with perceptions of the world and its components, such that these perceptions match the way the world is portrayed in the media. Because content analyses have shown that extreme thinness, coupled with average-bustedness, is the norm on television, it was predicted that:

H1. Exposure to ideal-body television images will be positively associated with women's and men's idealization of a slimmer female waist and hips, but not a smaller bust.

Regarding ideal bust size, a specific pattern of findings was predicted for female participants, based on the cultivation theory construct of "mainstreaming." Mainstreaming is described by cultivation theorists as the typical pattern of worldview change that cultivation, as a process, takes (Gerbner et al., 1994). Mainstreaming occurs when groups who are initially divergent in their worldviews come to hold similar views with greater television exposure. Their views converge to reflect the "reality" that is most commonly represented on television. If this media worldview is somewhere in the middle of a range of possibilities, extremists on either side should, according to theory, become less extreme and more moderate in their views with increased television exposure.

The television "worldview" of the ideal female waist and hips could be described as relatively extreme: thinner is better. In contrast, the television worldview of the ideal female bust is more moderate: medium is ideal. Thus, following the mainstreaming rationale, it was predicted that women starting from divergent personal realities regarding bust size would, with increased exposure to ideal-body television, converge upon a medium bust as their ideal.

H2. For larger-busted women, exposure to ideal-body television images should predict a smaller ideal bust size, whereas for smaller-busted women, exposure to ideal-body television images should predict a larger ideal bust size.

Because extremely thin waists and hips coupled with medium-sized breasts are the television norm, and because extreme measures are frequently required to attain this rather unnatural body shape, it was also predicted that exposure to ideal-body television images would be related to the approval of nondieting methods for changing the body. In particular, exposure to ideal-body television images was expected to predict approval of surgical methods of changing the breasts, waist, and hips, such as breast surgery (augmentation or reduction) and liposuction.

H3. Exposure to ideal-body television images should be positively associated with women's approval of using, and men's approval of women's use of, surgical body-alteration methods such as breast surgery and liposuction.

Finally, following the mainstreaming rationale, it was predicted that the bust-specific body-alteration methods women approved of would be a function of their own perceived bust size, so that ideal-body television exposure would be related to approval of different methods depending upon whether women perceived themselves to larger- or smaller-busted.

H4. For larger-busted women, exposure to ideal-body television images should predict approval of breast reduction surgery, whereas for smaller-busted women, exposure to ideal-body television images should predict approval of breast augmentation surgery.

Method

Participants

Undergraduates enrolled in introductory communication and psychology courses at a large Midwestern university were recruited with the offer of course credit in exchange for participation. The total sample consisted of 149 women (mean age 19.56) and 82 men (mean age 20.04). Most of the participants were White (68.5% of women and 73.2% of men), and their mean BMIs fell within the normal range, at 22.17 for women and 23.89 for men.

Measures

Whole-Figure Drawings. A set of nine adult female figure drawings was presented to each participant. The drawings were photocopies of those validated by Stunkard, Sorensen, and Schulsinger (1983), and they ranged from extremely thin to obese. Women were asked which of the nine figures looked most like their own figure, and which looked like the figure they would "most like to have" (i.e., their ideal figure). Men were asked which of the nine figures looked like the female figure they found most attractive (i.e., their ideal female figure).

The BodyBook. The whole-figure drawings by Stunkard et al. (1983) range from extremely thin (with small breasts) to obese (with large breasts), and offer no way to separate bust size from waist and hip sizes. To solve this problem, the BodyBook was constructed. The BodyBook is a spiral-bound, 9.5-by-11-in., hard-laminated, three-part flipbook that allows participants to choose separate bust, waist, and hip sizes. The top third of the book depicts stylized line drawings of nine different bust sizes, framed within a pair of shoulders that remain the same size in all drawings (100 mm wide). Below the breasts are two vertical lines that represent a ribcage that is 72 mm wide at its narrowest point, just above the waist panel. The only part of the bust drawings that varied was the size of the breasts. These drawings were arranged in random order within the book so that the first image was not necessarily the smallest or largest. There were two random orders for both the bust and hip drawings; subsequent analyses showed that there were no effects of order. The bottom third of the book depicted stylized line drawings of nine different hip widths. Hip width variation was a function of how widely the hip curves spread out from their starting points, just below the waist panel. The intervals between successive bust and hip drawings increased slightly with each size increase, in order to facilitate visual discrimination between the images.[1]

The middle section of the books consisted of blank panels for participants to draw in waists to connect their chosen bust and hip drawings. Participants used a wet-erase marker for this task; when they were finished, they handed their completed book to a research assistant, who measured the width of the drawn-in waists (in millimeters), recorded this measurement, and cleaned the ink off the books for reuse. Concave waist drawings were measured at their narrowest point, and convex drawings were measured at their widest point.

Women were first asked to indicate which figure looked most like their own by choosing the appropriate bust and hip drawings, and then drawing in the waist that connected these images in a way that reflected their own perceived body contours. They were then asked to repeat this procedure for their ideal bust, waist, and hips. Test-retest reliabilities for women's *own* bust, waist, and hip sizes were .95, .65, and .79.[2] For women's ideal bust, waist, and hip sizes, these coefficients were .74, .85, and .75, respectively. Men were asked to indicate which of the nine bust and hip drawings looked like the female figure they found most attractive, and then to draw in the waist that completed that figure. Test-retest reliability coefficients for men's ideal bust, waist, and hip sizes were .74, .95, and .75, respectively.

Approval of Body-Alteration Methods. Women were presented with the following item: "If cost were not an issue, how likely would you be to do each of the following to improve your appearance?" Response options ranged from 0 (*highly unlikely*) to 5 (*I have already done this*). There were 12 methods listed, including leg-length surgery, rib removal, liposuction, breast reduction surgery, breast augmentation surgery (implants), diet, exercise, and wearing a shaper/girdle, wearing control-top pantyhose, wearing a padded bra, wearing a minimizing bra, and wearing height-altering shoes. Men were presented with the same 12 methods, preceded by the following question: "To what extent do you approve or disapprove of the following measures women can take to improve their appearance?" Response options ranged from 0 (*strongly disapprove*) to 5 (*I have urged a woman in my life to do this*).

Exposure to Ideal-Body Television Images.

The procedure described by Harrison (2000) was followed for measuring and calculating exposure to ideal-body television images. This procedure has three steps: First, participants report their habitual exposure to popular television shows. Second, a separate, impartial sample of coders (not research participants) rates each program according to how thin they perceive its female main characters to be. Third, the mean ratings supplied by the coders are multiplied by participants' frequency-of-viewing scores for each show, and the crossproducts for all of the shows are added for each participant, which creates a single variable that reflects both frequency of viewing and extremity of thinness in the programs viewed.

Frequency of viewing (0 = *never* to 4 = *regularly*) was measured for 36 Nielsen top-rated programs for the winter/spring season of 2000. These programs were chosen because they were popular among young adults and because they contained a diverse sampling of the body types featured among characters in popular television entertainment. Following Harrison's three-step procedure (Harrison, 2000), 64 college undergraduates (61% women) in a research course were recruited to code the body sizes of the female main characters in each of the 36 programs. Ratings were made on a 7-point scale that ranged from 1 (*conspicuously fat*) to 7 (*conspicuously thin*); the midpoint was designated "average." Coders were told to consider a character's body size "conspicuous" if characters on the show periodically made reference to it as part of the character's identity, or if the character's body size was regularly adorned in such a way as to draw viewer attention to its size. There were no differences in the ratings by sex of coder, so mean ratings were calculated for the entire coder sample.[3]

Along with exposure, interest in television topics related to the attainment of an ideal body shape was measured following the rationale of Harrison and Cantor (1997), who argued that significant correlations between exposure to ideal-body images in the media and the tendency to favor a thin body type might simply reflect the fact that people who already embrace the thin ideal seek out media that reflect this ideal. By measuring and controlling interest in these media topics, then, one is able to discount this alternative explanation for the findings. Participants were asked how interested they would be in a hypothetical new television show if it covered each of nine separate topics. Among the topics listed were dieting, nutrition, fitness, and exercise, all of which are related to the attainment of an ideal body shape. Scores for these four topics were summed to create one measure of interest (a = .86 for women, a = .85 for men).

Procedure

Participants were asked to come at their convenience to a large campus laboratory, where they were tested in groups of 5–10. A research assistant gave each participant a complete testing packet, and allowed him or her to complete it undisturbed. Half of the participants received the figure drawings measure first, followed by the BodyBook measures; the other half received the BodyBook measures first. There were no effects of order. On average, participants required about 30 min to complete the questionnaire. A week later, participants were asked to return to complete only the BodyBook measure, so that test-retest reliability estimates could be obtained. All except four participants (two women and two men) returned.

Results

Figure Ideals

Women's and men's figure ratings are displayed in Table 24.1. Women desired a significantly smaller figure than their own, yet if thinness were the only body dimension that mattered, one should observe a desire to be smaller all over. The BodyBook measures showed that this was not the case. Women desired a waist and hips significantly smaller than their own, but at the same time wanted a significantly *larger* bust. When asked which of the nine whole-figure drawings they found most attractive, men chose a larger ideal than did women. However, examination of the Body-Book measures showed that men's idealization of a larger female body was rooted in their choice of a larger waist and bust; men's and women's ideal hip size ratings did not differ.

Table 24.1
Mean Whole-Figure, Bust, Waist, and Hip Size Ratings

Variable	Ratings [M(SD)]		
	Women's Own	*Women's Ideal*	*Men's Ideal*
Whole figure	3.78_b (1.08)	2.76_a (0.75)	3.32_b (0.65)
BodyBook bust	3.63_a (1.83)	4.95_b (1.39)	5.72_c (1.12)
BodyBook waist	69.39_b (7.75)	65.57_a (6.87)	69.40_b (5.61)
BodyBook hips	3.91_b (1.58)	2.82_a (1.31)	2.98_a (1.14)

Note: Whole-figure, bust, and hip size ratings ranged from 1 to 9. Waist size ratings were measured in millimeters. Within rows, means with different subscripts differ at $p < .05$ by the Tukey procedure.

Television Viewing and Ideal Body Proportions

To test the hypothesis that thin-ideal television exposure would be linked to the desire for a smaller waist and hips, multiple regression analyses were conducted with BMI and interest in television topics related to the attainment of an ideal body shape entered on the first step and exposure to ideal-body television images entered on the second step. To provide a benchmark for comparison, the first criterion variable was the ideal whole-figure rating. As expected, exposure to ideal-body television images predicted women's desire for a smaller figure, $\beta = -.20$, $\Delta R^2 = .04$, $p < .01$. What the whole-figure measure fails to reveal, however, is exactly which bodily proportions women wanted reduced. This question was answered with the BodyBook measures as criteria. With ideal hips, waist, and bust as separate criterion variables, regression analyses revealed that exposure to ideal-body television images significantly predicted women's desire for a smaller waist, $\beta = -.17$, $\Delta R^2 = .03$, $p < .05$, and hips, $\beta = -.17$, $\Delta R^2 = .03$, $p < .01$, but not a smaller bust, $\beta = -.06$, $\Delta R^2 = .01$, *ns*. To test the same hypothesis for men, identical multiple regression analyses were conducted without controlling for BMI.[4] Although the coefficients were in the predicted direction for overall figure size ($\beta = -.13$), hip size ($\beta = -.11$), waist size ($\beta = -.05$), and bust size ($\beta = .08$), none of these results were significant. The first hypothesis was therefore supported for women but not for men. The fact that exposure to ideal-body television images predicted a smaller whole-body rating for women may be due to the fact that the whole-figure scale forces women who want to choose a thinner figure to choose one that has a smaller bust as well.

The purpose of this study was not to single out specific television shows, but it is interesting that, in spite of the fact that exposure to ideal-body television images in general was unrelated to men's ideal figure ratings, viewing certain programs *was* related to men's ideals. For instance, viewing of the program *Felicity,* whose main character is small-busted, was correlated with the idealization of a smaller bust, $r = -.28$, $p < .01$. In contrast, viewing of *Baywatch,* known for its large-busted lifeguards, was associated with the idealization of a larger bust, $r = .29$, $p < .01$. The idealization of a smaller figure overall was linked with viewing of both *Ally McBeal,* $r = -.36$, $p, < .001$, and *Beverly Hills 90210,* $r = -.35$, $p < .001$, both of which have been criticized for portraying women who are extremely thin.

Differences Based on Own Perceived Bust Size. Depending on whether their own bust was larger or smaller to begin with, women's exposure to ideal-body television images was expected to be linked to their idealization of either a smaller or larger bust. The lack of significant findings in the above regression analyses for women's ideal bust size could be due to different processes occurring among smaller- and larger-busted women, processes that cancel each other out when the sample is combined as a whole. To test for this interaction between own perceived bust size and exposure to ideal-body television images, an ANOVA was performed with ideal bust size as the

Figure 24.1
Ideal-Body TV Viewing

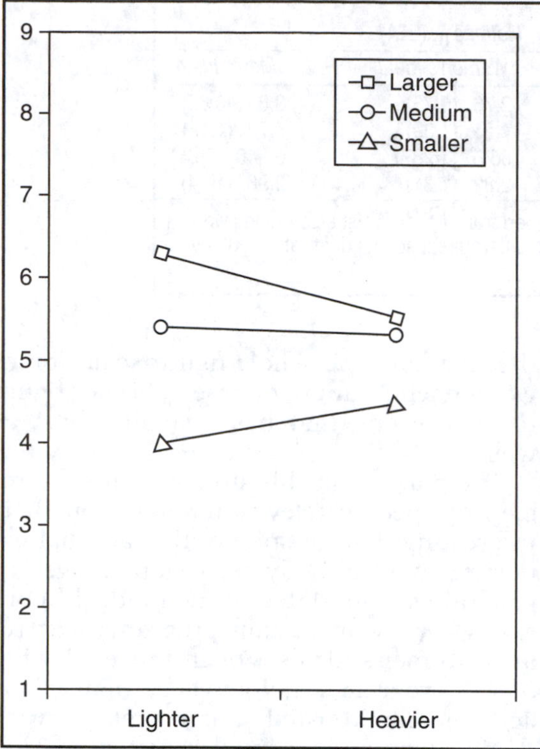

Note. Mainstreaming of Ideal Bust Size by Exposure to Ideal-Body Television Images, for Women of Smaller, Medium, and Larger Bust Sizes. Among the lighter TV viewers, ideal-bust scores M = 6.29, SD = 0.99, for larger-busted women; M = 5.41, SD = 0.83, for medium-busted women; and M = 4.00, SD = 1.30, for smaller-busted women. Among the heavier TV viewers, ideal-bust scores were M = 5.53, SD = 1.46, for larger-busted women; M = 5.53, SD = 1.09, for medium-busted women; and M = 4.50, SD = 1.23, for smaller-busted women.

dependent measure and exposure to ideal-body television images (split at the median into lighter and heavier viewing categories) and own perceived bust size (split by thirds into lowest, middle, and highest size categories) as factors. The main effects were not significant but, in support of hypothesis two, the predicted interaction was significant, $F(2,142) = 3.29$, $p < .05$, $n^2 = .05$. A clear mainstreaming pattern can be seen in Fig. 24.1. This pattern reflects the converging of divergent groups upon a similar belief, attitude, or ideal with greater television use. The ideal here is medium-bustedness. The more ideal-body television women viewed, the more both larger- and smaller-busted participants desired a medium bust. Medium-busted women, in contrast, maintained the medium-busted ideal regardless of amount of television viewing.

Approval of Body-Alteration Methods

It was predicted that exposure to ideal-body television images, with their emphasis on female bust, waist, and hip proportions (to the exclusion of other aspects of body build), would be positively correlated with acceptance of surgical methods for altering the bust, waist, and hips. To test this for women, semi-partial correlations were computed between exposure to ideal-body television images and the body-alteration methods; BMI and interest in television topics related to the attainment of an ideal body shape were controlled. Exposure to ideal-body television images was positively related to women's approval of breast surgery, $sr = .28$, $p < .001$, liposuction, $sr = .31$, $p < .001$, and wearing a special bra to change the appearance of bust size, $sr = .20$, $p < .05$, but was not significantly correlated with women's approval of leg-length surgery, $sr = .12$, rib removal, $sr = .09$, diet, $sr = .08$, exercise, $sr = .07$, or wearing a shaper/girdle, $sr = .14$, control-top pantyhose, $sr = .13$, or height-altering shoes, $sr = .07$. For men, semipartial correlations between exposure to ideal-body television images and approval of body-alteration methods were tabulated, and interest in television topics related to the attainment of an ideal body shape was controlled. Exposure to ideal-body television images significantly predicted men's approval of breast augmentation, $sr = .21$, $p < .05$, and liposuction, $sr = .23$, $p < .05$, but did not predict approval of breast reduction, $sr = -.12$, leg-length surgery, $sr = .14$, rib removal, $sr = -.07$, diet, $sr = .00$, exercise, $sr = .13$, or wearing a padded bra, $sr = .04$, minimizing bra, $sr = .00$, shaper/girdle, $sr = .10$, control-top pantyhose, $sr = .07$, or height-altering shoes, $sr = .09$. The third hypothesis was therefore supported for both women and men.

Differences by Own Perceived Bust Size. When the sample of women was split at the median of their own perceived bust size into small-to-medium-busted and medium-to-large-busted groups, different correlations emerged for breast surgery and wearing a special bra. For the small- to medium-busted group, television viewing was significantly correlated with approval of breast augmentation, $sr = .22$, $p < .05$, and wearing a padded bra, $sr = .19$, $p < .05$, but not correlated with approval of breast reduction, $sr = .04$, or wearing a minimizing bra, $sr = .03$. In contrast, for the medium-to-large-busted group, television viewing was significantly correlated with approval of breast reduction surgery, $sr = .27$, $p < .05$, and wearing a minimizing bra, $sr = 26$, $p < .05$, but not correlated with approval of breast augmentation, $sr = .07$, or wearing a padded bra, $sr = -.03$. These findings provide sound support for the fourth hypothesis. Exposure to ideal-body television images predicted acceptance of both surgical and cosmetic methods to change the bust size. This change was in the direction of an increase for women who perceived themselves to be smaller-busted and a decrease for women who perceived themselves to be larger-busted.

Discussion

In summary, exposure to ideal-body television images predicted women's idealization of a smaller waist, smaller hips, and a medium-sized bust, but it did not significantly predict men's perceptions of the ideal female figure. However, exposure to ideal-body television images predicted *both* men's and women's approval of surgical body-alteration methods such as breast surgery and liposuction. For larger-busted women, exposure to ideal-body television images predicted approval of breast-reduction methods, whereas for smaller-busted women, the same variable predicted approval of breast-augmentation methods.

The cultivation theory of media effects, including the pattern of mainstreaming, was supported by the findings of this study, but more so for women than for men. One of the assumptions of cultivation theory is that the mass media, and television in particular, present similar systems of stories, so that cultivation researchers usually downplay genre differences (Gerbner et al., 1994). However, the lack of findings for men suggests that there may be other genres that are more important in influencing men's perceptions of the ideal female body proportions. Table 24.1 shows that men, like women, preferred a thin lower body paired with a full bust, but unlike women, men's ideals were unrelated to their general exposure to ideal-body television images. It may be that media images do not play a major role in shaping young men's perceptions of the ideal female figure. It may also be that less mainstream media genres, such as soft-core erotica or pornography, contribute more to men's notions of the ideal female body than do the popular prime-time television programs measured here. Indeed, there is reason to suspect that this is the case. Harrison and Cantor (1997) found that men's exposure to "men's entertainment" magazines (e.g., *Playboy*) predicted their anticipated disappointment in meeting a blind date who turned out to be overweight, $r = .16$, $p < .01$. It is also possible that individual portrayals may be particularly important for men. Viewing of specific programs such as *Baywatch* and *Felicity* was related to men's female-body preferences, whereas the more comprehensive television exposure measure was not. Thus, perhaps there is a sort of "drench" effect (Greenberg, 1988) for men, such that individual portrayals make a disproportionately strong impact on their ideals. Certain female characters or media personalities may function as modern "pin-up girls" and set or change men's standards for the ideal female proportions. It is important, though, that exposure to mainstream television did predict men's acceptance of breast augmentation and liposuction for women. This is problematic because men's approval of these methods may encourage the women in their lives to use them.

The findings in the present study support those of other studies that show that ideal-body media exposure is linked to women's idealization of thinness, but here this idealization is limited to waist and hip size. Overall thinness is not necessarily desired; the ideal waist and hips are small, but the ideal bust is medium-sized. Further, the fact that exposure to ideal-body television images predicted approval of surgical body-alteration methods suggests that eating disorders are not the only potential adverse outcome of exposure to thin-ideal media images. Feeling pressured to change their bodies surgically could put young women at risk for doing "double damage" to themselves, by pairing extreme dieting and disordered eating with potentially risky medical procedures.

Also noteworthy is the fact that the only body-alteration methods predicted by exposure to ideal-body television images were those that directly change the body's proportions. Methods that change overall size (e.g., dieting) or height (e.g., shoes) were unrelated to media exposure. One might argue, then, that rib-removal surgery should also have been related to media exposure. The lack of a relationship here is likely due to a floor effect, because only a few participants reported any degree of approval for rib-removal surgery. Perhaps rib-removal surgery is an idea whose time has yet to come; it will be interesting to see if any future media trends in small-waistedness are accompanied by an increase in public interest in rib-removal surgery. In the meantime, liposuction will probably continue to function as the preferred surgical waist-whittler.

Limitations and Future Directions

This cross-sectional study was meant to uncover relationships between variables rather than to demonstrate cause and effect relationships. Implicit in my theoretical arguments is the assumption that media images of the ideal female body influence viewers' own body ideals, rather than the reverse: body ideals influence media viewing. However, the latter causal chain is not only possible but probable, which is why interest in television topics related to the attainment of an ideal body shape was measured and controlled. The findings therefore demonstrate that even for people who claim to have no interest in such television topics, exposure to ideal-body television images was still linked to thinness-favoring attitudes and approval of surgical body-alteration methods. Still, there is no substitute for experimental research as a follow-up strategy. Researchers interested in extending these findings would contribute much to our understanding by conducting experiments on the impact of ideal-body media images on perceptions of the ideal female bust, waist, and hip sizes. Moreover, the definition of ideal-body media images should be investigated further in light of the gender differences reported here. Perhaps standard commercial media have an effect on women, whereas men respond mainly to female body portrayals in "male-oriented" entertainment fare such as Comedy Central's *The Man Show*.

In summary, this study replicates others by showing that exposure to ideal-body television images is linked to the idealization of female thinness. Internalization of the thin ideal has been linked to disordered eating (Harrison & Cantor, 1997; Stice et al., 1994), which wreaks tremendous havoc on women's health. But the present study furthers our knowledge by suggesting that there is another potential adverse outcome of exposure to ideal-body media images: approval of risky surgical procedures to obtain the "curvaceously thin" female body ideal. Exposure to ideal-body media images may thus contribute to women's tendency to do "double damage" to their bodies through both extreme dieting *and* surgery.

Notes

1. A sample page from the BodyBook is available from the author.
2. The lower test-retest reliability coefficient for perceived own waist size might be explained by week-to-week fluctuations in abdominal girth that results from changes in eating patterns, the menstrual cycle, or other factors.
3. Starting with the "thinnest," the programs and their corresponding ratings were *Ally McBeal, M* = 6.84; *Melrose Place, M* = 6.77; *Baywatch, M* = 6.62; *Popular, M* = 6.60; *Friends, M* = 6.48; *Beverly Hills 90210, M*= 6.28; *Charmed, M* = 6.13; *Moesha, M* = 6.12; *Felicity, M* = 5.98; *Buffy the Vampire Slayer, M* = 5.88; *Just Shoot Me, M* = 5.78; *Suddenly Susan, M* = 5.76; *Dharma and Greg, M* = 5.60; *Jesse, M* = 5.45; *Once and Again, M* = 5.39; *Sabrina the Teenage Witch, M*=5.31; *Third Rock from the Sun, M* = 5.21; *Dawson's Creek, M* = 5.20; *Two Guys and a Girl, M* = 5.11; *Frasier, M* = 4.98; *Veronica's Closet, M*=4.98; *Will and Grace, M* = 4.94; *The Practice, M* = 4.92; *Stark Raving Mad, M* = 4.79; *Get Real, M* = 4.72; *Law and Order, M* = 4.67;

ER, M = 4.25; *Third Watch, M* = 4.09; *Judging Amy, M* = 3.76; *X Files, M* = 3.67; *Chicago Hope, M* = 3.41; *Everybody Loves Raymond, M* = 3.38; *JAG, M*=3.20; *King of Queens, M* = 3.09; *Touched by an Angel, M* = 2.44; and *Drew Carey, M* = 1.79.

4. BMI was not controlled in analyses involving men because there was no reason to expect men's own BMI to act as a confound between their media exposure and their ideal proportions for women.

References

Barber, N. (1998). Secular changes in standards of bodily attractiveness in American women: Different masculine and feminine ideals. *Journal of Psychology, 132,* 87–94.

Cattarin, J. A., Thompson, J. K., Thomas, C. & Williams, R. (2000). Body image, mood, and televised images of attractiveness: The role of social comparison. *Journal of Social and Clinical Psychology, 19,* 220–239.

Fouts, G., & Burggraf, K. (1999). Television situation comedies: Female body images and verbal reinforcements. *Sex Roles, 40,* 473–481.

Fouts, G., & Burggraf, K. (2000). Television situation comedies: Female weight, male negative comments, and audience reactions. *Sex Roles, 42,* 925–932.

Garner, D. M., Garfinkel, P. E., Schwartz, D., & Thompson, M. (1980). Cultural expectations of thinness in women. *Psychological Reports, 47,* 483–491.

Gerbner, G, Gross, L., Morgan, M., & Signorielli, N. (1994). Growing up with television: The cultivation perspective. In J. Bryant & D. Zillmann (Eds.), *Media effects: Advances in theory and research* (pp. 17–41). Hillsdale, NJ: Erlbaum.

Gleaves, D. H., Miller, K. J. Williams, T J., & Summers, S. A. (2000). Eating disorders: An overview. In K. J. Miller & J. S. Mizes (Eds.), *Comparative treatments for eating disorders* (pp. 1–49). New York: Springer.

Greenberg, B. (1988). Some uncommon television images and the drench hypothesis. *Applied Social Psychology Annual, 8,* 88–102.

Harrison, K. (2000). The body electric: Thin-ideal media and eating disorders in adolescents. *Journal of Communication, 50,* 119–143.

Harrison, K., & Cantor, J. (1997). The relationship between media consumption and eating disorders. *Journal of Communication, 47,* 40–67.

Henderson-King, E., & Henderson-King, D. (1997). Media effects on women's body esteem: Social and individual difference factors. *Journal of Applied Social Psychology, 27,* 399–417.

Irving, L. M. (1990). Mirror images: Effects of the standard of beauty on the self- and body-esteem of women exhibiting varying levels of bulimic symptoms. *Journal of Social and Clinical Psychology, 9,* 230–242.

Jourard, S. M., & Secord, P. F. (1955). Body-cathexis and personality. *British Journal of Psychology, 46,* 130–138.

Katch, V. L., Campaigne, B., Freedson, P., Sayd, S., Katch, F. L., & Behnke, A. R. (1980). Contribution of breast volume and weight to body fat distribution in females. *American Journal of Physical Anthropology, 53,* 93–100.

Kenrick, D. T. & Gutierres, S. E. (1980). Contrast effects and judgments of physical attractiveness: When beauty becomes a social problem. *Journal of Personality and Social Psychology, 38,* 131–140.

Koff, E., & Benavage, A. (1998). Breast size perception and satisfaction, body image, and psychological functioning in Caucasian and Asian American college women. *Sex Roles, 38,* 655–673.

McCreary, D. R., & Sadava, S. W. (1999). Television viewing and self-perceived health, weight, and physical fitness: Evidence for the cultivation hypothesis. *Journal of Applied Social Psychology, 29,* 2342–2361.

Sherwood, L. (1993). *Human physiology: From cells to systems.* St. Paul, MN: West Publishing.

Silverstein, B., Perdue, L., Peterson, B., & Kelly, E. (1986). The role of the mass media in promoting a thin standard of attractiveness for women. *Sex Roles, 14,* 519–532.

Silverstein, B., Perdue, L., Peterson, B., Vogel, L., & Fantini, R. (1986). Possible causes of the thin standard of bodily attractiveness for women. *International Journal of Eating Disorders, 5,* 907–916.

Spitzer, B. L., Henderson, K. A., & Zivian, M. T. (1999). Gender differences in population versus media body sizes: A comparison over four decades. *Sex Roles, 40,* 545–565.

Stice, E., Schupak-Neuberg, E., Shaw, H. E., & Stein, R. I. (1994). Relation of media exposure to eating disorder symptomatology: An examination of mediating mechanisms. *Journal of Abnormal Psychology, 103,* 836–840.

Stice, E., & Shaw, H. E. (1994). Adverse effects of the media portrayed thin-ideal on women and linkages to bulimic symptomatology. *Journal of Social and Clinical Psychology, 13,* 288–308.

Stunkard, A. J., Sorensen, T. I., & Schulsinger, F. (1983). Use of the Danish Adoption Register for the study of obesity and thinness. In S. Kety (Ed.), *The genetics of neurological and psychiatric disorders* (pp. 115–120). New York: Raven.

Turner, S. L., Hamilton, H., Jacobs, M., Angood, L. M., & Dwyer, D. H. (1997). The influence of fashion magazines on the body image satisfaction of college women: An exploratory analysis. *Adolescence, 32,* 603–614.

Wiseman, C. V., Gray, J. J., Mosimann, J. E., & Ahrens, A. H. (1992). Cultural expectations of thinness in women: An update. *International Journal of Eating Disorders, 11,* 85–89.

Discussion Questions

1. What specific health outcomes are influenced by viewing television images of idealized bodies?
2. What other than televised images may contribute to the practice of idealizing certain body types?
3. How do we balance the interests of free speech and freedom of expression with images that encourage risky health practices and general dissatisfaction with average-sized bodies? ✦

Chapter 25
Believing Is Seeing
The Co-Construction of Everyday Myths in the Media About College Drinking

Linda C. Lederman, Joshua B. Lederman, and Robert D. Kully

Chapter 25 also addresses the impact of the media on health issues by examining the ways in which media often perpetuate myths about social norms, particularly those related to health practices and outcomes. The authors focus particularly on the role of television in portraying a health issue and how the impact is a product of both the medium and the minds of its users. This chapter takes on myths about dangerous college drinking to demonstrate the co-constructed meanings between mediated images and the individuals who consume them. The authors argue that individuals cannot simply blame the media for fueling misperceptions. Rather, communication scholars must attend to the ways in which individuals make mediated images meaningful as they transfer those images into their own everyday realities.

Related Topics: alcohol prevention, college drinking, culture, media

Sometimes attitudes or beliefs slip into our unconscious mind without our ever realizing it, shaping our very perceptions of reality. Walsh (2004) claimed that television has the power to contribute to this shaping of our beliefs by silently influencing many of our perceptions. As a result, a dialectic relationship is created between our own internal belief system and real life experiences and the meanings evoked by the electronic images of television or film and the photos and words in print journalism. In addition, many of these unmonitored perceptions are not really correct but in fact, are misperceptions and distortions of some aspect of reality. Those distortions of reality, or myths, become so much a part of our sense of what is real that we bring them with us in our media consumption.

Elizabeth Thoman (1996) advocated that the cure for the influence of the media on our perceptions is the effective use of the media, or media literacy. She has said it involves learning how to become more wary of what we view and learning to ask the questions that allow us to watch mediated electronic images with a more mindful eye. Thoman referred to this as the development of our conscious awareness.

There are times, however, when even those of us who have developed more conscious awareness let down this critical guardedness. Topics slide under our critical-thinking radar screens, topics that are so mundane and ordinary that they are little noticed and simply taken as true. According to George Gerbner (2002), most of the images and information about lifestyles, relationships, and social interactions—most of the information we receive—does not come from our families or even from our friends and neighbors. He wrote that most of the stories that people incorporate into their sense of the world, the real world, are told by a few global conglomerates that have something to sell.

Two of the powerful industries that have stories they want told, especially to children, are the tobacco industry and the liquor industry. Although limits have been set on both in recent years in terms of advertising, no sophisticated, well-funded industry is without an army of extremely well-trained and effective media experts who know how to create and maintain images that serve their industry well despite the scrutiny of the Federal Communications Commission. Let us take as a case in point the use of alco-

From "Believing Is Seeing: The Co-Construction of Everyday Myths in the Media About College Drinking," Linda C. Lederman, Joshua B. Lederman, and Robert D. Kully, 2004, *American Behavioral Scientist*, Vol 48:1, pp. 130–136.

hol. In fact, let us narrow that down to the use of alcohol by college students.

No myth in the media has been more pervasive and more sustained than the image of college drinking as inevitable (Lederman, 1993), with the exception of the myth of romantic love as the basis of happiness (Galician, 2004) (evoked even in so "contemporary" a drama as *Sex and the City*). Burns and Goodstadt (1989) found that students view drinking alcohol as an adult thing to do and feel that they are now expected to act more like adults and are given more responsibility with less guidance. These images are reinforced for them by alcohol advertising, media messages, and sports events in which beer/alcohol sponsorship is evident and specific, as well as alcohol-related promotions for particular times of the academic year, such as spring break. But these studies indicate that students' perceptions of drinking behaviors are distorted (Burns, Ballou, & Lederman, 1991; Burns & Goodstadt, 1989). Students often do not recognize their drinking as excessive because their perception is relative to those around them—and they believe that the people around them are drinking excessively as well. For every student who drinks, there is another who seems to drink more frequently and to have more drinks per occasion.

This perception exists, in part, because the high-risk drinkers are drinking quite visibly. And these images are fueled by the mediated images of films such as *Animal House*, television shows such as *The Real World* that depict college as a drinking fest, and news reports of college drinking that emphasize the extreme as the norm (Lederman, 1993; Lederman & Stewart, in press). But in fact, Burns et al. (1991) found that more than half the students in their study were low-risk drinkers or abstained from drinking altogether, findings echoed in numerous other studies (Baer, Stacy, & Larimer, 1991; Berkowitz & Perkins, 1986, 1987; Haines & Spear, 1996; Lederman, 1993). A merger of meanings, a co-construction of realities, takes place when students interpret their selected experiences through these pervasive mediated images of drunkenness as the college norm. These all become merged in a way that makes it seem as if what they know, they know from their own experiences. Instead, they may well be shaping their own experiences by their beliefs, because believing is seeing.

As we discuss the issue of college students and their perceptions of themselves as co-constructed by their interaction with the media, it may help to look back at a text that we often have these same students read. Is not Plato's (2003) Allegory of the Cave a forerunner of what we now call media literacy? And if so, it seems that there may be a lesson for us to learn, because perhaps this phenomenon is not a product of what we call *media* at all but may instead be a built-in human response to any stimulus that we can regard as "the truth."

Most of us are familiar with the scenario: Plato described a cave where masses of prisoners are chained to a back wall and are able to see only the wall in front of them. In the back of the cave, a fire burns, and in front of this fire, statues are carried back and forth, and these statues create shadows on the wall that these prisoners are unable to look away from. Because they have never known anything else, these shadows are what the prisoners consider to be the real world. They have no idea that they are in a cave, or that there is a fire or statues, or that they are so far removed from the real outside world filled with actual objects rather than the shadows of imitation of these objects.

Although Plato created this allegory about 2,200 years before television and the Internet were invented, the similarities are eerie and describe the same phenomenon: Part of our nature is to take the information that is available to us (often failing to question its accuracy) and unconsciously synthesize it with what we already know so that we feel we have a sense of reality. In the case of college drinking, many students on college campuses reify these images through their selected perceptions of their socially situated learning experiences (Lederman et al., 2001; Lederman & Stewart, in press).

Part of Plato's wisdom in the allegory he created is that it is so clearly an exaggeration. When we present it to our students, it is easy for them to scoff at how foolish these people are. "I wouldn't stay in that cave!" is a common response. And that is the link that may be the key in helping us straighten out our own relationship to the "real world" as we understand it to be, primarily through our perceptions of the media. In the attempt to help our students understand the message of the allegory, we tell those who condemn the foolishness of the ignorant prisoners that the prisoners do not know they are prisoners, and that if they did, they might have a chance to escape (as one, of course, does). The value here is that if they do not know they are prisoners, it is because they are so wrapped up in their sense of reality (for several reasons that we sometimes explain, including comfort/complacency, fear of the unknown, or difficulty of abandoning any given belief system) that it would never occur to them unless it was pointed out. But we tell our students these things and have them read the allegory so that we can raise the questions: Are we any different? What do we really know about the world? and How do we know it? (And therefore, if we could see ourselves from the outside, would we pity ourselves and our obvious predicament the same way we pity Plato's prisoners?) Plato's allegory gives us a powerful doorway through which to explore the notion that if we, too, just sit and watch the shadows on the wall in front of us (now equipped with surround sound, of course), we may be just as ignorant of the reality of our situation as were those prisoners in the cave. Thus, the allegory becomes a way to address everyday-life media images, and media images become a way to lead students into better understanding Plato's allegory. We can use both to examine the co-construction of meaning that takes place when images and the meanings they have for viewers are both taken into account as part of the process of creating a sense of what is real.

We may ask our students what they would do if they were those prisoners. And we might encourage them to examine the ways in which the same ideas apply now with regard to media literacy. Plato's prisoners did not even know what they looked like. And how many college students really know what they look like?

Because our prime focus is on the myths of dangerous drinking in college, we can ask questions of ourselves as teachers, too. How many of us see our students walk into a noontime class clearly hung over? Some, true, but not a majority. We see these students every day, and it is easy to see firsthand that some of them do drink "dangerously," and that some of them are even proud of this. But it is equally clear that what we see firsthand is nowhere near what we would assume had we only been aware of media portrayals of college students. In fact, a semester may pass without seeing students during or after bouts of heavy drinking. But that is true not only for faculty who lack access to students around the clock but also for students themselves. How many of them perceive themselves in ways that are myth based? And then, of course, we must ask, How many actually seek to make these myths become reality, sometimes with disastrous effects? By believing that everyone in college drinks excessively, and wanting to fit in, dangerous drinking as a norm—the myth—becomes dangerous drinking as the norm—the reality. Students selectively "see" the visible drunkenness and use these observations to generalize and correspond with the images they already have from television shows, movies, and news stories,

Simply "blaming the media" for fueling us with misperceptions of the extensiveness of college drinking is too simplistic an answer to the perpetuation of the myth of the culture of college drinking. Instead, the answer lies in a co-construction of the meaning of the mediated images—the transference onto the screens of the images that we have of our realities. Sometimes these very images of reality come from previously mediated messages that have become part of our consciousness, albeit unnoticeably. For example, although few of us have been in police stations or participated in jury deliberations, based on our mediated images of these contexts, many of us nonetheless sense that we have or at least that we know how these contexts function. The lesson from Plato would be that this is part of the innate desire to make the world an understandable place, even if this has terrible consequences. Seen through the eyes of Plato's teachings, we recognize that this is not a situation unique to the modern era.

So if this is truly a part of the human condition, and not simply a by-product of our media-saturated society, then maybe we can take away a lesson from Plato in regard to what we have to do if we are to approach a less-distorted view of ourselves and of others. This lesson relates to one of the major skills that we encourage all of our students to develop: critical thinking. Perhaps Plato's prisoners' fates were sealed by their inability to think critically about their situation. They had grown up under a given regime—never knowing anything different— and had no skills or experience to enable them to analyze, question, or in any way consciously interact with what they thought to be reality. If they had, they would not have been prisoners for long. For what happens when they do critically analyze their situation and realize that they are indeed prisoners?

As Plato clearly showed us, the one man who escapes is never able to go back to his life of staring at the wall again. He would never again believe that those shadows were his reality. In fact, we argue that the moment he simply turned around and saw the fire and the statues, the moment that he realized he was in chains, he could never believe in those shadows again. So Plato's work is an example to us that an approach based on critical thinking may be the first but tremendously important step toward freeing ourselves from the myths we live by.

It is this habit of challenging everyday assumptions, especially those that result from the merger of mediated images and selective interpretations of experiences, that frees viewers from slavery to mediated images. As consumers of mediated messages, empowerment lies in the development of both our critical-thinking skills and our ability to examine and to question even those things we think we see for ourselves. To ask the questions that media literacy advocates such as Thoman (1996) have raised about evidence, viewpoint, connections/patterns, acts of supposition, and relevance is the beginning. These questions are grounded in the kinds of critical-thinking skills that are foundational in curricular offerings in literature, rhetoric, and public address that must now be applied to our understanding of all media in our lives.

The failure to question the inclination to take reality presented in the media as if it is reality rather than a construction of reality seems to be a dangerous thing, whether it relates to college-drinking norms, news reports on weapons of mass destruction, or even scientific reports. The profound similarity between the prisoners staring at a wall and any of us as we sit in front of our television sets only helps to underscore the importance of the issue of media literacy and the need to think critically about what is presented to us as the truth.

If this habit of noncritical absorption of images as if they are real is a hardwired human condition, perhaps media literacy really begins not with critical thinking about mediated images but with the examination of our responses to the media. Perhaps we can learn how much our own images of reality—our own ways of seeing, together with our need to form an understandable reality—have to do with the misperceptions we so readily accept. There is much that can be brought to bear in understanding this co-construction of what is real from the literature of communication and theories of the nature and derivation of the meanings people bring to messages (Deetz & Mokros, 2000; Gerbner, 2002; Littlejohn, 1999).

A co-constructionist view suggests that the meanings of these images are the coproductions of the viewers and media. Thus, rather than simply learning how to decode the messages put into the media by those who control these electronic pathways to information and entertainment, we need to learn about our own creation of reality or misperceptions of reality as well as the role of mediated messages in that reality creation. Failure to do both is what has the potential to make us the prisoners of the electronic images that dance on our walls.

References

Baer, J., Stacy, A., & Larimer, M. (1991). Biases in the perception of drinking norms among college students. *Journal of Studies on Alcohol, 52,* 580–586.

Berkowitz, A. D., & Perkins, H. W. (1986). Problem drinking among college students: A review of recent research. *Journal of American College Health, 35,* 21–28.

Berkowitz, A. D., & Perkins, H. W. (1987). Current issues in effective alcohol education programming. In J. Sherwood (Ed.), *Alcohol policies and practices on college and university campuses* (pp. 69–85). Columbus, OH: National Association of Student Personnel Administrators.

Burns, W. D., Ballou, J., & Lederman, L. (1991). *Perceptions of alcohol use and policy on the college campus: Preventing alcohol/drug abuse at Rutgers University.* Unpublished conference paper, U.S. Department of Education Fund for the Improvement of Post Secondary Education.

Burns, W. D., & Goodstadt, M. (1989). *Alcohol use on the Rutgers University campus: A study of various communities.* Unpublished conference paper, U.S. Department of Education Fund for the Improvement of Post Secondary Education.

Deetz, S., & Mokros, H. (2000). What counts as real. In L. Lederman & D. Gibson (Eds.), *Communication theory* (pp. 67–89). Dubuque, Iowa: Kendall/Hunt.

Galician, M. L. (2004). *Sex, love and romance in the mass media.* Mahwah, NJ: Lawrence Erlbaum.

Gerbner, G. (2002). Education and the challenge of mass culture. In M. Morgan (Ed.), *Against the mainstream: The selected works of George Gerbner* (pp. 63–79). New York: Peter Lang.

Haines, M., & Spear, S. F. (1996). Changing the perception of the norm: A strategy to decrease binge drinking among college students. *Journal of American College Health, 45,* 134–140.

Lederman, L. C. (1993). Friends don't let friends beer goggle: A case study in the use and abuse of alcohol and communication among college students. In E. B. Ray (Ed.), *Case studies in health communication* (pp. 161–174). Hillsdale, NJ: Lawrence Erlbaum.

Lederman, L. C., & Stewart, L. P. (in press). *Changing the culture of college drinking: A socially situated prevention campaign.* Creskill, NJ: Hampton Press.

Lederman, L., Stewart, L., Barr, S., Powell, R., Laitman, L., & Goodhart, F. (2001). RU SURE? Using communication theory to reduce dangerous drinking on a college campus. In R. E. Rice & C. Atkin (Eds.), *Public communication campaigns* (3rd ed., pp. 295–299). Thousand Oaks, CA: Sage.

Littlejohn, S. (1999). *Theories of human communication.* Belmont, CA: Wadsworth.

Plato. (2003). *Plato unmasked: Plato's Dialogues made new* (K. Quincy, Trans.). Spokane: Eastern Washington University Press.

Thoman, E. (1996). *Beyond blame: Challenging violence in the media* [Kit]. Los Angeles: Center for Media Literacy.

Walsh, B. (2004, March). *Influencing our attitudes and perceptions.* Available from www.medialit.org

Discussion Questions

1. What does it mean to participate in a co-constructed reality?
2. The authors suggest that greater media literacy might help us deal with some of the problems associated with media misperceptions. How does a person become more media literate, especially when it comes to health issues? What else might be useful in fixing media misperceptions?
3. How does critical thinking figure into the authors' argument? How do you teach individuals to be more critically aware? ✦

Chapter 26
Perceptions of Latinos, African Americans, and Whites on Media as a Health Information Source

Mollyann Brodie, Nina Kjellson, Tina Hoff, and Molly Parker

In the final chapter in this volume, Mollyann Brodie, Nina Kjellson, Tina Hoff, and Molly Parker explore the ways in which there is a need for accurate and effective mass media coverage of health topics and concerns for racially and ethnically diverse audiences. Even with the high reliance on mass media as a source of public health information, whites, African Americans, and Latinos have little trust in this source. In this chapter, Brodie and her colleagues document the significant role that mass media currently has in informing the public about health. However, despite this role, it is suggested that access to health information from mass media is fundamentally different for African Americans and Latinos when compared to whites. There is a need for accurate and effective mass media coverage of health topics for racially and ethnically diverse audiences. Each of the chapters in Part VII of this anthology provides a set of issues to consider when we realize that much of what we know about health is communicated to us through the mass media and the Internet. These chapters have shown how important it is for citizens today to be literate in their use of all the mass media, including the Internet.

Related Topics: culture, drug use, e-health, health campaigns, health-care behaviors, HIV/AIDS, Internet, media, patients' perspectives

Disparities in health outcomes and access to health care services between the White and non-White populations in this country are well documented (see, for example, Bullough & Bullough, 1982; Collins & Hawkes, 1997; Keil, Sutherland, Knapp, Tyroler, & Pollitzer, 1992; Mayberry et al., 1995; Mayberry & Stoddard-Wright, 1992; Sorlie, Rogot, Anderson, Johnson, & Backlund, 1992). African Americans and Latinos,[1] in particular, face health disparities ranging from heightened risk for certain medical conditions to worse outcomes from a range of diagnoses (Baker, Stevens, & Brook, 1996; Bartman, Moy, & D'Angelo, 1997; Blendon, Aiken, Freeman, & Corey, 1989; Molina & Aguirre-Molina, 1994). African Americans and Latinos are also more likely to lack health insurance and often face more barriers than Whites when seeking health care treatments and services (Brett, Schoendorf, & Kiely, 1994; Carlisle, Leake, Brook, & Shapiro, 1996; Carlisle, Leake, & Shapiro, 1997; Giles, Anda, Casper, Escobedo, & Taylor, 1995; Hayward, Shapiro, Freeman, & Corey, 1988; Langkamp, Foye, & Roghmann, 1990; Mort, Weissman, & Epstein, 1994; Peterson, Shaw, DeLong, Pryor, Califf, & Mark, 1997; Trevino, Moyer, Valdez, & Stroub-Benham, 1991).

Numerous and complex factors have been implicated in these differences in health status and health care access (most significantly economic, educational, and logistical barriers as well as cultural, attitudinal, and interpersonal constraints). Access to health news and information is believed to be critical to the advancement of public health and the elimination of disparities in health ac-

From "Preceptions of Latinos, African Americans, and Whites on Media as a Health Information Source," Mollyann Brodie, Nina Kjellson, Tina Hoff, and Molly Parker, 1999, *The Howard Journal of Communication*, Vol. 10:3, pp. 147–187. Reproduced by permission of Taylor & Francis Group, LLC., http://taylorandfrancis.com.

cess and outcomes.[2] However, the public's use of various sources of health information and its perceptions of the relevance and appropriateness of the information provided are poorly understood, especially across subgroups of the total population. Although research has explored general public perceptions of media as a health information resource, as well as the nature and amount of health coverage by general market mass media, less attention has been devoted to how well the media, among other sources, are meeting health information needs and preferences of minority populations. Even less attention has been turned to how general market health coverage compares with coverage by media directed primarily to minority audiences, such as Black-oriented and Spanish-language, Latino-oriented media.

In three nationally representative surveys of Latinos, African-Americans, and Whites from a general population sample, we measured public use of different health information sources and public opinion about the effectiveness of the media, in particular, as a source of news and information about health and health care. In addition, we assessed the extent to which different resources are used and trusted for health information to better understand the role and effectiveness of mass media sources. Through a series of measures, we evaluated the perceived usefulness and relevance of the health information conveyed by the media: Is the health news reported in the media seen by all audiences as accurate, detailed, and fair? Is health information presented in such a way as to be relevant to racially and ethnically diverse audiences? To what extent do the preferences and perceptions of African Americans, Latinos, and Whites differ? How are Black- and Latino-oriented media used and viewed, as compared with general market media, with respect to health coverage?

Theoretical Framework

This study examines the sources of health information used by African Americans, Latinos, and Whites in this country with a particular focus on mass media sources of health news and health information. Key measures include use and trust of different information sources as well as perceptions of the effectiveness, fairness, and personal or community relevance of media health coverage. As such, this study intersects two broad research domains: public health information and mass media, and mass media and race (including coverage of minority-relevant issues and media's treatment of minorities, in general).

In terms of the first broad research area, mass media, in particular, have been shown to play a pivotal role in informing the public about health and medical issues (for a comprehensive review, see Brown & Walsh-Childers, 1994; Atkin & Arkin, 1990). However, there is competing evidence about the nature of this role and the short- and long-term effects of different types of media health messages. Points of contention include whether messages are actively or passively received by audiences, the influence of format—news, advertising, entertainment—on message transmission, and the relationship between media-delivered health messages and public attitudes and behaviors. In addition, effects have been shown to vary by audience attributes, such as demographic composition or patterns of utilization, as well as the different mediums, ranging from print to broadcast (Brown & Walsh-Childers, 1994; see also Brown, Walsh-Chiders, & Waszak, 1990; Culbertson & Stempel, 1985; Dejong & Winsten, 1990; Freimuth et al., 1985; Jeffres & Hur, 1981; Korzenny, Neuendorf, Burgoon, Burgoon & Greenberg, 1983; Meyer, 1990; Pettegrew & Logan, 1987; Wallack, 1981, 1990; Winett & Wallack, 1996; Winsten, 1985). What remains less clear is how diverse audiences use mass media, specifically, as a health information source and, especially, whether preferences, use patterns, and qualitative assessments of media health coverage differ across racial and ethnic groups and, if these differences exist, whether they lead to differential access to health news and information.

Some analysis of media programming imperatives suggests that such differences do exist. Although media play a role in delivering health information, there is concern that media coverage of health and medical topics is targeted primarily at the health concerns of mainstream White audiences and overlooks the information interests of racial minorities (Klaidman, 1990). Many of the same imperatives that determine general news content (reporting quickly, accurately, and with sufficient "hook" about events judged current and important) also set the agenda for coverage of health and health care. But, because health reporting often extends beyond coverage of "breaking" health and medical news, other imperatives can also drive what is covered by the "health beat." As Klaidman (1990) argues, media organizations report on what they think the audience wants and needs to know about health, based on who their audience is. In so doing, he posits, media organizations judge health stories by more subjective tests of relevance and usefulness for target audiences. This, in turn, biases coverage toward informing and featuring the majority audience segment with little or no attention to the health needs and interests of narrower audience segments. This study specifically examines whether audiences perceive such a lack of inclusiveness and relevancy in health reporting and, if so, what underlying causes are implicated.

In terms of the second broad area of communications study—race and ethnicity in the media—research (ranging from content analyses and effects studies to analyses of the representation of minority individuals on the staffs of media organizations[3] suggests that mainstream media coverage often under- or misrepresents minorities or promulgates negative stereotypes of minority subgroups or both. Specifically, studies have shown significant deficits in the amount of minority-relevant coverage as well as disproportionately few depictions of minority individuals or groups in news, entertainment, and other reporting or programming (Nardi, 1993; Poindexter & Stroman, 1981; Quiroga, 1994). Other research has documented unfair treatment of minorities by the media, including unfavorable depictions and inappropriate or excessive associations of minority groups with social or political ills (Barlow, 1998; Entman, 1994; Entman, 1992; Entman, 1990; Gerbner, Gross, & Signorelli, 1984; Gilens, 1996; Romer, Jamieson, & de Coteau, 1998; Signorelli, 1985; Turk, Richard, Bryson, & Johnson, 1989). Studies have also shown a lack of minority journalists and editors across the print and broadcast media workforce, with numbers out of proportion with the minority composition of the population (Freeman, 1997; Shipler, 1998). Underrepresented in the research is a comparison of the subjective experiences and assessments of minority audiences to the objective findings about the shortcomings of media coverage with respect to minority individuals and issues.

The documented shortcomings of mainstream mass media for minority audiences make Black media and Latino-oriented media important foci of this research. Although these media have a longstanding market presence, recent years have brought a marked growth in the minority-oriented media market (Wilson & Gutierrez, 1995). With the changing racial and ethnic composition of the U.S. population, there has been radical growth of new and existing media (print, broadcast, and cable) that cater primarily to racial, ethnic, and cultural minorities (Chang, Shoemaker, Reese, & Danielson, 1987; Charlesworth & Hudes, 1997; Greenberg & Brand, 1994; Subervi-Vélez, 1994).

This study builds upon the first area of communications research by examining public access to health information, including that delivered by the media. Particularly, it contributes to the general understanding of how diverse audiences perceive mass media (both general market and Black and Latino oriented) as a health information source; whether assessments and utilization differs by racial and ethnic composition of audiences; and whether diverse audiences see their health information needs bring met by media health reporting.

It builds upon the second area of study by examining whether diverse audiences perceive the media to underrepresent or misrepresent minorities in their health reporting and by explicitly exploring the role of Black- and Latino-oriented media compared with general market sources.

This study asks the following questions: (1) What sources do African Americans, Latinos, and Whites turn to for information and news about health, health care, and health policy? (2) What is the role of mass media as a health information source? (3) Do African Americans, Latinos, and Whites differ in their assessments of media health coverage in terms of quality, usefulness or relevance, and fairness? (4) Do disparities exist in Latinos', African Americans', and Whites' access to desired health information?

Method

Three nationally representative telephone surveys were conducted in the spring of 1998: (1) a national survey of 2,006 Latino adults; (2) a national survey of 804 African American adults; and (3) a national general population companion survey of 874 adults, including 664 Whites.

Results from the Latino survey are based on 2,006 random-sample telephone interviews with Latino adults, aged 18 years and older, who live in the continental United States (Alaska, Hawaii, and Puerto Rico were not included). To ensure adequate representation of the role of Latino-oriented media, the final sample included oversampling from three regional markets with heavy Spanish-Language, Latino-oriented media penetration: the New York, Los Angeles, and Miami metropolitan areas.[4] Respondents were included in the survey if they self-identified as being Hispanic or Latino. To maximize participation of Spanish-speaking Latinos and to minimize the effects of a language barrier on the findings, every respondent was *explicitly* offered the option of being interviewed in Spanish. A specialist in qualitative research among Latinos reviewed the Spanish-language instrument to ensure that the vocabulary and phraseology was appropriate to the major Latino ethnic groups in the United States—Mexicans, Cubans, and Puerto Ricans. The interviews were conducted between February 23 and April 12, 1998. The margin of error for the total Latino sample is plus or minus 4 percentage points.

The African American sample is based on random-sample telephone interviews with 804 adults (18 years or older) who self-describe as Black and not of Hispanic or Latino origin. The interviews were conducted between June 9 and July 2, 1998. The margin of error for the African American sample is plus or minus 4 percentage points.

The general population sample is based on 875 random-sample telephone interviews with adults (ages 18 and older), including 664 Whites. The interviews were conducted between June 9 and July 7, 1998. The margin of error for the general population sample, as well as the subset of White respondents, is plus or minus 4 percentage points.

The three questionnaires were designed by researchers at the Kaiser Family Foundation and Princeton Survey Research Associates (PSRA) in conjunction with the National Association of Black Journalists (NABJ) with contributions from the National Association of Hispanic Journalists (NAHJ). Interviews were conducted by PSRA. Data from each of the samples were standardized to reflect probabilities of each case selection and to standardize samples to match U.S. census estimates of age, sex, education, and regional distributions of Latinos, African Americans, and the general population in the United States. Statistical tests of differences were performed using SAS software to compare responses across groups of respondents to test the null hypothesis that the mean response for two groups do not differ significantly.

In addition to sampling error, surveys are subject to other forms of errors from nonresponse, question wording, and context effects. Every effort was made to minimize these effects, including careful interviewer training, outside-expert evaluation of the Spanish-language questionnaire, and pretesting and subsequent modification of all three instruments.

The surveys of African Americans and Whites were conducted as companion studies using near-identical survey instruments and wording. The Latino study addresses a majority of the research questions posed in the other surveys, but on some items question wording differs. Wherever possible in our analysis, we make comparisons and tests of significance across the three groups. When there is no corresponding question on the Latino survey or wording differs sufficiently to preempt three-way analysis, our reporting is delimited to a comparison between African American and White responses and noncomparative presentation of Latino responses.[5]

Results

Survey respondents were interviewed about their health-related concerns; interest in health information; and reliance on and perceptions of mass media as a health information resource.

Sources of Health Information

Table 26.1 represents reported sources of information about health and health care in the year prior to the surveys for the three samples. Although respondents identified many sources as having provided at least *some* health information in the past year, mass media in general, and television in particular, dominated as the most abundant provider of information about health and health care.

Among Whites, equally high proportions (about 9 in 10) named television (92%), friends/family (88%), and newspapers (86%) as having provided any health information in the past year, followed closely by doctors/health providers (83%) and magazines (82%). Majorities also named radio, outdoor media (billboards), their church, and their employer. More named television (24%) than any other source as having provided the *most* information in the past year; the second most abundant source was doctor/health provider (15%).

Table 26.1
Sources of Health Information in Past Year; Top Two Most Important Sources in Past Year

	Whites saying they received health information (net: a lot, some, only a few) from each source in the past 12 months	*African Americans saying they received any information (net: a lot, some, only a few) from each source in the past 12 months*	*Latinos saying they received any information about health or health care from each source in the past year or so*
Television	92bb	92cc	80^{bb}_{cc}
Radio	74bb	73cc	55^{bb}_{cc}
Newspapers	86bb	84cc	59^{bb}_{cc}
Magazines	82bb	78cc	58^{bb}_{cc}
Street signs, flyers, or billboards	60^{aa}_{bb}	70^{aa}_{cc}	48^{bb}_{cc}
Employer/job	50	50	45
Church/place of worship	51^{aaa}_{bb}	68^{aaa}_{ccc}	40^{bb}_{ccc}
Doctor/health provider	83bb	86cc	75^{bb}_{cc}
Internet	30	35	n/acc
Family/friends†	88bbb	86ccc	50^{bbb}_{ccc}
One source providing the most information about health and health care[2]	Whites	African Americans	Latinos
Television	24	25	31
Doctor/health provider	15	20	27

†Latino survey asked about "husband/wife or other family members" and "friends" separately; responses were 46% and 50%, respectively.
[2] Latino survey asked about "most important source of health information in the past year."
a $p < 0.05$ for White versus African American.
b $p < 0.05$ for White versus Latino.
c $p < 0.05$ for African American versus Latino.
aa $p < 0.01$ for White versus African American.
bb $p < 0.01$ for White versus Latino.
cc $p < 0.01$ for African American versus Latino.
aaa $p < 0.001$ for White versus African American.
bbb $p < 0.001$ for White versus Latino.
ccc $p < 0.001$ for African American versus Latino.

Most African Americans also reported getting health information in the past year from television (92%), friends/family (86%), and doctors/health providers (86%), followed by newspapers (84%), radio (73%), and church (68%). African Americans, however, were about as likely to name television (25%) as doctor/health provider (20%) when asked which source provided the *most* health information in the past year.

Latinos were much more likely to report getting information from television (80%) and doctor/health provider (75%) than from any other source. These two sources were also named as having provided the *most* health information in the last year (31% television, 27% doctor/health provider). Majorities said they received health information from newspapers (59%), magazines (58%), radio (55%), and friends/family (50%); fewer than half named outdoor media/billboards (48%), employers (45%), or their church (40%) as recent sources.

Table 26.2
Health- and Health Care-Related Problems of Concern

	Whites saying each is major problem affecting people in this country today	*African Americans saying each is major problem affecting black people or African Americans in this country*	*Latinos saying each is a big problem for Hispanics in [their] area*
Being able to afford the cost of health insurance and necessary medical care†	75	78cc	71cc
The poor and elderly not getting enough help from Medicare and Medicaid to pay medical bills	62aa	75^{aa}_{cc}	66cc
Having enough good doctors and other health care providers near where they live	30^{aaa}_{bb}	45^{aaa}_{cc}	39^{bb}_{cc}
Having difficulty getting necessary medical care because of (African Americans and Whites: racial discrimination; Latinos: language barriers)	22aaa	45aaa	58
Alcoholism and drug addiction	83^{aa}_{bbb}	90^{aa}_{ccc}	71^{bbb}_{cc}
Cancer	90^{aa}_{bbb}	78^{aa}_{ccc}	56^{bbb}_{ccc}
Asthma	50a	57a	n/a
Sickle cell anemia	24aaa	53aaa	n/a
Lupus	17aaa	33aaa	n/a
AIDS or HIV, the virus that causes AIDS	82bbb	81ccc	53^{bbb}_{ccc}
Sexually transmitted diseases other than AIDS	58^{aaa}_{bb}	71^{aaa}_{ccc}	51^{bb}_{ccc}
Unplanned teenage pregnancies	79aa	89aa	80cc

†Latino survey asked about affordability of health insurance and affordability of necessary medical care separately; responses were 64% and 71%, respectively.
‡Latino survey asked about alcoholism and drug addiction separately; responses were 71% and 69%, respectively.
a $p < 0.05$ for White versus African American.
b $p < 0.05$ for White versus Latino.
c $p < 0.05$ for African American versus Latino.
aa $p < 0.01$ for White versus African American.
bb $p < 0.01$ for White versus Latino.
cc $p < 0.01$ for African American versus Latino.
aaa $p < 0.001$ for White versus African American.
bbb $p < 0.001$ for White versus Latino.
ccc $p < 0.001$ for African American versus Latino.

Preferred Health Information Source

Across all groups, television was not only the most common health information source but also the most preferred outlet among all media health sources. Half of African Americans and Latinos (55% and 50%, respectively) and somewhat fewer Whites (40%, $p < 0.001$) said television is their most preferred outlet when using the media to get "information on important health and health care issues." Magazines were named next most often (by 24% of Latinos, 23% of Whites, and 15% of African Americans, $p < 0.01$).

Health Issues of Concern and Call for Media to Do More

Comparisons across the groups showed high levels of concern about a range of public health issues as depicted in Table 26.2. Overall, more African Americans rated specific health and medical concerns as major problems compared with Whites, and the two groups differed somewhat with respect to the health problems viewed with greatest urgency. (The Latino survey included a related but differently worded item.) Concern among African Americans was highest over the impact of alcoholism and drug addiction (90%), HIV/AIDS (81%), and unplanned teenage pregnancies (89%) on African Americans in this country. By comparison, concern among Whites was highest for cancer (90%), followed by alcoholism and drug addiction (83%), and unplanned teenage pregnancies (79%). Not surprising given higher rates among African Americans, more African Americans than Whites said sickle cell anemia (53%) and lupus (33%) are major problems (compared with 24% and 17% of Whites). For Latinos, unplanned teenage pregnancies and alcohol and drug addiction also ranked high and were named by most as major problems for Latinos *in their area*. In addition, many health care access problems were named as significant concerns across groups (also Table 26.2).

These concerns about health and health care issues, combined with a strong reliance on media for health information, suggest a prominent role for media in meeting health information needs. However, survey findings document a general perception that media should be doing more stories on health and health care topics, especially those rated as of strong concern to respondents (Table 26.3). For every health topic asked about, majorities of African Americans and Latinos said the media were not providing enough coverage and that they and their families are not getting the information they need.[6] Lower but substantial percentages of Whites concurred. African Americans (71%) were more likely than both Whites (63%, $p < 0.01$) and Latinos (62%, $p < 0.01$) to say there were not enough stories about changes in government policies and the health care industry. Large proportions of African Americans and Latinos said there was not enough coverage of government health programs such as Medicaid and Medicare (73% and 74%, respectively, compared with 61% of Whites, $p < 0.001$). Seven in 10 African Americans (74%) and Latinos (69%), and only about half (49%) of Whites, said the media were not doing enough stories on the illnesses most likely to affect their communities.[7] African Americans (60%) and Latinos (63%) also proved more likely than Whites (45%, $p < 0.001$) to say that there was not enough media attention paid to "steps families can take to prevent illnesses." Latinos were most likely to say the media are not doing enough stories for parents about how to talk with children about difficult topics such as AIDS, violence, or drugs (69% compared with 53% of African Americans, $p < 0.05$, and 45% of Whites, $p < 0.01$).

Underscoring the power of media health information, respondents indicated that media health information influences their personal behaviors. Large proportions reported taking action in response to "something reported in the media about health or health care." Over 7 in 10 Whites (74%) and African Americans (71%) affirmed having talked with friends or family. Many others, but even greater proportions of African Americans than Whites, changed eating or exercise habits (55% and 45%, respectively, $p < 0.01$), and talked with sexual partners about issues such as birth control or sexually transmitted diseases (49% and 30%, respectively, $p < 0.001$) as a result of something reported in the media.

Table 26.3
Perceptions of Adequacy of Media Coverage of Health Topics

	Whites saying media are not doing enough stories on each topic	*African Americans saying media are not doing enough stories on each topic*	*Latinos saying media they use most often are not doing enough stories on each topic†*
Changes in government policies and health care industry that might affect your health care or health insurance	63aa	71^{aa}_{cc}	62cc
Medicare and Medicaid	61^{aa}_{bb}	73aa	74‡bb
Illnesses and medical conditions more likely to affect (African Americans; Black people; Whites; people like you; Latinos; Hispanics)	49^{aaa}_{bbb}	74^{aaa}_{c}	69^{bbb}_{c}
Steps families can take to prevent illnesses	45^{aaa}_{bb}	60aaa	63bb
How to talk with children about topics such as sexuality, AIDS, violence, or drugs	55^{aa}_{bb}	63^{aa}_{c}	69^{bb}_{c}
Testing, treatment, and prevention of HIV and other sexually transmitted diseases	43^{a}_{bb}	50a	54bb

ns = not statistically significant.
†On Latino survey, "media doing enough stories on topic" posed as follow-up to those respondents saying they have not been getting all the information they and their families need about topic.
‡On Latino survey, Medicare and Medicaid were asked about separately; responses were 74% and 75%, respectively.
¶On Latino survey, HIV and other sexually transmitted diseases were asked about separately; responses were 54% and 62%, respectively.
a $p < 0.05$ for White versus African American.
b $p < 0.05$ for White versus Latino.
c $p < 0.05$ for African American versus Latino.
aa $p < 0.01$ for White versus African American.
bb $p < 0.01$ for White versus Latino.
cc $p < 0.01$ for African American versus Latino.
aaa $p < 0.001$ for White versus African American.
bbb $p < 0.001$ for White versus Latino.
ccc $p < 0.001$ for African American versus Latino.

Perceptions of Media Coverage of Health; Adequacy of Minority Representation; Fairness of Minority Portrayals

On both African American and White surveys, respondents were asked for their assessments of the reliability of a range of health information sources. Also, respondents were asked to give their perceptions of general market and minority-oriented media's treatment of racial and ethnic minorities in coverage of health topics as well as other issues. (These questions were not asked on the Latino survey.)

Trust of Health Information Sources

To assess perceived credibility of sources, respondents on the African American and general population surveys were asked to quantify their trust of different health information sources. We found that although media is heavily relied upon for health information and preferred by most as a source of health information, media is not held as a highly trustworthy source. Using a 5-point scale, respondents assessed whether they trusted the source always, most of the time, only sometimes, hardly ever, or never.

Doctors and health providers are the only source of health information to be rated highly trustworthy by a majority of African Americans and Whites. Importantly, however, Whites (79%) were significantly more likely than African Americans (63%, $p < 0.001$) to report trusting health providers always or most of the time as reliable sources of health information. For all other sources, fewer than half of African Americans and Whites reported a high degree of trust.

Forty-six percent of African Americans named churches/religious organizations as highly trustworthy sources and 4 in 10 (44%) said friends/family could be trusted always or most of the time. Whites were approximately as trusting of friends and family (46%) but a little less trusting of churches/religious organizations (37%, $p < 0.05$). Neither group reported high trust of government agencies or holistic healers who promote alternative medicines; African Americans found these sources even less credible as providers of health information than did Whites (31% of Whites and 22% of African Americans trust the government always/most of the time, $p < 0.001$; 14% and 10%, respectively, trust holistic healers, $p < 0.01$).

Despite media's popularity as a source of health information, trust of the media as a health information source was moderate to low for both groups. About half of African Americans said the Black-oriented media (50%) are credible when it comes to health information; only 1 in 3 (34%) reported trusting general market media always or most of the time. Whites reported slightly higher trust of mainstream media for health information (41%, $p < 0.05$). However, the majority trust it only sometimes or hardly ever (54%). Overall, trust of media proved lower than might be expected in light of high reported reliance on, and preference for, the media as a source of health information.

Minority Relevance of Media Health Coverage

We used several measures to capture respondents' assessments of media health coverage in terms of its relevance to racially diverse audiences. On the Latino survey, 58% said they had not been getting information about "illnesses and medical conditions that are more likely to affect Hispanics" and, of those, 69% said the media are not doing enough stories to meet their need for health information. Similarly, on the African American survey, many reported marked dissatisfaction with how the general market media addresses health problems affecting Blacks as well as with how the media represents and portrays Blacks. Only 3 in 10 (31%) said that in all the media health coverage they consume, there is enough coverage of how Blacks are affected by health and health care problems; and 78% said health coverage fails to feature enough Black people and Black families. Whites also said media lacks in coverage relevant to minorities: only 31% said coverage adequately addresses the impact of different health problems for minorities. But far fewer Whites than African Americans (42% versus 76%, $p < 0.01$) said that minorities are underrepresented in health stories. (See Figure 26.1.)

However, African Americans' dissatisfaction with media health coverage appears to stem more from the underrepresentation of Blacks and the lack of coverage that is relevant to Blacks overall than with the media's failure to provide health information that is useful or relevant to them personally. As shown in Table 26.3, more African Americans said the media were doing a good job providing coverage of "the health and health care issues [they] deal with in [their] day" (40%) than said the media were doing a good job providing coverage of health issues Blacks face (31%, $p < 0.01$). Overall, 54% said the media were doing a "good job" telling them and their families what they needed to know about health and health care, and 40% said there was enough "practical information about what you can do to deal with specific health and health problems."

White respondents were about equally satisfied with the personal relevance and personal usefulness of media health coverage as they were with the job the media were doing to address the overall health information needs of "people in this country." Fifty-five percent of Whites said the media were doing a good job telling *people in this country* what they need to know about health and health care. Fifty-eight said the media were doing a good job meeting their personal health information needs. Whites were divided on whether or not there was enough media attention paid to "practical health information" (49% "enough," 49% "not enough"). Slight majorities said there was enough coverage of their day-to-day health issues as well as sufficient attention paid to

Figure 26.1
Perceptions of Minority Representation in General Media Coverage by Type of Stories

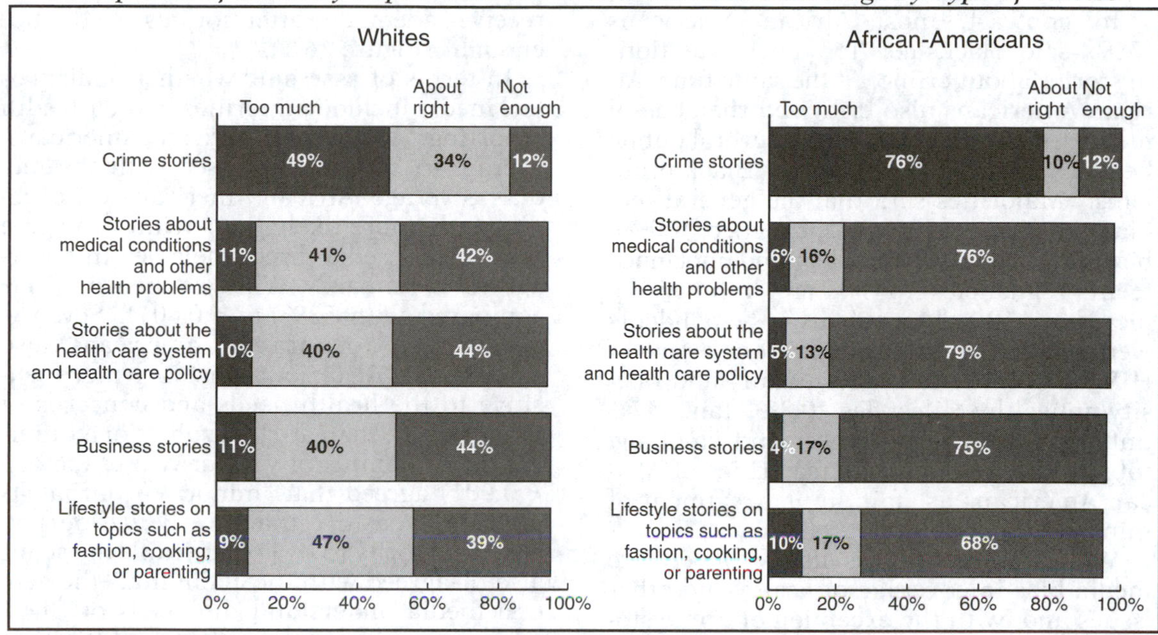

Percent saying (Whites: *members of minority groups*; African Americans: *Blacks*) get *too much*, *not enough* or *about the right amount* of attention in the general media's coverage of each story type.

Source: Kaiser Family Foundation/National Association of Black Journalists National Survey on Blacks, Media, and Health.

how people like themselves are affected by specific health and health care problems (on both items: 52% "enough," 45% "not enough").

Reasons Cited for Inadequate Minority-Relevant Health Coverage

Respondents who said general media coverage of minority health problems was inadequate were subsequently asked to categorize a set of reasons as relevant or irrelevant to this perception. Eight out of 10 African Americans who were dissatisfied with coverage named each of three reasons as relevant. The reason identified by the largest proportion (93%), and also named by a plurality (39%) as *most* important, was: "Most news organizations are not aware of—or interested in—the health problems of minorities." Other reasons proposed to respondents were, "There isn't enough data and research about the health problems of minorities" (named by 82% of those who said coverage of minority health was inadequate) and "There are not enough minority journalists reporting on health and health care" (identified by 84%).

While many Whites (54%) agreed that "minority" interests are under-represented in media health coverage, they attributed cause in slightly smaller numbers. Eighty-one percent named lack of interest or awareness, 75% named lack of minority journalists, and 72% named lack of research as possible explanations for inadequate minority-relevant health coverage.

Representations and Portrayals

As described above, 78% of African Americans reported a perception that "Black people and Black families" are underfeatured in media health stories. In addition, questions about a range of specific stories showed strong perceptions of under-representation across media content. African Americans said Blacks get "too little attention" in coverage of medical conditions and other health problems (76%); stories about the health care system and health policy (79%) ; stories about business (75%); and stories about lifestyle issues such as fashion, cooking, or parenting (68%).

In contrast, most African Americans (76%) said Blacks get "too much attention" in stories about crime. At the same time, African Americans also criticized the general media for biased portrayals of several public health and social problems as "Black problems." Majorities said that the general media's stories, welfare dependence (70%), births to single mothers (61%), and unplanned teen pregnancies (55%), are unfairly depicted as "Black problems." Respondents were divided on assessments of coverage of HIV/AIDS (48% fair, 48% unfair) and obesity/unhealthy lifestyles (48% fair, 47% unfair). Coverage of cancer and smoking/tobacco use was seen by majorities of African Americans as "fair" in its treatment of minorities.

Whites were far less likely to perceive media bias in coverage of health and other issues and, with the exception of crime stories, Whites were as likely to say minority representation in different stories is adequate as they were to say representation is lacking. While half (50%) of Whites agreed that welfare stories "unfairly portray welfare as a minority problem," strong majorities said coverage of other issues is generally fair (see Table 26.4). Half (49%) of Whites said that minorities get too much attention in crime; approximately a third (34%) said coverage is "about right."

Representation in lifestyle stories was seen by a plurality (47%) as "about right," and in stories about medical conditions, the health care system, and business issues, equal numbers of Whites said minorities receive adequate attention as said "not enough" (Figure 26.1).

In terms of assessing whether audiences feel media include minorities in their health reporting, we found African Americans, overall, to be less impressed with the media's coverage. African Americans were significantly more likely than Whites to agree that "most media direct their health coverage to a primarily White audience" (71% compared with 53%, $p < 0.001$). Seventy-two percent of African Americans also agreed that "Black journalists are more sensitive to the health needs and concerns of Black people than are journalists of a different race;" significantly fewer Whites (56%, $p < 0.001$) agreed that "minority" journalists are more sensitive than are *White* journalists. A majority (57%) of African Americans also disagreed with the claim that "the general media understand the needs of Black audiences" (compared with 42% of Whites,[8] $p < 0.001$).

Minority-Oriented Media Sources

Although general market media predominates as a source of health information, and news in general, we also found a strong reported role of minority-oriented media. In addition, Latinos and African Americans gave consistently favorable ratings of the health coverage of these media on a range of quality measures.

African Americans reported a strong preference for general market media over Black-

Table 26.4
Perceptions of Unfair Portrayals of Health Problems as "Black" or "Minority" Problems in Media Coverage

	Whites Saying Media's Coverage of Each Problem Unfairly Portrays It as a Problem Among Blacks, Latinos, and Other Minorities	African Americans Saying Media's Coverage of Each Problem Unfairly Portrays It as a "Black" Problem	
Unplanned teenage pregnancies	37	55	$p < 0.001$
Smoking and tobacco use	24	40	$p < 0.001$
Cancer	15	30	$p < 0.001$
HIV or AIDS	30	48	$p < 0.001$
Obesity and unhealthy lifestyles	30	47	$p < 0.001$
Welfare dependency	50	70	$p < 0.001$
Births to single mothers	37	61	$p < 0.001$

oriented media for news in general (72% versus 11%, $p < 0.001$) and general media was named by twice as many than Black-oriented media as a source of news and information about health and health care in the past year (56% versus 26%, $p < 0.001$). More African Americans also named general media as the *preferred* source when having to use media to get health information (48% compared with 28%, $p < 0.001$).

Despite this preference for general market media, African Americans reported high use of specific Black media for health information: 82% reported getting health information from "radio news or news talk shows directed to Black listeners" and from "magazines directed to Black readers, such as *Essence, Ebony,* or *Jet*" Seventy-nine percent said they got information about health or health care from "TV news or talk shows directed specifically to Black viewers, like those on *BET,* the cable network" and 69% from "newspapers directed to Black readers."

Latinos also reported heavier utilization of general market media sources for news as well as health information, although, not surprisingly, primary language influenced their preference. More Latinos (52%) reported getting news mainly from English-language general media than from Latino-oriented sources (39%, $p < 0.01$) and, overall, general market media was said to have provided more health news in the past year than Latino-oriented sources. Broken out by specific venue, Latinos were equally likely to say Spanish-language radio provided more health coverage as they were to say English-language radio provided more (26% and 23%, respectively). For television (40% versus 27%, $p < 0.001$) as well as newspapers and magazines (38% versus 16%, respectively, for both, $p < 0.001$), more Latinos reported getting most of their health information from English-language sources. In addition, 2 out of 5 Latinos reported a preference for general media when having to use media to get information about health and health care; 31% said they prefer Latino-oriented, Spanish-language sources.

Importantly, Latinos' preferences differed by primary language (in the survey, 39% reported being predominately Spanish speaking, 31% were mainly bilingual, and 30% reported speaking primarily English). Latinos who mainly speak Spanish (68%) showed a strong preference for Latino-oriented media as a resource for health information, while those who primarily speak English (88%) or are mostly bilingual (73%) said they prefer to learn about health issues from general market media sources.

On direct comparisons between Black media and general media health coverage, African Americans rated both equally in terms of addressing health issues of *personal* concern but rated Black media much more favorably in terms of addressing health concerns and information needs of Blacks, overall. More than half said Black media do a good job meeting the health information needs of Blacks in this country; fewer than 1 in 3 said the same of the general media. Latinos, however, reported no major differences in ratings of Latino-oriented versus general market media health coverage on any of the specific qual-

Table 26.5
Latino Ratings of General Market versus Latino-Oriented Media Health Coverage

	General Market Media	Latino-Oriented Media	
Doing a good job of telling you and your family what you need to know about health and health care	59	54	$p < .01$
Doing enough stories about the health and health care issues that are most important to you and your family	50	44	$p < .01$
Coverage of important health issues is usually accurate	67	60	$p < .01$
Reporting on health is usually clear and easy to understand	61	56	$p < .01$
Reporting on health usually goes into enough detail	45	44	ns

ns = not statistically significant

ity dimensions (see Table 26.5). On 4 out of 5 measures, ratings of general market media coverage were marginally higher than ratings of Latino-oriented media coverage, consistent with higher reliance on mainstream sources for health information among Latinos overall.

Discussion and Conclusions

The results reported here suggest that a majority of African Americans, Latinos, and Whites are relying heavily on the media compared with other sources for information about health and health care. At the same time, most African Americans and Latinos and many Whites voice a personal interest in *more* information on health and health care topics, and Latinos and African Americans call for *more relevant coverage* of minority health issues by the media. In addition, the surveys reveal important differences among African American, Latinos, and Whites with respect to assessments of media health coverage, particularly in terms of relevancy and credibility of coverage and sources.

African Americans and Latinos reported more regular use of general market versus Black- or Latino-oriented media for all news as well as health information. In addition, they reported a personal preference for general market media when seeking information about health and health care. However, it is important to recognize that Black- and Latino-oriented media sources also figured strongly in these audiences' access to health information and were rated equally high as general media on specific measures of adequacy, level of detail, and personal relevance of health coverage.

Whether reflective of a greater market presence of general media or more health coverage by general market sources, the use and preference of Latinos and African Americans is striking when considered with the finding that Latinos and African Americans found general market media reporting lacking in minority-relevant coverage. African Americans, in particular, criticized general media coverage for a lack of stories on Black health issues; underrepresentation of African Americans in health, business, and lifestyle stories; overrepresentation in stories about crime; and unfair portrayals of health and social issues as "Black problems." Moreover, only a third of African Americans surveyed reported trust of the general market media as a health information source, and strong majorities said that general media direct their coverage to primarily White audiences with inadequate sensitivity to the needs of Blacks and other minorities.

However, these surveys also document the power of mass media as a health information resource, standing out among institutional and interpersonal sources. Mass media are named as the number one provider of health news in the past year as well as being the sought-out source when specific health information is wanted. Still, African Americans, Latinos, and Whites, alike, see room for improvement in the breadth, depth, and regularity of media health coverage and look to the media to provide more information on the health issues of greatest personal and community concern. For African Americans and Latinos, the call for more and better is particularly strong in light of perceived exclusion from general market media coverage while at the same time relying most heavily on these general market sources.

The implications of this study place a heavy burden on both the media and the public health community. The media must recognize their potent role in communicating health information to the public and should strive to offer more coverage of minority health concerns as well as more inclusive treatment of racially diverse audiences in general. The public health community, in turn, has a responsibility to work with the media to educate an increasingly diverse population about health and health care, especially those segments of the population shouldering a disproportionate share of the nations' health concerns. Many opportunities exist for both groups if they accept these challenges. The media will find an attentive audience ready and willing to tune in and seek health coverage while the public health community gains access to dissemination mechanisms that reach far and wide across diverse populations.

Notes

1. The term Latino is used inclusively in this report to refer to U.S. residents who self-identify with the indigenous or Spanish-speaking cultures of Mexico, Puerto Rico, Central America, Cuba, or South America and is used inclusively to refer also to Hispanics of European Spanish origin. The use of this general term is not intended to slight the ethnicity of Latinos who self-identify in relation to country or group of origin or who identify more strongly with Anglo-American culture. African American and Black are used interchangeably to refer to Americans of African or Caribbean descent who self-identify as Black. White American or White is used to represent non-Hispanic White persons who self-identify as White and not of Hispanic origin.
2. A recent example of such an initiative is a 6-issue health improvement strategy commitment of $400 million initiated by the Department of Health and Human Services and the Clinton Administration to eliminate racial and ethnic disparities in health. This initiative emphasizes the critical importance of disseminating minority-relevant health information and highlights the pivotal role of the media in channeling this information to the public (*www.raceandhealth.hhs.gov*).
3. For a comprehensive review of research on representations and portrayals of minorities by the mass media, readers should refer to Greenberg & Brand (1994).
4. Mass media in different markets can vary significantly in content and audience reach. These differences, along with the demographic composition of audiences, have significant bearing on patterns of media utilization as well as assessments of media performance. Presentation of findings from regional subsamples in the Latino study is beyond the scope of this paper but are summarized in "What's the Diagnosis? Latinos, Media and Health," a Kaiser Family Foundation report (1998).
5. The tables reflect precise question wording. Complete survey questionnaires may be obtained by contacting the authors.
6. Question wording: On the Latino survey, adequacy of media coverage of list of health topics was assessed as a follow-up to those respondents saying they wanted more information about the topic on a previous item.
7. African Americans were asked about illnesses affecting Blacks; Latinos were asked about illness affecting Hispanics; Whites were asked about illnesses affecting "people like you").
8. Wording on the general population (GP) survey asked about the general media understanding and meeting the needs of "Blacks, Latinos, and other minorities."

References

Atkin, C. & Arkin, E. B. (1990). Issues and initiatives in communicating health information to the public. In C. Atkin & L. Wallack (Eds.), *Mass communication and public health* (pp. 13–40). Newbury Park, CA: Sage.

Barlow, M. H. (1998). Race and the problem of crime in Time and Newsweek cover stories, 1946 to 1995. *Social Justice, 25*(2), 149 (35). (Summer 1998 issue).

Baker, D. W., Stevens, C. D., & Brook, R. H. (1996). Determinants of emergency department use: Are race and ethnicity important? *Annals of Emergency Medicine, 28,* 677–682.

Bartman, B. A., Moy, E., & D'Angelo, L. J. (1997). Access to ambulatory care for adolescents: The role of a usual source of care. *Journal of Health Care for the Poor and Underserved, 8,* 214–226.

Blendon, R. J., Aiken, L. H., Freeman H. E., & Corey, C. R. (1989). Access to medical care for Black and White Americans. *Journal of the American Medical Association, 261,* 278–281.

Brett, K. M., Schoendorf, K. C. & Kiely, J. L. (1994). Differences between black and white women in the use of prenatal care technologies. *American Journal of Obstetrics and Gynecology, 170,* 41–46.

Brown, J. D., Walsh-Childers, K., & Waszak, C. S. (1990). Television and adolescent sexuality. *Journal of Adolescent Health Care, 11,* 62–70.

Brown, J. D., & Walsh-Childers, K. (1994). Effects of media on personal and public health. In J. Bryant & D. Zillman (Eds.), *Media effects: Advances in theory and research* (pp. 389–415). Hillsdale, NJ: Erlbaum.

Bullough, V. L., & Bullough, B. (1982). *Health care for the other Americans.* New York: Appleton-Century-Crofts.

Carlisle, D. M., Leake, B. D., Brook, R. H., & Shapiro, M. E. (1996). The effect of race and ethnicity on the use of selected health care procedures: A comparison of south central Los Angeles and the remainder of Los Angeles county. *Journal of Health Care for the Poor and Underserved, 7,* 308–322.

Carlisle, D. M., Leake, B. D., & Shapiro, M. F. (1997). Racial and ethnic disparities in the use of cardiovascular procedures: Associations with type of health insurance. *American Journal of Public Health, 87,* 263–267.

Chang, T., Shoemaker, P. J., Reese, S. D., & Danielson, W. A. (1987). Sampling ethnic media use: The case of Hispanics. *Journalism Quarterly, 64*(2), 189–191.

Charlesworth, E., & Hudes, K. (1997). Hispanic market sparks influx, outcry. *Folio: The Magazine for Magazine Management, 26,* 20.

Collins, J. W., & Hawkes, E. S. (1997). Racial differences in post-neonatal mortality in Chicago: What risk factors explain the black infant's disadvantage? *Ethnic Health, 2*(1–2), 117–125.

Culbertson, H. M., & Stempel, G. H. (1995). Media malaise—explaining personal optimism and societal pessimism about health care. *Journal of Communication, 35*(2), 180–190.

Dejong, W., & Winsten, J. A. (1990). The use of mass-media in substance abuse prevention. *Health Affairs, 9*(2), 30–46.

Entman, R. M. (1990). Modern racism and the images of blacks in local television news. *Critical Studies in Mass Communication, 7*(4), 332–345.

Entman, R. M. (1992). Blacks in the news: Television, modern racism and cultural change. *Journalism Quarterly, 69*(2), 341–361.

Entman, R. M. (1994). Representation and reality in the portrayal of blacks on network television news. *Journalism Quarterly, 71*(3), 509–520.

Freeman, G. (1997). Media put a black face on poverty. *St. Louis Journalism Review, 28*(200), 7–8.

Gerbner, G., Gross, L., Morgan, M., & Signorelli, N. (1984). Political correlates of television viewing. *The Public Opinion Quarterly, 48*(1B), 283–300.

Gilens, M. (1996). Race and poverty in America: Public misperceptions and the American news media. *Public Opinion Quarterly, 60*(4), 514–541.

Giles, W. H., Anda, R. F., Casper, M. L., Escobedo, L. G., & Taylor, H. A. (1995). Race and sex differences in rates of invasive cardiac procedures in US hospitals. *Archives Internal Medicine, 155,* 318–324.

Greenberg, B. S., & Brand, J. E. (1994). Minorities and the mass media: 1970s to 1990s. In J. Bryant & D. Zillman, *Media effects: Advances in theory and research* (pp. 273–314). Hillsdale, NJ: Earlbaum.

Grossman, L. (1979). The pattern of organized health care: Non-response to differing health beliefs and behavior. In E. L. Watkins & A. E. Johnson (Eds.), *Removing cultural and ethnic barriers to health care.* Chapel Hill: NC: University of North Carolina Press.

Hayward, R. A., Shapiro, M. F., Freeman, H. E., & Corey, C. R. (1998). Inequities in health services among insured Americans. Do working-age adults have less access to medical care than the elderly? *New England Journal of Medicine, 318,* 1507–1512.

Jeffres, L. W., & Hur, K. K. (1981). Communication channels within ethnic groups. *International Journal of Intercultural Relations, 5*(2), 115–132.

Kaiser Family Foundation. (1998). What's the Diagnosis? Latinos, Media, and Health.

Keil, J. E., Sutherland, S. E., Knapp, R. G., Tyroler, H. A., & Pollitzer, W. S. (1992). Skin color and mortality. *American Journal of Epidemiology, 136*(11), 1295–1302.

Kim, Y. Y. (1989). Intercultural adaptation. In M. K. Asante & W. B. Gudykunst (Eds.), *Handbook of international and intercultural communication* (pp. 275–294). Newbury Park, CA: Sage.

Klaidman, S. (1990). How well the media report health risks. *Daedalus,119*(4), 119–134.

Korzenny, F., Neuendorf, K., Burgoon, M., Burgoon, J. K., & Greenberg, B. S. (1983). Cultural identification as a predictor of content preferences of Hispanics. *Journalism Quarterly, 60*(2), 329–333.

Langkamp, D. L., Foye, H. R., & Roghmann, K. J. (1990). Does limited access to NICU services account for higher neonatal mortality rates among Blacks? *American Journal of Perinatology, 7,* 227–231.

Marin, G, & VanOss Marin, B. (1990). Perceived credibility of channels and sources of AIDS information among Hispanics. *AIDS Education and Prevention, 2*(2), 154–161.

Martindale, C. (1986). *The White press and Black America.* New York: Greenwood.

Mayberry, R. M., Coates, R. J., Hill, H. A., Click, L. A., Chen, V. W., Austin, D. F., Redmond, C. K., Fenoglio-Preiser, C. M., Hunter, C. P., Haynes, M. A., Muss, H. B., Wesley, M. N., Greenberg, R. S., & Edwards, B. K. (1995). Determinants of black/white differences in colon cancer survival. *Journal of the National Cancer Institute, 87,* 1686–1693.

Mayberry, R. M., & Stoddard-Wright, C. (1992). Breast cancer risk factors among black women and white women: Similarities and differences. *American Journal of Epidemiology, 136*(12), 1445–1456.

Meyer, P. (1990). News media responsiveness to public health. In C. Atkin & L. Wallack (Eds.), *Mass communication and public health* (pp. 52–59). Newbury Park, CA: Sage.

Molina, C. W., & Aguirre-Molina, M. (1994). *Latino health in the U.S.: A growing challenge.* Washington, DC: American Public Health Association.

Mort, E. A., Weissman, J. S., & Epstein, A. M. (1994). Physician discretion and racial variation in the use of surgical procedures. *Archives of Internal Medicine, 154,* 761–767.

Nardi, P. M. (1993). *The issue of diversity on prime time television.* Claremont, CA: Pitzer College Press.

Navarrete, L., & Kamasaki, C. (1994). *Out of the picture: Hispanics in the media—State of Hispanic American 1994.* Washington, DC: National Council of La Raza.

Newkirk, P. (1998, March 16). Whitewash in the newsroom: Thirty years after Kerner, the media still reflects biases of white America. *The Nation, 266*(10), 21–25.

Nuell, T. (1998). Blacks turn to black press for credibility. *St. Louis Journalism Review, 28*(204), 1–3.

Oddone, E. Z., Horner, R. D., Diers, T., Lipscomb, J., Mclntyre, L., Cauffman, C, Whittle, J., Passman, L. J., Kroupa, L., Heaney, R., & Matchar, D. (1998). Understanding racial variation in the use of carotid endarterectomy: The role of aversion to surgery. *Journal of the National Medical Association, 90,* 25–33.

Peterson, E. D., Shaw, L. K., DeLong, E. R., Pryor, D. B., Califf, R. M., & Mark, D. B. (1997). Racial variation in the use of coronary-revascularization procedures. Are the differences real? Do they matter? *New England Journal of Medicine, 336,* 480–486.

Pettegrew, L. S., & Logan, R. (1987). The health care context. In C. R. Berger & S. H. Chaffee (Eds.), *Handbook of communication science* (pp. 675–710). Newbury Park, CA: Sage.

Poindexter, P. M., & Stroman, C. (1981). Blacks and television: A review of the research literature. *Journal of Broadcasting, 25*(2), 103–122.

Quiroga, J. (1994). Hispanic voices: Is the press listening? *Havard Journal of Hispanic Policy, 7,* 67–94.

Romer, D., Jamieson, K. H., & de Coteau, N. J. (1998). The treatment of persons of color in local television news: Ethnic blame discourse or realistic group conflict? *Communication Research, 25*(3), 286–306.

Shipler, D. K. (1998). Blacks in the newsroom: progress? Yes, but. . . . *Columbia Journalism Review, 38*(1), 26–34.

Shoemaker, P. J., Reese, S. D., & Danielson, W. A. (1985). Spanish language print media use as an indicator of acculturation. *Journalism Quarterly, 62*(4:), 734–740.

Signorelli, N. (1985). *Role portrayal and stereotyping on television : An annotated bibliography of studies relating to women, minorities, aging, sexual behavior, health and handicaps.* Westport, CT: Greenwood Press.

Sorlie, P., Rogot, E., Anderson, R., Johnson, N. J., & Backlund, E. (1992). Black-white mortality differences by family income. *Lancet, 340*(8815), 346–350.

Stempel, G. H., & Westley, B. H. (1989). *Research methods in mass communication.* Englewood Cliffs, NJ: Prentice-Hall.

Subervi-Vélez, F. A. (1986). The mass media, ethnic assimilation and pluralism: A review and research proposal with special focus on Hispanics. *Communication Research, 13*(1), 71–89.

Subervi-Vélez, F. A. (1994). Mass communication and Hispanics. In F. Padilla, N. Kanellos, & C. Esteva-Fabregat (Eds.), *Handbook of Hispanic cultures in the United States: Sociology* (pp. 304–357). Houston, TX: Arte Publico Press.

Trevino, F. M., Moyer, M. E., Valdez, R. B., & Stroub-Benham, C. A. (1991). Health insurance coverage and utilization of health services by Mexican Americans, mainland Puerto Ricans, and Cuban Americans. *Journal of the American Medical Association, 265,* 233–237.

Turk, J. V., Richard, J., Bryson, R. L., Jr., & Johnson, S. M. (1989). Hispanic Americans in the news in two southwestern cities. *Journalism Quarterly,* 66(1), 107–113.

Wallack, L. (1981). Mass media campaigns: The odds against finding behavior change. *Health Education Quarterly, 8,* 209–260.

Wallack, L. (1990). Mass media and health promotion: Promise, problem, and challenge. In C. Atkin & L. Wallack (Eds.), *Mass communication and public health* (pp. 41–51). Newbury Park, CA: Sage.

Wilson, C. C., & Gutierrez, F. (1995). *Race, multiculturalism, and the media: From mass to class communication* (2nd ed.). Thousand Oaks, CA: Sage.

Winett, L. B., & Wallack, L. (1996). Advancing public health goals through the mass media. *Journal of Health Communication, 7*(3), 173–196.

Winsten, J. A. (1985). Science and the media: The boundaries of truth. *Health Affairs, 4*(1) 5–23

Witte, K. (1992). Preventing AIDS through persuasive communications: A framework for constructing effective culturally specific health messages. In F. Korzenny & S. Ting-Toomey (Eds.), *Mass media effects across cultures* (pp. 67–86). Newbury Park, CA: Sage.

Worsley, A. (1989). Perceived reliability of sources

of health information. *Health Education Research, 49*(3), 367.

Discussion Questions

1. The research presented in this chapter found that many people prefer the media as a source of health information and receive much of their information about health from the media. However, they do not believe the media is highly trustworthy. What are some possible explanations for this contradiction?
2. To what degree should the media be responsible for providing health information and to what audiences?
3. What are some ways that the public health community and mass media could work together to educate diverse communities on health care? ✦

A Final Word

Framing the Future of Health Communication

Linda C. Lederman, Marianne LeGreco, Tara J. Schuwerk, and Emily T. Cripe

Health communication is a complex and multi-faceted endeavor, and *Beyond These Walls* has included chapters that illustrate how the field of health communication has changed and continues to change. Now we reflect a bit beyond the materials covered in this reader. In this final word, we want to focus on the variety of topics, epistemological positions, and methodologies that in all likelihood will frame the future of health communication scholarship and practice. We realize that communication about health reaches us across a number of levels—from institutions to individuals, from macro-discourses (i.e., large social narratives and institutionalized ways of thinking, like capitalism and democracy) to micro-practices (i.e., personal behaviors, like the foods you choose to eat). As such, we have chosen to organize this chapter both topically and methodologically.

First, we will consider some of the larger structural issues at play in the future of health communication. By looking at important institutions, social discourses, and policies involved in the construction and delivery of health, we attend to the macro side of topics that link health and communication. Second, we will examine some of the less formal features that remain vital to the study of health communication. With a focus on topics like health disparities, alternative medicine, and stigmatized diseases, we hope to illustrate the micro-processes in need of further study. Finally, we conclude with some reflections on the methods used to study health topics both now and in the future. Given the proliferation of methods used to examine the role of communication in health issues, we see an increasingly significant role that researchers will play by doing critical/interpretive and participatory research. We also see an even stronger emphasis than already exists on applied projects that reach a wide array of individuals, groups, and institutions.

Scaling New Walls

Although *Beyond These Walls* encourages the reader to explore communication beyond the walls of traditional health-care research and delivery, there are still important structural elements to consider as we think about what the future holds. The future of health communication will develop more sophisticated understandings of the complex processes and practices that construct major health institutions, policies that guide health initiatives, and macro-discourses of health and wellness.

Social and medical institutions including managed care, the American Medical Association, and the U.S. Department of Agriculture play significant parts in the construction of health. These institutions provide health producers and consumers with rules and resources used to structure health-care interactions. In Chapter 2 of this reader, for example, Katherine Miller and Daniel Ryan illustrate the organizational and health concerns that communication scholars must address when working within a system of managed care. With the advent of institutions such as health maintenance organizations (HMOs) and preferred provider organizations (PPOs), communication about health has changed in structurally significant ways. Managed care organizations have altered interpersonal relationships between doctors and patients, organizational relationships between hospitals and insurance providers, and governmental relationships between health legislators and health citizens. Thus, promoting research that examines the structures that ensure goals like cost-effectiveness and patient satisfaction will be an important part of understanding these systems. We see this development as increasingly apparent over time.

In addition to managed care organizations, there are a variety of other important social and medical institutions that communication scholars will consider. Of particular interest to communication should be the relatively understudied institutions of Medicare and Medicaid. These government institutions construct how health should be conceptualized, delivered and evaluated for millions of senior citizens and the economically disadvantaged. In her analysis of Medicaid and managed care organizations, Gillespie (2001) argued that an emphasis on rationality and procedure contributed to the further marginalization of asthma patients in the Medicaid system. Therefore, it is important to illustrate the ways in which health-care institutions might reproduce the health disparities that they attempt to overcome. Moreover, while Gillespie examined practices and procedures within the Medicaid system, she stopped short of comparing experiences across social insurance and social assistance programs. Social insurance programs, such as Medicare and Social Security, are contribution-based programs. Usually, a portion of our paychecks goes to fund social insurance programs on the good faith that funds will be available when we retire to pay for things like health care and even prescription medications. Social assistance programs, by contrast, are means-based programs such as Medicaid or Temporary Assistance for Needy Families. These programs are in place for those individuals, primarily women and children, who cannot afford them otherwise. In his comparison of these programs, Soss (2002) documented the differences in interview procedures, case worker relationships, and stigmas between Medicare and Medicaid. Specifically, because of the conditions of participation, recipients of social insurance programs are treated with greater respect and dignity than recipients of social assistance programs.

Managed care, Medicare, and Medicaid represent only a handful of key institutions to which communication scholars must pay greater attention. Scholars in other fields such as nutrition and public health policy have examined communication phenomena including nutrition messages and external communication with regard to institutions. For example, Nestle's (2002) critique of the USDA Food Pyramid illustrated how discourses that encourage us to "Eat More" and "Eat Less" have actually contributed to the growing obesity epidemic in the United States. Additionally, in his analysis of health-based interest groups, the AMA in particular, Peterson (2001) used concepts such as rhetoric of commitment, trust, and power to explain how interest groups protect their own economic self-interests. Ultimately, these institutions raise important communication questions for us to examine with greater complexity.

One way to study these institutions with greater depth and sophistication in the future is to consider the role that policy plays in organizing and implementing health practices. Policy has been conceptualized as the documented posture that an organization takes in order to communicate the rules and resources available to consumers (Peterson & Albrecht, 1999). As Trethewey, Scott, & LeGreco (2006) clarified, "Policies pertaining to health insurance, workers' compensation, and parental leave provide employees with a framework to interpret their experiences when they fall ill, get hurt, or choose to have children" (p.136). Although most individuals encounter some sort of health-related policy over the course of their lives, the topic of *policy* remains relatively understudied in communication at this time. The small body of communication research about policy has focused on topics like work-family policy (e.g., Buzzanell & Liu, 2005; Kirby & Krone, 2002; Peterson & Albrecht, 1999) or organizational influences on public health policy (Conrad, 2004; Conrad & McIntush, 2003). At the same time, the majority of these studies give policy a secondary status, favoring concepts like public/private and strategic rhetoric.

The study of policy holds great promise for communication scholars, particularly those interested in the organization of health practice. Individuals negotiate a variety of health-related decisions based on their relationship to specific health policies. For example, the Dietary Guidelines for

Americans is a federal policy that provides citizens with updated nutrition information every five years. This policy provides the basis for health promotional materials including the USDA My Pyramid, as well as state and local nutrition policies for public schools. Additionally, Petronio's (2005) work on HIPAA and the policy of privacy offers another example of how consumers establish and manage boundaries in health-care relationships. Other policies such as employment-based health insurance, worker's compensation, and family leave, construct the relationship between organizations and individuals with regard to specific health states, risks, and outcomes. Thus, communication scholars are increasingly likely to examine how health policies are formulated through dialogue and deliberation, negotiated between producer and consumer, and resisted in everyday health communication practices.

Finally, the future of health communication will consider macro-discourses of health and wellness that incorporate trans-disciplinary perspectives and multi-methodological approaches. Communication scholars can make significant contributions to our understanding of health by illustrating how macro-discourses influence health-care decision making, stage health-care interactions, and reproduce health disparities across populations. In part, this trend has already begun as health communication researchers have sought external funding for their grants. Not only have researchers such as Parrott and Lemieux (2003) addressed health issues such as skin cancer, but also health communication researchers like Lederman and Stewart (2005) have sought and won funding from federal agencies, such as National Institute of Drug Abuse (NIDA) and U.S. Department of Education (DoE) to address alcohol abuse in college students by working in trans-disciplinary teams with psychologists, sociologists, and alcohol researchers. Federal, state, and local funding agencies, as well as special interest foundations that have supported health communication research, are funding trans-disciplinary research in increasing numbers. As federal agencies, such as the National Institutes for Health (NIH), the National Institute for Drug Abuse (NIDA), and the National Institute for Alcoholism and Alcohol Abuse (NIAAA), give preference in funding to trans-disciplinary projects, the future of health communication will progressively be comprised of cross-disciplinary approaches to health issues. Thus, these funding agencies and others like them will have an increasing role in shaping health communication and the directions of health communication research in the years to come. And given the emphasis placed by those funding agencies on trans-disciplinarity, it is most likely that the future of health communication will be characterized by widespread interdisciplinary teams working together across areas of specialization on funded research projects.

Myriad discourses could play out in this trans-disciplinary arena, and we offer the following three as examples: consumption, technology, and innovation. First, the topic of consumption grows out of a re-examination of the communicative-role relationship between doctors and patients. Historically, discourses of paternalism dominated most discussions of health and wellness (Conrad & McIntush, 2003; Longest, 2002; Patel & Rushefsky, 1999). Because most health information is controlled by gatekeepers, including doctors, policy makers, and health-care organizations, paternalistic discourses suggest that health decisions should be made by the individuals and institutions with the most information. In other words, we should all listen to our doctors because they know what is best for us. Critiques of paternalism in health systems, such as Foucault's (1975) theorizing on the "expert gaze" of medical experience, indicate that access to privileged knowledge reproduces our dependence on authorities to decipher complicated health information. Recently, discourses of consumption have begun to play a prevalent role in empowering the consumers of health information.

Discourses of consumption suggest that individual consumers have agency, or the capacity to make a difference, in their ability to make artifacts, practices, and discourses meaningful (Du Gay, Hall, Janes, Mackay, & Negus, 1997). In other words, the doctor can give a patient all the advice he or she wants; however, this advice will not be meaningful until the patient (the consumer) makes it so. As we have developed more nuanced understandings of human agency and the unintended consequences of hoarding health information in hospital records and doctors' brains, some health scholars have called for more consumer-based models of healthcare (Kreps, 2006). By emphasizing the consumer and the role that he or she plays in the access and application of health information, health communication will consider insights and needs from multiple and trans-disciplinary perspectives, including communication, psychology, information systems, media literacy, as well as the individuals and groups who are served.

A significant development in consumer-oriented health-care delivery involves the implementation of electronic medical records. Hospitals and clinics have begun to experiment with electronic medical records as a way to coordinate healthcare across sites and allow consumers access to their health information (Rosati & Harris-Salamone, 2006). This example illustrates the macro-discourses of technology that will continue to change in relation to the future of health communication. Moreover, this example also highlights the trans-disciplinary perspectives, including those from health-care providers and information systems, which inform how we use health information. Online access to health information via websites, including WebMD and MDChoice, has created new communication possibilities and problems as individuals are allowed to participate more fully in the management of their health. Discourses of technology emphasize the promise that the Internet, electronic medical records, and other advancements hold. At the same time, these discourses both enable and constrain individuals who might or might not want to become more proactive with their health. Concerns like the digital divide and health literacy are still very real, and their communication implications are an important part of the future agenda of health communication that will be examined as technology continues to progress.

Technological progress is also a major feature of discourses of innovation. Ever since Rogers' (1962/2003) publication of *Diffusion of Innovations,* discourses of innovation have been an important part of health communication. In the present and future, innovation will continue to play a major role in communication research, now from more trans-disciplinary perspectives. In a recent special issue of *The Journal of Health Communication,* Scott Ratzan (2004) assembled multiple essays on the diffusion of innovations theory and its significance to communication. Contributors ranged from university professors in communication and public health to non-profit organizations to Everett Rogers himself. This special issue demonstrated how the concept of innovation has become a lucrative idea across disciplines that deal with health issues. Another example is the nation's first Master's Program in Health Innovation. This program, recently launched by Arizona State University's College of Nursing, is a multidisciplinary endeavor between the schools of nursing, communication, and health policy and administration. These examples illustrate how studies in innovation and change have already begun and will continue to frame the future of health communication as a trans-disciplinary enterprise. Discourses of innovation remind us that health is not a fixed concept or state of being. Rather, new developments in science and technology, information systems, and relational communication will raise new communication questions for us to address using a variety of perspectives.

From this more structural, macro-oriented perspective on health communication's future, it is apparent that topics like formal institutions, public health policy, and innovation elicit intriguing challenges for communication scholars. As we move beyond the walls of traditional health communication scholarship and practice, health communication researchers will also continue to examine the ways in which these formal features frame health-care interactions. At the same time, the future of health communication will include looking beyond the institutions and formal rules of health communication to illustrate how health is negotiated culturally and what health alternatives are available.

Bridging New Cultures

Just as the future of health will pay greater attention to the macro-features of communication, scholars will also address the micro-practices of health that often manifest culturally. For example, in their analysis of personal responsibility in health campaigns, Guttman and Ressler (2001) noted that culture often enables and constrains our ability to pursue health. More specifically, it is difficult to blame an individual for failing to eat more fruits and vegetables, especially when those foods are not readily available in that individual's neighborhood. Within these culturally specific spaces, health communication scholars can make great contributions to the study of disadvantaged populations, health-care disparities, practices of resistance, and alternative approaches. To make such advances, the future of health communication is likely to focus on the role of culture in constituting health, the health disparities faced across numerous populations, and alternative approaches to both medicine and health promotion.

Cultures and minorities. Racial and ethnic minorities currently comprise approximately 35% of the population and will comprise about 50% of the population of the U.S. by 2050 (U.S. Census Bureau, 2004). Co-cultural diversity will increasingly bring fresh, new ideas, perspectives, and energy to the United States. Cultures define health differently, and individual cultures outline what health means for their members. The idea of culture "determines the etiology of diseases, establishes the parameters within which distress is defined and signaled, and prescribes the appropriate means to treat the disorder, both medically and socially" (Kagawa-Singer & Kassim-Lakha, 2003, p. 578). Health communication research has not been blind to the role that culture plays in constituting health-care interactions and health outcomes, as seen in Chapter 22 and Chapter 26. Research has focused most explicitly on discussions of race and ethnicity. Indeed, scholars have recently become more inclusive of different ages, sexual orientations, and genders in health communication research, as seen throughout this text. As encounters between people from different cultures become more frequent in health settings, health communication is likely to address the explicit link between culture and health. As health communication researchers, we have the opportunity to reduce potential cross-cultural miscommunication and to generate knowledge that is and will continue to be more applicable to the multi-cultural society in which we live. Approaching health communication research within a context of culture will allow us the potential to improve health outcomes across a variety of populations.

Although some scholarship has seriously considered the role of culture in constituting health, both communication scholars and those outside our discipline will begin to incorporate greater diversity in terms of topics and research participants. Many of the studies conducted in both clinical and social settings have used white males as a research base. As such, these researchers have developed nuanced understandings of conditions like sexual dysfunction and heart disease in males; however, we have developed less-than-stellar understandings of similar conditions in their female counterparts. Our future will demand new strategies of health-care interaction and delivery that manage cultural diversity in both clinical encounters between providers and patients and public health initiatives designed for specific communities.

Responsive health care will require competent communication among all involved: the provider, client, family, community, and nation. Culture is an undeniably important factor in communication (Martin & Nakayama, 2004) and Tseng (2004) posits that:

> Communication between the healer and the client is one of the most crucial aspects of therapeutic work. This is particularly true in intercultural therapy, in which the therapist and the patient do not share the same language or culture . . . a caution is needed even when the therapist and the patient share a common language, because the meanings behind words and the values embedded in language need careful attention and clarification, and may vary from one person to another. (p.153)

The importance of communication in these clinical settings in increasingly noteworthy. Each client has a different background, and each encounter has its own context. While the current research already notes that it is vital for practitioners to not only understand the intricacies of different cultures (Arthur, Chan, Fung, Wong, & Yeung, 1999), but to be interculturally competent communicators. In the future, these intercultural challenges will become increasingly incorporated into health communication.

To illustrate this point, consider the assertion by Singh, McKay, & Singh (1998) that "mental health professionals need to understand the cultural context of communication because it provides the basis for understanding and appreciating the behavior of people seeking mental health services" (p.404). In other words, classifications of "mentally ill" and "mentally well," as well as standards for treatment, are often culturally prescribed. Therefore, effective communication about health cannot commence without a detailed understanding of the cultural rules and resources that often abide by the structural rules and resources. Mental health, in particular, provides an intriguing context within which to study the influence of culture on health-care interactions and outcomes. By focusing on health disparities, such as those that surface in mental health cases, communication scholars can direct the future of health in more inclusive and democratic ways.

The U.S. Department of Health and Human Services, DHHS, (2001b) note that co-cultural contributions:

> Like those of all [U.S.] Americans rest on a foundation of mental health. Mental health is fundamental to overall health and productivity. It is the basis for successful contributions to family, community, and society. Throughout the lifespan, mental health is the wellspring of thinking and communication skills, learning, resilience, and self esteem. (p.11)

About 21% percent of adults and children in the United States have a mental disorder (DHHS, 1999). According to DHHS (2001a), based on available research, the occurrence of mental disorders among co-cultures living in the community is at least similar to the prevalence among the dominant culture (whites). Although clinical trials have been used to create treatment guidelines for several mental disorders, an investigation conducted for the Surgeon General (DHHS, 2001a) discovered that the researchers conducting these trials did not perform any specific analyses for any racial or ethnic co-cultural group.

Current research supports the argument that many disparities exist in mental healthcare between the dominant culture and co-cultures within the United States (DHHS, 2001a). The major disparities co-cultures face, reported by DHHS (2001a), are underrepresentation in mental health research, less access to and availability of mental health services, less likelihood of receiving needed mental health services, and receipt of poorer quality mental healthcare. For example, Arthur et al. (1999) indicate that mental health nurses are often trained and educated on "western" theories and strategies using Eurocentric communication. This is a perfect illustration of a situation that could be aided by solid health communication research of mental health and culture. Another example might be taken from the personal experiences of a graduate student. According to Michael Uvanile, a clinical psychology graduate student at Nova Southeastern University, students of psychodynamic psychotherapy take only one specialized class in multicultural psychology to earn their Doctor of Psychology degree (personal communication, October 21, 2006). Feminist and minority perspectives have only been recently introduced into the remaining coursework. The rest of their concepts and methodology course-load is mainly based on upper-middle class Northern European males. Uvanile also explains that in the past, practitioners had not been trained much about the culture of the minorities they would be working with, and they were usually too overloaded to research the cultural nuances of their clients once they entered the field. He explains, "this is extremely important. If a person makes a joke, you have to be paying attention to their culture to know what type of emotion is being expressed. The difference between true humor and a display of anger or despair can make all the difference."

The disparities in knowledge, access, utilization, and quality of mental healthcare (DHHS, 2001a) for racial and ethnic co-cultures are also devastating. In addition to these obstacles, co-cultures also contend with racism, discrimination, mistrust, fear of treatment, language barriers, and differences in communication (DHHS, 2001a). When the history of racial and ethnic discrimination is added to the disparities previously mentioned, miscommunication could lead to misdiagnosis, inappropriate treatment, mistrust, and the deepening of mental illness, which could possibly lead to death. Even though the problem of disparities is currently being addressed by the office of the Surgeon General, it is clear that health communication researchers need to address this issue as well, especially since disparities related to communication have been specifically identified.

In light of the fact that all of the proposed solutions to the existing disparities require competent communication at some level, especially between practitioner and client, it seems odd that this aspect has not been studied in depth. This affects not only mental health, but other health conditions including obesity, heart disease, diabetes, HIV/AIDS, and alcoholism, in which it is apparent that further communication-based research on health disparities is needed. By concentrating on communication for underserved populations, such as racial and ethnic minorities, women and children, and the elderly, health communication researchers will provide the research needed to not only further the discipline, but also to aid those in our society who are in need. In the current literature on alcoholism, for example, it has been found that senior citizens are both the most at risk and yet the most underreported segment of the population suffering from alcoholism (Lederman, Stewart, & Kully, 2001). In fact, Lederman (2006) refers to alcoholism among senior citizens as the silent epidemic. By paying careful attention to culture and health disparities among segments of the population as we move forward, we may be able to avoid backtracking to understand the important role that culture plays in constructing who is and who is not healthy. We will also be able to address the power imbalances reflected in the importance placed on one individual's health over another's. This issue raises itself both in the selection of those who receive vital health care, such as organ transplants, and populations for whom funding is more readily available for research.

Alternative Medicine

With an increased focus on culture, the future of health communication will continue to explore options other than those offered by Western medicine and biomedical perspectives of health. These perspectives have traditionally dominated the field of health in both clinical and social settings. Recently, however, researchers and practitioners have started to place an emphasis on alternative approaches to health. Both alternative medicine, sometimes called *holistic* or *complementary* medicine, and new approaches to health promotion have generated communication phenomena in need of greater attention. We consider each of these alternative approaches in turn.

Alternative medicine is not a new fad (Udani, 1998), and Eisenberg et al. (1998) report that visits to alternative medicine practitioners in the late 1990s increased from earlier that decade by 47.3%, with approximately 629 million visits in 1997. This number exceeds the total visits to all primary care physicians in the United States during the same year. Similarly, the budget for the National Institute of Health's National Center for Complementary and Alternative Medicine increased from $50 million in 1999 to $122.7 million in 2006 (National Institute of Health, 2006). Taking this into consideration, as well as the fact that people are using alternative medicines and spending increasingly more money on holistic approaches (Eisenberg et al., 1998), it is surprising that the health communication research on the topic has been so limited until now.

This statement does not discount the fact that some communication research is being done. Ho (2003), for example, is looking into holistic medicine using discourse analysis, or the study of language used by a specific community. The analysis included printed material available at a holistic health fair and identified discourses that create distinctive forms of legitimate health care. Unfortunately, Ho's research is an exception to the norm, and too few communication scholars have engaged holistic therapies despite their growing popularity in the United States.

The health communication literature, as it stands, tends to focus on the biomedical approaches that are prevalent within the dominant culture of the United States. Schreiber (2005) deftly points out that if we are to understand both healthcare and communication in the U.S., all the medical practices and systems should be considered. "Given that the discipline is committed to equality and listening to voices from the margins, research on holistic medicine . . . must be addressed in its own right" (Schreiber, 2005, p.174). Going deeper into the subcategories of alternative medicine, as listed in Schreiber's article (2005), research in health communication will reflect developments in alternative therapies. Food, diet, and vitamin therapies, such as nutritional supplements or fasting, could be studied taking into account how to communicate information about them to members of diverse cultural backgrounds. Exercise and movement therapies such as yoga and Tai Chi already enjoy some familiarity in the United States, but the benefits of these forms of exercise may not be widely shared. Health communication research might again enlighten others to this possibility for improving or maintaining health. In addition to specific therapies, we can also capitalize on health communication research opportunities in alternative systems of medicines. Several examples might include African medicine, Ayurvedic medicine, Chinese medicine, Islamic medicine, and Native American medicine. Health communication research concerning many of these therapies is desperately needed as the U.S. population and the rest of the world continue to look for alternatives to biomedical approaches.

Alternative approaches to health care hold great promise with numerous possibilities for health communication research. Schreiber (2005) notes that, "patient education and public health campaigns, mass mediated messages, consumer satisfaction and compliance, cultural differences, the illness experience, and spirituality and healing as they relate to holistic medicine are also ripe areas of study from a communication perspective" (p. 174). As such, future health communication scholarship and practice will also consider alternative approaches to health promotion. These new strategies for health promotion often take an innovative spin on traditional public health campaigns and mediated messages by promoting increased participation and awareness on the part of the consumer.

Health Promotion

Along with patient/provider communication, the topic of health promotion accounts for a significant portion of health communication research. The design of messages that prompt predictable behaviors has long interested health communication scholars (Murray-Johnson & Witte, 2000). Research has spotlighted such health issues as smoking and drug prevention (Borland, 1997; Hahn, Simpson, & Kidd, 1996; Hawkins & Hane, 2000; Stephenson et al., 1999), HIV awareness (Singhal & Rogers, 2000; Witte, 1992), alcohol abuse prevention (Lederman, 1993; Lederman and Stewart, 2005) and reproductive health (Meyerowitz & Chaiken, 1987; Morman, 2000). The majority of this research has focused on specific features in the design of a message such as persuasive fear appeals and uncertainty reduction. Furthermore, much of this research has limited its scope to commercial advertisements, public service announcements, and some community outreach programs. More recent research, particularly from organizational perspectives, has emphasized additional features important in the design of health promotion messages. These alternatives to television campaigns and public service announcements can be seen in the rise of workplace health promotion.

Workplaces have made health promotion part of their business. Organizations realize that healthy workers mean more productive workers; therefore, some workplaces have begun to implement wellness programs, onsite fitness centers, and health counseling as part of the average workday (Farrell & Geist-Martin, 2005; Zoller, 2003a, 2003b). As workplace health promotion programs become more prevalent in contemporary organizations, health communication scholars will continue to examine workplaces as alternatives to traditional media in the dissemination of health information. Considering that we spend a significant portion of our days at work, the use of workplace health promotion programs could have a considerable influence on how we construct and encourage individual health practices.

Other health campaigns have addressed environmental management issues such as college campuses and the impact of the environment on college drinking. As illustrated in Chapter 20, Lederman and Stewart (2005) have focused on the role of language in creating such a cultural environment and the need to bring interpersonal interaction and intervention into the cultural discourse to change the culture of college drinking. Likewise, Yanovitzky, Stewart, and Lederman (2006) have worked to identify variables associated with campaign effectiveness.

Stigmatized Illness

One last area that we see changing as more health communication researchers address an increasingly wide range of health issues is the role of communication in stigmatized diseases. While much research has been done in this area to date on HIV/AIDS, more will be done. The arena in which communication scholars have only begun to examine the role of health communication is in alcoholism and drug dependency. Literature that is sorely lacking in health communication research concerns the interface between family communication and issues of chronic and stigmatized diseases, such as alcoholism. The literature on alcoholism recognizes it as a family disease and the self-help literature is filled with common wisdom on the impact of alcoholism on family members. Health communication scholars are beginning to address the study of these topics, and a likely trend of the future is more cross disciplinary work in addressing issues such as alcoholism, a disease that affects 1 in every 10 Americans today. Attention to these new directions will give rise to new trends regarding how we do research. As such, we will finally consider some of the emerging trends in our approaches to research.

Charting New Research

Research in health communication has traditionally reflected the scientific approach that focuses on controlling the variables that produce predictable health outcomes. Increasingly, however, health communication researchers are using rhetorical methods, interpretive and ethnographic research, critical perspectives, and participatory methods. These methodologies allow for researchers to access the lived experiences of practitioners and patients in a wide variety of contexts. Furthermore, they have helped move health communication beyond the hospital or physician's office and into the everyday realms where health practices are shaped. The walls between them are blurry. Researchers will often utilize a critical perspective while conducting ethnographic research, but in whatever combination, they represent important directions in which health communication scholarship is moving. We see these trends continuing, as they have shaped our understandings in different ways through the variety of reporting styles used and the different kinds of data collected.

Rhetorical Studies

Health rhetoricians thus far have focused on political discourse about health communication, controversy over health-related issues such as the abortion debate or euthanasia, and media coverage of health. However, in the future we see them moving to broader analyses of the various discourses of health in society. For instance, as patients and providers increasingly communicate electronically via email and other media, rhetorical analyses will help us to understand how these media affect interactions and relationships. In addition to examining the new directions mentioned earlier in this chapter, such as new health technologies and modes of health communication, rhetorical scholars will expand research into discourses of health among specific communities. By gaining a greater understanding about the ways health can be rhetorically shaped and constituted, we will learn new or better ways of communicating about health.

Interpretive/Ethnographic Research

Interpretive and ethnographic work in health communication has helped researchers to better understand how health functions in multiple settings and as a layered practice, involving teamwork, complex interactions, and sometimes power struggles (e.g., Ellingson in Chapter 14). Additionally, narrative reports of ethnographic research (e.g., Hirschmann in Chapter 6) provide us with unique insights into researchers' (and participants') experiences. Geist and Gates (1996), for instance, discuss important issues in recovering patient identities through a narrative of one of the authors' own experiences in a health-care setting. Hearing more direct patient and participant voices, such as in these examples, is an important and growing trend in health communication research.

Communication researchers are reflecting more critically about issues such as patient voice, and will likely continue to do so in the future. This shift is particularly important, for as Geist and Gates (1996) discuss, there is a "crisis of representation" in health care where patients' voices are lost. They argue that "the 'science-ing' (of our research, our medicine, our lives) is silencing in the sense that it marginalizes aspects of our identities that we attempt to incorporate in our interactions with others" (p. 219-220). Possessing an expanded understanding of patients' lives could facilitate helping other patients to understand the ways they may be affected by a procedure besides the obvious side effects. At the same time, patients can learn that their experiences are not abnormal, thus improving communication about health. Shifts towards understanding how patients live with diseases and illness, as well as how others within their social networks are affected, will be an important direction to take.

Critical Approaches

Lupton (1994) and others have called for greater critical inquiry into health communication. While that call is starting to be answered, there is still much that health communication scholars can and will continue to contribute to our critical understanding of health discourses. Critical approaches can ask important questions that might change the ways we see, do, and practice health. For instance, thus far critical scholars in health communication have examined issues with physician socialization and stress, women in medicine, minority groups and cultural understandings of health, and patient empowerment. Critical approaches can be insightful methods for looking at health communication because of the personal nature of health care and the inherent issues of power and politics associated with health care and health problems, and as researchers continue to increasingly adopt critical frames when looking at health issues (especially as health and health policy changes rapidly) our understanding and careful consideration of all of the issues entailed by health practices will be greatly enriched.

Participatory Research Methods

Participatory research methods have helped to bring health communication research into communities directly affected by it. Using participatory methods involves inviting research participants to contribute to the research process. Researchers can incorporate participant voices by asking them to identify the problems that they face, aid in analyzing data, check researcher interpretations, and formulate solutions to their problems right there in the field. Participatory research can also involve asking participants to co-create health campaigns that would be more effective in reaching members of their community. Zoller's (2005) discussion of health activism provides scholars with a useful theoretical approach to assisting in the development of more health campaigns and greater public involvement in health issues.

By working within communities, not only do researchers gain greater stakeholder participation in health campaigns, but those campaigns also end up being ultimately more effective because they are tailored to the people they are designed to target. Additionally, stakeholders are invested in the campaign and its success. Looking at broader communities and cultures through more participatory methods is also a growing focus among some researchers. For instance, Dutta-Bergman (2004) conducted ethnographic research among the Santalis in rural Bengal. By focusing on the local culture and interpretations of members, both the researcher and participants identified discourses of resistance and revolution. Dutta-Bergman's research concluded that agency, a characteristic often located in community members themselves, is necessary for improved health outcomes. These results provide further support for other researchers who wish to do similar research (in addition to emphasizing the necessity of doing such research in the first place).

On a slightly more micro-level, studying the families and social systems that have an impact on individual health (e.g., informal networks such as the play group discussed by Tardy and Hale in Chapter 16) is crucial to understanding how health practices play out in everyday life. For instance, physicians can advise patients who are diabetic, have heart conditions, or have high blood pressure to change their diet. However, if that change means eating differently from the rest of their family, or giving up foods with important cultural significance, there is a considerable chance that patients will not comply and will end up back in their doctor's offices months later with the condition worsened. However, to study how to fix these problems, patients' experiences must be sought, and the entire family or community system needs to be studied and understood first. One example of this is DeSantis' (2002) study of cigar shop customers and culture, which revealed patrons' collectively developed pro-smoking beliefs and messages. Understanding these beliefs is essential if, for instance, a health campaign is to reach these participants. Health communication researchers will continue to expand their research into broader, disparate contexts affecting health, and this kind of research can improve health-care experiences for patients and providers alike.

Methods of Representation

Finally, and perhaps most importantly, health communication scholars are starting to and will continue to make their research more accessible to wider ranges of audiences through publication in non-traditional outlets (e.g., magazines and other publications). For instance, Lynn Harter and her colleagues' work with Passion Works is an example of this innovative approach to sharing our research (Harter, Scott, Novak, Leeman, and Morris, 2006). Passion Works is an organization that provides creative opportunities for people with and without recognized disabilities to collaborate on artistic works. In terms of communication research, Harter and her colleagues' work has included creating documents for this organization, such as fliers with stories of participant experiences developed from fieldnotes in addition to publishing their results in more scholarly outlets. This serves both as a way of giving back to the community participants and as a form of research report, which is accessible and useful to people beyond communication scholars. By making our work more accessible (i.e., publishing in alternative outlets), we can broaden both the conversations we are having and the impact of our research. Researchers will hopefully continue this trend to increase the impact of our scholarship and enrich the conversations we have about our research. Hopefully, one day soon it will not be at all uncommon for health communication research to be reported widely, so that patients in waiting rooms may find themselves flipping through a popular magazine and reading about ways that they can communicate with their provider more effectively. As Goodall (2004) notes, if we fail to communicate our research in ways that reach out to the populations to which it is relevant, then we end up simply talking to each other. This deprives health consumers of the valuable knowledge that they often need much more than we do.

A Final Word

Health communication began in the early 1980s, and the first journal dedicated to health communication matters has recently published its 75th issue. While much has changed over that time, the trends we see happening suggest a burgeoning of change during the next 20 years. Theories have begun to drive more work in health communication, and it is likely that the years to come will see the emergence of theory-building in health communication. As researchers such as Cline (2003) examine conversations about health in everyday life and others such as Floyd (2006) examine the impact of expressions of affection on cortisol levels, we see the vastness of the landscape for health communication that exists outside those walls that once separated it from much of the world beyond. Those of us contributing to this area of study have new vistas, and this volume, *Beyond These Walls,* has been compiled to contribute to the growing need to examine the role of communication in health issues across and beyond the foci of its origins.

References

Arthur, D., Chan, H. K., Fung, W. Y., Wong, K. Y., & Yeung, K. W. (1999). Therapeutic communication strategies used by Hong Kong mental health nurses with their Chinese clients. *Journal of Psychiatric and Mental Health Nursing, 6,* 29–36.

Borland, R. (1997). Tobacco health warnings and smoking-related cognitions and behaviours. *Addiction, 92,* 1427–1435.

Buzzanell, P. M., & Liu, M. (2005). Struggling with maternity leave policies and practices: A poststructuralist feminist analysis of gendered organizing. *Journal of Applied Communication Research, 33,* 1–25.

Cline, R. J. (2003). Everyday interpersonal communication and health. In T. L. Thompson, A. M. Dorsey, K. I. Miller, & R. Parrott (Eds.), *Handbook of health communication* (pp. 285–313). Mahwah, NJ: Lawrence Erlbaum Associates, Inc.

Conrad, C. (2004). Organizational discourse analysis: Avoiding the determinism-volunteerism trap. *Organization, 11,* 427–439.

Conrad, C., & McIntush, H. G. (2003). Organizational rhetoric and healthcare policymaking. In T. L. Thompson, A. M. Dorsey, K. I. Miller, R. Parrott (Eds.) *Handbook of health communication* (pp. 403–443). Mahwah, NJ: Lawrence Erlbaum Associates.

DeSantis, A. D. (2002). Smoke screen: An ethnographic study of a cigar shop's collective rationalization. *Health Communication. 14,* 167–198.

Du Gay, P., Hall, S., Janes, L., Mackay, H., & Negus, K. (1997). *Doing cultural studies: The story of the Sony Walkman.* Thousand Oaks, CA: Sage Publications.

Dutta-Bergman, M. J. (2004). The unheard voices of Santalis: Communicating about health from the margins of India. *Communication Theory, 14,* 237–263.

Eisenberg, D. M., Davis, R. B., Ettner, S. L., Appel, S.,Wilkey, S., Van Rompay, M., & Kessler, R. C. (1998). Trends in alternative medicine use in the United States, 1990–1997: Results of a national follow-up study. *Journal of the American Medical Association, 280,* 1569–1575.

Geist, P., & Gates, L. (1996). The poetics and politics of re-covering identities in health communication. *Communication Studies, 47,* 218–228.

Gillespie, S. R. (2001). The politics of breathing: Asthmatic Medicaid patients under managed care. *Journal of Applied Communication Research, 29,* 97–116.

Goodall, H. L., Jr. (2004). Narrative ethnography as applied communication research. *Journal of Applied Communication Research, 32,* 185–194.

Guttman, N., & Ressler, W. (2001). On being responsible: Ethical issues in appeals to personal responsibility in health campaigns. *Journal of Health Communication, 6,* 117–136.

Farrell, A., & Geist-Martin, P. (2005). Communicating social health: Perceptions of wellness at work. *Management Communication Quarterly, 18,* 543–592.

Floyd, K. (2006). Human affection exchange: XII. Affectionate communication is associated with diurnal variation in salivary free cortisol. *Western Journal of Communication, 70,* 47–63.

Foucault, M. (1975). *The birth of the clinic.* New York: Random House.

Hahn, E., Simpson, M. R., & Kidd, P. (1996). Cues to parent involvement in drug prevention and school activities. *The Journal of School Health, 66,* 165–181.

Harter, L. M., Scott, J. A., Novak, D. R., Leeman, M., & Morris, J. F. (2006). Freedom through flight: Performing a counter-narrative of disability. *Journal of Applied Communication Research, 34, 3–29.*

Hawkins, K., & Hane, A. C. (2000). Adolescents' perceptions of print cigarette advertising: A case for counteradvertising. *Journal of Health Communication, 5,* 83–96.

Ho, E. (2003). 'Have you seen your aura lately?': *Understanding the discourses of health in holistic health pamphlets.* Paper presented at the 2003 Annual meeting of the International Communication Association, San Diego, CA.

Kagawa-Singer, M., & Kassim-Lakha, S. (2003). A strategy to reduce cross-cultural miscommunications and increase the likelihood of improving health outcomes. *Academic Medicine, 78* (6), 577–587.

Kirby, E., & Krone, K. J. (2002). "The policy exists but you can't really use it": Communication and the structuration of work-family policies. *Journal of Applied Communication Research, 24,* 217–239.

Kreps, G. (2006). *Information based healthcare practice as transformational tools: Separating rhetoric from reality.* Presentation at the national symposium Transforming American Healthcare over the Next Decade: Pathways to Change. Phoenix, AZ.

Lederman, L. C. (2003). Friends don't let friends beer goggle: A case study in the use and abuse of alcohol and communication among college students. In E. B. Ray (Ed.), *Case Studies In Health Communication.* Hillsdale, NJ: Lawrence Erlbaum.

Lederman, L. C. (2006). *And nobody notices: Alcoholism among older adults as an "invisible epidemic."* Keynote Address. Emeritus and Retired Faculty Association, California State University at Northridge, Northridge, California.

Lederman, L. C., & Stewart, L. P., (2005). *Changing the culture of college drinking: A socially situated prevention campaign.* Cresskill, NJ: Hampton Press.

Lederman, L. C., Stewart, L. P., & Kully, R. D. (2001). *Lessons learned from the myths and misperceptions about college drinking: Do they apply to alcoholism among older adults?* National Communication Association, Atlanta, GA.

Longest, B. B. (2002). *Health policymaking in the United States.* Chicago: Health Administration Press.

Lupton, Deborah. (1994). Toward the development of critical health communication praxis. *Health Communication, 6*(1), 55–67.

Martin, J. N., & Nakayama, T. K. (2004). *Intercultural Communication in Context* (3rd ed.). Boston, MA: McGraw-Hill.

Meyerowitz, B. E., & Chaiken, S. (1987). The effect of message framing on breast self-examination attitudes, intentions and behaviors. *Journal of Personality and Social Psychology, 52,* 500–510.

Morman, T. (2000). The influence of fear appeals, message design, and masculinity on men's motivation to perform the testicular self-exam. *Journal of Applied Communication Research, 28,* 91–116.

Murray-Johnson, L., & Witte, K. (2000). Looking toward the future: Health message design strategies. In T. L. Thompson, A. M. Dorsey, K. I. Miller, & R. Parrott (Eds.), *Handbook of health communication* (pp. 473–496). Mahwah, NJ: Lawrence Erlbaum Associates.

National Institute of Health National Center for Complementary and Alternative Medicine. (2006). *NCCAM funding: Appropriations history.* Retrieved on October 21, 2006 from http://nccam.nih.gov/about/appropriations/index.htm

Nestle, M. (2002). *Food politics: How the food industry influences nutrition and health.* Berkeley: University of California Press.

Parrott, R., & Lemieux, R. (2003). When the worlds of work and wellness collide: The role of familial support on skin cancer control. *The Journal of Family Communication, 3,* 95–106.

Patel, K., & Rushefsky, M. E. (1999). *Health care politics and policy in America* (2nd ed). Armonk, NY: M.E. Sherman.

Peterson, L. W., & Albrecht, T. (1999). Deconstructing organizational maternity leave policy. *Journal of Management Inquiry, 8,* 168–181.

Peterson, M. A. (2001). From trust to political power: Interest group, public choice, and health care. *Journal of Health Politics, Policy and Law, 26,* 1145–1163.

Petronio, S. (2005) HIPAA Regulation of patient privacy: Does it really protect consumers from their perspective? IARR Conference on Exploring Relationships in Health or Health Relationships (with Kinney ED). IUPUI, Indianapolis, IN.

Ratzan, S. C. (2004). Editor's note. *Journal of Health Communication, 9* (Supplement 1), 1-1.

Rogers, E. (1962/2003). *Diffusion of innovations.* London: Free Press.

Rosati, K. B., & Harris-Salamone, K. D. (2006). *Health information technology and Arizona innovation.* Presentation at the national symposium Transforming American Healthcare over the Next Decade: Pathways to Change. Phoenix, AZ.

Schreiber, L. (2005). The importance of precision in language: Communication research and (so-called) alternative medicine. *Health Communication, 17*(2), 173–190.

Singh, N. N., McKay, J. D., & Singh, A. N. (1998). Culture and mental health: Nonverbal communication. *Journal of Child and Family Studies, 7*(4), 403–409.

Singhal, A., & Rogers, E. M. (2000). *Entertainment-education: A communication strategy for social change.* Mahwah, NJ: Lawrence Erlbaum Associates.

Soss, J. (2002). *Unwanted claims: the politics of participation in the U.S. welfare system.* Ann Arbor: University of Michigan Press.

Stephenson, M., Palmgreen, P., Hoyle, R. H., Donohew, L., Lorch, E. P., & Colon, S. E. (1999). Short-term effects of an anti-marijuana media campaign targeting high sensation seeking adolescents. *Journal of Applied Communication Research, 27,* 175–195.

Trethewey, A., Scott, C., & LeGreco, M. (2006). Constructing embodied organizational identities: Commodifying, securing and servicing professional bodies. In B. Dow & J. Wood (Eds.). *The Handbook of Gender and Communication* (pp. 123–143). Thousand Oaks, CA: Sage Publications.

Tseng, W. (2004). Culture and psychotherapy: Asian perspectives. *Journal of Mental Health, 13* (2), 151–161.

Udani, J. (1998). Integrating alternative medicine into practice. *Journal of the American Medical Association, 280,* 1620.

U.S. Census Bureau. (2004). U.S. interim projections by age, sex, race, and Hispanic Origin. Retrieved December 1, 2004, from http://www.census.gov/ipc/www/usinterimproj/

U.S. Department of Health and Human Services (1999). *Mental health: A report of the Surgeon General.* Rockville, MD: U.S. Department of Health and Human Services, Substance Abuse and Mental Health Services Administration, Center for Mental Health Services, National Institutes of Health, National Institute of Mental Health.

U.S. Department of Health and Human Services (2001a). *Mental health: Culture, race, and ethnicity—A supplement to mental health: A report of the Surgeon General.* Rockville, MD: US Department of Health and Human Services, Public Health Service, Office of the Surgeon General.

U.S. Department of Health and Human Services. (2001b). *Mental health: Culture, race, and ethnicity—A supplement to mental health: A report of the Surgeon General—Executive summary.* Rockville, MD: US Department of Health and Human Services, Public Health Service, Office of the Surgeon General.

Vanderford, M. L., Jenks, E. B., and Sharf, B. (1997). Exploring Patients' Experiences as a Primary Source of Meaning. *Health Communication, 9,* 13–26.

Witte, K. (1992). Preventing AIDS through persuasive communications: A framework for constructing effective, culturally-specific, preventative health messages. *International and Intercultural Annual, 16,* 67–86.

Yanovitzky, I., Stewart, L. P., & Lederman, L. C. (2006) Social distance, perceived drinking by peers, and alcohol use by college students. *Health Communication, 19*(1), 1–10.

Zoller, H. M. (2003a). Health on the line: Identity and disciplinary control in occupational health and safety discourse. *Journal of Applied Communication Research, 31,* 118–139.

Zoller, H. M. (2003b). Working out: Managerialism in workplace health promotion. *Management Communication Quarterly, 17,* 171–205.

Zoller, H. M. (2005). Health activism: Communication theory and action for social change. *Communication Theory, 15,* 341–364. ✦